Oxford Textbook of

Anaesthesia for the Obese Patient

OXFORD TEXTBOOKS IN ANAESTHESIA

Oxford Textbook of Anaesthesia for the Elderly Patient
Edited by Chris Dodds, Chandra Kumar, and Bernadette Veering

Oxford Textbook of Anaesthesia for Oral and Maxillofacial Surgery
Edited by Ian Shaw, Chandra Kumar, and Chris Dodds

Principles and Practice of Regional Anaesthesia, Fourth Edition
Edited by Graeme McLeod, Colin McCartney, and Tony Wildsmith

Oxford Textbook of Cardiothoracic Anaesthesia
Edited by R. Peter Alston, Paul Myles, and Marco Ranucci

Oxford Textbook of Transplant Anaesthesia and Critical Care
Edited by Ernesto A. Pretto, Jr, Gianni Biancofiore, Andre DeWolf, John R. Klinck, Claus Niemann, Andrew Watts, and Peter D. Slinger

Oxford Textbook of Obstetric Anaesthesia
Edited by Vicki Clark, Marc Van de Velde, and Roshan Fernando

Oxford Textbook of Neuroscience and Anaesthesiology
Edited by George A. Mashour and Kristin Engelhard

Oxford Textbook of Anaesthesia for the Obese Patient
Edited by Ashish C. Sinha

Oxford Textbook of

Anaesthesia for the Obese Patient

EDITED BY

Ashish C. Sinha, MD, PhD, DABA, MBA, FASA

Professor, University of California Riverside, Designated Institutional Official and Founding Program Director (Anesthesiology), Riverside Community Hospital/ University of California Riverside, Riverside, CA, USA

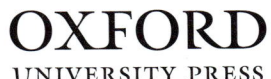

OXFORD

UNIVERSITY PRESS

OXFORD
UNIVERSITY PRESS

Great Clarendon Street, Oxford, OX2 6DP,
United Kingdom

Oxford University Press is a department of the University of Oxford.
It furthers the University's objective of excellence in research, scholarship,
and education by publishing worldwide. Oxford is a registered trade mark of
Oxford University Press in the UK and in certain other countries

First Edition published in 2021

Impression: 1

Published in the United States of America by Oxford University Press
198 Madison Avenue, New York, NY 10016, United States of America

British Library Cataloguing in Publication Data
Data available

Library of Congress Control Number: 2020943920

ISBN 978–0–19–875714–6

DOI: 10.1093/med/9780198757146.001.0001

Printed in Great Britain by
Bell & Bain Ltd., Glasgow

Acknowledgements

First off, I have to acknowledge the support of my single biggest supporter, from birth and before, my mother, Prity Sinha. As soon as I could hold a spoon she put a pencil in my hand and taught me the three Rs. She was, and continues to be, my biggest supporter, especially when I was a young sapling and needed a support for my growth—she was there every time. Next of course is dad, my hero. I guess I always wanted to be him; for smarts, wit, one-line zingers, dint of purpose, and inability to accept the first, second, or even the third time when told, 'No, it cannot be done'. Many of his one-liners like 'If it's worth doing, it's worth doing right!', 'Many can buy an elephant; not all of those can feed an elephant' still pepper my lexicon. And for the lesson that '3 No Trump' is a closing bid! After attending a lecture that I was delivering, and me having acknowledged him from the lectern, he commented afterwards that in the audience he was thrilled by the role reversal—to be identified as my father; in most past settings I was recognized as his son. Dad and mom inspired me and had unwavering confidence in yours truly; who looked at me and saw something bigger, way bigger, than I could ever see in me.

Next is my brother, for his strength of character and focus on the 'right' thing to do. Many hot summer days playing cricket (broken bulbs and windows!) and many warm evenings spent during summer vacations staring at chess boards. My friend and confidante, sometimes disapproving of my escapades but always supportive. In medical school, when I needed, nay wanted, to have a motorcycle and our father had said a firm 'No', he bought it for me and said dad shouldn't find out! Well, sorry brother, he just did!

My next acknowledgement is for my children, Kavita, Ishan, and Anamika. I hope I make you proud and that you, in turn, exceed my accomplishments, and whatever they may be, in every way. That is the, sometimes silent, prayer of every parent.

Then I wish to acknowledge people who were in my life in certain roles and have moved on: friends, partners, and family. I thank you for your support at those times when you were with me and I was engrossed in this project, and I wish you well in the future because our past had some amazing times!

To my favourite cousin Sharad and his best friend ABS, who have guided and supported this 'wayward' cousin of theirs!

In academic medicine one has to have focus and I have to thank my mentor, Lee A. Fleisher, who convinced me to focus a majority of my academic effort on obesity. This is what has ultimately culminated in this book!

A few years ago, when I had my first interaction with Oxford University Press and was invited to edit a textbook on this subject, I had possibility underestimated the time and effort that would be expended in this endeavour, but I am thrilled to be at this point in the project. The people who I have to singularly recognize from Oxford University Press are Geraldine Jeffers, Rachel Goldsworthy, Fiona Sutherland, Helen Cook, Karen Moore, and Sean McLeod.

Last, and most importantly, I wish to thank all my contributors; you are what made this book possible! I apologize for harassing you for drafts and edits. You own the glory of this book and I will take credit for anything less than perfect.

Ashish C. Sinha

Contents

SECTION 6
Other important aspects

Abbreviations

ABW	adjusted body weight
AB	axillary block
ABG	arterial blood gas
ACCP	American College of Chest Physicians
AEC	airway exchange catheter
AF	atrial fibrillation
AgRP	agouti-related peptide
AHA	American Heart Association
AKI	acute kidney injury
AMG	acceleromyography
ARC	arcuate nucleus
ASA	American Society of Anesthesiologists
ASPEN	American Society for Parenteral and Enteral Nutrition
BiPAP	bi-level positive airway pressure
BIS	bispectral index
BMI	body mass index
BNP	brain natriuretic peptide
BPD	biliopancreatic diversion
BPD-DS	biliopancreatic diversion with duodenal switch
BSA	body surface area
BV	blood volume
CABG	coronary artery bypass graft
CAD	coronary artery disease
CART	cocaine- and amphetamine-regulated transcript
CCK	cholecystokinin
CNS	central nervous system
CO	cardiac output
CO_2	carbon dioxide
COX	cyclooxygenase
CPAP	continuous positive airway pressure
CPB	cardiopulmonary bypass
CPN	common peroneal nerve
CPR	cardiopulmonary resuscitation
CRP	C-reactive protein
CT	computed tomography
CTPA	computed tomography pulmonary angiography
CVC	central venous catheter
CVD	cardiovascular disease
DBMV	difficult bag-mask ventilation
DLCO	carbon monoxide diffusion capacity
DM	diabetes mellitus
DSE	dobutamine stress echocardiography
DVT	deep vein thrombosis
ECG	electrocardiogram
EE	energy expenditure
EPAP	expiratory positive airway pressure
ERAS	enhanced recovery after surgery
EWL	excess weight loss
FDA	Food and Drug Administration
FEV_1	forced expiratory volume in 1 second
FFM	fat-free mass
FG	fat group
FI	inspired partial pressure
FiO_2	fraction of inspired oxygen
FOB	flexible fibreoptic bronchoscopy
FRC	functional residual capacity
Fv	partial pressure in mixed-venous blood
FVC	forced vital capacity
GORD	gastro-oesophageal reflux disease
GWAS	genome-wide association study
HR	hazard ratio
IAP	intra-abdominal pressure
IBW	ideal body weight
ICB	infraclavicular block
ICU	intensive care unit
IDF	International Diabetes Federation
IPAP	inspiratory positive airway pressure
ITDG	inter-tissue diffusion group
IV	intravenous
IVC	inferior vena cava
LAGB	laparoscopic adjustable gastric band
LBM	lean body mass
LBW	lean body weight
LCD	low-calorie diet
LCOS	low cardiac output syndrome,
LMWH	low-molecular-weight heparin
LSG	laparoscopic sleeve gastrectomy
LV	left ventricle/ventricular
LVH	left ventricular hypertrophy
MAC	minimal alveolar concentration
MetS	metabolic syndrome
MG	muscle group
MHO	metabolically healthy obese
MRI	magnetic resonance imaging
MSH	melanocyte-stimulating hormone
MUO	metabolically unhealthy obese
N_2O	nitrous oxide
NAFLD	non-alcoholic fatty liver disease
NASH	non-alcoholic steatohepatitis
NIRS	near-infrared spectroscopy
NIV	non-invasive ventilation

NMB	neuromuscular blockade	SAP	safe apnoea period
NMDA	N-methyl-D-aspartate	SCB	supraclavicular block
NPY	neuropeptide Y	SCCM	Society of Critical Care Medicine
NVM	nerve to the vastus medialis	$ScvO_2$	central venous oxygen saturation
O_2	oxygen	SGA	supraglottic airway
OFA	opioid-free anaesthesia	SNP	single nucleotide polymorphism
OHS	obesity hypoventilation syndrome	SPECT	single-photon emission computed tomography
OLV	one-lung ventilation	SSI	surgical site infection
OSA	obstructive sleep apnoea	$StPO_2$	tissue oxygen saturation
OSAS	obstructive sleep apnoea syndrome	T2D	type 2 diabetes
PAC	pulmonary artery catheter	TBW	total body weight
PACU	post-anaesthesia care unit	TEA	thoracic epidural analgesia
PaO_2	arterial partial pressure of oxygen	TEE	total energy expenditure
PCA	patient-controlled analgesia	TLC	total lung capacity
PCO_2	partial pressure of carbon dioxide	TN	tibial nerve
PCV	pressure-controlled ventilation	TOE	transoesophageal echocardiography
PE	pulmonary embolism	tPO_2	tissue oxygen tension
PEEP	positive end-expiratory pressure	TPVB	thoracic paravertebral block
PET	positron emission tomography	UFH	unfractionated heparin
PO_2	partial pressure of oxygen	US	ultrasonography *or* United States
POAF	postoperative atrial fibrillation	V/Q	ventilation/perfusion
POMC	pro-opiomelanocortin	VA	alveolar ventilation
PSV	pressure support ventilation	VATS	video-assisted thoracoscopic surgery
PTC	post-tetanic count	VBG	vertical banded gastroplasty
PVR	pulmonary vascular resistance	VC	vital capacity
PYY	peptide YY	VCO_2	carbon dioxide production
REE	resting energy expenditure	VCV	volume-controlled ventilation
RML	rhabdomyolysis	Vd	volume of distribution
RML	recruitment manoeuvre	VLCD	very-low-calorie diet
RR	relative risk	VO_2	oxygen consumption
RSI	rapid sequence induction	VRG	vessel-rich group
RV	right ventricle/ventricular	VTE	venous thromboembolism
RYGB	Roux-en-Y gastric bypass	WHO	World Health Organization
SAH	subarachnoid haemorrhage	WHR	waist-to-hip ratio

Contributors

Hawa Abubakar, MD Fellow, Anesthesiology Critical Care Medicine, Vanderbilt University Medical Center, Nashville TN, USA

Muhammad Ahmed, MD Assistant Professor of Clinical Anesthesiology, Temple University Hospital, Lewis Katz School of Medicine, Philadelphia, PA, USA

Fahad Aman, MD Clinical Research Associate, Interventional Pain Medicine, Advocate Aurora Health, Oshkosh, WI, USA

Mansoor M. Aman, MD, DABA Interventional Pain Medicine Specialist, Advocate Aurora Health, Oshkosh, WI, USA

Aditee P. Ambardekar, MD, MSEd Associate Professor and Residency Program Director, Department of Anesthesiology and Pain Management, UT Southwestern Medical Center, Dallas, TX, USA

Ajisha Aravindan, MD, DNB Assistant Professor, Department of Anaesthesiology, Pain Medicine and Critical Care, All India Institute of Medical Sciences, New Delhi, India

Eugenia Ayrian, MD Associate Professor of Anesthesiology, Director of Division of Neuroanesthesiology, Director of Neuroanesthesiology Fellowship, Keck School of Medicine of the University of Southern California, Los Angeles, CA, USA

Christian Balabanoff-Acosta, MD Assistant Professor, Department of Anesthesiology and Perioperative Medicine, The University of Alabama at Birmingham, Birmingham, AL

Abiona Berkeley, MD, JD Professor of Clinical Anesthesiology, Director, Anesthesiology Residency Program, Department of Anesthesiology, Temple University School of Medicine, Philadelphia, PA, USA

Sara Bowman, MD Consultant Anaesthetist, Homerton University Hospital NHS Foundation Trust, Hackney, London, UK

Jerrad R. Businger, DO Assistant Professor of Anesthesiology and Critical Care, Chief, Division of Anesthesia Critical Care, Fellowship Director, Anesthesia Critical Care, University of Louisville Hospital, Louisville, KY, USA

Stephanie Rayos Callison, MD Clinical Assistant Professor, Department of Anesthesiology, University of Michigan, Ann Arbor, MI, USA

Andres Castellanos†, MD, FACS Associate Professor and Executive Vice Chairman, Department of Surgery, Drexel University College of Medicine, Philadelphia, PA, USA

Frances Chung, MBBS, FRCPC Professor, Department of Anesthesia and Pain Medicine, Toronto Western Hospital, University Health Network, University of Toronto, Canada

Michelle Cole, MBChB, FRCA Consultant Anaesthetist, University College London Hospitals, London, UK

Scott R. Coleman, DO Assistant Professor, Section on Cardiothoracic Anesthesiology, Wake Forest Baptist Medical Center, Winston-Salem, NC, USA

Jeremy Collins, MB, ChB, FRCA Executive Vice Chair, Department of Anesthesiology, Emory University, Atlanta, GA, USA

Luc De Baerdemaeker, MD, PhD, DEAA Academic Anesthesiologist, University Hospital Ghent, Ghent, Belgium

Andre M. De Wolf, MD Professor of Anesthesiology, Department of Anesthesiology, Feinberg School of Medicine, Northwestern University, Chicago, IL, USA

Alissa Doll, MD Assistant Professor, Department of Anesthesiology and Pain Management, Children's Health/UT Southwestern Medical Centre, Dallas, TX, USA

Clint Fleckenstein, DO Anesthesiology specialist, Temple Health, Philadelphia, PA, USA

Alvaro Galvez, MD Resident, Department of Surgery, Drexel University College of Medicine, Philadelphia, PA, USA

Akshat Gargya, MBBS, MD Assistant Professor, Department of Anesthesiology, University of Vermont Medical Center, Burlington, Vermont, USA

Eric Gewirtz, MD Professor of Anesthesiology, Temple Health, Philadelphia, PA, USA

Mahmood Ghazanwy, MD Anaesthesia Specialist, Princess Marina Hospital, Gaborone, Botswana

David Gilhooly†, MD Consultant Anaesthetist, University College Hospital, London, UK

Marc Goldberg, MD Associate Professor of Anesthesiology, Associate Vice Chair for Clinical Operations, Department of Anesthesiology, Lewis Katz School of Medicine, Temple University, Philadelphia, PA, USA

Karla Greco MD, MHS Chief Anesthesiologist, Exeter Hospital, Exeter, NH, USA

Jan Hendrickx Professor of Anesthesiology and Perioperative Medicine, Department of Basic and Applied Medical Sciences, Ghent University, Ghent; and Staff Anesthesiologist, Department of Anesthesiology, OLV Hospital, Aalst, Belgium

Rainer Lenhardt, MD Associate Professor, Clinical Director, Neuroscience-Anesthesia Intensive Care Unit, Department of Anesthesiology and Perioperative Medicine, University of Louisville, Louisville, KY, USA

Jon Livelsberger, DO Assistant Professor, Temple University Hospital, Philadelphia, PA, USA

Kelly A. Machovec, MD, MPH Associate Professor of Anesthesiology, Duke University Medical Center, Durham, NC, USA

Ammar Mahmoud, MD Interventional Pain Management Specialist, Northern Light Health, Eastern Maine Medical Center, Bangor, ME, USA

Dipty Mangla, MD Medical Director, APG Pain Management, Atlanticare Regional Medical Center, Galloway, NJ, USA

Maureen McCunn, MD, MIPP, FCCM, FASA Professor, University of Maryland School of Medicine, Department of Anesthesiology, Divisions of Trauma Anesthesia and Surgical Critical Care, Baltimore, MD, USA

Gabriel Mekel, MD Resident in General Surgery, Drexel University College of Medicine/ Hahnemann University Hospital, Philadelphia, PA, USA

Brita M. Mittal, MD Clinical Assistant Professor of Anesthesiology, Stanford University School of Medicine, Stanford, CA, USA

Tiffany Sun Moon, MD, FASA Associate Professor, Department of Anesthesiology & Pain Management, UT Southwestern Medical Center, Dallas, TX, USA

S. R. Moonesinghe, MD(Res), MRCP, FRCA, FFICM Professor of Perioperative Medicine, Consultant Anaesthetist, University College London (UCL) and UCL Hospitals, London, UK

Jan P. Mulier, MD, PhD Bariatric Anesthesiologist, Department of Anesthesiology, Intensive Care and Reanimation, Brugge; and University of Leuven, Leuven, Belgium

Patrick J. Neligan, MA, MD, FFARCSI, FJFICM Honorary Senior Lecturer NUI Galway, Galway; Consultant Anaesthetist, Galway University Hospitals, Galway; and Medical Director Critical Care, University College Hospital, Galway, Ireland

Detlef Obal, MD, PhD, DESA Assistant Professor, Medical Center Line, Department of Anesthesiology, Perioperative, and Pain Medicine, Stanford Cardiovascular Institute, Stanford University, Stanford, CA, USA

Babatunde O. Ogunnaike, MD, FASA Professor, Department of Anesthesiology and Pain Management, University of Texas Southwestern Medical Center, Dallas, TX, USA

Onyi C. Onuoha, MD, MPH Director, Obstetric Anesthesiology Fellowship; Chief, Preoperative Medicine and Consultation Service; Assistant Professor of Clinical Anesthesiology and Critical Care, Hospital of the University of Pennsylvania, Philadelphia, PA, USA

Peter J. Papadakos, MD, FCCM, FAARC Director of Critical Care Medicine, University of Rochester, NY, USA

Ajintha Pathmanathan, MD Anaesthesiologist, Visiting Scholar, Stanford University, Stanford, CA, USA

Matthew E. Pontell, MD Resident, Department of Surgery, Drexel University College of Medicine, Philadelphia, PA, USA

Jahan Porhomayon, MD, FCCP, FCCM Professor of Anesthesiology, Director of Critical Care Medicine, Department of Anesthesiology & Perioperative Medicine, University at Buffalo, Buffalo, NY, USA

Hemkumar Pushparaj, MD Clinical Fellow, Department of Anesthesia, Toronto Western Hospital, Toronto, Canada

Raviraj Raveendran, FANZCA Consultant Anaesthetist, Department of Anaesthesia, Palmerston North Hospital, Midcentral District Health Board, Palmerston North, New Zealand

Elizabeth Renza-Stingone, MD, FACS, FASMBS Associate Professor of Clinical Surgery, Lewis Katz School of Medicine, Temple University, Philadelphia, PA, USA

Justin Richards, MD Assistant Professor of Anesthesiology, R. Adams Cowley Shock Trauma Center, University of Maryland School of Medicine, Baltimore, MD, USA

Chase D. Rose, MD Anaesthesiologist, Anesthesiology Department, Mayo Clinic, Phoenix, AZ, USA

Bhavna Saxena, DNB Senior Anaesthesiologist and Critical Care Specialist, Department of Anaesthesiology and Critical Care, Deen Dayal Upadhyay Hospital, New Delhi, India

Roman Schumann, MD Associate Chief of Anesthesia for Research and Development, Professor of Anesthesiology, Professor of Surgery (Sec), Tufts University School of Medicine, VA Boston Healthcare System, West Roxbury, MA, USA

Prashant Singh, MBBS Assistant Professor, Department of Anesthesiology, Division of Obstetric Anesthesiology, University of Michigan, Ann Arbor, MI, USA

Preet Mohinder Singh, MD Assistant Professor, Department of Anesthesia, Washington University in Saint Louis, St. Louis, MO, USA

Shubhangi Singh, MBBS, MD Assistant Professor, Department of Anesthesiology, Division of Obstetric Anesthesiology, University of Michigan, Ann Arbor, MI, USA

Ashish C. Sinha, MD, PhD, DABA, MBA, FASA Professor, University of California Riverside, Designated Institutional Official and Founding Program Director (Anesthesiology), Riverside Community Hospital/University of California Riverside, Riverside, CA, USA

Sunil Sinha, MD, MBA Vice President and Chief Medical Officer, BJC Medical Group, St. Louis, MO, USA

Jose Sosa-Herrera, MD Assistant Professor, Temple Health, Philadelphia, PA, USA

Alla Spivak, DO Assistant Professor Anesthesiology, Westchester Medical Center, Valhalla, NY, USA

Eric Stander, MD Assistant Professor, Drexel University College of Medicine, Philadelphia, PA, USA

Paul Stewart, MBBS, FANZCA Clinical Associate Professor, Sydney Medical School, The University of Sydney, Sydney, Australia

Rajeshwari Subramaniam, MD Professor and Head of Department, Anaesthesiology, Pain Medicine and Critical Care, All India Institute of Medical Sciences, New Delhi, India

Adrian Sultana, MD, FRCP, FANZCA Specialist Anaesthesiologist, St. Luke's Care, Sydney, Australia

Anurag Tewari, MD Medical Director, Evokes LLC, Mason, OH, USA

Matthew Troum, DO Anesthesiologist, Morristown Medical Center, Morristown, New Jersey, USA

Andrea L. Tsai, MD Assistant Professor, Department of Anesthesiology and Perioperative Medicine, Tufts Medical Center, Boston, MA, USA

Deepu S. Ushakumari, MD, MHCDS, FASA, CPE Chief of Anesthesiology, Atrium Health Central Division, Scope Anesthesia of North Carolina, Charlotte, NC, USA

Elizabeth A. Valentine, MD Chief, Anesthesia for Vascular Surgery and Endovascular Therapy, Associate Professor of Clinical Anesthesiology and Critical Care, Hospital of the University of Pennsylvania, Philadelphia, PA, USA

Ranjani Venkataramani, MD Clinical Assistant Professor, Department of Anesthesiology and Critical Care, University of New Mexico, Albuquerque, NM, USA

Anupama Wadhwa, MBBS, MSc, FASA Clinical Professor in Anesthesiology, University of California, San Diego, CA, USA

Ruben Wouters, MD Anesthesiologist/Intensive Care Physician, AZ Sint Jan Bruges, Bruges, Belgium

SECTION 1
Foundations

Obesity
A global epidemic

Bhavna Saxena and Ashish C. Sinha

Introduction

The French lawyer and politician who gained fame as an epicure and gastronome, Jean Anthelme Brillat-Savarin, wrote in his much applauded book *The Physiology of Taste*, 'tell me what you eat, and I will tell you what you are', from which derives the old adage 'you are what you eat'. Considering that not only does food nourish our bodies but also affects the quality of our lives, weight, energy, the ageing process, and our overall health and well-being, this statement is literally true.

Since the beginning of civilization, chronic food shortage and malnutrition have been the bane of humankind [1]. The modern emergence of a steady food supply with a lesser need for physical exertion, in combination with lower dietary quality, provided an environment in which diseases flourished and life expectancy decreased. [2].

According to the World Health Organization (WHO), obesity is one of today's most blatantly visible, yet most neglected, public health problems; an escalating global epidemic of overweight and obesity—'globesity'—is taking over many parts of the world [3]. This global 'fat epidemic' is no longer the exclusive problem of rich countries—many poorer nations are now facing the same threat [3]. For the first time, the number of overweight individuals in the world rivals those who are underweight. WHO global estimates show that:

> In 2016, more than 1.9 billion adults (39% of the adult population) aged 18 years and older were overweight. Of these, over 650 million adults were obese (13% of the world's adult population). The worldwide prevalence of obesity nearly tripled between 1975 and 2016. Unfortunately, this trend is not limited to adults alone. In 2016, an estimated 41 million children under the age of 5 years were overweight or obese and over 340 million children and adolescents aged 5–19 were overweight or obese in the same year, a dramatic rise from just 4% in 1975 to just over 18% in 2016. [4]

The decision to define obesity as a disease

Until the mid to late twentieth century, undernourishment and hunger were considered as greater public health concerns than obesity [5], which was considered more of a cosmetic issue caused by overeating and poor self-control. In spite of recognizing the problems associated with obesity, medical societies vacillated in their opinions on the classification of obesity as a disease. This was probably due to the lack of a clear, objective, and widely accepted definition of what constitutes a 'disease'. In their paper, Dr G. A. Bray and colleagues use the 'epidemiological model' of disease for this purpose [6]. In this model, there is 'an environmental agent that acts on a host to produce a disease', and the disease is 'related to the virulence of the agent and the susceptibility of the host' [6,7]. The authors state that food may be considered the primary environmental agent and that the decline in physical activity is a secondary cause of obesity [6–8].

In 1950, the first medical society was formed for the clinical management of obesity, the National Obesity Society—now the Obesity Medicine Association [5]. Since 1977 (when the American Health Care Financing Administration decided obesity was not a disease), a gradual movement has been seen towards acceptance of the proposition that obesity is a 'disease process' [5,7]. In 2010, the Scottish Intercollegiate Guidelines Network [9] described obesity as 'a disease process characterized by excessive body fat accumulation with multiple organ-specific consequences' [7,9]. In 2013, the American Medical Association's Council on Science and Public Health opined that obesity should not be considered a disease. They reasoned that the use of the body mass index (BMI) to define obesity was simplistic and flawed, and since there were no specific symptoms associated with obesity, it was more a risk factor leading to other conditions than a disease in its own right [10]. However, the American Medical Association's House of Delegates rejected the Council's conclusion arguing that 'The suggestion that *obesity* is not a disease but rather a consequence of a chosen lifestyle exemplified by overeating and/or inactivity is equivalent to suggesting that lung cancer is not a disease because it was brought about by an individual choice to smoke cigarettes' [11].

Thus, this age-old controversy culminated in more and more health organizations agreeing to recognize obesity as a disease, including the Food and Drug Administration (FDA) and the National Institutes of Health in the United States, and the WHO—which recognizes obesity as a 'condition of abnormal or excessive fat accumulation in adipose tissue, to the extent that health may be impaired' [12]. The World Obesity Federation takes the position that obesity is a chronic, relapsing, progressive disease process requiring immediate action for prevention and control [7,13].

Body weight regulation and energy balance

Understanding body weight regulation requires an understanding of energy balance [14]. According to the first law of thermodynamics, our body weight should remain stable if energy intake (EI) and energy expenditure (EE) remain equal over time [15]. The body's energy balance is, in effect, the difference between the amount of energy taken in as food and the amount expended in metabolism and physical activity. When EI is greater than EE, a state of positive balance occurs, resulting in an increase in weight gain, 60–80% of which usually consists of body fat. On the other hand, when EE is more than EI, a state of negative energy balance occurs with resulting weight loss, 60–80% of which is, again, body fat [12,15,16]. EE has three main components:

1. The resting/basal metabolic rate—this is the amount of energy needed to fuel the body at rest.
2. Dietary thermogenesis or the thermic effect of food—this is the energy cost of absorbing and metabolizing food.
3. Energy spent in physical activity [12].

Resting/basal metabolic rate is a tightly controlled variable, proportional to the amount of fat-free body mass [15]. In a sedentary individual this is approximately 60% of the EE, with activity accounting for around 30%. Dietary thermogenesis appears to remain constant at around 10% [12,15,17,18]. Physical activity is the key variable component of EE [12].

The overall stability of body weight is proof that energy balance is subject to physiological control [15]. Our body appears to be able to actively regulate energy balance since altering any one component can affect the others [14,19]. For example, chronic changes in the amount of food consumed lead to changes in metabolism which in turn oppose changes in body weight. Similarly, chronic changes in physical activity can affect intake of food. These compensatory physiological changes, however, are not enough to prevent changes in body weight when there is persistent positive or negative energy balance [14,20,21]. Our physiology seems to protect us more against weight loss than against weight gain, that is to say it regulates energy balance best under conditions in which physical activity 'pulls' appetite [14]. This makes sense, because historically starvation has always been a greater problem than obesity [22].

Studies addressing the association between EE and weight gain found a low resting energy expenditure (REE) to be a predictor of weight gain [23,24]. This finding fuelled a discussion about whether obesity is due to high EI or low EE [25,26]. As most obese subjects tended to have a high rather than a low EE [27], the focus of research had shifted from EE to EI as the major determinant of a positive energy balance and obesity [13,28]. The assessment of EI, however, is inaccurate and biased in overweight subjects [29,30]. Mathematical modelling of energy balance revealed that pharmacological inhibition of sodium-glucose co-transporter 2 (SGLT2), used for metabolic control of patients with type 2 diabetes mellitus, led to an increase in EI whereas EE remained unchanged. This is in

line with genetic studies showing that defects in the EI underlies all known causes of obesity. However, a second look at the SGLT2-inhibition data, showed that the increase in EI was lesser than the energy losses, leading to an energy gap, resulting in an involuntary weight loss. The increase in EI could not match EE. EE, on the other hand, was kept constant suggesting that it is tightly controlled. This experience showed that there is no tight feedback control of EI by EE, giving credence to the idea that EE and not EI is under tight control and is therefore the major determinant of energy balance [17].

Under steady-state conditions food is metabolized and used to fuel basal metabolism, thermogenesis, and physical activity. Any excess is stored as fat in adipose cells for later use [31]. Though genetics plays a role in body weight determination [31,32], the gradual weight gain of the population cannot be attributed primarily to genetic factors [14]. There are three main factors that affect and maintain energy balance and a steady body weight by interacting with each other— the homoeostatic, environmental, and behavioural processes [33,34]. Alterations in any of these may lead to weight gain [33].

Homoeostatic processes

Body weight is regulated by a complex neurohormonal system [33,35]. Inputs from this system are integrated in the arcuate nucleus of the hypothalamus [31,36], the caudal brainstem, and parts of the cortex and limbic system [31]. The hypothalamus processes signals from both the centre and the periphery [31]. Centrally acting appetite regulators may be divided into orexigenic (hunger stimulating), for example, neuropeptide Y (NPY) and agouti-related peptide (AgRP); and anorexigenic (hunger suppressing), for example, pro-opiomelanocortin (POMC) and cocaine- and amphetamine-regulated transcript [31,33]. Peripheral signals to the hypothalamus convey information about short-term food intake (i.e. nutrient availability) or long-term energy balance (i.e. energy stores) [33,36]. These signals are conveyed either by (1) orexigenic hormones—ghrelin and gastric inhibitory polypeptide, or (2) anorexigenic hormones— from (a) the gastrointestinal tract: glucagon-like peptide-1 (GLP-1), peptide YY (PYY or peptide tyrosine tyrosine), and cholecystokinin (CCK); (b) the pancreas: pancreatic polypeptide (PP), amylin, and insulin; and (c) adipocytes: leptin [31,33,36,37].

A feedback loop is created between the brain and periphery (gastrointestinal tract, pancreas, liver, muscle, and adipose tissue) by these signals [31,34]. Peripheral signals about energy stores and nutrient availability are received by the brain, which then accordingly adjusts energy balance to meet the requirements of energy homeostasis [34]. The response to these inputs originates in the paraventricular nucleus and lateral hypothalamus and is expressed via behavioural, autonomic, and endocrine output pathways [31]. An adaptation takes place in this feedback system when EI is restricted, promoting a positive energy imbalance [34]. Insulin is unique since it reduces food intake centrally but causes weight gain when used peripherally to treat diabetes [34]. Leptin and insulin are responsible for long-term regulation of energy balance. Conversely, ghrelin, CCK, GLP-1, amylin, PP, and PYY are responsible for short-term, meal-to-meal regulation [36].

The hypothalamus additionally receives inputs from the cortex and limbic system via 'hedonic' pathways. These pathways are linked not only to the sight, smell, and taste of food, but also emotional and social factors. The hedonic pathways increase the craving for palatable energy-rich food even when our body has ample energy stores and can override the homeostatic pathways [36]. This is evidenced by the fact that we eat for reasons other than just to meet our nutritional requirements.

Glial cells too have been postulated to have an important role in the regulation of body weight. Diets with large amounts of saturated fat may cause inflammation, gliosis, and neuronal stress in the medio-basal hypothalamus [38]. Chronic activation of glial cells results in disturbances to leptin responsiveness and has been linked to the development of obesity [39,40]. Energy homeostasis thus suggests that obesity is a disorder of a regulated system and not merely a result of deficiency of discipline and self-control [41].

Environmental processes

The extent to which the body's physiological regulatory mechanisms are capable of maintaining body weight depends on the environment [14]. We may partly attribute the current levels of obesity to an 'obesogenic' environment which effects the corticolimbic areas of the brain [33,42]. Easy availability coupled with aggressive marketing of high-calorie foods provides ample opportunity to indulge in large portions of high-fat, high-calorie fare [43,44]. This increase in EI along with decreases in physical activity, which have arisen unintended as a result of societal progress, are the main factors forming an obesogenic environment. Basically, our biology tells us to eat whenever food is available and to rest whenever physical activity is not required. Throughout history this simple physiological control was sufficient to maintain body weight, without undue effort. However, in the present-day environment, this physiological regulation appears to be insufficient [14]. Weight gain increases resting metabolic rate and energy cost of physical activity; this increase in energy output thus balances the higher EI [15]. Becoming obese then is a 'trade-off' for maintaining a low level of physical activity and appears to represent a new 'settling point'. Indeed, this may be the only way to achieve energy balance when living a sedentary lifestyle [14,15]. Under such conditions, weight gain can only be prevented with conscious efforts to eat less or to be physically active without the need to be physically active [14]. McAllister et al. [44]

postulated that many other environmental factors, such as epigenetics, increased maternal age, sleep debt, endocrine disruptors, and pharmaceutical iatrogenesis, were contributory in the development of obesity. Though lifestyle modifications are important we should try to understand how the brain deals with environmental stimuli and develop behavioural strategies to cope with them [42]. Table 1.1 shows the environmental factors which potentially influence body weight.

Behavioural processes

Behavioural patterns are important aetiological factors leading to obesity development, hence, behavioural therapy is often a fundamental part of management [45]. Personal motivation for weight loss can play a radical role in modifying unhealthy habits and lifestyle [33]. 'Behaviour therapy' is a set of principles and techniques meant to help obese individuals modify eating habits, physical activity, and thought processes likely contributing to their condition [45,46]. The main component of behaviour therapy is to set specific goals, taking into account that factors other than behaviour (e.g. genetics, metabolism, and hormonal influences) can predispose to obesity. The goals set should therefore be realistic and achievable [47]. An example of such a goal for exercising more would be: 'I will walk on the track at the local high school for 30 minutes at a brisk pace Monday to Saturday at 7 am. If it rains, I will exercise in the den using my walking DVD' [57]. Patients are asked to keep detailed records of their food intake, physical activity, and body weight; these records are reviewed by the physician and amendments are made accordingly in areas needing improvement. Record-keeping has now expanded to include information about times, places, thoughts, and feelings associated with eating and physical activity [45]. Frequent self-monitoring can consistently predict both short- and long-term weight losses. Behavioural treatment in addition to diet, exercise, and self-monitoring also includes slowing the rate of eating, stimulus control, problem-solving, cognitive restructuring, and relapse prevention training [45].

Table 1.1 Environmental factors potentially influencing body weight

Obesogenic environment	• Increased availability of large portions of energy-dense foods with a decrease in physical activity constitute the obesogenic environment
Infection	• Adipose tissue has been shown to have a role in activating the immune system • Certain immune cells, macrophages, and adipocytes are functionally similar, and pre-adipocytes can differentiate into macrophages. Also, adipose tissue has the potential to expand in response to infection leading to surplus energy • Adenovirus AD-36 has been shown to cause obesity in non-human primates, and humans with antibodies to AD-36 are more obese
Intrauterine and intergenerational effects	• The perinatal environment can change metabolic programming in the fetus, resulting in persistent pathological consequences • Progeny of obese mothers/those with excessive gestational weight gain are at an increased risk of obesity
Epigenetics	• Epigenetic modifications potentially lead to 'metabolic programming' resulting in long-term metabolic changes
Increasing maternal age	• Mean maternal age has steadily increased over the years and has been associated with the development of obesity • Comorbidities, such as obesity, insulin resistance, and hypertension, are common
Sleep debt	• Circadian desynchrony resulting from shift work and sleep disruption has been implicated in metabolic pathologies • Studies have shown a relationship between disrupted or decreased amounts of sleep and the increase in obesity across diverse ages and ethnicities
Iatrogenic effects of pharmacotherapies	• Some of the most commonly prescribed drugs have been associated with significant weight gain

Physiological adaptations leading to weight regain after weight loss

Although weight loss can usually be achieved through restriction of caloric intake and/or increased physical activity, most individuals have a tendency to regain the lost weight over time [36]. This is a result of certain biological changes, which take place in appetite regulation, energy storage, and utilization of energy—see **Fig. 1.1** [36]. These changes affect the neurohormonal system regulating energy homoeostasis, levels of circulating appetite-related hormones, alterations in nutrient metabolism, and subjective appetite [33]. A plausible hypothesis for this tendency to regain lost weight, may be that body weight is maintained at a particular set level, and deviations from this set point are resisted and minimized by a feedback control system [47–50].

Changes in the neurohormonal system

Following weight loss, hormonal changes occur, leading to weight regain by increasing hunger and promoting energy storage [33,37]. Diet-induced weight loss has been associated with increases in ghrelin [51] and gastric inhibitory peptide [32,36,37] and decreases in leptin [37,52], PYY [53,54], CCK [36,37,53,55], amylin [37,53], insulin [33,37], and GLP-1 levels [53]—all hormones decrease food intake [56–61], except ghrelin, which stimulates hunger [62,63], and gastric inhibitory peptide, which plays a role in energy storage [53]. Normally, ghrelin levels increase prior to meals and are suppressed postprandially [48,62]. Apart from stimulation of appetite, administration of exogenous ghrelin leads to a decrease in metabolic rate and fat catabolism [48]. Thus, higher levels of ghrelin after weight loss promote weight regain by two mechanisms: an increase in EI combined with a decrease in EE [48].

Leptin reduces food intake and increases EE by stimulating POMC and reducing AgRP and NPY, by acting on the hypothalamus [36]. Leptin levels decrease during reductions in diet and are decreased more during dynamic weight loss than during weight loss maintenance [36]. 'Replacement' of leptin to levels existing prior to weight loss reverses most of the adaptive physiological changes which occur

[36,64]. Sumithran et al. showed that these changes are not transient and can persist for up to 1 year [37]. Another study, however, showed that those who regained at least 10% of the lost weight had higher leptin and lower ghrelin levels compared to those who maintained their body weight. This was contrary to expectation, thus suggesting a disruption in the sensitivity to these hormones, leading to weight regain [65].

Increased cortisol levels such as in Cushing syndrome lead to weight gain, especially central adiposity. A significant correlation was found between increases in appetite and fasting plasma cortisol after a weight-loss programme in obese patients [66]. Rodent studies have shown that cortisol inhibits the suppressive action of leptin on food intake and body weight [36,67]. Decreased EI has been shown to increase circulating levels of cortisol [36,68], which returns to normal on resumption of normal feeding [69].

Thyroid hormones have an important role in EE. Increased levels lead to upregulation of REE, postulated to be due to mitochondrial uncoupling in skeletal muscles [36]. Energy restrictions have been shown to suppress the hypothalamic–pituitary–thyroid axis, leading to reduced secretion of thyroid-stimulating hormone in response to thyrotropin-releasing hormone (TRH), decreased triiodothyronine and increased reverse triiodothyronine, with variable effects on total and free thyroxine [36], leading to regain of lost weight, by increasing hunger, decreasing satiety, and enhancing energy storage.

Obesity is also associated with resting sympathetic nervous system overactivity. This chronic overactivity may lead to blunting of sympathetic nervous system responsiveness due to reduced sensitivity or downregulation of adrenoreceptors [36,70,71], possibly impairing EE, postprandial thermogenesis, and fat oxidation [36,72]. Diet-induced weight-loss has been shown to be accompanied by decreased sympathetic activity and increased cardiac parasympathetic activity [71,73].

Energy homeostasis

Maintenance of the body weight post diet-induced weight loss is associated with compensatory changes in EE favouring weight gain [19]. Leibel et al. showed that after weight gain, total energy expenditure (TEE) increased but REE did not change much. An increase in the non-REE accounted for this difference [19,48]. A major component of non-REE is skeletal muscle activity. After weight gain, muscle utilizes more energy to accomplish the same task, becoming less metabolically efficient [19,74]. Weight loss leads to a decrease in TEE, REE, and non-REE [19,34], to a level unaccounted for solely due to decreased body weight and altered body composition [19,75]. It has been proposed that this is due largely to an enhanced metabolic efficiency of skeletal muscles, especially at low workloads [34,74,76]. The body becomes more metabolically efficient, and so needs less energy than before at rest, and also expends less energy during exercise. This protects against additional weight loss [48]. The energy cost of moving less total body mass, at similar levels of physical activity, is lower, resulting in a decrease in non-REE [33]. It has been shown that there is a disproportionate slowing of REE during weight loss, in spite of relative preservation of fat-free mass. Unless high levels of physical activity or caloric restriction are maintained, this decrease in REE predisposes individuals to weight regain [77]. Changes in skeletal muscles leading to alterations in EE occurring with weight loss may be the reason exercise is helpful in maintaining a reduced body weight [19].

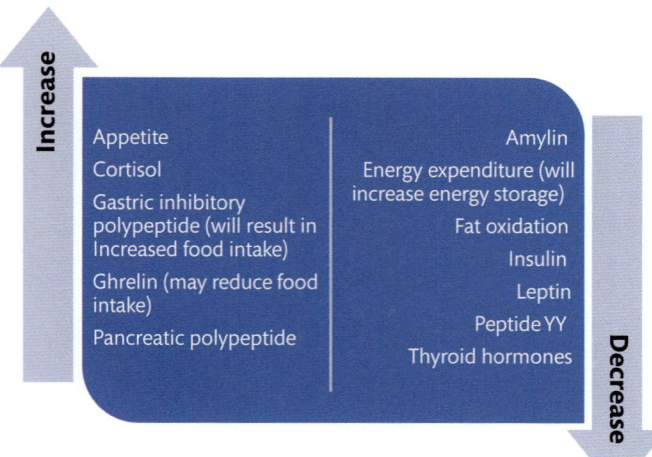

Increase		Decrease
Appetite		Amylin
Cortisol		Energy expenditure (will increase energy storage)
Gastric inhibitory polypeptide (will result in Increased food intake)		Fat oxidation
		Insulin
Ghrelin (may reduce food intake)		Leptin
		Peptide YY
Pancreatic polypeptide		Thyroid hormones

Fig. 1.1 Physiological changes after diet-induced weight loss.
Source: data from Sumithran, P. and Proietto, J. (2012) The defence of body weight: a physiological basis for weight regain after weight loss. *Clinical Science*, 124(4): 231–241.

Decreased EE after weight loss would matter little if EI was proportionately reduced [33,75]; however, there is an apparent disconnect between EI and energy output [33]. In fact, maintenance of decreased body weight is accompanied by an increase in EI above that required to maintain it. This increased EI in response to decreased energy output is a result of decreases in satiety and perception of amount of food consumed, along with changes in neuronal signalling in response to food. Together these factors keep energy (fat) stores of the body above the defined threshold. Most of these biological changes in response to diet-induced weight loss are proposed to be mediated by the hormone leptin [75]. The adaptive metabolic response to exercise-induced weight loss leading to decreased REE along with increased EI, indicates that both physiological and behavioural components of energy balance are affected [78]. These findings may explain the problem of not being able to lose the 'last few pounds' of a set weight-loss goal [48].

Nutrient metabolism

The composition of the diet used for weight loss may influence subsequent weight regain [79,80]. Ebbeling et al. compared patients receiving low-fat, low-glycaemic index, and very-low-carbohydrate diets and observed that the low-fat diet group showed the greatest decrease in TEE and REE, whereas the very-low-carbohydrate group showed the least. They suggested that reducing carbohydrate rather than dietary fat diet may help in maintaining weight loss [81].

Studies in rodents have shown that diet-induced weight loss is initially accompanied by preferential utilization of lipids over carbohydrates [33,82]. However, maintenance of weight loss leads to a shift towards carbohydrates as fuel [34,82]. Increased carbohydrate utilization spares dietary fat from oxidation, predisposing its deposition and storage in adipose tissue [82]. A low rate of fat oxidation in obese individuals may explain the tendency towards weight regain [83,84].

Subjective appetite

Since eating is pleasurable and rewarding, it stimulates associated brain centres, explaining the urge to eat in spite of satiety. Overeating is probably due to an imbalance between hypothalamic control and reward circuits, and/or a shift in the hedonic set point for food reward [85,86]. Obese individuals have been shown to have decreased dopamine D_2 receptors. Since dopamine is responsible for modulation of motivation and reward circuits, dopamine deficiency may lead to overeating as a compensatory phenomenon [33,87]. Hormonal adaptations to weight reduction lead not only to sustained increases in subjective appetite following diet-induced weight loss [37,66] but also in the perceived rewarding properties of food and a preference for calorie-rich food [36]. Food cravings are a component of the hedonic response [33]. Though dieting tends to increase the likelihood of food cravings, over time it has been shown to actually reduce the desire for high-fat, high-carbohydrate foods. Studies have also shown that mobilization of neural circuits responsible for executive control to resist food cravings may be the reason for the successful outcome of gastric bypass surgeries [88,89].

If the obesogenic environment is an important factor in the rise in obesity, then the obvious solution is to change it. Since we are not likely to go back in time and give up our convenient modern lifestyles, the challenge lies in engaging in physical activity and healthy eating in a way that is compatible with our current way of life.

Unfortunately, dietary strategies and physical activity by themselves are not always sufficient, and just like with other chronic illnesses, pharmacotherapy and surgical management too are required to treat obesity.

Management of obesity

Prior to counselling for weight-loss management and starting treatment, all patients need to be screened and evaluated. A focused, obesity-related history and physical examination are important, along with relevant laboratory assessments. Although behavioural factors relating to diet and physical activity are mainly responsible for weight gain, secondary causes of obesity, such as polycystic ovarian syndrome, hypothyroidism, Cushing's syndrome, and hypothalamic disease, should be ruled out. A history should also be taken of treatment with medications which promote weight gain [90]. Drugs implicated in weight gain and their alternatives are given in **Table 1.2** [91,92]. These have been taken from a systematic review commissioned by The Endocrine Society, in which a list of 54 commonly used drugs were compared to placebos in randomized controlled trials [91]. It is equally important to take a history of comorbidities, such as hypertension, coronary artery disease, metabolic syndrome, type 2 diabetes, osteoarthritis, and obstructive sleep apnoea, which are commonly, associated with obesity (**Table 1.3**) [90,93]. Other factors causing obesity may be genetics, smoking cessation, sleep disorders, or chronic stress.

Physical examination for degree and type of obesity

This includes assessment of parameters such as BMI and waist circumference or waist-to-hip ratio (WHR) [90]. See **Table 1.4** [12] for BMI risk categories. BMI is calculated by dividing weight (in kilograms) by squared height (in metres)—kg/m². Studies have shown that BMI has high specificity in diagnosing obesity but low sensitivity in identifying adiposity, thus missing many individuals with excess fat [94,95], especially the elderly, in whom a reduced lean body mass might be mistaken for a healthy BMI [96–98]. BMI can also overestimate body fat in muscular individuals [96]. Waist circumference can be used as a measure of visceral abdominal fat, which has been shown to carry a higher health risk than peripheral fat [96,99]. It is measured at the top of the right iliac crest with the tape held parallel to the floor at normal respiration, as per National Heart, Lung, and Blood Institute guidelines [96]. WHO, however, recommends measuring waist circumference at the midpoint between the lowest rib and the iliac crest, at the end of a normal expiration. For women and men, a waist circumference of at least 88 cm (35 inches) and at least 102 cm (40 inches), respectively, indicates an elevated risk of complications from obesity [96,99]. Such patients are at risk of type 2 diabetes, dyslipidaemia, hypertension, and cardiovascular disease [96]. The WHR is the ratio of a person's waist circumference to hip circumference. Based on WHR people may be categorized as 'apple shaped'—carrying weight around the middle—and 'pear shaped'—carrying weight around the hips. A WHR of at least 1.0 increases the risk of heart disease and other associated comorbidities [96]. A ratio of 0.90 or less for men and 0.80 or less for women is considered safe [96]. Hip circumference should be measured around the widest portion of the buttocks, with the tape parallel to the floor [100]. Body composition can be measured by various non-invasive methods such

Table 1.2 Drugs associated with weight gain and suggested alternatives (where evidence is mixed or reports are of a few cases, a '?' has been added)

Category	Drug class	Weight gain	Alternatives – weight reducing in parentheses
Psychiatric agents	Antipsychotic	Clozapine Risperidone Olanzapine Quetiapine Haloperidol Perphenazine Quetiapine	Ziprasidone Aripiprazole
	Antidepressants/mood stabilizers: tricyclic	Amitriptyline Doxepin Imipramine Nortriptyline Trimipramine	(Bupropion) Nefazodone Fluoxetine (short term) Sertraline (<1 year)
	Antidepressants/mood stabilizers: SSRIs	Mirtazapine Fluoxetine? Sertraline? Paroxetine Fluvoxamine	
	Antidepressants/mood stabilizers: MAO inhibitors	Phenelzine Tranylcypromine	
	Lithium		
Neurological agents	Anticonvulsants	Carbamazepine Gabapentin Valproate	Lamotrigine? (Topiramate) (Zonisamide)
Endocrinological agents	Diabetes drugs	Insulin (weight gain differs with type and regimen used) Sulfonylureas Thiazolidinediones Sitagliptin? Metiglinide	(Metformin) (Acarbose) (Miglitol) (Pramlintide) (Exenatide) (Liraglutide)
Gynaecological agents	Oral contraceptives	Progestational steroids Hormonal contraceptives containing progestational steroids	Barrier methods IUDs
	Endometriosis treatment	Depot leuprolide acetate	Surgical methods
Cardiological agents	Antihypertensives	α-blocker? β-blocker?	ACE inhibitors Calcium channel Blockers Angiotensin-2 receptor antagonists
Infectious disease agents	Antiretroviral therapy	Protease inhibitors	None
General	Steroid hormones	Corticosteroids Progestational Steroids	NSAIDs
	Antihistamines/anticholinergics	Diphenhydramine? Doxepin? Cyproheptadine?	Decongestants Steroid inhalers

ACE, angiotensin-converting enzyme; IUDs, intrauterine devices; MAO, monoamine oxidase; NSAIDs, non-steroidal anti-inflammatory drugs; SSRIs, selective serotonin reuptake inhibitors.
Source: Data from Domecq, J.P., Prutsky G., Leppin A., et al. Drugs commonly associated with weight change: a systematic review and meta-analysis. *The Journal of Clinical Endocrinology & Metabolism*, 100(2): 363–370, 2015 The Endocrine Society and Oxford University Press; Data from Apovian, C.M., Aronne, L.J., Bessesen, D.H., et al. Pharmacological management of obesity: an Endocrine Society clinical practice guideline. *The Journal of Clinical Endocrinology & Metabolism*,100(2): 342–362, 2015. The Endocrine Society and Oxford University Press.

as dual-energy X-ray absorptiometry, bioimpedance analysis, air-displacement plethysmography (BOD POD®), and body scanning procedures such as computed tomography and magnetic resonance imaging [101,102]. These methods have made it easy to classify individuals based on the degree of body fat, independent of BMI.

Body composition measurement is useful in determining fat and lean mass before and after treatment [101]. In clinical settings, due to cost, availability, time, and technical skills required for imaging methods, anthropometric measurements may be used as estimates of adipose tissue distribution [103]. Anthropometric measurements

Table 1.3 Diseases and symptoms linked to obesity

Cardiovascular	• Hypertension • Congestive heart failure • Cor pulmonale • Varicose veins • Pulmonary embolism • Coronary artery disease
Respiratory	• Dyspnoea • Obstructive sleep apnoea • Hypoventilation syndrome • Pickwickian syndrome • Asthma
Endocrine	• Metabolic syndrome • Type 2 diabetes • Dyslipidaemia • Polycystic ovarian syndrome
Gastrointestinal	• Gastro-oesophageal reflux disease • Non-alcoholic fatty liver disease • Cholelithiasis • Hernias • Colon cancer
Musculoskeletal	• Hyperuricaemia and gout • Immobility • Osteoarthritis (knees and hips) • Low back pain • Carpal tunnel syndrome
Genitourinary	• Urinary stress incontinence • Obesity-related glomerulopathy • Hypogonadism (male) • Breast and uterine cancer • Pregnancy complications
Psychological	• Depression/low self-esteem • Body image disturbance • Social stigmatization
Neurological	• Stroke • Idiopathic intracranial hypertension • Meralgia paresthetica • Dementia
Integument	• Striae distensae • Stasis pigmentation of legs • Lymphoedema • Cellulitis • Intertrigo, carbuncles • Acanthosis nigricans • Acrochordons (skin tags) • Hidradenitis suppurativa

Reproduced with permission from Kasper, D.L., Hauser, F.A. et al. *Harrison's Principles of Internal Medicine*, 19th Edition. New York: McGraw-Hill Education. Copyright © 2015 McGraw-Hill Education.

include limb circumference measurements and skinfold thickness of various parts of the body [103]. However, the drawback remains of obtaining reliable readings in older people with loose connective tissue and even in the extremely obese, with large skin folds [103].

Treatment criteria

According to the European guidelines for obesity management in adults (2015), the following are the minimum data required prior to starting treatment [101]:

• Fasting blood glucose
• Serum lipid profile (total, triglycerides, high-density lipoprotein, and low-density lipoprotein)
• Uric acid

• Thyroid function (thyroid-stimulating hormone level)
• Liver function (hepatic enzymes)
• Cardiovascular assessment, if indicated
• Endocrine evaluation if Cushing syndrome or hypothalamic disease suspected
• Liver investigation (ultrasound, biopsy) if abnormal liver function tests suggest non-alcoholic fatty liver disease or other liver pathology
• Sleep laboratory investigation for sleep apnoea.

Although sustained weight loss of as little as 3–5% of body weight can lead to clinically meaningful reductions in cardiovascular risk factors, larger weight losses produce greater benefits [104]. The American College of Cardiology (ACC), the American Heart Association (AHA), and The Obesity Society (TOS), in their 2013 guideline, recommend as an initial goal the loss of 5–10% of body weight within 6 months [104]. Since permanent weight loss is difficult to attain exclusively with diet and exercise, pharmacotherapy becomes an important adjunct. Medications act to potentiate the effect of behavioural changes, encouraging consumption of fewer calories [92]. In people trying to lose weight, there are often repeated cycles of weight loss and regain called weight cycling, which is associated with negative health outcomes and makes future weight loss more difficult [12,101]. It is usually associated with depression and psychological distress and requires appropriate therapy [105]. The Endocrine Society, in January, 2015, released new guidelines on the treatment of obesity [92] emphasizing that diet, exercise, and behavioural modification should be a part of all obesity management, with adjunctive pharmacotherapy as necessary.

Lifestyle management

Diet therapy

Food consists of more than just calories; selecting healthy yet palatable and tasty food improves the chances of sticking to the diet. Guidelines from the National Heart, Lung, and Blood Institute recommend initiating treatment with a calorie deficit of 500–1000 kcal/day compared with the patient's normal diet. This reduction is consistent with a goal of losing 1–2 pounds per week (0.5–1 kg) [90,96]. The 2013 AHA/ACC/TOS guidelines for the management of overweight and obesity in adults advocate estimating the individual energy requirements according to either the Harris–Benedict equation, or the Mifflin–St Jeor equation (a modification of the Harris–Benedict equation) given in Table 1.5 and Table 1.6 [106,107]. They advise an energy deficit of 500–750 kcal/day or 30% of the daily requirement [104].

This calorie deficit can be instituted through dietary substitutions or alternatives. It is important that dietary counselling remains patient centred and that the goals set should be practical, realistic, and achievable [101]. Diets which provide 1200 kcal/day or more are called hypocaloric balanced diets or balanced deficit diets. They result in significant weight loss regardless of which macronutrient is emphasized, can be tailored to individual needs, and hence have the best chance for long-term success [101]. An emphasis on the proportions of macronutrients in different diets (e.g. low fat, low carbohydrate, or high protein contents) did not prove better than

Table 1.4 Classification of overweight and obesity by BMI, waist circumference, and associated disease risk

	BMI (kg/m²)	Obesity class	Disease risk[a] relative to normal weight and waist circumference	
			Men ≤102 cm (≤40 in)	Men >102 cm (>40 in)
			Women ≤88 cm (≤35 in)	Women >88 cm (>35 in)
Underweight	<18.5		–	–
Normal[b]	18.5–24.9		–	–
Overweight	25.0–29.9		Increased	High
Obesity	30.0–34.9	I	High	Very high
	35.0–39.9	II	Very high	Very high
Extreme obesity	≥40	III	Extremely high	Extremely high

[a] Disease risk for type 2 diabetes, hypertension, and cardiovascular disease.

[b] Increased waist circumference can also be a marker for increased risk even in persons of normal weight.

Reproduced with permission from *Obesity: preventing and managing the global epidemic. Report of a WHO Consultation* (WHO Technical Report Series 894). Copyright © 2000, World Health Organization. https://www.who.int/nutrition/publications/obesity/WHO_TRS_894/en/

hypocaloric balanced diets, except for low glycaemic load diets (carbohydrate content of the diet × glycaemic index) in the short term [79,108–111]. In fact, all reduced-energy diets, with varying macronutrient composition, have a similar effect on body-fat loss in the short term, though little is known about their long-term effects [111]. Diets providing less than 1200 kcal/day may cause micronutrient deficiencies, requiring the use of dietary supplements. Low-calorie diets (LCDs), provide between 800 and 1500 kcal/day [96]. An appropriate nutrient composition for an LCD diet according to the NHLBI is less than 30% fat (saturated fatty acids, 8–10%; mono-unsaturated fatty acids, up to 15%; polyunsaturated fatty acids up to 10%), carbohydrates 55% or more and proteins approximately 15% [96]. Very-low-calorie diets (VLCDs) provide less than 800 kcal/day [96,101] by providing large amounts of dietary protein, usually 0.8–1.5 g protein/kg ideal body weight, up to 80 g carbohydrate/day and 15 g fat/day, along with 100% of the recommended daily allowance of essential vitamins and minerals, to avoid nutritional inadequacies [112]. Replacing one or two daily meal portions by a VLCD may give a nutritionally better-balanced diet [101]. VLCDs should be used strictly under the supervision of an obesity specialist. Since the given definition does not take into account the REE or energy requirement of the patient, an alternative definition of a VLCD is a diet that provides less than 50% of an individual's predicted REE [112]. Vitamin deficiency, starvation ketosis, and electrolyte derangements are potential complications to look for in any LCD.

Depending on the nutrient composition, the four best known diets are low-carbohydrate, low-fat, Mediterranean, and low glycaemic load diets [45]. Low-carbohydrate diets (e.g. the Atkins diet [113]),

advocate as little as 20 g/day of carbohydrate and have high protein and fat content. Higher protein intake is associated with greater satiety [79]. Low-fat diets, such as recommended by the AHA, advocate 10–20% of calories from fat and recommend greater portions of grains, fruits, and vegetables [114]. These are low-energy-density diets which allow larger amounts of food to be consumed and provide greater satiety [45,114]. Mediterranean-type diets advise higher consumption of unsaturated fats (such as from olive oil, nuts, and fish) rather than saturated fats (such as from red meat and butter) [115]. They also encourage an increased intake of fruits, vegetables, and whole grains. Portion-controlled diets or meal replacements are another option. They provide a fixed portion of food, usually a high-protein, liquid diet [45].

The glycaemic index (GI) is a relative ranking of carbohydrate in foods according to how they affect blood glucose levels. Accordingly, food can be divided into those with a low (≤55), moderate (56–69), or high glycaemic index (≥70). Low glycaemic load diets are based on the principle that foods with a lower glycaemic index favourably affect blood sugar (decrease glycated haemoglobin). Meals with a high glycaemic index cause a rapid spike in glucose which results in a shift of metabolic processes from oxidation to nutrient storage. This causes blood sugar levels to drop below the normal range, resulting in increased hunger and ultimately weight gain. Conversely, foods with a low glycaemic index are digested, absorbed, and metabolized slowly, thus inducing satiety [45,116,117].

Another concept is that of energy density. The energy density of a food is the energy content of that food divided by the amount of food. For example, the energy density of 80 g of grapes = 0.75 (i.e. 60 kcal per 80 g) and for 80 g cheese = 4.0 (320 kcal per 80 g). Thus,

Table 1.5 Harris–Benedict equation

BMR calculation for men (metric)	BMR = 66.5 + (13.75 × weight in kg) + (5.003 × height in cm) – (6.755 × age in years)
BMR calculation for women (metric)	BMR = 655.1 + (9.563 × weight in kg) + (1.850 × height in cm) – (4.676 × age in years)

BMR, basal metabolic rate.

Reproduced from Harris, J.A., Benedict, F.G. A biometric study of human basal metabolism. *Proceedings of the National Academy of Sciences,* 4(12): 370–373. Copyright © 1918, Authors.

Table 1.6 Mifflin–St Jeor equation

Men	BMR = (10 × weight in kg) + (6.25 × height in cm) – (5 × age in years) + 5
Women	BMR = (10 × weight in kg) + (6.25 × height in cm) – (5 × age in years) – 161

BMR, basal metabolic rate.

Reproduced with permission from Mifflin, M.D., St Jeor, S.T., Hill, L.A. et al. A new predictive equation for resting energy expenditure in healthy individuals. *The American Journal of Clinical Nutrition,* 51(2):241–247. Copyright © 1990, Oxford University Press on behalf of the American Society for Clinical Nutrition.

food with higher fat content will be more energy dense than others for a similar weight [116]. Since we tend to eat a constant volume of food, decreasing the energy density of a diet is an effective weight-loss strategy. Increasing the water and fibre content of food decreases the total energy density without affecting caloric content of a diet, at the same time giving it greater volume, thereby influencing satiety [90,116]. Weight loss, it must be remembered, is not linear as predicted by Max Wishnofsky's rule ('the caloric equivalent of one pound of body weight lost or gained will be 3500') [118,119] but curvilinear, tending to be rapid initially then slowing down until a plateau is reached [108,120,121]. The initial decrease in caloric intake leads to compensatory mechanisms, increasing the food intake and reducing weight loss [37]. Adherence to the dietary programme is the key to the success of any dietary therapy. To achieve weight loss over long term, obese individuals need to consciously decrease EI, by reducing portion sizes, decreasing the energy density of the diet, counting calories, or combining any of these [46].

Physical activity therapy

Exercise alone is only moderately effective for weight loss; however, the combination of diet and exercise is an effective behavioural approach for the treatment of obesity. Its most important role is in the maintenance of the weight loss [45,90]. Physical activity increases cardiorespiratory fitness independent of weight loss, thereby reducing the risk for cardiovascular disease [96,122,123]. It also leads to improvements in risk factors of other comorbidities such as metabolic syndrome, insulin resistance, type 2 diabetes, dyslipidaemia, hypertension, and pulmonary disease [123]. Aerobic training is the optimal mode of exercise for reducing fat mass and body mass while resistance training is needed for increasing lean mass, especially in middle-aged and overweight/obese individuals [101,124], and for increasing resting metabolic rate [45,108]. By itself, resistance exercise results only in minimal reductions in body weight [108]. The 2008 Physical Activity Guidelines for Americans recommend 150 minutes of moderate-intensity or 75 minutes of vigorous-intensity aerobic physical activity per week, performed in episodes of at least 10 minutes and preferably spread throughout the week, for adults; this should be combined with muscle-strengthening activities that involve all major muscle groups on two or more days a week [125]. A consensus statement of the International Association for the Study of Obesity in 2002 says that such population guidelines, however, are more effective for promoting health and primarily preventing risk factors for chronic diseases rather than for the treatment or reversal of established obesity, for which they are clearly insufficient [126]. Moderate intensity activity of approximately 45–60 minutes per day is recommended as a requirement to prevent the transition to overweight or obesity. The prevention of weight regain in formerly obese individuals on the other hand requires 60–90 minutes of moderate intensity activity or lesser amounts of vigorous intensity activity per day [126].

The American College of Sports Medicine recommendations for physical activity to maintain health [127] and promote weight loss [128] can be summarized as follows [129]:

- For maintaining and improving health: 150 min/week
- For prevention of weight gain: 150–250 min/week
- To promote clinically significant weight loss: 225–420 min/week
- For prevention of weight gain after weight loss: 200–300 min/week.

Physical activity has been shown by investigators to be critical for long-term weight management [130–133]. The probable explanation for how physical activity facilitates the maintenance of lost weight is that increased physical activity helps in maintaining the energy balance. Walking 3–4 miles a day may help to compensate for indiscretions of diet which are occasionally committed and which are associated with weight regain. Another explanation is that exercise spares the loss of fat-free mass during diet-induced weight reduction [45,46,134]. High levels of physical activity seem to be essential in compensating for the increase in energy efficiency after weight loss [45]. Rosenbaum et al., in their study of obese individuals who had lost 10% of initial weight, showed that maintenance of reduced body weight was associated with a decrease in TEE, approximately 300 to 500 kcal/day more than that predicted by changes in body mass and composition. This decrease in TEE was mainly due to a decrease in non-REE, showing increased work efficiency of skeletal muscle. Paradoxically, successful weight losers may have to nearly double their physical activity to make up for their increased energy efficiency [45,135]. The overweight, the obese, and even individuals of average weight often do not exercise, citing lack of time. It should be emphasized that, for weight control, physical activity at moderate intensity, even in short bouts of 10 minutes, can be effective [45]. It has been shown that as part of a comprehensive weight-loss programme, weight loss can be achieved just as effectively with multiple short bouts of activity throughout the day as with a single long bout (>40 minutes) [136]. Studies have also shown that activities involving increased EE throughout the day, without any emphasis on the intensity or duration of the activity, are as effective for weight control as more traditional activities such as jogging, swimming, cycling, and so on [45,137].

Behavioural therapy

Behaviour therapy is a set of principles and techniques which are employed to help obese individuals in modifying their eating habits, physical activity, and thought processes contributing to their obesity [45]. Key components of behaviour therapy include setting specific goals for behaviour change that specify what an individual will do, and when, where, and for how long he/she will engage in that behaviour [45,47]. Self-monitoring is the most important component of behavioural treatment [46] and has been shown to consistently predict both short- and long-term weight loss [138]. Cognitive behavioural therapy is used to help change and reinforce new dietary and physical activity behaviours. Stress management techniques, stimulus control (e.g. using smaller plates, not eating in front of the television), social support, problem-solving, and cognitive restructuring may help patients develop more positive and realistic thoughts about themselves [90,96].

Behavioural approaches are based on the classical principle of conditioning, which states that behaviours are often based on previous or simultaneous events, which on repetition become strongly linked. For example, eating may be triggered by negative emotions, long periods of dietary restriction, watching a favourite television show, or socializing with friends. The cognitive approach recognizes the importance of thinking patterns which cause behaviour change. The assumption is that thoughts directly affect feelings and behaviours. Put simply, what a person thinks about a situation determines how they feel and what they will do. These thought processes are important for behaviour changes and this basic premise is the foundation of cognitive therapy [47].

New technologies, including wi-fi scales, smart phones, and tablets (with weight-loss applications) have made it easier and convenient to monitor food intake, physical activity, and weight behaviours [45]. Programmes that are delivered from a distance by call centres, text messaging, or social networking sites can benefit a greater number of people by increasing ease of participation [45].

It has been shown that sleep patterns also play a role in obesity. Adequate and healthy sleep patterns help in the maintenance of fat-free mass during periods of reduced caloric intake, and therefore are an important component in harnessing weight-loss benefits from various interventions. Insufficient sleep, conversely, detracts from the body's ability to maintain the weight lost. An optimal period of sleep would be 7–9 hours. Shorter or longer periods are associated with weight gain [139,140].

Pharmacotherapy

Pharmacotherapy is justified only when the benefit outweighs the risk, since all medications inherently have more risks than diet and exercise. Pharmacotherapy is recommended with a BMI of 30 kg/m² or greater, or a BMI of 27 kg/m² or greater with comorbidity, as an adjunct to caloric restriction, increased physical activity, and behaviour modification [90,96,141]. The efficacy of pharmacotherapy should be evaluated after the first 3 months. If satisfactory weight loss is achieved (>5% in non-diabetic and >3% in diabetic patients), treatment should be continued [92,101,141,142].

Medications for obesity have traditionally been divided into two major categories: appetite suppressants (anorexiants) and gastro-intestinal fat blockers. Appetite suppressants are centrally acting drugs, which primarily target the noradrenergic, dopaminergic, and serotonergic receptors in the hypothalamus. Gastrointestinal fat blockers are peripherally acting drugs which reduce the absorption of selective macronutrients, such as fat, from the gastrointestinal tract [90,143]—for details of all these medications, see Table 1.7 [101]. FDA-approved medication can also be divided into two groups based on treatment term [108]:

- Agents approved for long-term treatment: these include orlistat, lorcaserin, liraglutide, the combination of phentermine/topiramate extended release, and the combination of naltrexone and bupropion sustained release.
- Agents approved for short-term use (<12 weeks): these include phentermine, diethylpropion, benzphetamine, and phendimetrazine.

Medications approved by the FDA for long-term use

Centrally acting anorexiant medications

Anorexiants increase satiety and decrease hunger, thus they are successful in reducing caloric intake without a sense of deprivation. The biological effect of these agents on appetite

Table 1.7 Pharmacotherapy for obesity

Drugs	Status	Mechanism	Dosing	Response evaluation	Warnings	Contraindications	Side effects
Orlistat	FDA & EMA approved	Pancreatic, gastric lipase inhibitor	120 mg tid 60 mg tid (OTC)	2.9–3.4% 1 year	Hepatitis, liver failure (rare), concomitant, multivitamin advised	Pregnancy, breast feeding, chronic malabsorption syndrome, cholestasis	Decreased absorption of fat-soluble vitamins, steatorrhoea, faecal urgency
Lorcaserin	FDA approved	5HT2c-R agonist	10 mg bid	3.6% 1 year Stop if <5% weight loss at 12 weeks	Serotonin syndrome, cognitive impairment, depression, valvulopathy, hypoglycaemia, priapism	Pregnancy, breast feeding, use with caution: MAOIs, SSRIs, SNRIs	Headache, nausea, dry mouth, dizziness, fatigue, constipation
Phentermine/ topiramate	FDA approved	NE release (P) GABA Modulation (T)	Starting dose: 3.75/23 qd Recommended dose: 7.5/46 qd * high dose: 15/92 qd	6.6% (recommended dose) 1 year 8.6% (high dose) 1 year Stop if <%5 weight loss at 12 weeks	Fetal toxicity, acute myopia, cognitive dysfunction, metabolic acidosis, hypoglycaemia	Pregnancy, breast feeding, glaucoma, hyperthyroidism, use with caution: MAOIs	Insomnia, dry mouth, constipation, paraesthesia, dizziness, dysgeusia
Bupropion/ naltrexone	FDA & EMA approved	DA/NE reuptake inhibitor (B) Opioid antagonist (N)	8/90 mg tb 2 tb bid	4.8% 1 year Stop if <5% weight loss at 12 weeks	Fetal toxicity, increased seizure risk, glaucoma, hepatoxicity	Uncontrolled hypertension, seizure, anorexia nervosa/bulimia, drug or alcohol withdrawal, use with caution: MAOIs	Nausea, constipation, headache, vomiting, dizziness
Liraglutide	FDA & EMA approved	GLP-1 agonist	3 mg SC	5.8 kg 1 year Stop if <4% weight loss at 14 weeks	Acute pancreatitis, acute gall bladder disease	Medullary thyroid cancer history, MEN type 2 history	Nausea, vomiting, pancreatitis

* Careful observation.

5HT2c-R, 5 hydroxytryptamine 2c receptor; bid, twice daily; DA, dopamine; EMA, European Medicinal Agency; FDA, Food & Drug Administration; GABA, gamma-aminobutyric acid; GLP-1, glucagon-like peptide-1; MAOIs, monoamine oxidase inhibitors; MEN, multiple endocrine neoplasia; NE, norepinephrine; OTC, over the counter; qd, four times daily; SC, subcutaneous; SNRI, serotonin norepinephrine reuptake inhibitor; SSRI, selective serotonin reuptake inhibitor; tb, tablet; tid, three times daily

regulation is produced by augmentation of the neurotransmission of three monoamines: norepinephrine, serotonin, and dopamine [90,96,143]. They work by increasing the secretion of these monoamines into the synaptic neural cleft, by inhibiting their reuptake back into the neuron, or by both mechanisms [96,143]. The target site for the actions of anorexiants is the ventromedial and lateral hypothalamus [90].

Lorcaserin

This is a selective 5-hydroxytryptamine $(HT)_{2C}$ receptor agonist. It is thought to decrease food intake through the POMC system of neurons, present in the arcuate nucleus of the hypothalamus, which acts on anorexigenic melanocortin-4 receptors by cleaving to α-MSH [90,144]. The selectivity of lorcaserin at the $5-HT_{2C}$ receptors is an advantage, in that it avoids the cardiovascular effects (valvulopathy) of other non-selective serotonergic medications [145]. However, in higher doses, lorcaserin also acts on $5-HT_{2B}$ and $5-HT_{2A}$ receptors [144,145]. Lorcaserin is 70% protein bound, it is metabolized in the liver, and 92% is excreted renally. It has a half-life of 11 hours [144,146]. The recommended dosage is 10 mg twice daily [90,145]. The most common side effects seen with lorcaserin treatment are headache, dizziness, tiredness, nausea, dry mouth, and constipation, and in diabetics, hypoglycaemia, headache, back pain, cough, and fatigue [147]. Since lorcaserin affects serotonin receptors, serotonin syndrome and neuroleptic malignant syndrome-like reactions may be precipitated if used in conjunction with other serotonergic agents. It should, therefore, be used with caution, in combination with norepinephrine reuptake inhibitors, selective serotonin reuptake inhibitors, monoamine oxidase inhibitors, tramadol, meperidine, and dopamine antagonists [145,147]. Serotonin syndrome presents with the classical triad of (1) changes in mental status (e.g. hallucinations, coma, agitation), (2) autonomic dysfunction (e.g. tachycardia, labile blood pressure, hyperthermia), and (3) neuromuscular excitation (e.g. incoordination, hyperreflexia). Lorcaserin inhibits cytochrome P450 and may increase the bradycardiac effects of beta blockers metabolized by the same enzyme (metoprolol, propranolol) [146]. However, since lorcaserin is metabolized via multiple pathways, serotonin syndrome and not increased drug effect is the main concern [146]. Patients on long-term treatment, especially diabetics, are at an increased risk of hypoglycaemia and require blood sugar monitoring [144,147]. Lorcaserin is a schedule IV substance, since it has potential for abuse [148]. It is contraindicated in pregnancy (pregnancy category X drug) [144,145].

Phentermine/topiramate extended release

This is a combination of two drugs based on the principle of synergism, that a lower dose of both will provide efficacy with lesser toxicity [101]. This combination contains a catecholamine releaser (phentermine) and an anticonvulsant (topiramate). Topiramate is approved by the FDA as an anticonvulsant. Weight loss was identified as an unintended side effect of topiramate during its clinical trials for epilepsy. The mechanism of weight loss is thought to be mediated via augmentation of gamma-aminobutyric acid receptors, inhibition of carbonic anhydrase, and antagonism of glutamate [90]. Phentermine is a sympathomimetic amine pharmacologically similar to amphetamines, which induces anorectic effects by the release of catecholamines (norepinephrine) in the hypothalamus, causing appetite suppression by increasing blood leptin

concentration [108,146,149]. The recommended starting dose is 3.75 mg/23 mg four times daily for at least 2 weeks; if tolerated, it is increased to 7.5 mg/46 mg [92]. Common side effects are dry mouth, constipation, insomnia, palpitations, dizziness, paraesthesias, and disturbances in attention [142,146]. Disturbances in bicarbonate, potassium, and creatinine have been observed with phentermine/topiramate treatment. Prior clinical trials with topiramate monotherapy showed that it may cause metabolic acidosis by inhibiting carbonic anhydrase. Similar results were observed in the 1- and 2-year safety cohort studies with high-dose phentermine/topiramate. The consequences of untreated chronic metabolic acidosis may include hyperventilation, fatigue, anorexia, and an increased risk of osteomalacia or osteoporosis. Reductions in potassium values are a known effect of topiramate's carbonic anhydrase inhibition, though a dose-related increase in serum creatinine has been observed, suggesting a decline in renal function; however, the cause and clinical significance of this increase has not been definitively established [150]. The combination is contraindicated during pregnancy due to its teratogenic potential (increased risk of cleft lip/cleft palate) [108]. Glaucoma is a rare side effect of topiramate. Other potential issues include risk of kidney stones (associated with topiramate) and increased heart rate in patients susceptible to phentermine [108].

Bupropion/naltrexone (Contrave®)

This combines two centrally acting medications. Bupropion is a dopamine and norepinephrine reuptake inhibitor. Naltrexone is a mu-opioid receptor antagonist [90,92,101]. The anorectic effect of bupropion is due to activation of POMC neurons in the arcuate nucleus. POMC neurons cleave into alpha-melanocyte-stimulating hormone (α-MSH), which is a potent anorectic neuropeptide [101,108,146]. It also releases beta-endorphin which creates a negative feedback loop; this loop is suppressed by naltrexone [108,146]. It is available as an 8 mg/90 mg combination tablet recommended as follows: one tablet in the morning to begin with; after 1 week, one tablet added before the evening meal; then increased progressively to a maximum of two tablets twice daily by the fourth week [92,151,152]. The most common adverse effects are nausea, headache, dizziness, insomnia, and vomiting [151,153]. An increase in systolic and/or diastolic blood pressure as well as an increase in resting heart rate, is an important side effect, mandating careful monitoring [151,152]. Naltrexone/bupropion should be used with caution in patients with renal disease and is contraindicated in those with severe hepatic disease [146]. The naltrexone component of this drug has the potential to cause problems with concomitant opioid medications. Shehebar et al., in the first published case of naltrexone/bupropion complicating perioperative anaesthetic and analgesic management, concluded that as naltrexone (an opioid antagonist) has a half-life of 5 hours, the combination should be discontinued at least 24 hours prior to anaesthesia [154]. Attempting to overcome the antagonistic effects of naltrexone, by administering high doses of opioids to manage postoperative pain, however, may cause an abrupt offset of the drug, leading to delayed respiratory depression in the postoperative period [154]. In cases of long-term opioid usage, the combination should be restarted 7–10 days after discontinuation of opioids, to prevent precipitation of opioid withdrawal [151,152].

The concomitant use of naltrexone/bupropion with a monoamine oxidase inhibitor is associated with increased chances of hypertensive reactions. A 14-day gap is recommended between discontinuation of a monoamine oxidase inhibitor and starting treatment with this combination [152]. Bupropion is a strong inhibitor of cytochrome P450 and can increase concentrations of selective serotonin reuptake inhibitors, antipsychotics (e.g. haloperidol and risperidone), beta-blockers (e.g. metoprolol), and type 1C antiarrhythmics (e.g. propafenone and flecainide); hence, dose reduction when used together should be considered [151,152]. Additionally, it has a dose-related propensity to cause seizures [152]. Extra caution should be exercised when administering naltrexone/bupropion to patients with predisposing factors which increase seizure risk such as history of head injury, epilepsy, stroke, arteriovenous malformation, central nervous system tumour or infection, or metabolic disorders (e.g. hypoglycaemia, hyponatraemia, severe hepatic impairment, and hypoxia). Care must also be taken during concomitant administration of drugs which may lower the seizure threshold (e.g. antipsychotics, tricyclic antidepressants, theophylline and systemic steroids). The use of bupropion with levodopa or amantadine, due to combined dopamine agonistic effects, has been reported to cause restlessness, agitation, tremor, ataxia, gait disturbance, vertigo, and dizziness [151,152]. Naltrexone/bupropion carries a boxed warning for suicidal thoughts and behaviours, and neuropsychiatric reactions. Though it is not approved for the treatment of major depressive disorder or other psychiatric disorders, it may increase the risk of suicidal thoughts and behaviour. Similarly, though not approved for smoking cessation it may cause serious neuropsychiatric reactions in these patients [151].

Liraglutide

Liraglutide has a dual mechanism of action, that is, on the gastrointestinal tract and the brain [155]. This is a GLP-1 receptor agonist, an analogue of the endogenous hormone incretin, approved for the treatment of type 2 diabetes with independent weight loss effects due to hypothalamic neural activation causing appetite suppression [90]. Slowing of gastric emptying is an important effect of GLP-1 activity. This leads to gastric stretching which sends vagal afferent signals to the solitary nucleus of the medulla and hypothalamic appetite centres, inducing satiety; signals to the area postrema induce nausea [156]. Delayed gastric emptying may result from enhanced pyloric tone or diminished duodenal motility and should be borne in mind during preoperative preparation of the patient [157]. Long-term use of liraglutide has been associated with a decrease in glycated haemoglobin levels and systolic blood pressure [155,158]. Treatment is started at a dose of 0.6 mg daily by subcutaneous injection and increased by 0.6 mg per week up to a maximum of 3.0 mg [92]. Commonly seen side effects are nausea, vomiting, and change in bowel habits. Liraglutide is contraindicated in people with a family history of medullary thyroid carcinoma or multiple endocrine neoplasia syndrome type 2. It has been also been associated with the development of pancreatitis, cholelithiasis, and cholecystitis. There is an increased risk of hypoglycaemia when used together with insulin, and oral hypoglycaemics such as sulfonylureas in patients with type 2 diabetes, therefore regular blood sugar monitoring is required [108,159].

Peripherally acting medications

Orlistat

Orlistat is a synthetic derivative of lipostatin, a potent inhibitor of pancreatic, gastric, and carboxyl ester lipases and phospholipase A_2, needed for the hydrolysis of dietary fat into free fatty acids which decreases its epithelial absorption. It acts in the lumen of the stomach and small intestine, blocking the digestion and absorption of approximately 30% of dietary fat by forming a covalent bond with the active serine sites of these lipases [90,160]. It is associated with modest improvements in risk factors of obesity-related comorbidities, such as hypertension, glycaemic profile, and lipid parameters [155,161]. The recommended dose is 120 mg three times daily [92]. Most adverse events related to orlistat treatment are due to malabsorption of fat. Serum concentrations of the fat-soluble vitamins A, D, E, and K and beta-carotene may be reduced, necessitating vitamin supplements to prevent potential deficiencies [90,161,162]. It should be borne in mind that decreased absorption of vitamin K may increase warfarin's anticoagulant effect [161]. The absorption of certain fat-soluble drugs (amiodarone, ciclosporin, warfarin, and thyroxine) has also been shown to be affected [163]. Cases of severe liver injury have been reported [164]; therefore, it should be considered in case of itching, jaundice, pale colour stools, or anorexia [108,165]. Isolated cases of severe hypertension have also been reported, though a causal relationship has not been established [166,167]. Psyllium mucilloid taken concomitantly helps mitigate orlistat-induced gastrointestinal side effects such as faecal urgency, fatty/oily stool, and increased defecation [90].

Cetilistat

The undesirable gastrointestinal side effects of orlistat have led to the search for a peripherally acting drug with equal or greater efficacy to orlistat, while generating fewer adverse effects [168]. Cetilistat (ATL-962) 120 mg, developed by Alizyme in collaboration with Takeda Pharmaceutical and marketed as OBLEAN®, has been used in Japan since 2013 for the treatment of obesity and related diabetes or dyslipidaemia [169,170]. Cetilistat is a pancreatic lipase inhibitor which absorbs fat from the diet as efficiently as orlistat does, leading to weight loss but with 30% less gastrointestinal side effects [169,170]. It acts peripherally to reduce the appetite and does not affect the brain, similar to orlistat [169,170]. Studies have shown that cetilistat is well tolerated, significantly reduces body weight, and improves glycaemic control (modest improvement in in Hba1c) and the gastrointestinal side effects are significantly fewer compared with orlistat [171,172,173].

Medications approved by the FDA for short-term use

Four drugs have FDA approval for short-term (8–12 weeks) treatment of obesity as adjuncts to diet and physical therapy: phentermine, diethylpropion, benzphetamine, and phendimetrazine [108]. Phentermine is a sympathomimetic drug, producing central excitation, manifested as dry mouth, insomnia, or nervousness. Since sympathomimetic drugs increase heart rate and blood pressure, they should be used with caution in patients with cardiovascular disease [92]. Being advocated only for short-term use presents a conundrum for clinicians, as weight regain is likely after medication is stopped. Phentermine is currently widely prescribed, probably due to its low cost, and it is likely that much of this prescription is off label [92]. According to the Endocrine Society Clinical Practice Guideline, it seems reasonable for clinicians to prescribe phentermine long term as long as the patient:

- Has no evidence of serious cardiovascular disease
- Does not have serious psychiatric disease or a history of substance abuse

- Has been informed about FDA-approved weight-loss medications for long-term use and has been told that these have been documented
- Does not demonstrate a clinically significant increase in pulse or blood pressure
- Demonstrates a significant weight loss while using phentermine.

These points are to be documented in the patient's medical record along with the off-label nature of the prescription, at each visit. Medication is started at 7.5 or 15 mg/day initially and increased if the patient does not demonstrate significant weight loss. Follow-up should be done monthly during increase in dosage and later every 3 months when on a stable dose.

Other medications

Several medications approved for other indications may also promote weight loss and are used off-label for obesity such as:

- Metformin: this is a biguanide that is approved by the FDA for the treatment of diabetes mellitus. It decreases hepatic glucose production and glucose absorption from the gastrointestinal tract while enhancing insulin sensitivity [142]. Metformin has been associated with weight neutrality or mild weight loss [174].
- Exenatide: this is a GLP-1 receptor agonist, which has been approved by the FDA for treatment of type 2 diabetics inadequately controlled on metformin or sulfonylureas. Exenatide reduces glucose levels both during fasting and postprandially, slows gastric emptying, and decreases food intake [142]. Vilsbøll et al. found in their study that treatment with GLP-1 receptor agonists (exenatide and liraglutide) resulted in weight loss among overweight or obese patients [175].
- Pramlintide: this is another antidiabetic drug and synthetic analogue of the pancreatic hormone amylin. It has also been reported to cause weight loss and improve glycaemic control in patients with diabetes [142,176].
- Catechin: this is a flavonoid found in green tea, which may aid in weight loss [177].

The following agents are still under investigation and may be useful in the treatment of obesity in the future:

- Ghrelin antagonists
- Alpha-MSH analogues
- Enterostatin
- Neuropeptide YY antagonists
- Beta-3-adrenergic agonists.

Tagatose is a low-calorie sugar substitute, suggested for use in foods and beverages that is undergoing trials. It is a potential antidiabetic drug with weight-loss benefits and beneficial effects on postprandial hyperglycaemia and hyperinsulinaemia [178].

Olestra is a fat substitute made from fatty acids esterified to sucrose and is approved for use as a supplement or replacement for fat in the preparation of food. Olestra provides zero calories and may help in weight loss. Fat-soluble vitamins may need to be supplemented in such diets [179].

Bariatric surgery

Surgical therapy for obesity (bariatric surgery) is a therapeutic option associated with clinically significant and sustained weight loss in patients with morbid obesity. Bariatric surgery substantially decreases the risks of comorbidities and improves existing ones. The National Institutes of Health Consensus Development Conference Panel recommends bariatric surgery as the best alternative treatment for patients with extreme obesity (BMI ≥40 or ≥35 kg/m² with comorbidities). This topic will be dealt with elsewhere in this book [180].

REFERENCES

1. Eknoyan G. A history of obesity, or how what was good became ugly and then bad. Advances in Chronic Kidney Disease. 2006;**13**(4):421–27.
2. Gardner G, Halweil B, Peterson JA. Underfed and Overfed: The Global Epidemic of Malnutrition. Washington, DC: Worldwatch Institute; 2000.
3. World Health Organization. Controlling the global obesity epidemic. 2018. http://www.who.int/nutrition/topics/obesity/en/
4. World Health Organization. Obesity and overweight. 2018. http://www.who.int/en/news-room/fact-sheets/detail/obesity-and-overweight
5. Kyle TK, Dhurandhar EJ, Allison DB. Regarding obesity as a disease: evolving policies and their implications. Endocrinology and Metabolism Clinics. 2016;**45**(3):511–20.
6. Paddock C. Experts define obesity as a disease. 2017. https://www.medicalnewstoday.com/articles/317442.php
7. Bray G, Kim K, Wilding J, World Obesity Federation. Obesity: a chronic relapsing progressive disease process. A position statement of the World Obesity Federation. Obesity Reviews. 2017;**18**(7):715–23.
8. Bray GA. Obesity: the disease. Journal of Medicinal Chemistry. 2006;**49**(14):4001–4007.
9. Scottish Intercollegiate Guidelines Network (SIGN). Management of Obesity: A National Clinical Guideline. Edinburgh: SIGN; 2010.
10. Fryhofer S. Report of the Council on Science and Public Health (CSAPH). American Medical Association House of Delegates 2013 Annual Meeting (Resolution 115-A-12). Report 3-A-13. 2013.
11. Martin DW (Chair). Report of the Council on Science and Public Health. American Medical Association House of Delegates. Recognition of Obesity as a Disease. Resolution 420(A-13). 2013.
12. World Health Organization (WHO). Obesity: Preventing and Managing the Global Epidemic. Report of a WHO Consultation. Geneva: WHO; 2000.
13. Müller M, Geisler C. Defining obesity as a disease. European Journal of Clinical Nutrition. 2017;**71**(11):1256–58.
14. Mitchell NS, Catenacci VA, Wyatt HR, Hill JO. Obesity: overview of an epidemic. Psychiatric Clinics. 2011;**34**(4):717–32.
15. Hill JO, Wyatt HR, Peters JC. Energy balance and obesity. Circulation. 2012;**126**(1):126–32.
16. Hill JO, Commerford R. Physical activity, fat balance, and energy balance. International Journal of Sport Nutrition. 1996;**6**(2):80–92.
17. Müller M, Geisler C. From the past to future: from energy expenditure to energy intake to energy expenditure. European Journal of Clinical Nutrition. 2017;**71**(3):358–64.
18. Woo R, Daniels-Kush R, Horton ES. Regulation of energy balance. Annual Review of Nutrition. 1985;**5**(1):411–33.
19. Leibel RL, Rosenbaum M, Hirsch J. Changes in energy expenditure resulting from altered body weight. New England Journal of Medicine. 1995;**332**(10):621–28.
20. Blundell JE, Stubbs RJ, Hughes DA, Whybrow S, King NA. Cross talk between physical activity and appetite control: does physical

activity stimulate appetite? Proceedings of the Nutrition Society. 2003;**62**(3):651–61.

21. Epstein LH, Paluch RA, Consalvi A, Riordan K, Scholl T. Effects of manipulating sedentary behavior on physical activity and food intake. Journal of Pediatrics. 2002;**140**(3):334–39.

22. Prentice AM. Fires of life: the struggles of an ancient metabolism in a modern world. Nutrition Bulletin. 2001;**26**(1):13–27.

23. Ravussin E, Lillioja S, Knowler WC, et al. Reduced rate of energy expenditure as a risk factor for body-weight gain. New England Journal of Medicine. 1988;**318**(8):467–72.

24. Roberts SB, Savage J, Coward W, Chew B, Lucas A. Energy expenditure and intake in infants born to lean and overweight mothers. New England Journal of Medicine. 1988;**318**(8):461–66.

25. Wells J. Is obesity really due to high energy intake of low energy expenditure? International Journal of Obesity. 1998;**22**(11):1139–40.

26. Roberts S, Leibel R. Excess energy intake and low energy expenditure as predictors of obesity. International Journal of Obesity. 1998;**22**(5):385–86.

27. Carneiro IP, Elliott SA, Siervo M, et al. Is obesity associated with altered energy expenditure? Advances in Nutrition. 2016;**7**(3):476–87.

28. Friedman JM. Leptin at 14 y of age: an ongoing story. American Journal of Clinical Nutrition. 2009;**89**(3):973S–79S.

29. Dhurandhar NV, Schoeller D, Brown AW, et al. Energy balance measurement: when something is not better than nothing. International Journal of Obesity. 2015;**39**(7):1109–13.

30. Dhurandhar NV, Brown AW, Thomas D, Allison DB. We agree that self-reported energy intake should not be used as a basis for conclusions about energy intake in scientific research. Journal of Nutrition. 2016;**146**(5):1141–42.

31. Lenard NR, Berthoud HR. Central and peripheral regulation of food intake and physical activity: pathways and genes. Obesity. 2008;**16**(S3):S11–22.

32. O'Rourke RW. Metabolic thrift and the genetic basis of human obesity. Annals of Surgery. 2014;**259**(4):642–48.

33. Greenway F. Physiological adaptations to weight loss and factors favouring weight regain. International Journal of Obesity. 2015;**39**(8):1188–96.

34. MacLean PS, Bergouignan A, Cornier M-A, Jackman MR. Biology's response to dieting: the impetus for weight regain. American Journal of Physiology-Regulatory, Integrative and Comparative Physiology. 2011;**301**(3):R581–R600.

35. Karatsoreos IN, Thaler JP, Borgland SL, Champagne FA, Hurd YL, Hill MN. Food for thought: hormonal, experiential, and neural influences on feeding and obesity. Journal of Neuroscience. 2013;**33**(45):17610–16.

36. Sumithran P, Proietto J. The defence of body weight: a physiological basis for weight regain after weight loss. Clinical Science. 2013;**124**(4):231–41.

37. Sumithran P, Prendergast LA, Delbridge E, et al. Long-term persistence of hormonal adaptations to weight loss. New England Journal of Medicine. 2011;**365**(17):1597–604.

38. Valdearcos M, Robblee MM, Benjamin DI, Nomura DK, Xu AW, Koliwad SK. Microglia dictate the impact of saturated fat consumption on hypothalamic inflammation and neuronal function. Cell Reports. 2014;**9**(6):2124–38.

39. García-Cáceres C, Fuente-Martín E, Argente J, Chowen JA. Emerging role of glial cells in the control of body weight. Molecular Metabolism. 2012;**1**(1–2):37–46.

40. Jastroch M, Morin S, Tschöp MH, Yi C-X. The hypothalamic neural–glial network and the metabolic syndrome. Best Practice & Research Clinical Endocrinology & Metabolism. 2014;**28**(5):661–71.

41. Morton G, Cummings D, Baskin D, Barsh G, Schwartz M. Central nervous system control of food intake and body weight. Nature. 2006;**443**(7109):289–95.

42. Zheng H, Lenard N, Shin A, Berthoud H-R. Appetite control and energy balance regulation in the modern world: reward-driven brain overrides repletion signals. International Journal of Obesity. 2009;**33**(S2):S8–13.

43. Wadden TA, Brownell KD, Foster GD. Obesity: responding to the global epidemic. Journal of Consulting and Clinical Psychology. 2002;**70**(3):510–25.

44. McAllister EJ, Dhurandhar NV, Keith SW, et al. Ten putative contributors to the obesity epidemic. Critical Reviews in Food Science and Nutrition. 2009;**49**(10):868–913.

45. Wadden TA, Webb VL, Moran CH, Bailer BA. Lifestyle modification for obesity: new developments in diet, physical activity, and behavior therapy. Circulation. 2012;**125**(9):1157–70.

46. Wadden TA, Butryn ML, Wilson C. Lifestyle modification for the management of obesity. Gastroenterology. 2007;**132**(6):2226–38.

47. Wadden TA, Foster GD. Behavioral treatment of obesity. Medical Clinics of North America. 2000;**84**(2):441–61.

48. Dokken BB, Tsao T-S. The physiology of body weight regulation: are we too efficient for our own good? Diabetes Spectrum. 2007;**20**(3):166–70.

49. Keesey RE, Hirvonen MD. Body weight set-points: determination and adjustment. Journal of Nutrition. 1997;**127**(9):1875S–83S.

50. Leibel RL, Hirsch J. Diminished energy requirements in reduced-obese patients. Metabolism-Clinical and Experimental. 1984;**33**(2):164–70.

51. Cummings DE, Weigle DS, Frayo RS, et al. Plasma ghrelin levels after diet-induced weight loss or gastric bypass surgery. New England Journal of Medicine. 2002;**346**(21):1623–30.

52. Ahima RS. Revisiting leptin's role in obesity and weight loss. Journal of Clinical Investigation. 2008;**118**(7):2380–83.

53. Zhao X, Han Q, Gang X, et al. The role of gut hormones in diet-induced weight change: a systematic review. Hormone and Metabolic Research. 2017;**49**(11):816–25.

54. Essah P, Levy J, Sistrun S, Kelly S, Nestler J. Effect of weight loss by a low-fat diet and a low-carbohydrate diet on peptide YY levels. International Journal of Obesity. 2010;**34**(8):1239–42.

55. Chearskul S, Delbridge E, Shulkes A, Proietto J, Kriketos A. Effect of weight loss and ketosis on postprandial cholecystokinin and free fatty acid concentrations. American Journal of Clinical Nutrition. 2008;**87**(5):1238–46.

56. Muurahainen N, Kissileff HR, Derogatis AJ, Pi-Sunyer FX. Effects of cholecystokinin-octapeptide (CCK-8) on food intake and gastric emptying in man. Physiology & Behavior. 1988;**44**(4–5):645–49.

57. Flint A, Raben A, Astrup A, Holst JJ. Glucagon-like peptide 1 promotes satiety and suppresses energy intake in humans. Journal of Clinical Investigation. 1998;**101**(3):515–20.

58. Batterham RL, Cowley MA, Small CJ, et al. Gut hormone PYY 3–36 physiologically inhibits food intake. Nature. 2002;**418**(6898):650–54.

59. Woods SC, Lutz TA, Geary N, Langhans W. Pancreatic signals controlling food intake; insulin, glucagon and amylin. Philosophical Transactions of the Royal Society of London B: Biological Sciences. 2006;**361**(1471):1219–35.

60. Loh K, Zhang L, Brandon A, et al. Insulin controls food intake and energy balance via NPY neurons. Molecular Metabolism. 2017;**6**(6):574–84.

61. Batterham R, Le Roux C, Cohen M, et al. Pancreatic polypeptide reduces appetite and food intake in humans. Journal of Clinical Endocrinology & Metabolism. 2003;**88**(8):3989–92.

62. Cummings DE, Shannon MH. Roles for ghrelin in the regulation of appetite and body weight. Archives of Surgery. 2003;**138**(4):389–96.

63. Wren A, Seal L, Cohen M, et al. Ghrelin enhances appetite and increases food intake in humans. Journal of Clinical Endocrinology & Metabolism. 2001;**86**(12):5992.

64. Rosenbaum M, Sy M, Pavlovich K, Leibel RL, Hirsch J. Leptin reverses weight loss-induced changes in regional neural activity responses to visual food stimuli. Journal of Clinical Investigation. 2008;**118**(7):2583–91.

65. Crujeiras AB, Goyenechea E, Abete I, et al. Weight regain after a diet-induced loss is predicted by higher baseline leptin and lower ghrelin plasma levels. Journal of Clinical Endocrinology & Metabolism. 2010;**95**(11):5037–44.

66. Doucet E, Imbeault P, St-Pierre S, et al. Appetite after weight loss by energy restriction and a low-fat diet–exercise follow-up. International Journal of Obesity. 2000;**24**(7):906–14.

67. Zakrzewska K, Cusin I, Sainsbury A, Rohner-Jeanrenaud F, Jeanrenaud B. Glucocorticoids as counterregulatory hormones of leptin: toward an understanding of leptin resistance. Diabetes. 1997;**46**(4):717–19.

68. Tomiyama AJ, Mann T, Vinas D, Hunger JM, DeJager J, Taylor SE. Low calorie dieting increases cortisol. Psychosomatic Medicine. 2010;**72**(4):357–64.

69. Johnstone AM, Faber P, Andrew R, et al. Influence of short-term dietary weight loss on cortisol secretion and metabolism in obese men. European Journal of Endocrinology. 2004;**150**(2):185–94.

70. Smith MM, Minson CT. Obesity and adipokines: effects on sympathetic overactivity. Journal of Physiology. 2012;**590**(8):1787–801.

71. Thorp AA, Schlaich MP. Relevance of sympathetic nervous system activation in obesity and metabolic syndrome. Journal of Diabetes Research. 2015;**2015**: 341583.

72. Greenfield JR, Campbell LV. Role of the autonomic nervous system and neuropeptides in the development of obesity in humans: targets for therapy? Current Pharmaceutical Design. 2008;**14**(18):1815–20.

73. Arone L, Mackintosh R, Rosenbaum M, Leibel RL, Hirsch J. Autonomic nervous system activity in weight gain and weight loss. American Journal of Physiology-Regulatory, Integrative and Comparative Physiology. 1995;**269**(1):R222–25.

74. Rosenbaum M, Vandenborne K, Goldsmith R, et al. Effects of experimental weight perturbation on skeletal muscle work efficiency in human subjects. American Journal of Physiology-Regulatory, Integrative and Comparative Physiology. 2003;**285**(1):R183–92.

75. Rosenbaum M, Kissileff HR, Mayer LE, Hirsch J, Leibel RL. Energy intake in weight-reduced humans. Brain Research. 2010;**1350**:95–102.

76. Doucet E, Imbeault P, Sylvie S-P, et al. Greater than predicted decrease in energy expenditure during exercise after body weight loss in obese men. Clinical Science. 2003;**105**(1):89–95.

77. Johannsen DL, Knuth ND, Huizenga R, Rood JC, Ravussin E, Hall KD. Metabolic slowing with massive weight loss despite preservation of fat-free mass. Journal of Clinical Endocrinology & Metabolism. 2012;**97**(7):2489–96.

78. Hopkins M, Gibbons C, Caudwell P, et al. The adaptive metabolic response to exercise-induced weight loss influences both energy expenditure and energy intake. European Journal of Clinical Nutrition. 2014;**68**(5):581–86.

79. Larsen TM, Dalskov S-M, van Baak M, et al. Diets with high or low protein content and glycemic index for weight-loss maintenance. New England Journal of Medicine. 2010;**363**(22):2102–13.

80. Blomain ES, Dirhan DA, Valentino MA, Kim GW, Waldman SA. Mechanisms of weight regain following weight loss. ISRN Obesity. 2013;**2013**:210524.

81. Ebbeling CB, Swain JF, Feldman HA, et al. Effects of dietary composition on energy expenditure during weight-loss maintenance. JAMA. 2012;**307**(24):2627–34.

82. Jackman MR, Steig A, Higgins JA, et al. Weight regain after sustained weight reduction is accompanied by suppressed oxidation of dietary fat and adipocyte hyperplasia. American Journal of Physiology-Regulatory, Integrative and Comparative Physiology. 2008;**294**(4):R1117–29.

83. Frisancho AR. Reduced rate of fat oxidation: a metabolic pathway to obesity in the developing nations. American Journal of Human Biology. 2003;**15**(4):522–32.

84. Larson DE, Ferraro RT, Robertson DS, Ravussin E. Energy metabolism in weight-stable postobese individuals. American Journal of Clinical Nutrition. 1995;**62**(4):735–39.

85. Yu YH. Making sense of metabolic obesity and hedonic obesity. Journal of Diabetes. 2017;**9**(7):656–66.

86. Egecioglu E, Skibicka KP, Hansson C, et al. Hedonic and incentive signals for body weight control. Reviews in Endocrine and Metabolic Disorders. 2011;**12**(3):141–51.

87. Berthoud H-R, Münzberg H, Morrison CD. Blaming the brain for obesity: integration of hedonic and homeostatic mechanisms. Gastroenterology. 2017;**152**(7):1728–38.

88. Scholtz S, Miras AD, Chhina N, et al. Obese patients after gastric bypass surgery have lower brain-hedonic responses to food than after gastric banding. Gut. 2014;**63**(6):891–902.

89. Goldman RL, Canterberry M, Borckardt JJ, et al. Executive control circuitry differentiates degree of success in weight loss following gastric-bypass surgery. Obesity. 2013;**21**(11):2189–96.

90. Kasper DL, Fausi AS, Hauser SL, Longo DL, Jameson L, Loscalzo J. Harrison's Principles of Internal Medicine. 19th ed. New York: The McGraw-Hill Companies, Inc.; 2015.

91. Domecq JP, Prutsky G, Leppin A, et al. Drugs commonly associated with weight change: a systematic review and meta-analysis. Journal of Clinical Endocrinology & Metabolism. 2015;**100**(2):363–70.

92. Apovian CM, Aronne LJ, Bessesen DH, et al. Pharmacological management of obesity: an Endocrine Society clinical practice guideline. Journal of Clinical Endocrinology & Metabolism. 2015;**100**(2):342–62.

93. Karam JM. Secondary causes of obesity. Therapy. 2007;**4**(5):641–50.

94. Okorodudu D, Jumean M, Montori V, et al. Diagnostic performance of body mass index to identify obesity as defined by body adiposity: a systematic review and meta-analysis. International Journal of Obesity. 2010;**34**(5):791–99.

95. Romero-Corral A, Somers VK, Sierra-Johnson J, et al. Accuracy of body mass index in diagnosing obesity in the adult general population. International Journal of Obesity. 2008;**32**(6):959–66.

96. National Heart, Lung, and Blood Institute. Clinical guidelines on the identification, evaluation, and treatment of overweight and obesity in adults: the evidence report. NHLBI Obesity Education Initiative Expert Panel on the Identification, Evaluation,

and Treatment of Obesity in Adults (US). Obesity Research. 1998;Suppl 2:51S-209S.

97. Gill LE, Bartels SJ, Batsis JA. Weight management in older adults. Current Obesity Reports. 2015;**4**(3):379–88.

98. Romero-Corral A, Somers VK, Sierra-Johnson J, et al. Normal weight obesity: a risk factor for cardiometabolic dysregulation and cardiovascular mortality. European Heart Journal. 2009;**31**(6):737–46.

99. Aronne LJ. Classification of obesity and assessment of obesity-related health risks. Obesity Research. 2002;**10**(S12):105S–15S.

100. World Health Organization. Waist circumference and waist-hip ratio: report of a WHO expert consultation. 2008. http://www.who.int/iris/handle/10665/44583

101. Yumuk V, Tsigos C, Fried M, et al. European guidelines for obesity management in adults. Obesity Facts. 2015;**8**(6):402–24.

102. Silver HJ, Welch EB, Avison MJ, Niswender KD. Imaging body composition in obesity and weight loss: challenges and opportunities. Diabetes, Metabolic Syndrome and Obesity: Targets and Therapy. 2010;**3**:337–47.

103. Cornier M-A, Després J-P, Davis N, et al. Assessing adiposity: a scientific statement from the American Heart Association. Circulation. 2011;**124**(18):1996–2019.

104. Jensen MD, Ryan DH, Apovian CM, et al. 2013 AHA/ACC/TOS guideline for the management of overweight and obesity in adults: a report of the American College of Cardiology/American Heart Association Task Force on Practice Guidelines and The Obesity Society. Journal of the American College of Cardiology. 2014;**63**(25 Part B):2985–3023.

105. Marchesini G, Cuzzolaro M, Mannucci E, et al. Weight cycling in treatment-seeking obese persons: data from the QUOVADIS study. International Journal of Obesity. 2004;**28**(11):1456–62.

106. Harris JA, Benedict FG. A biometric study of human basal metabolism. Proceedings of the National Academy of Sciences. 1918;**4**(12):370–73.

107. Mifflin MD, St Jeor ST, Hill LA, Scott BJ, Daugherty SA, Koh YO. A new predictive equation for resting energy expenditure in healthy individuals. American Journal of Clinical Nutrition. 1990;**51**(2):241–47.

108. Bray GA, Heisel WE, Afshin A, et al. The science of obesity management: an Endocrine Society Scientific Statement. Endocrine Reviews. 2018;**39**(2):79–132.

109. Sacks FM, Bray GA, Carey VJ, et al. Comparison of weight-loss diets with different compositions of fat, protein, and carbohydrates. New England Journal of Medicine. 2009;**360**(9):859–73.

110. Radulian G, Rusu E, Dragomir A, Posea M. Metabolic effects of low glycaemic index diets. Nutrition Journal. 2009;**8**(1):5.

111. Hall KD, Sacks G, Chandramohan D, et al. Quantification of the effect of energy imbalance on bodyweight. Lancet. 2011;**378**(9793):826–37.

112. Tsai AG, Wadden TA. The evolution of very-low-calorie diets: an update and meta-analysis. Obesity. 2006;**14**(8):1283–93.

113. Atkins RD. Dr Atkins' New Diet Revolution. New York: HarperCollins; 2002.

114. Krauss RM, Eckel RH, Howard B, et al. AHA Dietary Guidelines: revision 2000: a statement for healthcare professionals from the Nutrition Committee of the American Heart Association. Circulation. 2000;**102**(18):2284–99.

115. Freedland SJ, Aronson WJ. Re: weight loss with a low-carbohydrate, Mediterranean, or low-fat diet. European Urology. 2009;**55**(1):249–50.

116. Makris A, Foster GD. Dietary approaches to the treatment of obesity. Psychiatric Clinics. 2011;**34**(4):813–27.

117. Foster-Powell K, Holt SHA, Brand-Miller JC. International table of glycemic index and glycemic load values: 2002. American Journal of Clinical Nutrition. 2002;**76**(1):5–56.

118. Wishnofsky M. Caloric equivalents of gained or lost weight. American Journal of Clinical Nutrition. 1958;**6**:542–46.

119. Hill J, Catenacci V, Wyatt H. Obesity: etiology. Modern Nutrition in Health and Disease. 2006:1024–25.

120. Thomas DM, Gonzalez MC, Pereira AZ, Redman LM, Heymsfield SB. Time to correctly predict the amount of weight loss with dieting. Journal of the Academy of Nutrition and Dietetics. 2014;**114**(6):857–61.

121. Heymsfield S, Thomas D, Nguyen A, et al. Voluntary weight loss: systematic review of early phase body composition changes. Obesity Reviews. 2011;**12**(5):e348–61.

122. Weiss EP, Albert SG, Reeds DN, et al. Effects of matched weight loss from calorie restriction, exercise, or both on cardiovascular disease risk factors: a randomized intervention trial. American Journal of Clinical Nutrition. 2016;**104**(3):576–86.

123. Klein S, Burke LE, Bray GA, et al. Clinical implications of obesity with specific focus on cardiovascular disease: a statement for professionals from the American Heart Association Council on Nutrition, Physical Activity, and Metabolism: endorsed by the American College of Cardiology Foundation. Circulation. 2004;**110**(18):2952–67.

124. Willis LH, Slentz CA, Bateman LA, et al. Effects of aerobic and/or resistance training on body mass and fat mass in overweight or obese adults. Journal of Applied Physiology. 2012;**113**(12):1831–37.

125. Physical Activity Guidelines Advisory Committee. Physical Activity Guidelines Advisory Committee Report, 2008. Washington, DC: US Department of Health and Human Services. 2008.

126. Saris W, Blair S, Van Baak M, et al. How much physical activity is enough to prevent unhealthy weight gain? Outcome of the IASO 1st Stock Conference and consensus statement. Obesity Reviews. 2003;**4**(2):101–14.

127. Haskell WL, Lee I-M, Pate RR, et al. Physical activity and public health: updated recommendation for adults from the American College of Sports Medicine and the American Heart Association. Circulation. 2007;**116**(9):1081–93.

128. Donnelly JE, Blair SN, Jakicic JM, Manore MM, Rankin JW, Smith BK. American College of Sports Medicine Position Stand. Appropriate physical activity intervention strategies for weight loss and prevention of weight regain for adults. Medicine and Science in Sports and Exercise. 2009;**41**(2):459–71.

129. Swift DL, Johannsen NM, Lavie CJ, Earnest CP, Church TS. The role of exercise and physical activity in weight loss and maintenance. Progress in Cardiovascular Diseases. 2014;**56**(4):441–47.

130. Catenacci VA, Wyatt HR. The role of physical activity in producing and maintaining weight loss. Nature Reviews Endocrinology. 2007;**3**(7):518–29.

131. Wing RR, Hill JO. Successful weight loss maintenance. Annual Review of Nutrition. 2001;**21**(1):323–41.

132. Tate DF, Jeffery RW, Sherwood NE, Wing RR. Long-term weight losses associated with prescription of higher physical activity goals. Are higher levels of physical activity protective against weight regain? American Journal of Clinical Nutrition. 2007;**85**(4):954–59.

133. Chaput J-P, Klingenberg L, Rosenkilde M, Gilbert J-A, Tremblay A, Sjödin A. Physical activity plays an important role in body weight regulation. Journal of Obesity. 2010;2011:360257.

134. Blair S, Leermakers E. Exercise and weight management. In: Wadden TA, Stunkard AJ, eds. Handbook of Obesity Treatment. New York: Guilford Press; 2002:283–300.

135. Rosenbaum M, Goldsmith R, Bloomfield D, et al. Low-dose leptin reverses skeletal muscle, autonomic, and neuroendocrine adaptations to maintenance of reduced weight. Journal of Clinical Investigation. 2005;115(12):3579–86.

136. Murphy MH, Blair SN, Murtagh EM. Accumulated versus continuous exercise for health benefit. Sports Medicine. 2009;39(1):29–43.

137. Andersen RE, Wadden TA, Bartlett SJ, Zemel B, Verde TJ, Franckowiak SC. Effects of lifestyle activity vs structured aerobic exercise in obese women: a randomized trial. JAMA. 1999;281(4):335–40.

138. Helsel DL, Jakicic JM, Otto AD. Comparison of techniques for self-monitoring eating and exercise behaviors on weight loss in a correspondence-based intervention. Journal of the American Dietetic Association. 2007;107(10):1807–10.

139. Nedeltcheva AV, Kilkus JM, Imperial J, Schoeller DA, Penev PD. Insufficient sleep undermines dietary efforts to reduce adiposity. Annals of Internal Medicine. 2010;153(7):435–41.

140. Thomson CA, Morrow KL, Flatt SW, et al. Relationship between sleep quality and quantity and weight loss in women participating in a weight-loss intervention trial. Obesity. 2012;20(7):1419–25.

141. Toplak H, Woodward E, Yumuk V, Oppert J-M, Halford JC, Frühbeck G. 2014 EASO Position Statement on the use of anti-obesity drugs. Obesity Facts. 2015;8(3):166–74.

142. Bray GA. Medical treatment of obesity: the past, the present and the future. Best Practice & Research Clinical Gastroenterology. 2014;28(4):665–84.

143. Kushner RF. Anti-obesity drugs. Expert Opinion on Pharmacotherapy. 2008;9(8):1339–50.

144. Brashier DB, Sharma A, Dahiya N, Singh S, Khadka A. Lorcaserin: a novel antiobesity drug. Journal of Pharmacology & Pharmacotherapeutics. 2014;5(2):175–78.

145. Gustafson A, King C, Rey JA. Lorcaserin (Belviq): a selective serotonin 5-HT2C agonist in the treatment of obesity. Pharmacy and Therapeutics. 2013;38(9):525–34.

146. Darnobid JA, Jones SB. The perioperative implications of new weight loss drugs. Advances in Anesthesia. 2016;34(1):1–11.

147. FDA Center for Drug Evaluation and Research. Belviq NDA 3151563 drug label. 27 June 2012. http://www.accessdata.fda.gov/scripts/cder/drugsatfda/index.cfm?fuseaction=Search.DrugDetails

148. Drug Enforcement Administration. Schedules of controlled substances: placement of lorcaserin into schedule IV. 2012. http://www.deadiversion.usdoj.gov/fed_regs/rules/2012/fr1219.htm

149. Fleming JW, McClendon KS, Riche DM. New obesity agents: lorcaserin and phentermine/topiramate. Annals of Pharmacotherapy. 2013;47(7–8):1007–16.

150. Roberts M, Center for Drug Evaluation and Research. Clinical review: complete response submission, NDA 22580 QSYMIA, Phentermine/Topiramate extended-release. Reference ID: 3159813.

151. Takeda Pharmaceuticals America Inc. Contrave (naltrexone HCl/bupropion HCl) prescribing information. 2014.

152. Sherman MM, Ungureanu S, Rey JA. Naltrexone/Bupropion ER (Contrave): newly approved treatment option for chronic weight management in obese adults. Pharmacy and Therapeutics. 2016;41(3):164–72.

153. Pucci A, Finer N. New medications for treatment of obesity: metabolic and cardiovascular effects. Canadian Journal of Cardiology. 2015;31(2):142–52.

154. Shehebar M, Khelemsky Y. (434) Considerations for perioperative Contrave (naltrexone HCl/bupropion HCl) administration. Journal of Pain. 2016;17(4):S83.

155. Ioannides-Demos LL, Piccenna L, McNeil JJ. Pharmacotherapies for obesity: past, current, and future therapies. Journal of Obesity. 2010;2011:179674.

156. Crane J, McGowan B. The GLP-1 agonist, liraglutide, as a pharmacotherapy for obesity. Therapeutic Advances in Chronic Disease. 2016;7(2):92–107.

157. Delgado-Aros S, Kim D-Y, Burton DD, et al. Effect of GLP-1 on gastric volume, emptying, maximum volume ingested, and postprandial symptoms in humans. American Journal of Physiology-Gastrointestinal and Liver Physiology. 2002;282(3):G424–31.

158. Nauck M, Frid A, Hermansen K, et al. Efficacy and safety comparison of liraglutide, glimepiride, and placebo, all in combination with metformin, in type 2 diabetes: the LEAD (liraglutide effect and action in diabetes)-2 study. Diabetes Care. 2009;32(1):84–90.

159. Food and Drug Administration. Full prescribing information, saxenda. reference id: 3989124. 2016. https://www.accessdata.fda.gov/drugsatfda_docs/label/2016/206321s003lbl.pdf

160. Guerciolini R. Mode of action of orlistat. International Journal of Obesity and Related Metabolic Disorders. 1997;21:S12–23.

161. Ballinger A, Peikin SR. Orlistat: its current status as an anti-obesity drug. European Journal of Pharmacology. 2002;440(2–3):109–17.

162. Sjostrom L, Rissanen A, Andersen T, et al. Randomised placebo-controlled trial of orlistat for weight loss and prevention of weight regain in obese patients. Lancet. 1998;352(9123):167–72.

163. Carter R, Mouralidarane A, Ray S, Soeda J, Oben J. Recent advancements in drug treatment of obesity. Clinical Medicine. 2012;12(5):456–60.

164. Federal Drug Administration. FDA Drug Safety Communication: completed safety review of Xenical/Alli (orlistat) and severe liver injury. 2018. https://www.fda.gov/drugs/postmarket-drug-safety-information-patients-and-providers/fda-drug-safety-communication-completed-safety-review-xenicalalli-orlistat-and-severe-liver-injury

165. Bray G, Ryan D. Medical therapy for the patient with obesity. Circulation. 2012;125(13):1695–703.

166. Persson M, Vitols S, Yue Q-Y. Orlistat associated with hypertension. BMJ. 2000;321(7253):87.

167. Ogunnaike B, Jones S, Jones D, Provost D, Whitten C. Anesthetic considerations for bariatric surgery. Anaesthesia Analgesia. 2002;95(6):1793–805.

168. Valentino M, Lin J, Waldman S. Central and peripheral molecular targets for antiobesity pharmacotherapy. Clinical Pharmacology and Therapeutics. 2010;87(6):652–62.

169. Cetilistat - Investigational Drug for Obesity - Clinical Trials Arena [Internet]. Clinicaltrialsarena.com. 2020 [cited 10 October 2020]. Available from: https://www.clinicaltrialsarena.com/projects/cetilistat/

170. Pilitsi E, Farr OM, Polyzos SA, et al. Pharmacotherapy of obesity: available medications and drugs under investigation. Metabolism. 2019;92:170–92.

171. Bryson A, de la Motte S, Dunk C. Reduction of dietary fat absorption by the novel gastrointestinal lipase inhibitor cetilistat in healthy volunteers. British Journal of Clinical Pharmacology. 2009;**67**(3):309–15.

172. Kopelman P, et al. Weight loss, HbA1c reduction, and tolerability of cetilistat in a randomized, placebo-controlled phase 2 trial in obese diabetics: comparison with orlistat (Xenical). Obesity. 2010;**18**(1):108–15.

173. Kopelman P, et al. Cetilistat (ATL-962), a novel lipase inhibitor: a 12-week randomized, placebo-controlled study of weight reduction in obese patients. International Journal of Obesity. 2007;**31**(3):494–9.

174. Desilets AR, Dhakal-Karki S, Dunican KC. Role of metformin for weight management in patients without type 2 diabetes. Annals of Pharmacotherapy. 2008;**42**(6):817–26.

175. Vilsbøll T, Christensen M, Junker AE, Knop FK, Gluud LL. Effects of glucagon-like peptide-1 receptor agonists on weight loss: systematic review and meta-analyses of randomised controlled trials. BMJ. 2012;344:d7771.

176. Dunican KC, Adams NM, Desilets AR. The role of pramlintide for weight loss. Annals of Pharmacotherapy. 2010;**44**(3):538–45.

177. Nagao T, Meguro S, Hase T, et al. A catechin-rich beverage improves obesity and blood glucose control in patients with type 2 diabetes. Obesity. 2009;**17**(2):310–17.

178. Lu Y, Levin G, Donner T. Tagatose, a new antidiabetic and obesity control drug. Diabetes, Obesity and Metabolism. 2008;**10**(2):109–34.

179. Eldridge A, Cooper D, Peters J. A role for olestra in body weight management. Obesity Reviews. 2002;**3**(1):17–25.

180. Grundy S, Barondess J, Bellegie N, et al. Gastrointestinal surgery for severe obesity. Annals of Internal Medicine. 1991;**115**(12):956–61.

Defining obesity

Sunil Sinha and Hawa Abubakar

Obesity: defining the problem

Obesity is defined by the World Health Organization (WHO) as excessive or abnormal accumulation of fat that presents a health risk. It can be measured using the body mass index (BMI)—weight in kilograms divided by height in metres squared (kg/m^2). A BMI greater than 30 kg/m^2 is considered diagnostic of obesity. Morbid obesity is defined as a BMI greater than 40 kg/m^2, or greater than 35 kg/m^2 and experiencing obesity-related health conditions such as hypertension, diabetes, hyperlipidaemia, cardiovascular disease, stroke, asthma, arthritis, or obstructive sleep apnoea.

In addition to BMI, other measures of obesity exist including densitometry, single-cut imaging of the abdomen using computed tomography scanning or magnetic resonance imaging, and dual-energy X-ray absorptiometry. Measurements of waist circumference, hip circumference, and waist-to-hip ratio are attempts at assessing abdominal obesity, which has been shown to be an independent predictor of several cardiovascular and cancer-related outcomes [1].

Obesity has now reached epidemic proportions globally. The epidemic is thought to have begun in the 1980s but did not get significant global attention until 1997. Obesity rates have continued to rise, affecting both developed and developing countries [2]. The WHO reports that in 1995 there were an estimated 200 million obese adults worldwide. In the 5-year period to 2000, this number increased by 100 million to an estimated 300 million obese adults worldwide. Several factors have contributed to the rising trend including urbanization, car dependence, as well as sedentary occupations. A study in 2015 has shown that increasing food energy supply may also be a driver of the global epidemic. In 81% of the countries analysed between 1971 and 2010, an increase in food energy supply paralleled increases in body weight, suggesting that an abundance of calories likely contributes to overconsumption leading to observed increases in weight [3].

The epidemiology of obesity confirms that, contrary to popular opinion, obesity does significantly affect developing nations with an estimated 115 million people suffering from obesity-related problems. The paradox in the developing world is that obesity routinely coexists with malnutrition [4]. In fact, the United Nations Food and Agriculture Organization predicts that by 2030 obesity will overtake undernourishment as the primary diet-related health issue in Central Asia and the Caucasus region [5].

When analysing the global prevalence of obesity, America has the highest rate whereas South East Asia has the lowest, 62% versus 14% respectively. Females are more affected than males, particularly when comparing prevalence rates in North Africa, South Africa, the South Pacific islands, and the Middle East. Higher-income countries have approximately double the prevalence of obesity when compared to their lower-income counterparts (**Fig. 2.1** and **Fig. 2.2**).

Epidemiology in the United States

More than one-third (34.9% or 78.6 million) of adults in the United States (US) are considered obese [6]. In the US, obesity has long been recognized as a public health concern with a reported 15.2% of preventable deaths attributable to obesity in the year 2000 [7]. As the rates of obesity continue to rise, there is concern that it may overtake smoking as the single leading cause of preventable death. Using data from the National Health and Nutrition Examination Surveys (NHANESs) between 1970 and 2004, it was predicted that if the rise in obesity continues at the same pace, approximately 51.1% of US adults would likely develop obesity by the year 2030 [8].

Data from the US Centers for Disease Control and Prevention suggest that at present no state has obesity prevalence rates below 20% with Southern and Midwestern states leading with rates of 30.2% and 30.1% respectively [9]. **Fig. 2.3** clearly depicts the progressive fattening of America over the course of 2011–2014. These data also show a difference in prevalence based on ethnicity with obesity rates being highest among non-black Hispanics (37.6%), followed by Hispanics (30.6%), and lastly non-Hispanic whites (26.6%) [6]. The prevalence of obesity appears to have increased at all income levels in the years 1988–1994 and 2007–2008. When looking at women in particular, 29% of women in high-income households (income ≥350% of the poverty level) are obese compared to 42% of women in low-income households (<130% of the poverty level). This suggests a correlation between low income and obesity although most obese women are not in the low-income bracket. A similar trend towards lower rates of obesity among highly educated women has also been observed [10]. According to the same data, there does not appear to be a relationship between income status and level of education among men; however, when specifically looking at non-Hispanic black and Mexican-American men, low-income men are less likely to be obese compared to their high-income counterparts [11].

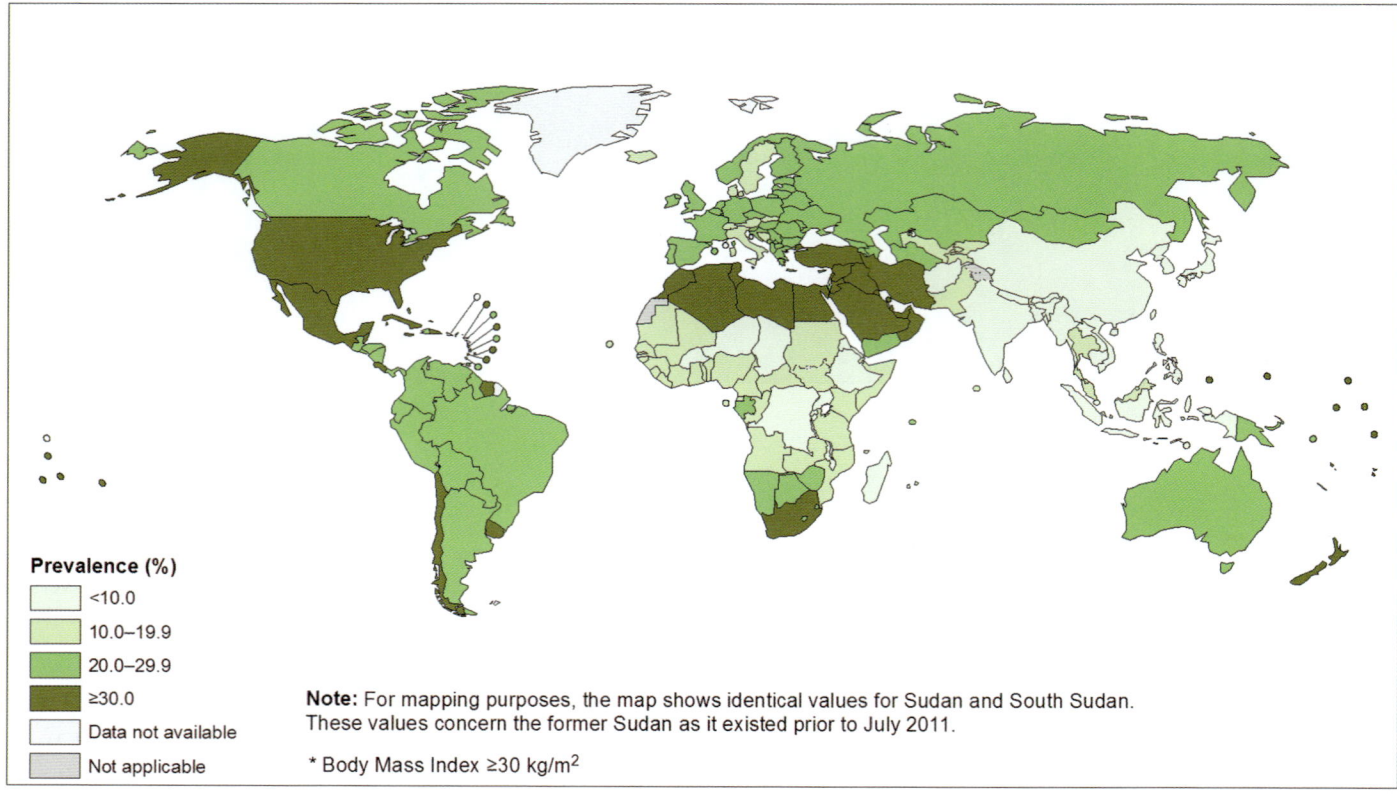

Prevalence (%)

<10.0

10.0–19.9

20.0–29.9

≥30.0

Data not available

Not applicable

Note: For mapping purposes, the map shows identical values for Sudan and South Sudan. These values concern the former Sudan as it existed prior to July 2011.

* Body Mass Index ≥30 kg/m²

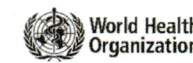

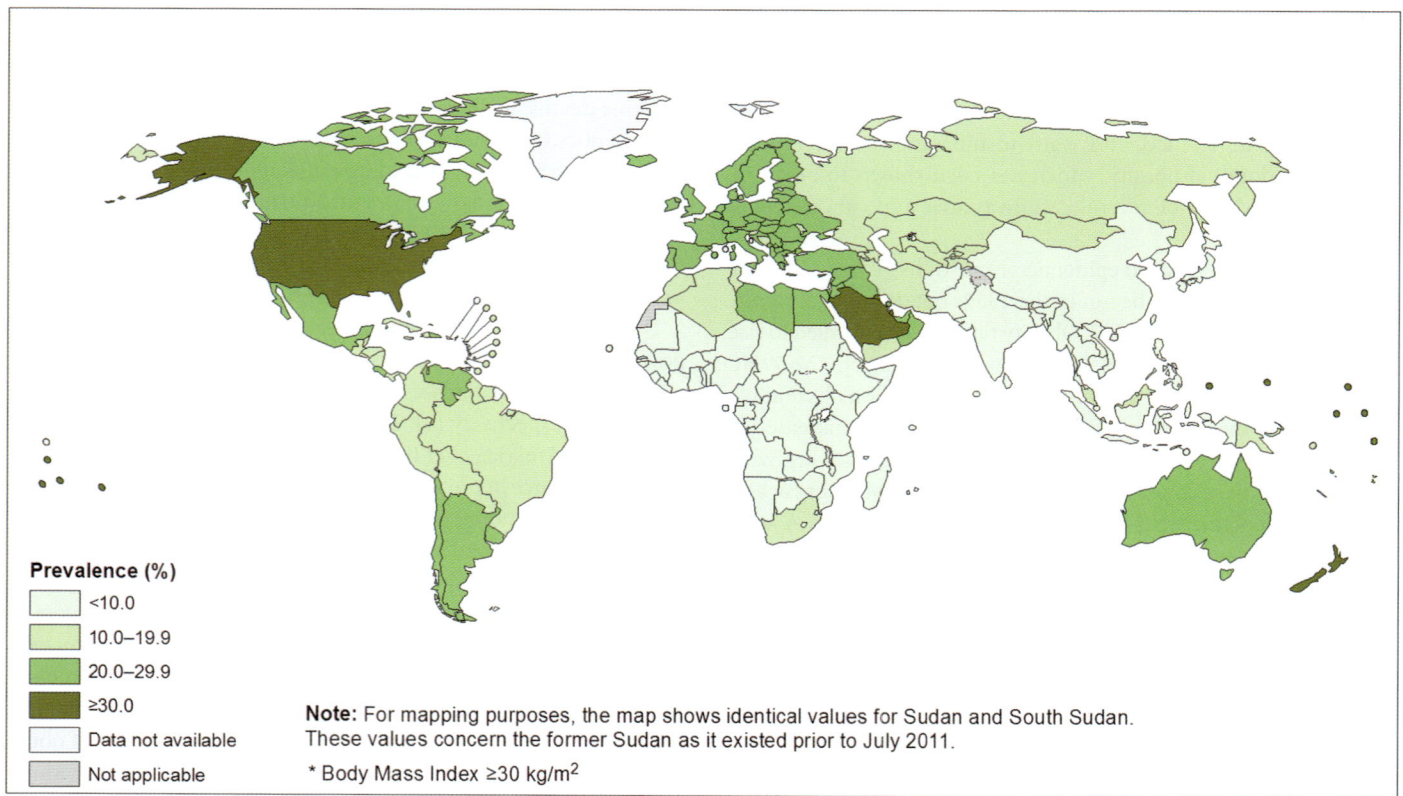

Prevalence (%)

<10.0

10.0–19.9

20.0–29.9

≥30.0

Data not available

Not applicable

Note: For mapping purposes, the map shows identical values for Sudan and South Sudan. These values concern the former Sudan as it existed prior to July 2011.

* Body Mass Index ≥30 kg/m²

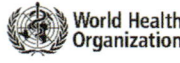

Fig. 2.1 Global maps showing the prevalence of obesity in (a) females and (b) males in 2016.

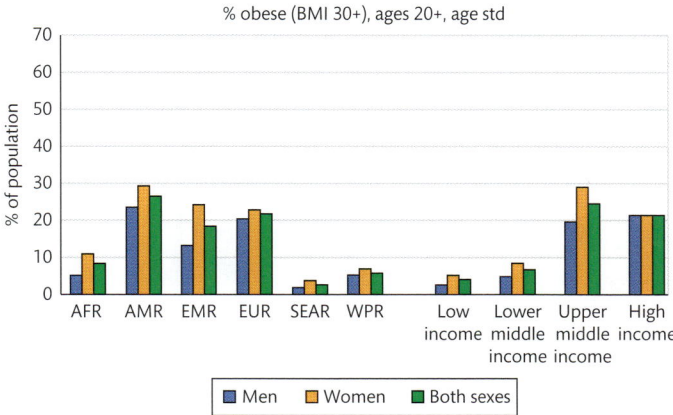

Fig. 2.2 Prevalence rates for obesity by WHO regions and income status. AFR, Africa; AMR, America; EMR, Eastern Mediterranean Region; EUR, Europe; SEAR, South East Asia; WPR, Western Pacific Region.

Reproduced with permission from Global Health Observatory Map Gallery and from Global Health Observatory (GHO) data. Copyright © World Health Organization. http://gamapserver.who.int/mapLibrary/app/searchResults.aspx and https://www.who.int/gho/ncd/risk_factors/bmi_text/en/

dose–response relationship with those more overweight having even greater risk of developing comorbidities [12]. When considering gastrointestinal health, obesity is known to increase the risk of a myriad of conditions (Table 2.1) [13]. Moreover, obesity is independently associated with an increase in the risk of death. In a 10-year prospective cohort study of approximately 520,000 AARP-registered US men and women aged between 50 and 71 years with control for smoking as a confounding factor, it was reported that the risk of death increased by two- to threefold in obese compared with normal-weight patients [14].

Most diseases associated with obesity are chronic illnesses; therefore, they pose an additional financial burden on the individual as well as national economies. For the year 2008, it is estimated that the medical cost of obesity was US $147 billion. When comparing the cost of healthcare between obese and non-obese patients, healthcare for obese people on average was greater by US $1429 or 42% compared to someone who was normal weight [15]. These financial considerations include direct medical costs, productivity costs, transportation costs, and human capital costs [16]. We will explore these further in the coming sections.

Impact on health

In recent years, it has become increasingly clear that increased adiposity is associated with multiple comorbidities. Obesity is a recognized risk factor for cardiovascular health and is associated with diabetes mellitus, hypertension, hyperlipidaemia, heart disease, obstructive sleep apnoea, and stroke. The association exhibits a

Defining the cost

It is projected that by 2030 there will be 65 million more obese adults in the US, leading to an increase in obesity-associated illness. Based on simulation models, it is expected that there will be an additional 6–8.5 million cases of diabetes, 5.7–7.3 million cases of vascular diseases such as stroke and heart disease, and 492,000–669,000 cases of cancer as

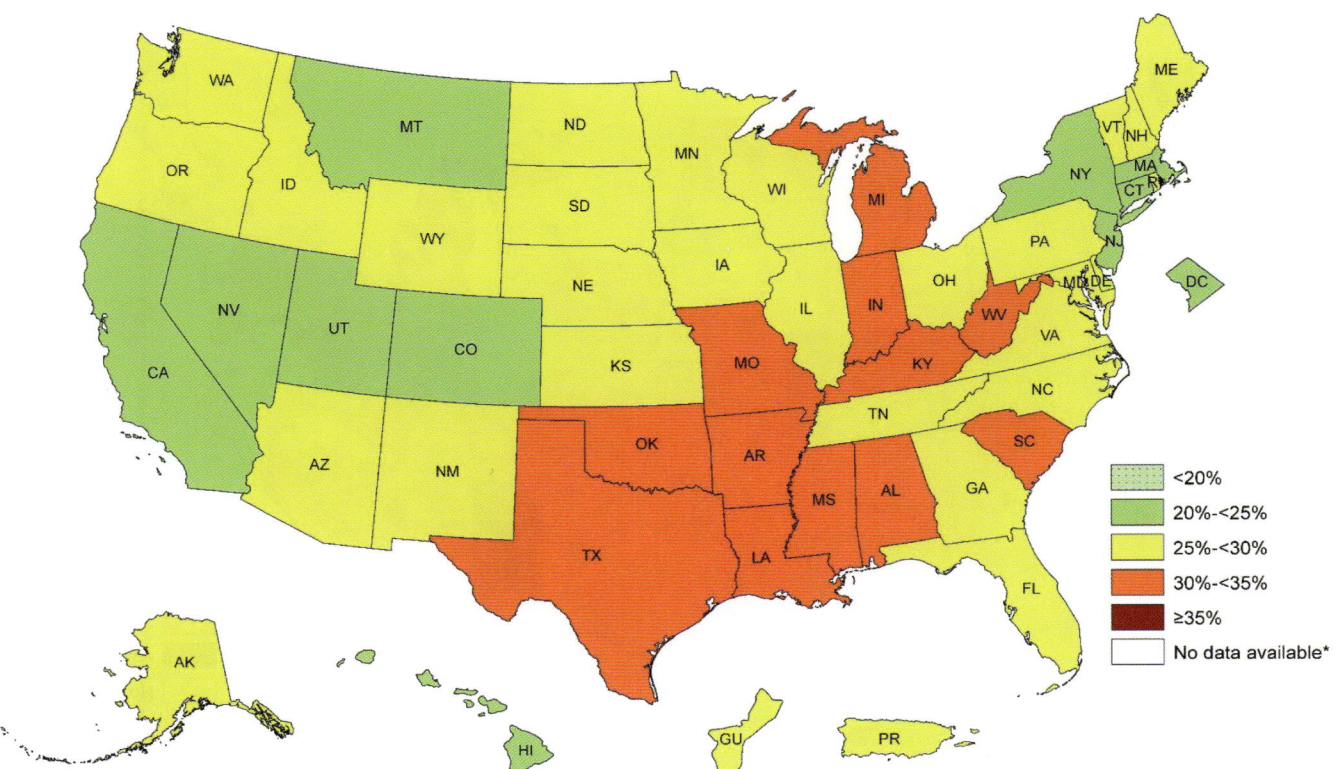

Fig. 2.3 Prevalence of self-reported obesity among US adults by state and territory; (a) 2011; (b) 2012; (c) 2013; (d) 2014. *Sample size <50 or the relative standard error (dividing the standard error by the prevalence) ≥30%.

Reproduced from Adult Obesity Prevalence Maps. Source: CDC; Materials developed by Behavioral Risk Factor Surveillance System (BRFSS) 2014. https://www.cdc.gov/obesity/data/prevalence-maps.html

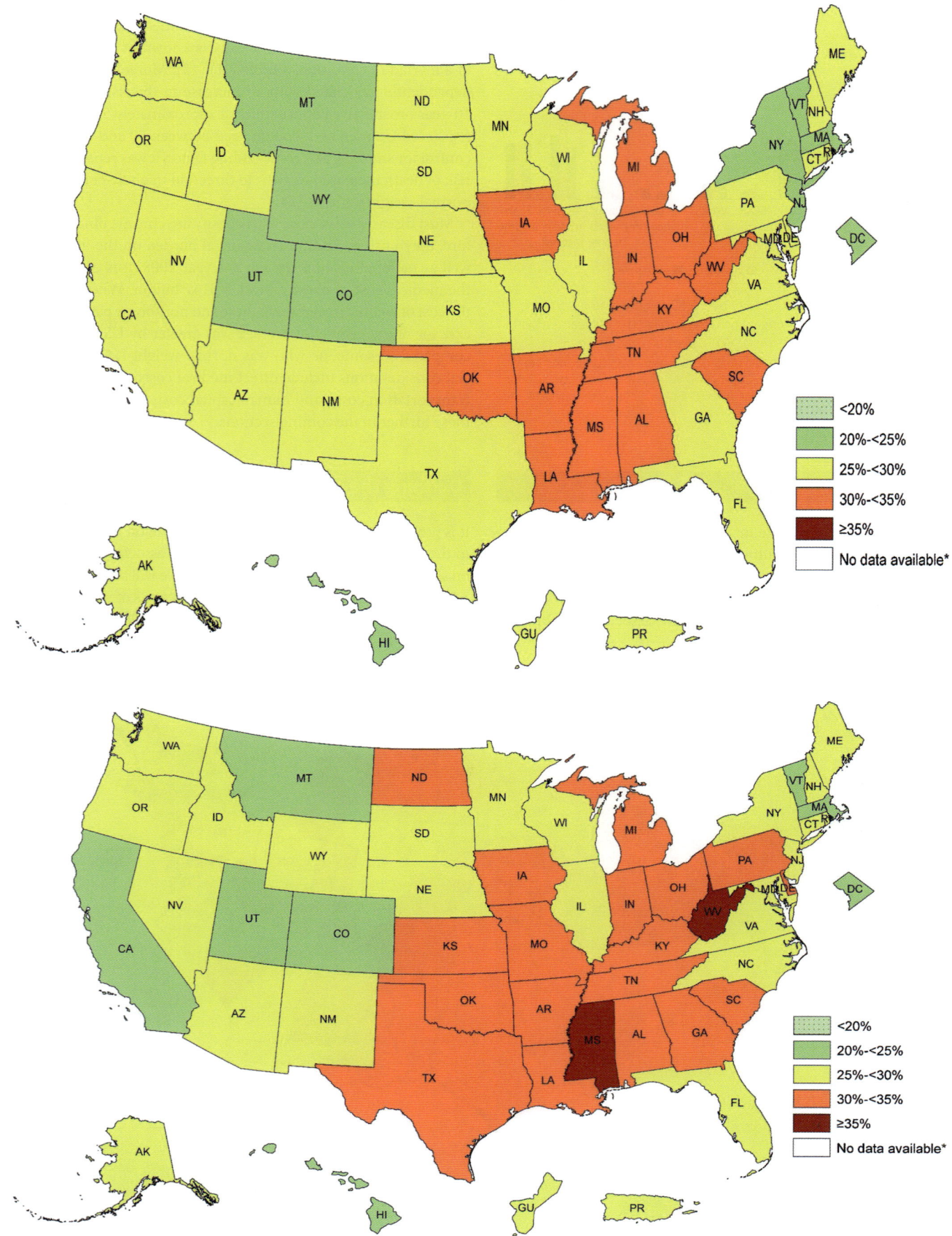

Fig. 2.3 *Continued*

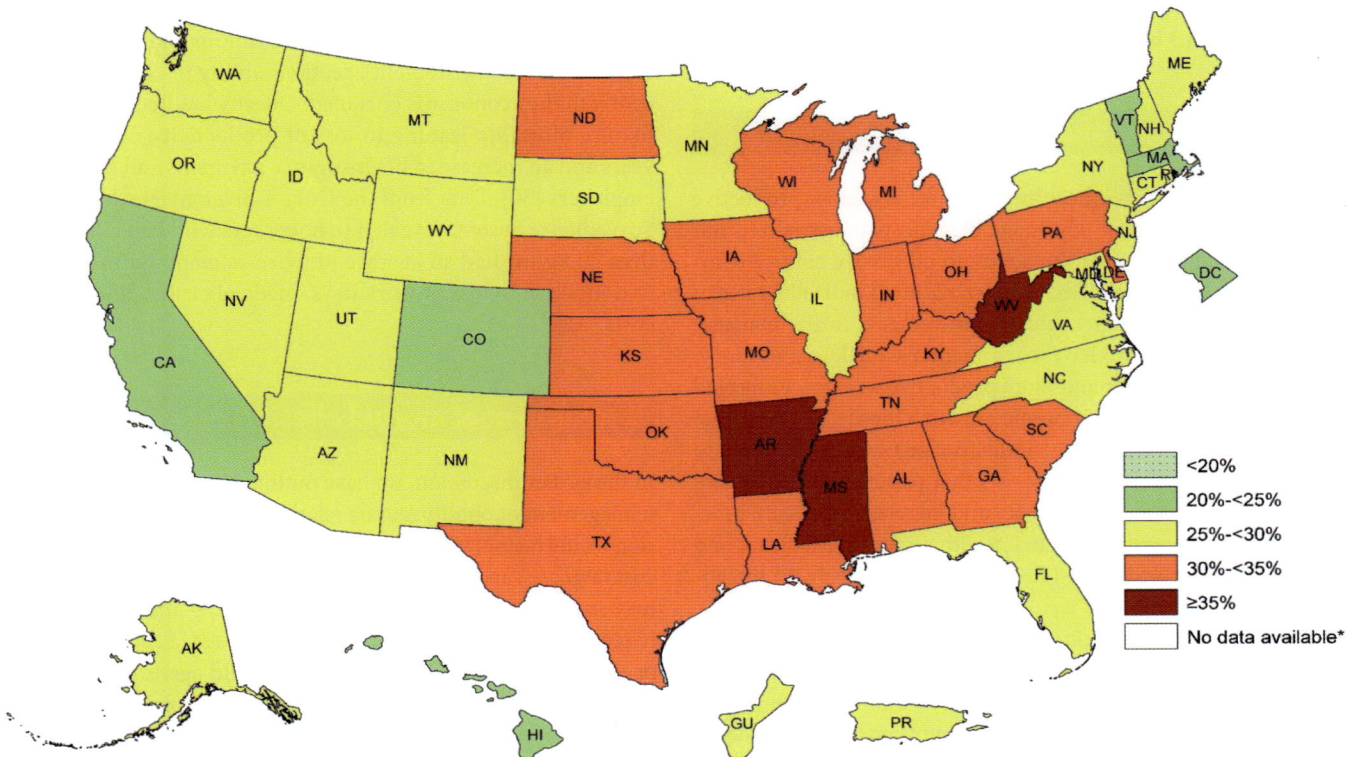

Fig. 2.3 *Continued*

a direct result of the increased prevalence of obesity. Quality-adjusted life years are expected to decrease by 26–55 million [17]. The health burden of obesity is significant; looking specifically at cancer risk, for every 5 kg/m² rise in BMI, the risk of developing oesophageal cancer goes up by 52% and that of colon cancer by 24% in men. In women, the risk of endometrial cancer increases by 59%, postmenopausal breast cancer by 12.5%, and gallbladder cancer by 59% [18].

Table 2.1 Gastrointestinal disease associated with obesity

	Magnitude of increased risk with obesity (compared to low or normal BMI)
Oesophagus	
GORD	50%
Erosive oesophagitis	50–100%
Barrett's oesophagus	2-fold
Oesophageal adenocarcinoma	2-fold
Gallbladder	
Stones	2–3-fold
Cancer	35–85%
Pancreas	
Cancer	35–85%
Acute pancreatitis	20–50%
Colon	
Adenoma (particularly advanced)	50–100%
Cancer	2-fold
Liver	
Non-alcoholic fatty liver disease	2–3-fold
Advanced HCV-related disease	50%
Cirrhosis	30–50%
Hepatocellular carcinoma	30–50%

GORD, gastro-oesophageal reflux; HCV, hepatitis C virus.
Adapted with permission from Obesity and Your GI Health: Do You Know Your Risks?, American College of Gastroenterology (ACG).

The connection between rising rates of obesity and rising medical spending is undeniable [15]. As the rate of obesity rises so do direct health costs. Annual healthcare expenditure directly attributable to obesity among full-time employees is estimated at approximately 73.1 billion. People with a BMI greater than 35 kg/m² account for 37% of the obese population; however, in terms of excess cost, they represent 61% of the added healthcare expenditure [19]. Globally, obesity is estimated to account for 0.7–2.8% of a given country's total healthcare expenditure. The medical costs for obese individuals are approximately 30% higher than their normal-weight peers; however, it is not entirely clear exactly how these excess costs are being accrued [20].

Studies have demonstrated that the risk of disease is associated with an increase in BMI. Relative to individuals with a BMI within the normal range (22.5 kg/m²), the risk of hypertension is approximately 40–60% greater in overweight people (BMI 27.5 kg/m²) and two times greater in obese people (BMI 32.5 kg/m²). The lifetime risk of coronary heart disease was 41.8% in obese men versus 34.9% in non-obese men. In women, this risk increased from 25.5% for non-obese to 32.4% for obese individuals [21]. When looking at cross-sectional data from NHANES II, the risk of developing hypertension and diabetes is increased by a factor of 3.0 and 2.9 in men and women respectively when compared to their normal-weight counterparts [22,23]. The majority of illness associated with obesity is preventable; therefore, the management and treatment of these ailments represents added costs. In 2008, the obesity-attributable drug costs to Medicare as part of the part D prescription benefit amounted to US $7 billion [15]. The management of preventable illness associated with obesity is projected to increase by US $48–66 billion per year in the US [17]. In fact, it has been postulated that obesity-related healthcare costs are greater than the costs associated with smoking, drinking, or poverty [24]. The increase in comorbidity associated with obesity was estimated to cost an excess of US $147 billion in adults and US $14.3 billion in children in 2008 [16].

Effects on business and industry

It is widely accepted that a healthy workforce is a more productive workforce. The significant advantage that most industrialized nations have benefited from is the ability to effectively control communicable diseases, thereby decreasing childhood mortality rates in addition to overall mortality rates. Improvements in the management of chronic conditions have led to an increase in life expectancy; this has resulted in a larger and more productive workforce engaged in building and sustaining economic growth. Obesity, a disease that has significant prevalence in the industrialized world, threatens to disrupt these benefits. Research shows that private payers bear the bulk of the costs as a result of obesity and its related illnesses; however, government spending in the US with regard to Medicare and Medicaid would be 8.5% and 11.8% lower, respectively, in the absence of obesity [15].

Accounting for race, smoking status, education level, age, and sex, BMI has been shown to predict both average annual healthcare costs and work absence hours [25]. With regard to work absence, two issues seem to be at play: absenteeism and presenteeism. Obesity is associated with increased rates of absenteeism; high-BMI employees are more likely to take more sick days and have longer periods of sick leave, thereby incurring greater productivity losses when compared to low-BMI counterparts [26]. Obesity also contributes to presenteeism (the concept of attending work while sick, resulting in an overall reduction in productivity). In a study looking at manufacturing employees, it was shown that those employees who were moderately to severely obese experienced greater health-related work limitations. These workers needed more time to complete assigned tasks and had a comparatively reduced ability to perform physically demanding activities. There was a 4.2% health-related loss in productivity in the moderately to extremely obese subset of workers compared to 3.02% in all other employees. This observed difference equates to US $506 worth of lost productivity per worker yearly [27]. From this study it appears that there is a threshold effect whereby mildly obese workers are not less productive. In a cross-sectional survey of the US workforce using data from telephone surveys, it was found that obese workers were more likely to report loss of productive time than normal-weight workers ($P < 0.0001$). Health status was the primary mediator between obesity and loss of productive time with those requiring more healthcare being less productive on the whole [28]. This study showed a similar threshold effect with those that were overweight not incurring a significant amount of lost productivity. It is estimated that obese workers contribute US $42.29 billion worth of losses in productive time. This represents an extra US $11.70 billion compared to normal-weight workers with presenteeism representing the greatest share of this cost, accounting for 67.8%. In fact, presenteeism is thought to cost employers more revenue than direct costs related to medical care [19]. Overall, it appears that obesity is linked to lost productivity with the costs associated with this being comparatively higher than direct health costs [29].

Another consideration is the loss of productive years. If someone is afflicted by significant comorbid conditions and rendered unable to work at a pre-retirement age, their ability to contribute significantly to the economy is curtailed. Obesity has been linked to premature mortality leading to loss of productivity during working years and an increase in life insurance payments and premiums for employers [30]. Data from the Duke University Health and Safety Surveillance System revealed that workers who had a BMI greater than 30 kg/m^2 had an average of twice as many claims and a tenfold increase in loss of work days, medical claims, and indemnity costs [31].

Is treatment of morbid obesity cost saving?

In the earlier discussion, we have outlined the costs associated with management of obesity and its related conditions. A logical conclusion would be that treatment or prevention of obesity would result in cost savings. Van Baal et al. predicted that a 20-year-old with obesity may incur lower costs for healthcare during their lifetime compared to a normal-weight adult of the same age [32]. This was driven primarily by shortened life expectancy. Old age is associated with age-related comorbidities; with an increased lifespan, one is more likely to develop conditions such as Alzheimer's disease, leading to comparatively increased lifetime healthcare spending. An obese individual with a shorter life expectancy is less likely to develop these illnesses and therefore will not require the additional expenditure. This suggests that savings accrued by preventing obesity should be looked at as reduced costs in terms of morbidity and mortality as opposed to overall decreased healthcare dollar spending over a given lifetime [32].

When looking at preventative measures, corporations, realizing the costs to them due to loss of productivity, have proactively devised programmes to incentivize their employees to maintain a healthy weight. These programmes range from providing easy access to exercise equipment by facilitating gym memberships to providing monetary rewards for achieving or maintaining an individualized target weight. Evidence suggests that current work environments encourage obesity, with job stress, shift work, and long hours as contributing factors [24]. Taking this evidence into consideration, it would follow that interventions within this environment would represent a cost-effective way of addressing the issue of obesity. To date, the evidence to suggest workplace interventions succeed remains scant. When examining large-scale attempts by corporations at controlling employee weight through financial incentives or penalties, no savings have been generated from long-term weight loss to date. Moreover, there was no reduction in the number of in-patient hospital stays associated with obesity. In fact, these programmes may promote ill health among the employees with added pressure to meet a certain target encouraging crash dieting and concomitant psychological ill health [33]. The pivotal issue is that voluntary weight loss is generally difficult to achieve and usually limited in extent and unsustainable or temporary even when achieved. This, in part, explains the great success the weight loss industry enjoys, generating revenue of approximately US $72 billion in 2018. In the morbidly obese category, the situation is slightly different as there is a well-established and effective treatment—bariatric surgery.

Bariatric surgery

Bariatric surgery has been identified as the most effective weight loss therapy for those suffering from morbid obesity. Given the significant costs associated with obesity, it would be logical to conclude that measures taken to reverse obesity would result in cost savings; however, we have so far established that this may not be the case when looking at mild obesity (BMI 30–34.9 kg/m²). According to the US National Institutes of Health, bariatric procedures on average cost from US $20,000 to $25,000 [34]. In the last decade, the rate of bariatric procedures has increased and plateaued at approximately 113,000 procedures annually. Open gastric bypass accounts for 3% of all procedures and costs US $4600 less than minimally invasive procedures. In the United Kingdom, similar procedures cost the National Health Service significantly less per patient, approximately £6000 (US $8660), suggesting that there may be even greater cost savings to be realized in the US market [35].

Laparoscopic surgery is the mainstay of current practice with laparoscopic-assisted gastric banding accounting for 37% of bariatric procedures [36]. When looking at morbidly obese patients with diabetes who underwent bariatric surgery in a 9-year period between 1999 and 2007 who had private insurance, on average, cost savings became evident to third-party payers at 3 months. The costs of the actual operation irrespective of whether the surgery was open or laparoscopic were recouped at 30 months. Comparing the overall cost of care between those who underwent bariatric surgery versus equally matched patients who had standard diabetic management, the overall cost in healthcare dollars was lower in the bariatric surgery group [36]. This would suggest that surgical therapy is a more cost-effective way to manage these patients. When looking at the impact of bariatric surgery on all patients with BMI greater than 35 kg/m² irrespective of whether or not they had diabetes as a comorbidity, it was found that the cost of laparoscopic procedures could be recovered at 25 months [37]. The mean investment in the US for bariatric surgery is between US $17,000 and $26,000, with the expectation that downstream savings related to decreased healthcare use with reduction of risk of hypertension, diabetes, arthritis, sleep apnoea, cardiovascular disease, and stroke estimated to offset the initial cost within 2–4 years. These savings exclude benefits resulting from potential quality of life and length of life benefits, reductions in disability claims, and loss of work [37].

Conclusion

Obesity is now a global epidemic and has significant costs associated with it. Whereas direct healthcare costs related to the treatment of obesity as well as its associated comorbidities such as diabetes, hypertension, and obstructive sleep apnoea play a major role, productivity costs are perhaps more significant when examining national economies. Bariatric surgery has been identified as a treatment for obesity and the cost savings associated with this procedure are only appreciable in the morbid obesity subgroup.

REFERENCES

1. Kumanyika SK, Obarzanek E, Stettler N, Bell R, Field AE, Fortmann SP, et al. Population-based prevention of obesity: the need for comprehensive promotion of healthful eating, physical activity, and energy balance: a scientific statement from American Heart Association Council on Epidemiology and Prevention, Interdisciplinary Committee for Prevention (formerly the expert panel on population and prevention science). Circulation. 2008;**118**(4):428–64.
2. James WPT. The epidemiology of obesity: the size of the problem. J Intern Med. 2008;**263**(4):336–52.
3. Vandevijvere S, Chow CC, Hall KD, Umali E, Swinburn BA. Increased food energy supply as a major driver of the obesity epidemic: a global analysis. Bull World Health Organ. 2015;**93**(7):446–56.
4. World Health Organization. Controlling the global obesity epidemic. http://www.who.int/nutrition/topics/obesity/en/
5. World Health Organization. Obesity problems ahead. Bull World Health Organ Bull. 2012;**90**:404–405.
6. Ogden CL, Carroll MD, Kit BK, Flegal KM. Prevalence of childhood and adult obesity in the United States, 2011–2012. JAMA. 2014;**311**(8):806–14.
7. Mokdad AH, Marks JS, Stroup DF, Gerberding JL. Actual causes of death in the United States, 2000. JAMA. 2004;**291**(10):1238–45.
8. Wang Y, Beydoun MA, Liang L, Caballero B, Kumanyika SK. Will all Americans become overweight or obese? estimating the progression and cost of the US obesity epidemic. Obesity (Silver Spring). 2008;**16**(10):2323–30.
9. Centers for Disease Control and Prevention. Adult obesity prevalence maps. 2016. http://www.cdc.gov/obesity/data/prevalence-maps.html
10. Ogden C, Lamb MM, Carroll MD, Flegal KM. Obesity and socioeconomic status in adults: United States, 2005–2008. Natl Cent Health Stat. 2010;**50**:1–8.
11. Centers for Disease Control and Prevention. Obesity and overweight for professionals: data and statistics. Adult obesity. 2015. http://www.cdc.gov/obesity/data/adult.html
12. Field AE, Coakley EH, Must A, Spadano JL, Laird N, Dietz WH, et al. Impact of overweight on the risk of developing common chronic diseases during a 10-year period. Arch Intern Med. 2001;**161**(13):1581–6.
13. American College of Gastroenterology. Obesity and your digestive health: do you know your GI risks? 2011. https://s3.gi.org/patients/obesity/pdfs/ACG_Obesity_Patient_Education_Pamphlet.pdf
14. Adams KF, Schatzkin A, Harris TB, Kipnis V, Mouw T, Ballard-Barbash R, et al. Overweight, obesity, and mortality in a large prospective cohort of persons 50 to 71 years old. N Engl J Med. 2006;**355**(8):763–78.
15. Finkelstein EA, Trogdon JG, Cohen JW, Dietz W. Annual medical spending attributable to obesity: payer-and service-specific estimates. Health Aff (Millwood). 2009;**28**(5):w822–31.
16. Hammond RA, Levine R. The economic impact of obesity in the United States. Diabetes Metab Syndr Obes Targets Ther. 2010;**3**:285–95.
17. Wang YC, McPherson K, Marsh T, Gortmaker SL, Brown M. Health and economic burden of the projected obesity trends in the USA and the UK. Lancet. 2011;**378**(9793):815–25.
18. Renehan AG, Tyson M, Egger M, Heller RF, Zwahlen M. Body-mass index and incidence of cancer: a systematic review and

meta-analysis of prospective observational studies. Lancet. 2008;**371**(9612):569–78.

19. Finkelstein EA, DiBonaventura MD, Burgess SM, Hale BC. The costs of obesity in the workplace. J Occup Environ Med. 2010;**52**(10):971–76.

20. Withrow D, Alter DA. The economic burden of obesity worldwide: a systematic review of the direct costs of obesity. Obes Rev. 2011;**12**(2):131–41.

21. Thompson D, Edelsberg J, Colditz GA, Bird AP, Oster G. Lifetime health and economic consequences of obesity. Arch Intern Med. 1999;**159**(18):2177–83.

22. Gorsky RD, Pamuk E, Williamson DF, Shaffer PA, Koplan JP. The 25-year health care costs of women who remain overweight after 40 years of age. Am J Prev Med. 1996;**12**(5):388–94.

23. Van Itallie TB. Health implications of overweight and obesity in the United States. Ann Intern Med. 1985;**103**(6 Pt 2):983–88.

24. Schulte PA, Wagner GR, Ostry A, Blanciforti LA, Cutlip RG, Krajnak KM, et al. Work, obesity, and occupational safety and health. Am J Public Health. 2007;**97**(3):428–36.

25. Bungum T, Satterwhite M, Jackson AW, Morrow JR. The relationship of body mass index, medical costs, and job absenteeism. Am J Health Behav. 2003;**27**(4):456–62.

26. Borak J. Obesity and the workplace. Occup Med (Lond). 2011;**61**(4):220–22.

27. Gates DM, Succop P, Brehm BJ, Gillespie GL, Sommers BD. Obesity and presenteeism: the impact of body mass index on workplace productivity. J Occup Environ Med. 2008;**50**(1):39–45.

28. Ricci JA, Chee E. Lost productive time associated with excess weight in the U.S. Workforce. J Occup Environ Med. 2005;**47**(12):1227–34.

29. Dee A, Kearns K, O'Neill C, Sharp L, Staines A, O'Dwyer V, et al. The direct and indirect costs of both overweight and obesity: a systematic review. BMC Res Notes. 2014;7:242.

30. Trogdon JG, Finkelstein EA, Hylands T, Dellea PS, Kamal-Bahl SJ. Indirect costs of obesity: a review of the current literature. Obes Rev. 2008;**9**(5):489–500.

31. Ostbye T, Dement JM, Krause KM. Obesity and workers' compensation: results from the Duke Health and Safety Surveillance System. Arch Intern Med. 2007;**167**(8):766–73.

32. van Baal PH, Polder JJ, de Wit GA, Hoogenveen RT, Feenstra TL, Boshuizen HC, et al. Lifetime medical costs of obesity: prevention no cure for increasing health expenditure. PLOS Med. 2008;**5**(2):e29.

33. Lewis A, Khanna V, Montrose S. Employers should disband employee weight control programs. Am J Manag Care. 2015;**21**(2):e91–94.

34. National Institute of Diabetes and Digestive and Kidney Diseases (NIDDK). Bariatric surgery for severe obesity. https://www.niddk.nih.gov/health-information/weight-management/bariatric-surgery

35. Gregory A. Two million obese Brits to get free gastric band operations on the NHS. The Mirror. 27 November 2014.

36. Klein S, Ghosh A, Cremieux PY, Eapen S, McGavock TJ. Economic impact of the clinical benefits of bariatric surgery in diabetes patients with BMI ≥35 kg/m². Obesity (Silver Spring). 2011;**19**(3):581–87.

36. Livingston EH. The incidence of bariatric surgery has plateaued in the U.S. Am J Surg. 2010;**200**(3):378–85.

37. Cremieux PY, Buchwald H, Shikora SA, Ghosh A, Yang HE, Buessing M. A study on the economic impact of bariatric surgery. Am J Manag Care. 2008;**14**(9):589–96.

Genetics of obesity

Chase D. Rose and Ajintha Pathmanathan

Introduction

Obesity is a global public health pandemic affecting over a third of the population in some regions [1]. Of significant concern for future generations is the rising trend and prevalence of obesity in children and adolescents aged 2–19 years, which has reached a prevalence rate of 17% in the United States [2].

We know that obesity results from an energy imbalance. As an individual's caloric intake increases, the amount of energy that can be utilized reaches a plateau and the rest is transitioned and stored as adipose tissue. The aetiology of obesity is complex, multifactorial, and polygenic. Only 2–5% of clinical obesity can be traced back to a single gene mutation [3].

Excessive body weight and obesity can have significant and detrimental medical, psychosocial, and economic consequences. There is strong clinical evidence of causal associations between obesity and numerous comorbidities including type 2 diabetes, cardiovascular disease, hypertension, obstructive sleep apnoea, stroke, and various forms of cancer [3]. Genetic studies of obese animals and humans have led to findings of multiple genes that confer risk of developing obesity. Individuals can be classified as having genetic obesity, strong or slight genetic predisposition, or genetic resistance to obesity [4]. The current evidence based on familial studies suggests that 40–80% of the variation between individual body mass indices (BMIs) has a genetic basis [3,4].

The genetic reference tool 'human obesity gene map' provides a global encyclopaedia for identified genes, mutations, and qualitative trait loci [5]. Studies such as genome-wide association studies (GWASs) have pointed researchers towards new pathways of neurohumoral mechanisms, other regulators of energy balance, and the interplay with the obesogenic environment.

Gene studies have also unmasked the presence and significance of human microbiomes (particularly gut microbiomes) in the pathogenicity of obesity. The likelihood or presence of clinical obesity can be predicted in an individual through the use of genetic susceptibility with 60% accuracy. When gut microbiomes are identified, the predictive accuracy increases to 90%.

The ultimate goal of genomic (genetic, epigenetic, and microbiome) science is to isolate, understand, and cultivate therapeutic and preventative mechanisms that may eventually be used to prevent the development of obesity and related comorbidities. The benefit to the healthcare system in delivering efficient, low-cost, accurate, personalized, therapeutic, and preventive healthcare is invaluable.

Fundamentals of the human genome, epigenetics, and microbiomes

The discovery of the structure of DNA as a double helix in 1953 by Watson and Crick was a landmark moment in human history. The DNA of a cell is an instruction manual that defines how it will function. This code represents an evolutionary timeline with humans having 99.9% identical genomes. Yet this 0.1% difference results in the large variability seen in phenotypic diversity across the human population [6,7]. There is only a 4% variation of a human genome when compared with that of a chimpanzee. The human nuclear genome consists of 3.2 billion base pairs containing approximately 20,000 genes. It is constructed only of four bases: adenine, thymine, cytosine, and guanine (A, T, C, and G). A single sequenced genome is equivalent to 200 GB of hardware space and can have as many data entry errors as standard computer software.

The mitochondrial genome follows a maternal inheritance pattern. *In utero* studies have suggested several embryogenic associations with obesity. In addition, the intrauterine atmosphere during specific developmental phases can alter the epigenetics of an individual and may work as a foundation for obesity and other phenotypes during later stages of life [8]. Several studies have also shown that various mitochondrial single nucleotide polymorphisms (SNPs) can have a positive association with the incidence of obesity in various human ethnic groups [8].

Epigenetic changes such as DNA methylation and histone modifications can activate the phenotypic expression of a gene. These alterations are believed to have regulatory roles in the inheritance of genetic susceptibility [8]. A recent study found that both mice and humans possess a network of genetic haploinsufficiency that acts as a phenotypic switch in causing obesity [9].

In concert with genes and epigenetic modulation, human microbiomes are thought to exert a co-founder effect [10]. Since the 1960s, researchers have identified a highly personalized metagenome that was formed through co-evolution of trillions of microbes in the human microbiome [6]. This results in a significantly greater biodiversity with 250–800 times (i.e. 2–20 million) more genes [6,11]. The 'healthy microbiome' core is a functional necessity for humans. However, dysbiosis in the microbiome has been associated with numerous diseases including obesity, diabetes, and cancer.

Neuroendocrine system and genetics

Gene discovery has aided our understanding of the complex pathways that regulate energy balance. Peripheral tissues, the gastrointestinal tract, and the pancreas are in constant communication with the brain about energy balance, engaging two main neuroendocrine systems, the *anorexigenic* and *orexigenic pathways* (**Fig. 3.1**) [12]. These homeostatic mechanisms alter behaviours such as energy expenditure, energy storage, hunger, and addiction (**Fig. 3.2**).

In 1994, a key anorexigenic hormone, *leptin*, was identified and shown to communicate the sensation of satiety, thus causing a decrease in food intake [13]. Synthesized and released mainly from adipose tissue, leptin crosses the blood–brain barrier to act on leptin receptors highly expressed at the arcuate nucleus of the hypothalamus [14,15]. The leptin axis is complex and not the sole key to obesity. However, serum leptin hormone levels are strongly correlated with

total body adipose tissue stores with levels decreasing after weight loss and increasing after weight gain [16].

The binding of leptin receptors (LEPRs) leads to activation of Janus kinase 2 (JAK2), by autophosphorylation and activation of a key signal transducer, STAT3. When phosphorylated, STAT3 translocates to the nucleus regulating the transcription of various genes, including neuropeptide Y (NPY), agouti-related peptide (AgRP), pro-opiomelanocortin (POMC), and the signalling inhibitor suppressor of cytokine signaling-3 (SOCS3). Activation of the POMC/cocaine- and amphetamine-regulated transcript (CART) neurons induces a catabolic effect on energy stores, while the leptin inhibition of NPY/AgRP stimulates the orexigenic pathways. SOCS3 forms an inhibitory feedback loop in leptin signalling, targeting the LEPR–JAK2 complex [12].

Starvation states result in the fall of serum leptin levels. This results in an absence of activation of the POMC/CART neurons and a loss of inhibition of the NPY/AgRP neuronal pathway [8,17]. The downstream effect of this process is the stimulation of food intake behaviours, anabolic effects on metabolism, and a decline in energy expenditure.

Many other hormones are also involved in this pathway, including ghrelin, insulin, and cholecystokinin (CCK). Ghrelin is secreted by the stomach and duodenum with levels of ghrelin increasing before

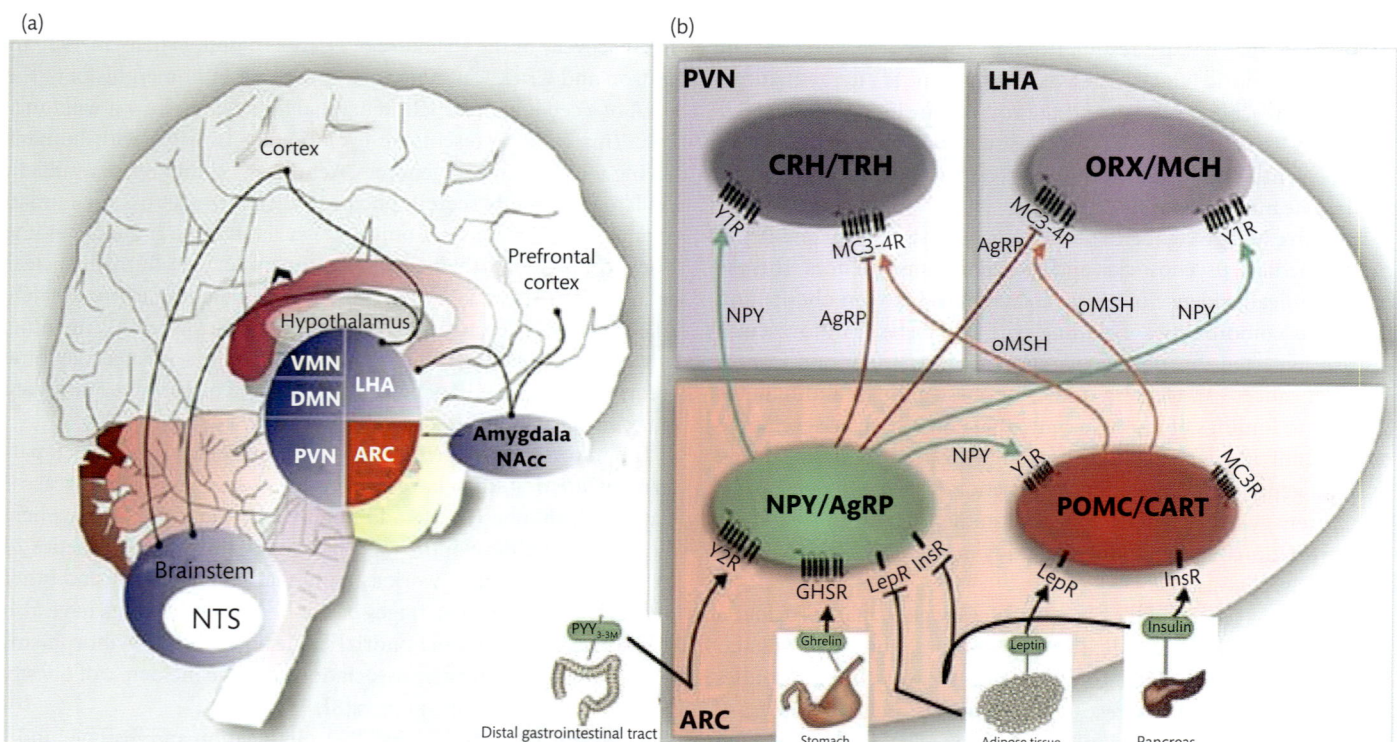

Fig. 3.1 The appetite control system in the brain. (a) The structural components of the system include the arcuate nucleus (ARC), paraventricular nucleus (PVN), lateral hypothalamus area (LHA), ventral medial nucleus (VMN), and dorsal medial nucleus (DMV) at the hypothalamus; the nucleus tractus solitarii (NTS) at the brainstem; the nucleus accumbens (NAcc) and amygdala in the prefrontal cortex; and the cortex. (b) The major appetite signal reception and integration occur in the hypothalamus. In the ARC, the NPY/AgRP neuron (green) produces NPY and AgRP while the pro-opiomelanocortin (POMC)/cocaine- and amphetamine-regulated transcript (CART) neuron (red) produces POMC and CART. These two types of neurons are activated or inhibited by many peripheral signals through cell surface receptors such as Y2R, GHSR, LepR and insR. The signals from these neurons are integrated in PVN and LHA to produce orexigenic or anorexigenic signals through the production of corticotropin-releasing hormone (CRH), thyrotropin-releasing hormone (TRH), orexin (ORX), melanin-concentrating hormone (MCH), etc. Leptin and insulin similarly activate POMC/CART and inhibit NPY/AgRP to cause satiety and increased energy expenditure. Ghrelin and peptide YY activate NPY/AgRP causing increased food intake and reduced energy expenditure.

Adapted with permission from Schellekens, H., Finger, B.C., Dinan, T.G., Cryan, J.F. Ghrelin signalling and obesity: at the interface of stress, mood and food reward. *Pharmacology & Therapeutics*, 135(3):316–26. Copyright © 2012 with permission from Elsevier. doi: 10.1016/j.pharmthera.2012.06.004

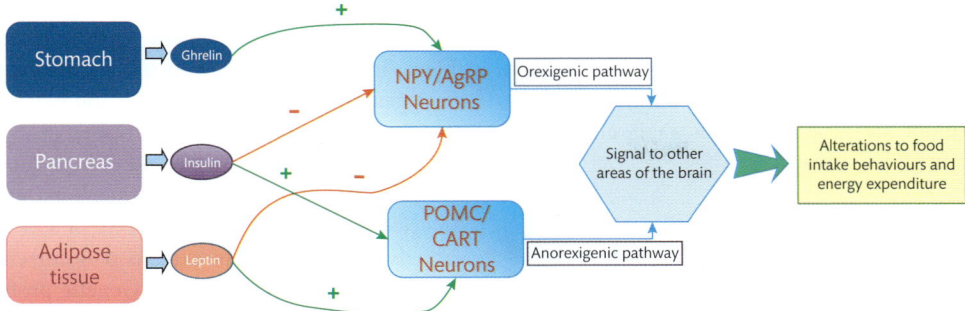

Fig. 3.2 Energy expenditure pathway.

a meal, and then declining after food has been consumed. When ghrelin is secreted during periods of low food intake, it acts at the hypothalamus through the activation of the orexigenic NPY/AgRP neurons, and thus creating a feeling of hunger [18].

Insulin has similar anorexigenic effects on the arcuate neurons to leptin. After being secreted by the pancreas, it can move to the hypothalamus and inhibit the NPY/AgRP neurons while activating the POMC/CART neurons [19]. Satiety is also controlled by various physiological systems such as gut extension, peptide YY, glucagon-like peptide-1, oxyntomodulin, gastric inhibitory peptide (GIP), and CCK release [20–22].

The arcuate nucleus processes the various signals and sends a downstream signal to different areas of the brain, including the melanin-concentrating hormone neurons of the lateral hypothalamus, the thyroid-releasing hormone neurons involved in the hypothalamic–pituitary–thyroid axis, and the gamma-aminobutyric acid neurons in the paraventricular nucleus. Certain neurotransmitters also have an effect on this hunger signal including serotonin, dopamine, and endocannabinoids [23].

Peroxisome proliferator-activated receptors (PPAR-α, PPAR-γ, PPAR-δ) belong to a nuclear hormone receptor superfamily and either promote or prevent gene transcription. Hypothalamic PPAR-γ has been found to cause weight gain [24]. However, peripherally they play a critical role in the regulation of weight, inflammation, lipoprotein metabolism, and glucose homeostasis (Fig. 3.3) [25]. Peripheral activity of these receptors results in decreased adipose tissue [26]. As a result, they have become targets for drug therapy for diseases such as diabetes, atherosclerosis, and obesity.

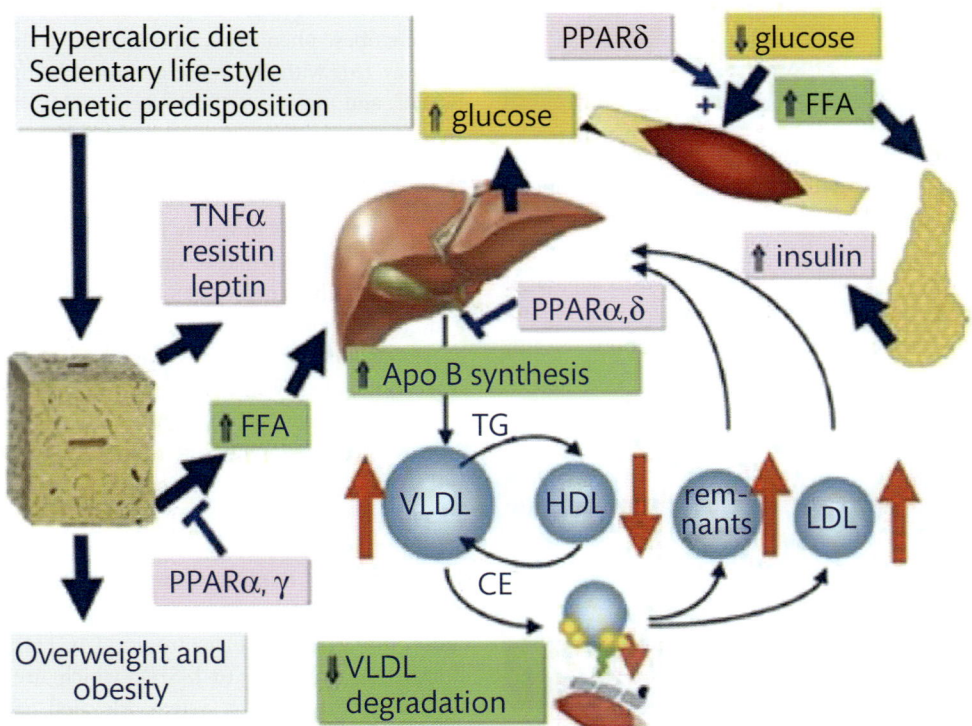

Fig. 3.3 All three PPAR subtypes counteract adverse effects on lipid and glucose metabolism resulting from elevated free fatty acids (FFAs) and glucose in the bloodstream. The most important role of PPARδ most likely is to significantly increase the capacity of skeletal and heart muscle for utilizing fatty acids for their energy metabolism. Furthermore, PPARδ together with PPARα inhibits glucose and very-low-density lipoprotein (VLDL) secretion from the liver. These effects are very important for preserving normal FFA, triglyceride, and high-density lipoprotein (HDL) levels as well as insulin sensitivity in the presence of high dietary fat intake.

Reproduced with permission from Seedorf, U., Aberle, J. Emerging roles of PPARδ in metabolism. *Biochimica et Biophysica Acta (BBA)—Molecular and Cell Biology of Lipids*, 1771(9):1125–1131. Copyright © 2007 Elsevier. https://doi.org/10.1016/j.bbalip.2007.04.017

These molecular, hormonal, and neuronal connections, once activated, affect body weight and energy balance through three main methods: behaviours (feeding and physical activity), metabolism, and neuroendocrine products such as cortisol, insulin, thyroid hormone, and growth hormone [20]. The shift in this fragile energy balance can result in obesity [27].

Influence of the obesogenic environment

The pandemic of obesity is predominantly non-syndromic and is attributed to the gene–environment interplay. Industrialization, urbanization, and sedentary lifestyle has resulted in a doubling of obesity between 1980 and 2014, by World Health Organization estimates.

In 1962, James Neel postulated the 'thrifty genotype' theory. He postulated that some of the genes that predispose humans to obesity provided the ability to efficiently store large amounts of dietary fats in energy-dense adipose tissue [28]. This physiology conferred a survival advantage during periods of famine in an era of the hunter-gatherer society. Over the past five decades, our genomes have changed very little but we have become increasingly exposed to an abundance of convenient, inexpensive, palatable, and energy-dense foods (Box 3.1).

The thrifty genotype theory may be explained by a classic study looking at an obese ethnic group, Pima Indians. The study revealed those living in a 'restrictive' environment of the remote Sierra Madre mountains of Mexico had a lower prevalence of obesity than those living in the industrialized 'obesogenic' environment of Arizona, United States [29].

Familial obesity

Familial risk has been identified as a significant contributor to the development of obesity. Monozygotic twins (genetically identical) have shown a correlation in fat mass of 70–90%. Similar studies looking at dizygotic twins (sharing half of their genetics) found a 35–45% correlation in fat mass [30]. Monozygotic twins separated at birth show a strong correlation in BMI while separated dizygotic twins have been shown to have no correlation [31]. National Health and Nutrition Examination Survey III (NHANES III) in the United States has demonstrated that the prevalence of obesity (BMI >30 kg/m²) was twice as high in families with an obese family member compared to the general population. A person with a severely obese family member (BMI >45 kg/m²) had a seven to eight times increase in the risk of developing obesity [32].

Box 3.1 Recent environmental changes involved in increasing obesity rates

- Processed, nutrient-poor foods have become a mainstay in children's diets.
- People are living a more sedentary life.
- Consumption of sugary beverages has increased dramatically.
- Animal products have become a bigger portion of our diet.
- Cheap, unhealthy fast-food chains have become abundant worldwide.

Using familial genetic risk information, behavioural modification therapies are being developed. A study evaluating mothers' food choices for their children from a virtual buffet proved that high-risk messages, coupled with risk-reduction education, led to more appropriate food choices for their children [33].

Ethnicity also plays a role. Studies have shown an increased likelihood of obesity for African Americans and Mexican/Hispanic Americans compared to their white or European-origin counterparts that cannot easily be explained by current lifestyle, diet, or environmental factors alone [34]. Genetic profiling of the fatty acid desaturase 1 (FADS1) gene, which affects fatty acid metabolism, suggests that the C allele (poor converters) is predominant in Native Americans, Latin Americans, and East Asians. These ethnicities have increased risk of hyperlipidaemia and insulin resistance when given high free fatty acid diets. However, those with the A allele (high converters) are at increased risk of coronary artery disease.

Monogenic forms of obesity

Mendelian disorders

Over 30 complex developmental disorders have been identified with obesity as a feature, most of which present early in childhood. The pattern of inheritance can be autosomal dominant, autosomal recessive, X-linked dominant, and X-linked recessive. See Table 3.1 for a list of some of the notable Mendelian disorders.

Single gene disorders

Monogenic genetic causes are implicated in 2–5% of obesity cases and are likely to present as early childhood obesity. To date, researchers have revealed 20 gene mutations in humans that result in a severe obese phenotype, all occurring in the leptin–melanocortin pathway [8], with the most common being leptin (LEP), LEPR, POMC, and melanocortin-4 receptor (MC4R). See Fig. 3.4 for examples of types of variations present in human genes [35].

Congenital leptin deficiency is characterized by hyperphagia starting at 4 months of age and hypogonadotropic hypogonadism. This suggests that leptin may not only have an effect on energy expenditure, but it also may be important in reproduction and puberty. This genetic abnormality, caused by a frameshift in the leptin protein, has only been documented in four people. These patients can be treated with subcutaneous injections of human leptin, which fully reverses the obesity and induces the beginning of puberty [36].

LEPR mutations are thought to have a pleiotropic effect with a more severe phenotype and show significant growth retardation and hypothalamic hypothyroidism in addition to the obesity phenotype [4].

Pro-opiomelanocortin (POMC) is post-transcriptionally spliced to form various hormones that participate in the hypothalamic–pituitary–adrenal axis. Some of these neuropeptides include B-endorphins, adrenocorticotropin (ACTH), and α-melanocyte stimulating hormone (α-MSH), which are heavily involved in the energy expenditure system. Elevated leptin levels induce the transcription of α-MSH, which then activates the MC4R in the hypothalamus. This signal produces behaviours associated with decreased food intake and increased energy expenditure [37]. Patients with the POMC gene deficiency will present with adrenal crisis at a younger age because of the loss of the ACTH hormone. The loss of the α-MSH hormone induces a state of hyperphagia and eventually

Table 3.1 Notable Mendelian disorders

Disorder	Epidemiology	Chromosomal abnormality	Phenotype
Prader–Willi syndrome (PWS)	Prevalence of 1 in 25,000	Autosomal dominant affecting chromosome 15 (15q11)	Obesity, reduced fetal activity, muscular hypotonia at birth, short stature, hypogonadism, mental retardation, small hands and feet, and hyperphagia that usually develops between 12 and 18 months
Albright hereditary osteodystrophy (AHO)	Reporting only in the Japanese population, 1 in 139,000	Autosomal disorder affecting the GNAS1 gene at chromosome 20q13.3	Obesity, round facies, short stature, brachydactyly, subcutaneous calcifications, intellectual disability in some cases, and pseudohypoparathyroidism (parathyroid hyperplasia with elevated parathyroid hormone and hypocalcaemia) and the milder pseudopseudohypoparathyroidism (no hormonal resistance observed)
Bardet–Biedl syndrome (BBS)	Prevalence of 1 in 1,60,000 in the British population and 1 in 13,500 in the Middle East due to consanguinity	Genetically heterogenous disorder linked to at least seven loci (on chromosomes 11, 15, and 16)	Primary disorder of the cilium involved in the kidney and eye. Features include obesity, intellectual disability, pigmentary retinopathy, polydactyly, and hypogenitalism
Cohen syndrome	Rare. High prevalence in older Amish and Finnish population	Autosomal recessive. Chromosome 8. Mutation of COH1 (VPS13B gene)	Encodes a transmembrane protein of unknown function. Microcephaly, intellectual disability, hypotonia, hypermobility of joints, retinal dystrophy. Distinctive facial features. Associated with childhood truncal obesity
Alström syndrome	Rare, <900 people diagnosed worldwide	Autosomal recessive. ALMS1 gene	Coding protein involved in the normal functioning of primary cilia. Normal birth weight but become obese during their first year, resulting in childhood truncal obesity
WAGR	1 in 500,000	Chromosome 11. PAX6 and WT1 genes	Wilm's tumour, aniridia, genitourinary anomalies, and intellectual disability

early-onset obesity. These patients also have pale skin and red hair because α-MSH is involved in the pigmentation of hair and skin. People with the POMC gene deficiency will need cortisol replacement therapy for the remainder of their lives [38].

MC4R (found on chromosome 18q22) deficiency is the most common inherited obesity syndrome with over 30 different types of mutations, including missense, nonsense, and frameshift [39]. These alterations are found in 1–6% of obese children [5]. Larsen et al. showed that 2.5% of the Danish population with a BMI greater than 30 kg/m² had a MC4R mutation. Patients with this genetic trait will have hyperphagia and increased bone density, possibly due to hyperinsulinaemia [40]. Currently, setmelanotide, a MC4R agonist has been developed but remains under evaluation [41].

The identification of single genes has enabled mapping of the energy expenditure pathway and has led to the development of genetic testing to identify and treat susceptible individuals.

Polygenic forms of obesity

Finding a candidate gene

Researchers use various methods to identify and study candidate genes that could be of importance in certain diseases. The functional approach utilizes current medical knowledge to study genes based on pathophysiology. Obesity studies using this method concentrated on genes involved in the energy balance pathway and adipose tissue biology. The positional approach uses knowledge of existing loci from established genomic studies to predict the importance of

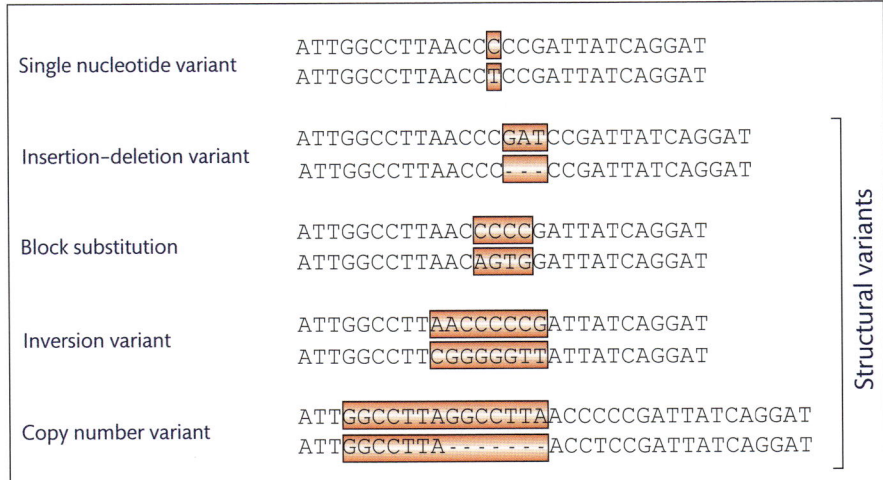

Single nucleotide variants in four human genomes

	(n)	In dbSNP (%)
J.Craig Venter's genome	3,213,401	91.0
James D. Watson's genome	3,322,093	81.7
Asian genome	3,074,097	86.4
Yoruban genome	4,139,196	73.6

Structural variants in the Venter genome

	(n)	length (bp)
Block substitutions	53,823	2–206
Indels (heterozygous)	851,575	1–82,711
Inversions	90	7–670,345
Copy number variants	62	8,855–1,925,949

Fig. 3.4 Types of variations present in human genome sequences.

Reproduced with permission from Frazer K.A., Murray, S.S., Schork, N.J., Topol, E.J., Human genetic variation and its contribution to complex traits. *Nature Reviews Genetics*, 10(4):241–51, Copyright © 2009 Springer Nature. doi: 10.1038/nrg2554

other nearby loci. The research outcomes with these methods have been inconsistent and relatively weak to date.

Some of the functional studies focused on *mitochondrial uncoupling proteins* (UCPs) due to their functional association with energy expenditure. UCP1 plays an important role in the thermogenesis of brown adipose tissue. UCP2 and UCP3 genes were found to be associated with altered BMI, waist-to-hip ratio, skinfold thickness, respiratory quotient, and resting metabolic rate [4].

The β_3-*adrenoreceptor (AR) gene* which is predominantly found in infant brown fat and at low levels in adult deep fat (such as perirenal and omental fat), has been studied for its thermogenic, anti-obesity, and antidiabetic properties in animals. In humans, a 20-week endurance-training programme resulted in a greater decrease in total and subcutaneous fat in individuals with β_2-AR and β_3-AR polymorphisms [4].

Genome-wide association studies

A GWAS is a non-hypothesis-driven method that was developed in response to limitation studies utilizing familial, single gene, candidate gene, and other modalities. The entire genome of an obese individual is assayed and compared to that of a lean individual. All variations in DNA, including those with low to rational penetrance that may or may not be functionally significant, are identified.

According to the 12th update of the human obesity gene map, there are 253 quantity trait loci for obesity-related phenotypes from a series of 61 genome-wide scan studies [8]. A large proportion of these loci possess genes that are expressed in the brain [36].

In 2007, the fat mass and obesity (FTO) gene was discovered in a study of diabetic individuals [42]. It was later identified that the FTO gene was causing diabetes through the stimulation of obesity [43,44]. Further, studies have shown that individuals with some of these SNPs (ESR1, FTO) are less likely to maintain the weight loss and glycaemic control that happen after surgery, while other genes (UCP2) confer greater weight reduction after surgery [45].

Several SNPs in the FTO loci have been shown to change the expression of promoters in a gene named Iroquois homeobox 3 (IRX3), resulting in the obese phenotype [46,47]. Mice that are deficient in the IRX3 gene have a 25–30% reduction in weight due to reduced body fat and increased metabolic rates (through a switch of white adipose tissue to brown adipose tissue).

In 2008, a GWAS examining 11,955 individuals of European and Indian heritage correlated variation in the loci near the MC4R gene with increased waist circumference and insulin resistance [48] (**Fig. 3.5**).

Another locus of interest that was found to have SNP variation in the obese population is near the GIP receptor (GIPR) gene. GIP

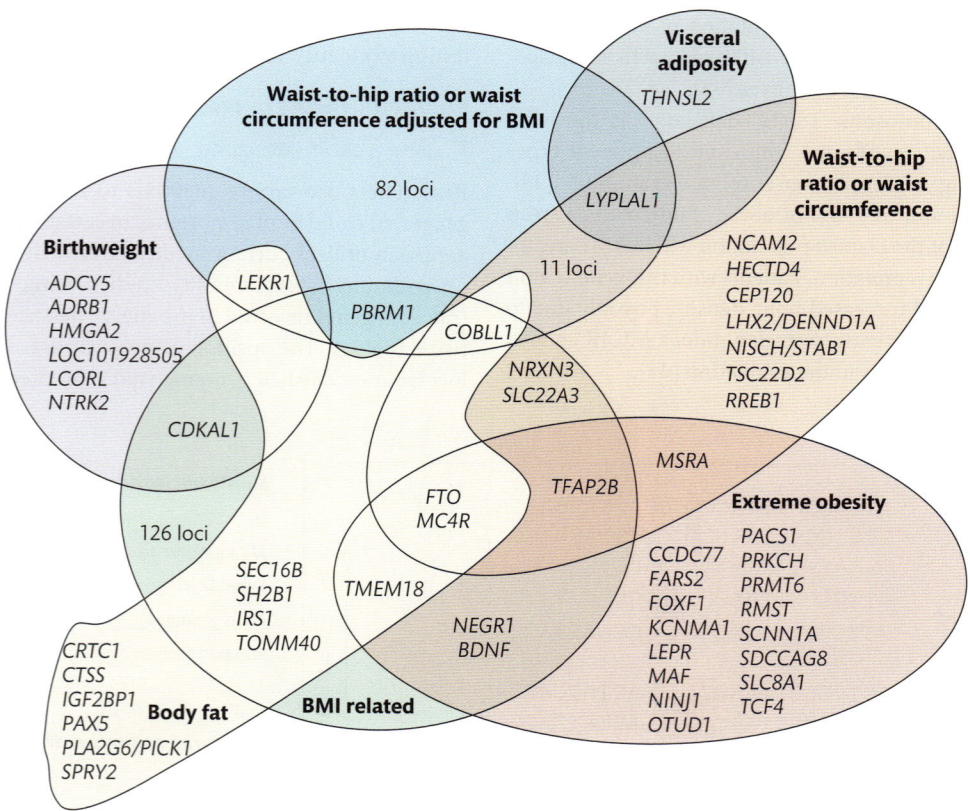

Fig. 3.5 Major GWAS discoveries for adiposity traits. For clarity of presentation, findings of GWASs, are grouped into seven categories: BMI related (includes GWAS for BMI, weight, overweight or obese status in adulthood, childhood BMI, childhood obesity, and BMI change over time; 141 loci); body fat (includes GWASs for body fat percentage and body fat mass; 15 loci); birthweight (eight loci); waist-to-hip ratio or waist circumference adjusted for BMI (97 loci); visceral adiposity (includes GWASs for visceral fat and visceral-to-subcutaneous adipose tissue ratio; two loci); waist-to-hip ratio or waist circumference (includes GWASs for waist-to-hip ratio and waist circumference not adjusted for BMI; 26 loci); and extreme obesity (includes GWAS for extreme childhood and extreme adult obesity; 23 loci).

is an incretin hormone secreted by the K cells of the duodenum and intestine that is involved in the release of insulin after glucose ingestion [49].

The success of the prior GWAS publications paved the way for the Genetic Investigation of Anthropometric Traits (GIANT) team to perform a series of meta-analysis studies. The most recent by this group looked at the association between BMI and millions of SNPs in a total of 322,154 individuals of European descent and 17,072 individuals of non-European descent from 125 studies [50]. The group found 97 different loci for BMI, of which 56 were novel. However, these 97 loci have been shown to explain only 2.7% of the variance in BMI [50,51].

With numerous identified variants and only modest effect size, there are challenges to the clinical application of GWAS-identified loci. One way of estimating their cumulative burden is to use the Genetic Risk Score (GRS). Some studies have found a high GRS to be associated with low physical activity and high BMI. Although the GRS is statistically significant at the population level, it does not take into account the gene–gene or gene–environment interplay [52].

Currently a number of commercial entities sell obesity gene testing for the unambiguous causal mutations. One such test has been adopted by a National Health Service Trust trust in the United Kingdom under a pilot programme in 2005. In the United States, pilot programmes have also commenced that combine genetic testing with coaching to develop personalized weight loss programmes. Some of the genes tested are FTO, MC4R, and dopamine receptor D_2 (DRD2) (which has been linked to addictive behaviours such as overeating).

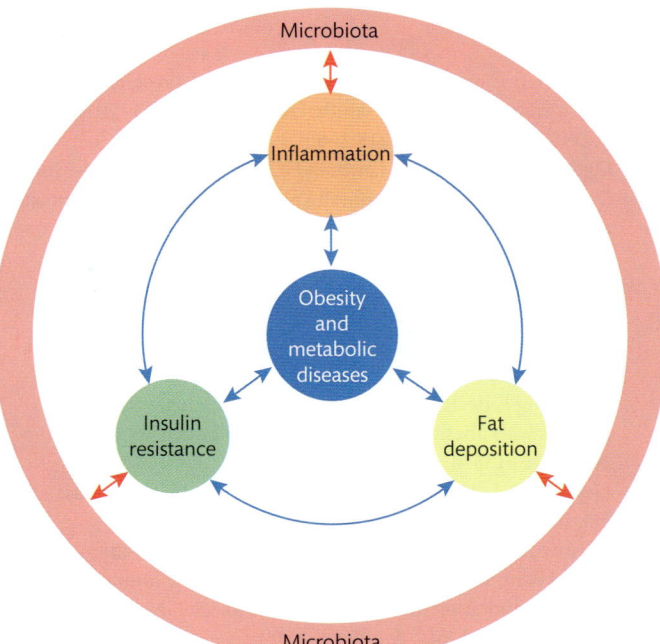

Fig. 3.6 Crosstalk between the gut microbiota and the mammalian host in inflammation and metabolism. The gut microbiota can contribute to host insulin resistance, low-grade inflammation, and fat deposition through a range of molecular interactions with the host and therefore can indirectly participate in the onset of obesity and metabolic diseases.

Reproduced from Boulangé, C.L., Neves, A.L., Chilloux, J., Nicholson, J.K., Dumas, M.E. Impact of the gut microbiota on inflammation, obesity, and metabolic disease. *Genome Medicine*, 8(42): 42. DOI: 10.1186/s13073-016-0303-2. This article is distributed under the terms of the Creative Commons Attribution 4.0 International License (CC BY 4.0), http://creativecommons.org/licenses/by/4.0/.

Obesity and microbiomes

Microbes have been shown to help educate the immune system, digest food, resist disease, and determine how we respond to drugs (**Fig. 3.6**). They also can increase obesogenic or anorexigenic behaviour. Further, if children are administered antibiotics in the first 6 months of life they are more likely to become obese later on in life.

One human study found gut biodiversity to be low in both obese individuals and those having lap band surgery. However, those with gastric bypass surgery had a restoration of high gut biodiversity and weight loss [53]. The therapeutic potential of using surgery and prebiotic/probiotic interventions has seen positive results in rodents and is being explored in human studies with some promising results [54]. Further, microbiome-generated therapeutic interventions may help induce improved food-intake behaviours.

Conclusion

We now know that obesity is inherited as much as height and more than almost any other studied condition [55]. The social, medical, and economic costs of obesity are steep. In 2014, the global economic impact study of obesity was estimated to be US $2 trillion or 2.8% of the global gross domestic product [56]. In 2008, the obese patients' annual medical costs were $1429 more than patients with normal weight In Australia, it was estimated in 2016 that the cost of childhood obesity of preschoolers was approximately Australian $17 million [57].

We are beginning to understand the numerous environmental and genetic factors that intricately control obesity. The World Health Organization has adopted the Global Strategy on Diet, Physical Activity and Health, but no health system is yet meeting the challenges of managing obesity. In addition, no society has enforced an effective strategy to prevent it [58,59]. Success in achieving the strategic goals requires strong governmental leadership, effective policymaking, urban and environment planning, and increasing availability of education and subsidized healthy food.

Addressing the obesity pandemic is likely to require a paradigm shift for which genomics may be a fundamental force. Our understanding of the pathophysiology of obesity is aided by genomic science, rapidly evolving technology, and data science.

The clinical utility of genetic profiling and risk information lies in the ability to develop individualized behavioural therapy, nutrition programmes, pharmacological interventions, gene treatments, and procedures. We will be able to screen an individual and predict how well a person will respond to a given procedure [60]. There is also hope of reducing the total cost of healthcare from these approaches due to rapid diagnosis and decreases in misdiagnoses, failed treatments, complications, and side effects [61].

Genomics technology in precision healthcare is not tomorrow— it's here today. However, global and country-specific ethical and strategic policies, relevant regulation (such as Equality, Data Protection, and Privacy Acts), social contracts, and workforce management need to be enacted before we can make full use of its capabilities.

REFERENCES

1. Ogden CL, Carroll MD, Fryar CD, Flegal KM. Prevalence of obesity among adults and youth: United States, 2011–2014. NCHS Data Brief. 2015;**219**:1–8.

2. Ogden CL, Carroll MD, Lawman HG, Fryar CD, Kruszon-Moran D, Kit BK, et al. Trends in obesity prevalence among children and adolescents in the United States, 1988–1994 through 2013–2014. JAMA. 2016;**315**(21):2292–99.

3. Haslam DW, James WPT. Obesity. Lancet. 2005;**366**(9492):1197–209.

4. Loos RJF, Bouchard C. Obesity—is it a genetic disorder? J Intern Med. 2003;**254**(5):401–25.

5. Phan-Hug F, Beckmann JS, Jacquemont S. Genetic testing in patients with obesity. Best Pract Res Clin Endocrinol Metab. 2012;**26**(2):133–43.

6. Lloyd-Price J, Abu-Ali G, Huttenhower C. The healthy human microbiome. Genome Med. 2016;**8**(1).

7. Harrow J, Frankish A, Gonzalez JM, Tapanari E, Diekhans M, Kokocinski F, et al. GENCODE: the reference human genome annotation for The ENCODE Project. Genome Res. 2012;**22**(9):1760–74.

8. Rao KR, Lal N, Giridharan NV. Genetic & epigenetic approach to human obesity. Indian J Med Res. 2014;**140**(5):589–603.

9. Dalgaard K, Landgraf K, Heyne S, Lempradl A, Longinotto J, Gossens K, et al. Trim28 haploinsufficiency triggers bi-stable epigenetic obesity. Cell. 2016;**164**(3):353–64.

10. Carbonero F. Human epigenetics and microbiome: the potential for a revolution in both research areas by integrative studies. Future Science OA. 2017;**3**(3):FSO207.

11. Komaroff AL. The microbiome and risk for obesity and diabetes. JAMA. 2017;**317**(4):355–56.

12. Schellekens H, Finger BC, Dinan TG, Cryan JF. Ghrelin signalling and obesity: at the interface of stress, mood and food reward. Pharmacol Ther. 2012;**135**(3):316–26.

13. Bell CG, Walley AJ, Froguel P. The genetics of human obesity. Nat Rev Genet. 2005;**6**(3):221–34.

14. Clément K, Vaisse C, Lahlou N, Cabrol S, Pelloux V, Cassuto D, et al. A mutation in the human leptin receptor gene causes obesity and pituitary dysfunction. Nature. 1998;**392**(6674):398–401.

15. Margetic S, Gazzola C, Pegg GG, Hill RA. Leptin: a review of its peripheral actions and interactions. Int J Obes Relat Metab Disord. 2002;**26**(11):1407–33.

16. Maffei M, Halaas J, Ravussin E, Pratley RE, Lee GH, Zhang Y, et al. Leptin levels in human and rodent: measurement of plasma leptin and ob RNA in obese and weight-reduced subjects. Nat Med. 1995;**1**(11):1155–61.

17. Friedman JM, Halaas JL. Leptin and the regulation of body weight in mammals. Nature. 1998;**395**(6704):763–70.

18. Barsh GS, Schwartz MW. Genetic approaches to studying energy balance: perception and integration. Nat Rev Genet. 2002;**3**(8):589–600.

19. Air EL, Strowski MZ, Benoit SC, Conarello SL, Salituro GM, Guan X-M, et al. Small molecule insulin mimetics reduce food intake and body weight and prevent development of obesity. Nat Med. 2002;**8**(2):179–83.

20. Spiegelman BM, Flier JS. Obesity and the regulation of energy balance. Cell. 2001;**104**(4):531–43.

21. Maier C, Riedl M, Vila G, Nowotny P, Wolzt M, Clodi M, et al. Cholinergic regulation of ghrelin and peptide YY release may be impaired in obesity. Diabetes. 2008;**57**(9):2332–40.

22. Goldstone AP, Miras AD, Scholtz S, Jackson S, Neff KJ, Pénicaud L, et al. Link between increased satiety gut hormones and reduced food reward after gastric bypass surgery for obesity. J Clin Endocrinol Metab. 2016;**101**(2):599–609.

23. Flier JS, Harris M, Hollenberg AN. Leptin, nutrition, and the thyroid: the why, the wherefore, and the wiring. J Clin Invest. 2000;**105**(7):859–61.

24. Lu M, Sarruf DA, Talukdar S, Sharma S, Li P, Bandyopadhyay G, et al. Brain PPAR-γ promotes obesity and is required for the insulin-sensitizing effect of thiazolidinediones. Nat Med. 2011;**17**(5):618–22.

25. Seedorf U, Aberle J. Emerging roles of PPARdelta in metabolism. Biochim Biophys Acta. 2007;**1771**(9):1125–31.

26. Blaschke F. Obesity, peroxisome proliferator-activated receptor, and atherosclerosis in type 2 diabetes. Arterioscler Thromb Vasc Biol. 2006;**26**(1):28–40.

27. Schwartz MW, Woods SC, Porte D Jr, Seeley RJ, Baskin DG. Central nervous system control of food intake. Nature. 2000;**404**(6778):661–71.

28. Neel JV. The 'thrifty genotype' in 1998. Nutr Rev. 1999;**57**(5 Pt 2):S2–9.

29. Ravussin E, Valencia ME, Esparza J, Bennett PH, Schulz LO. Effects of a traditional lifestyle on obesity in Pima Indians. Diabetes Care. 1994;**17**(9):1067–74.

30. Srivastava A, Srivastava N, Mittal B. Genetics of obesity. Indian J Clin Biochem. 2016;**31**(4):361–71.

31. Stunkard AJ, Harris JR, Pedersen NL, McClearn GE. The body-mass index of twins who have been reared apart. N Engl J Med. 1990;**322**(21):1483–87.

32. Lee JH, Reed DR, Price RA. Familial risk ratios for extreme obesity: implications for mapping human obesity genes. Int J Obes Relat Metab Disord. 1997;**21**(10):935–40.

33. McBride CM, Persky S, Wagner LK, Faith MS, Ward DS. Effects of providing personalized feedback of child's obesity risk on mothers' food choices using a virtual reality buffet. Int J Obes. 2013;**37**(10):1322–27.

34. Cossrow N, Falkner B. Race/ethnic issues in obesity and obesity-related comorbidities. J Clin Endocrinol Metab. 2004;**89**(6):2590–94.

35. Frazer KA, Murray SS, Schork NJ, Topol EJ. Human genetic variation and its contribution to complex traits. Nat Rev Genet. 2009;**10**(4):241–51.

36. Farooqi IS, O'Rahilly S. New advances in the genetics of early onset obesity. Int J Obes. 2005;**29**(10):1149–52.

37. Flier JS, Maratos-Flier E. Obesity and the hypothalamus: novel peptides for new pathways. Cell. 1998;**92**(4):437–40.

38. Farooqi IS. Monogenic human obesity syndromes. Prog Brain Res. 2006;**153**:119–25.

39. Hinney A, Schmidt A, Nottebom K, Heibült O, Becker I, Ziegler A, et al. Several mutations in the melanocortin-4 receptor gene including a nonsense and a frameshift mutation associated with dominantly inherited obesity in humans. J Clin Endocrinol Metab. 1999;**84**(4):1483–86.

40. Larsen LH, Echwald SM, Sørensen TIA, Andersen T, Wulff BS, Pedersen O. Prevalence of mutations and functional analyses of melanocortin 4 receptor variants identified among 750 men with juvenile-onset obesity. J Clin Endocrinol Metab. 2005;**90**(1):219–24.

41. Collet T-H, Dubern B, Mokrosinski J, Connors H, Keogh JM, de Oliveira EM, et al. Evaluation of a melanocortin-4 receptor (MC4R) agonist (setmelanotide) in MC4R deficiency. Mol Metab. 2017;**6**(10):1321–29.

42. Frayling TM. Genome-wide association studies provide new insights into type 2 diabetes aetiology. Nat Rev Genet. 2007;**8**(9):657–62.

43. Scuteri A, Sanna S, Chen W-M, Uda M, Albai G, Strait J, et al. Genome-wide association scan shows genetic variants in the FTO gene are associated with obesity-related traits. PLoS Genet. 2007;**3**(7):e115.

44. Speliotes EK, Willer CJ, Berndt SI, Monda KL, Thorleifsson G, Jackson AU, et al. Association analyses of 249,796 individuals reveal 18 new loci associated with body mass index. Nat Genet. 2010;**42**(11):937–48.

45. Liou T-H, Chen H-H, Wang W, Wu S-F, Lee Y-C, Yang W-S, et al. ESR1, FTO, and UCP2 genes interact with bariatric surgery affecting weight loss and glycemic control in severely obese patients. Obes Surg. 2011;**21**(11):1758–65.

46. Ragvin A, Moro E, Fredman D, Navratilova P, Drivenes Ø, Engström PG, et al. Long-range gene regulation links genomic type 2 diabetes and obesity risk regions to HHEX, SOX4, and IRX3. Proc Natl Acad Sci U S A. 2010;**107**(2):775–80.

47. Smemo S, Tena JJ, Kim K-H, Gamazon ER, Sakabe NJ, Gómez-Marín C, et al. Obesity-associated variants within FTO form long-range functional connections with IRX3. Nature. 2014;**507**(7492):371–75.

48. Chambers JC, Elliott P, Zabaneh D, Zhang W, Li Y, Froguel P, et al. Common genetic variation near MC4R is associated with waist circumference and insulin resistance. Nat Genet. 2008;**40**(6):716–18.

49. Saxena R, Hivert M, Langenberg C, Tanaka T, Pankow JS, Vollenweider P, et al. Genetic variation in GIPR influences the glucose and insulin responses to an oral glucose challenge. Nat Genet. 2010;**42**(2):142–48.

50. Locke AE, Kahali B, Berndt SI, Justice AE, Pers TH, Day FR, et al. Genetic studies of body mass index yield new insights for obesity biology. Nature. 2015;**518**(7538):197–206.

51. Goodarzi MO. Genetics of obesity: what genetic association studies have taught us about the biology of obesity and its complications. Lancet Diabetes Endocrinol. 2018;**6**(3):223–36.

52 Belsky, D. W., Moffitt, T. E., Sugden, K., Williams, B., Houts, R., McCarthy, J., & Caspi, A. (2013). Development and evaluation of a genetic risk score for obesity. Biodemography and social biology, **59**(1), 85–100. https://doi.org/10.1080/19485565.2013.774628

53. Boulangé CL, Neves AL, Chilloux J, Nicholson JK, Dumas M-E. Impact of the gut microbiota on inflammation, obesity, and metabolic disease. Genome Med. 2016;**8**(1):42.

54. Ilhan ZE, DiBaise JK, Isern NG, Hoyt DW, Marcus AK, Kang D-W, et al. Distinctive microbiomes and metabolites linked with weight loss after gastric bypass, but not gastric banding. ISME J. 2017;**11**(9):2047–58.

55. Friedman JM. Modern science versus the stigma of obesity. Nat Med. 2004;**10**(6):563–69.

56. Tremmel M, Gerdtham U-G, Nilsson PM, Saha S. Economic burden of obesity: a systematic literature review. Int J Environ Res Public Health. 2017;**14**(4):435.

57. Brown V, Moodie M, Baur L, Wen LM, Hayes A. The high cost of obesity in Australian pre-schoolers. Aust N Z J Public Health. 2017;**41**(3):323–24.

58. Lu J, Bi Y, Ning G. Curbing the obesity epidemic in China. Lancet Diabetes Endocrinol. 2016;**4**(6):470–71.

59. World Health Organization. Report of the Commission on Ending Childhood Obesity. Implementation Plan: Executive Summary. 2016. Geneva: World Health Organization.

60. Lin JS, Thompson M, Goddard KAB, Piper MA, Heneghan C, Whitlock EP. Evaluating genomic tests from bench to bedside: a practical framework. BMC Med Inform Decis Mak. 2012;**12**:117.

61. The Lancet. Public genomes: the future of the NHS? Lancet. 2017;**390**(10091):203.

Pharmacokinetics and pharmacodynamics in obesity

Tiffany Sun Moon and Babatunde O. Ogunnaike

Introduction

Over one-third of adults are obese (body mass index (BMI) ≥30 kg/m²) with 5% of the population being morbidly obese (BMI ≥40 kg/m²) [1]. The worldwide incidence of morbid obesity has tripled over the past three decades [2]. Obesity is a risk factor for several diseases including hypertension, coronary artery disease, obstructive sleep apnoea, and diabetes. Furthermore, obese patients have increased rates of morbidity and mortality compared to non-obese subjects [3]. These patients not only pose difficulties to physicians as a result of their anatomical differences, but changes in their body composition also impose differences in the pharmacokinetic and pharmacodynamic profiles of anaesthetic drugs.

Obesity increases both fat and lean muscle mass, but the amount of adipose tissue increases disproportionately, affecting the volume of distribution of drugs according to their lipid solubility. Changes in cardiac output, total blood volume, and regional blood flow also affect the peak plasma concentration, clearance, and elimination half-life of anaesthetic agents. Obese and morbidly obese individuals are frequently excluded from clinical trials therefore dosing information on package inserts may not be accurate when applied to obese and morbidly obese individuals [2]. Pathological changes that occur as a result of obesity and morbid obesity can lead to alterations in the pharmacokinetics and pharmacodynamics of drugs, which may require dose adjustments. Anaesthesiologists should be aware of how obesity affects the pharmacokinetics and pharmacodynamics of anaesthetic agents to avoid relative over- or underdosing of drugs with narrow therapeutic indices.

Measures of weight and obesity

Direct and indirect methods are available to evaluate the body composition of obese subjects. The goal is to determine the amount of lean tissue versus fat mass to appropriately dose drugs.

Direct measures of body composition

Total body water can be measured because water maintains a stable relationship to fat-free mass so that measured water-isotope dilution volumes can predict fat mass and fat-free mass (FFM) in non-obese patients [4]. However, this technique is limited in the obese because 15–30% of total body water is present in adipose tissue as extracellular fluid, which increases proportionally with the degree of adipose tissue accumulation [5].

Total (whole) body counting measures the amount of naturally radioactive potassium-40 in the body. Since potassium is almost all intracellular, it can provide an estimate of cell mass [6]. Generally, this method is reserved for research purposes.

Dual-energy X-ray absorptiometry is another method to quantify fat, lean tissue, and bone density. The scan exposes the subject to a very minute amount of radiation. Mathematical algorithms are then used to calculate separate components of the body [4]. Dual-energy X-ray absorptiometry may not be very reliable in extreme populations such as the morbidly obese [7]. Computed tomography and magnetic resonance imaging can also be used to directly assess body composition. However, some computed tomography and magnetic resonance imaging scanners may not be able to physically accommodate morbidly obese individuals. Furthermore, whole-body computed tomography delivers a large dose of radiation, and magnetic resonance imaging scans are time-consuming to perform [4].

Indirect measures of body composition

Anthropometry is one of the most basic methods of indirectly evaluating body composition. Measurements describe body mass, size, and shape and include weight, height, skinfold thickness, circumferences, and limb lengths [6]. Abdominal circumference, or more commonly, the ratio of abdominal circumference to hip circumference or waist-to-hip ratio, is sometimes used to describe fat distribution. A waist-to-hip ratio greater than 1.0 for men and 0.85 for women is associated with an increased risk for cardiovascular disease and diabetes [8]. Skinfold measurement using calipers can also be used to determine subcutaneous fat thickness and body fat percentage, but in morbidly obese patients can be technically difficult to perform.

Bioelectrical impedance measures the resistance of the body as a conductor to a very small alternating electric current and estimates the total body water, FFM, and fat mass of a subject. Although commercial bioelectrical impedance analysers are available, their use in clinical medicine is limited. Large errors can occur for individual measurements, especially among obese patients, thus limiting its clinical utility [4].

Body size descriptors for pharmacokinetic studies (dosing scalars)

Total body weight

Total body weight (TBW) is the actual body weight of an individual. TBW is often used to estimate the severity of obesity by determining the percentage increase of TBW from ideal body weight (IBW). Individuals are considered obese when the TBW exceeds 120% of the IBW [9]. Dosing recommendations for many drugs are based on TBW, which is appropriate for normal-weight individuals whose TBW, lean body weight (LBW), and IBW are comparable. In obese patients, fat mass and lean mass increase disproportionately because lean mass accounts for only 20–40% of the increased weight. Thus, in obese individuals, the ratio of LBW to TBW decreases. Blood flow to fat normally accounts for 5% of the total cardiac output but may decrease to only 2% in morbidly obese patients [10]. This decrease in perfusion to excess adipose tissue may explain why the volume of distribution of lipophilic agents does not increase proportionally to the amount of excess adipose tissue. Thus, drug dosages based on TBW may result in an overdose in obese individuals.

Body mass index

The most widely used descriptor of obesity is BMI, defined as TBW (kg)/height (metres squared). Obesity is frequently classified into subgroups according to BMI (**Table 4.1**). A BMI of 30 kg/m² or greater and 40 kg/m² or greater define obesity and morbid obesity, respectively. The main disadvantage is that BMI does not take into account the difference between fat mass and muscle mass so that individuals with a large muscle mass (e.g. athletic, heavily muscled individuals) will have the same BMI as individuals with a large amount of fat. Additionally, BMI is not sex specific.

Ideal body weight

IBWs were originally derived from height–weight tables collected by the Metropolitan Life Insurance Company and first published in 1943 [11]. The terms 'ideal' and 'desirable' body weight were used synonymously and were meant to indicate the weight that was associated with the lowest mortality. Although many formulas have been published, the most commonly used was derived by Devine in 1974 [11]:

$$\text{IBW men} = 50\,\text{kg} + 2.3\,\text{kg / inch above 5 feet}$$

Table 4.1 Classification of obesity

BMI (kg/m²)	Description	Obesity class
18.5–24.9	Normal	–
25.0–29.9	Overweight	–
30.0–34.9	Obesity	I
35.0–39.9	Obesity	II
>40	Extreme obesity	III

BMI, body mass index.

$$\text{IBW women} = 45.5\,\text{kg} + 2.3\,\text{kg/inch above 5 feet}$$

Using IBW for drug dosing does not account for the differing ratios of lean body mass to fat mass associated with obesity. Additionally, it proposes that all patients of the same sex and height receive the same dose of medication. In morbidly obese individuals, using the above-mentioned equations can result in a calculated IBW that is less than the patient's actual LBW and could result in underdosing [9].

Body surface area

Body surface area (BSA) is most commonly calculated with the Mosteller equation [12]:

$$\text{BSA(m}^2) = ([\text{height(cm)} \times \text{weight(kg)}]/3600)^{\frac{1}{2}}$$

Dosing drugs based on BSA has the same pitfalls as dosing drugs based on IBW because BSA does not differentiate between differing proportions of lean body mass and fat mass in obese patients. BSA is mainly used for dosing of chemotherapeutic agents and frequently limited to a maximum value of 2 m² [9]. It is not used to determine doses of anaesthetic drugs.

Fat-free mass

FFM is TBW minus fat mass. It consists of bones, muscles, organs, and extracellular fluid. FFM does not include lipids in cellular membranes, the central nervous system, and bone marrow, which are components of LBW [4]. However, in clinical practice, LBW and FFM are frequently used interchangeably. FFM can be measured using bioelectrical impedance analysis or dual-energy X-ray absorptiometry [13].

Lean body weight

LBW is defined as TBW minus fat mass. In obese patients, LBW increases in a non-proportional manner to TBW (**Fig. 4.1**). As an individual becomes more obese, the absolute LBW will increase, but the ratio of LBW/TBW actually decreases. LBW is a useful predictor of the pharmacokinetic behaviour of drugs that are highly water-soluble. It significantly correlates with cardiac output and clearance, which are important for determination of drug loading and maintenance doses [14]. LBW may be the ideal dosing scalar (**Table 4.2**) for drug administration in obese patients, but its usefulness is limited because under normal clinical conditions, there is

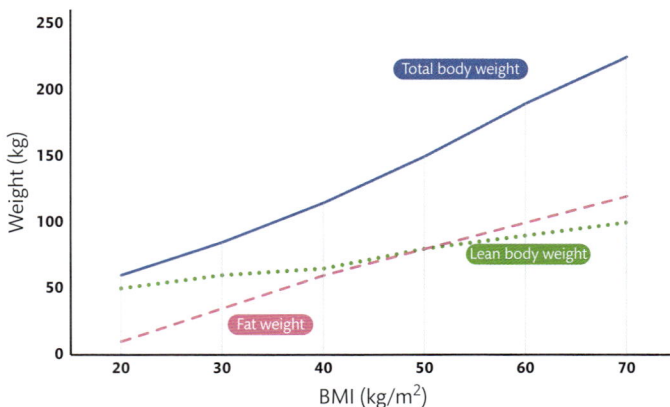

Fig. 4.1 Relationship of TBW, fat weight, and LBW to BMI in a standard height male.

Source: Data from Janmahasatian, S., Duffull, S. B., Ash, S., et al. Quantification of lean bodyweight. *Clinical Pharmacokinetics*, 44(10):1051–65, 2012.

Table 4.2 Dosing scalars and derivations

Dosing scalar	Derivation
BMI (kg/m²)	TBW (kg)/height (m²)
IBW (kg)	Men = 50 kg + 2.3 kg/inch above 5 feet Women = 45.5 kg + 2.3 kg/inch above 5 feet [11]
BSA (m²)	([Height (cm) × weight (kg)]/3600)^½ [12]
ABW (kg)	IBW + correction factor × (TBW – IBW) [16]
FFM (kg)	Men: (0.285 × TBW) + (12.1 × height (m²)) Women: (0.287 × TBW) + (9.74 × height (m²)) [17]
LBW (kg)	Men: (1.1 × TBW) – (0.0128 × BMI × TBW) Women: (1.07 × TBW) – (0.0148 × BMI × TBW) [17]

ABW, adjusted body weight; BMI, body mass index; BSA, body surface area; FFM, fat-free mass; IBW, ideal body weight; LBW, lean body weight; TBW, total body weight.

no practical or accurate way to measure it [9]. Equations have been derived to calculate LBW for patients with BMIs up to 43 kg/m² [15]. However, in patients whose TBW exceeds 120 kg, the formula starts to give a lower LBW, even reaching negative values in super morbidly obese patients. Since FFM and LBW can be considered interchangeable for purposes of clinical drug dosing, formulas derived for estimating FFM can be extrapolated to estimate LBW [13]. Using a semi-mechanistic model based on sex, height, and weight, equations have been derived to calculate LBW for males and females [13]. This equation has been shown to have accurate predictive properties when compared with body weights derived from dual-energy X-ray absorptiometry and bioelectrical impedance analysis.

As TBW increases, the increase in LBW and fat weight is not proportional so that the LBW/TBW ratio declines as obesity worsens [9].

Adjusted body weight

Adjusted body weight (ABW) is intended to correct the volume of distribution in obese patients. It is not a measured number but is derived using the patient's IBW and TBW. To calculate ABW, a correction factor is used to determine a fixed percentage of the TBW, which is then added to the patient's IBW. Some authors chose to use 40% of the patient's excess weight as a correction factor for calculating propofol infusion rates in obese patients [16]. However, the calculated ABW did not improve the accuracy of the predicted propofol plasma concentrations in the study. Since the volume of distribution and physiochemical properties of drugs differ, ABW should be determined for each drug [2]. ABW is not a frequently used dosing scalar for clinical anaesthesia but is used in pharmacokinetic experiments of specific drugs.

Percentage ideal body weight

Percentage IBW is the ratio of TBW to IBW. For example, a 163 cm (5′4″) woman who weighs 100 kg would have a percentage IBW of 180%, indicating that she is 80% over her IBW. Clinically, percentage IBW is not used as a dosing scalar but may be useful to indicate the degree to which a patient is in proportion to their IBW.

Predicted normal weight

Predicted normal weight is the sum of the LBW and predicted normal fat mass. This parameter was derived to better describe the pharmacokinetics of drugs, rather than for prediction of patient morbidity. It represents the expected normal weight of an obese individual as the sum of their LBW and their predicted 'normal' fat mass [2]. It is not a frequently used dosing scalar in clinical anaesthesia but may be useful as a comparative value.

Pathophysiology of obesity

Many pathophysiological changes that occur with obesity can affect the pharmacokinetic and pharmacodynamic profiles of anaesthetic drugs (**Box 4.1**). With obesity, there is an absolute increase in total blood volume and cardiac output. Although the absolute blood volume is increased, the calculation for total blood volume is decreased from 75 mL/kg for non-obese subjects to 50 mL/kg for morbidly obese subjects [18]. Formulas for estimating blood volume in obese and morbidly obese subjects have been described [19]. Normally, blood flow to fat accounts for 5% of the total cardiac output, whereas viscera and lean tissues receive 73% and 22% of cardiac output, respectively [20]. Obesity causes an increase in adipose tissue, but blood flow to adipose tissue may decrease to 2% of cardiac output [10].

Obesity also affects drug binding to plasma proteins, but the literature offers conflicting results. One study reported that the increased concentration of triglycerides, lipoproteins, and free fatty acids inhibit protein binding, thus increasing the free plasma concentrations of drugs [21]. Conversely, others found that increased concentrations of acute phase reactants such as alpha-1-acid glycoprotein increased the degree of protein binding, thus reducing the free plasma concentrations of drugs [22,23]. Serum levels of albumin and total protein are generally not affected by obesity. Low levels of albumin may be a better predictor of complications after surgery than obesity alone [24].

Obesity-induced changes in renal and hepatic function can alter drug metabolism and clearance, thereby affecting the pharmacokinetic profiles of anaesthetic drugs. Obesity has been found to decrease clearance of drugs metabolized by the cytochrome P450 (CYP) 3A4 pathway, which is important for metabolizing many drugs including fentanyl [25]. Obese patients have increased activity of CYP2E1, for which volatile anaesthetics are a substrate [26]. Steatosis of the liver, also called non-alcoholic steatohepatitis or non-alcoholic fatty liver disease, is common in obese patients and can further degenerate into liver fibrosis with reduced hepatic clearance [27]. Although up to 90% of morbidly obese patients have histological abnormalities of the liver, preoperative liver function tests may not reflect the severity of liver dysfunction [28]. Increased glucuronidation of acetaminophen in patients with non-alcoholic fatty liver disease may predispose these patients to acetaminophen toxicity [29].

Box 4.1 Pathophysiology of obesity

- Increased adipose tissue.
- Increased LBW.
- Decreased LBW/TBW ratio.
- Increased cardiac output.
- Decreased functional residual capacity and respiratory compliance.
- Increased renal blood flow and glomerular filtration rate.
- Non-alcoholic fatty liver disease.
- Altered protein binding.

Renal clearance in obesity is usually increased from the increased renal blood flow and glomerular filtration rate [30]. Creatinine clearance in otherwise healthy obese subjects is increased in proportion to the estimated fat-free mass. However, the presence of diabetes and hypertension, which frequently accompany long-standing obesity, may lead to glomerular injury and renal dysfunction [31]. In obese patients with renal dysfunction, the dosing of renally excreted drugs should be adjusted according to the measured creatinine clearance since the calculated creatinine clearance using the standard formula may be inaccurate [32].

The increase in circulating blood volume and higher cardiac output in obese patients can lead to hypertension. Up to 60% of obese patients have mild to moderate hypertension and 5–10% of obese patients have severe hypertension [33]. Hypertension is a risk factor for left ventricular hypertrophy, increased left ventricular wall stress, and atherosclerosis [34]. Patients with thickened myocardium are susceptible to subendocardial ischaemia perioperatively, especially if hypotension or tachycardia is present. In addition, patients who have obstructive sleep apnoea or obesity hypoventilation syndrome may have pulmonary hypertension and associated right heart dysfunction [35].

Pulmonary function is altered in obese patients and may be significantly so in morbidly obese patients. Obese patients have a decrease in respiratory compliance, functional residual capacity, total lung capacity, and expiratory reserve volume [36]. The higher resistance of the respiratory system can increase the work of breathing in obese patients and is worsened in the recumbent position. Morbidly obese patients have significantly lower arterial oxygen concentrations than their non-obese counterparts during open abdominal surgery [37]. In the postoperative period, obese patients, especially those with obstructive sleep apnoea, are at very high risk for postoperative hypoxia [38]. Obstructive sleep apnoea has a prevalence of 40–70% in obese patients [39]. The choice of anaesthetic drugs used and their correct dosing is critical to ensure a safe perioperative course.

Pharmacokinetic and pharmacodynamic concepts

Pharmacokinetics describes the relationship between the dose of a drug administered and the blood concentration. The systemic absorption and bioavailability of drugs is not changed with obesity, despite the increased splanchnic blood flow [14]. Volume of distribution is defined as the fluid volume that would be required to contain the amount of drug present in the body at the same concentration as in the plasma. It is more of an apparent volume rather than a physical volume and is the pharmacokinetic parameter that is most often altered with obesity [40]. In obese patients, TBW is the best descriptor of volume of distribution. For drugs where rapid attainment of maximum concentration is important (e.g. propofol), the volume of distribution determines the loading dose [9]. Although obesity increases both the lean muscle mass and fat mass, the increase in lean body mass represents only 20–40% of total excess body weight, thus leading to a decreased percentage of lean body mass [20]. For hydrophilic drugs, the volume of distribution is more likely to be linearly correlated with LBW rather than TBW. For lipophilic drugs,

the volume of distribution may be markedly increased in the obese [41]. Over 99% of metabolic processes occur within lean tissues [42]. Thus, clearance is linearly related to LBW rather than TBW [43]. The absolute clearance of drugs is greater in obese patients, assuming there is no concurrent hepatic or renal dysfunction.

Pharmacodynamics describes the relationship between organ concentration and therapeutic effect. The pathophysiological changes that occur with obesity can lead to altered pharmacodynamics and a different therapeutic window for drugs. Furthermore, the physiological, nutritional, and genetic changes associated with obesity can result in altered receptor expression or receptor affinity to drugs, further changing the pharmacodynamic profile. Many drugs may have a narrowed therapeutic window in the obese population. Consideration should be given to whether drugs should be given in fixed doses or titrated on the basis of drug-specific characteristics.

Anaesthetic drug dosing in obesity

Anaesthesia is a reversible state mediated by the central nervous system that produces unconsciousness, immobility, amnesia, analgesia, and suppression of reflexes [44]. To achieve this state, anaesthesiologists use an arsenal of different drugs. The physiological changes produced by obesity can drastically alter the distribution, binding, and elimination of many of these drugs. Knowledge of how obesity affects each drug is vital to avoiding potentially incorrect dosing and adverse events.

Table 4.3 shows the commonly used intravenous anaesthetic agents and the suggested dosing scalars with comments. Generally, most agents should be dosed according to LBW since cardiac output is significantly correlated with LBW. This does not apply to those with obesity cardiomyopathy who may need decreased doses of medications or adjustments in anaesthetic agents. Succinylcholine should be given dosed on TBW, especially in circumstances where rapid control of the airway is critical (i.e. rapid sequence induction). The non-depolarizing muscle relaxants should be dosed based on IBW to prevent a prolonged duration of action and possibly an increased risk of postoperative respiratory complications.

Propofol

Propofol is the most commonly used induction agent in obese patients. It is highly lipophilic with a fast onset and short duration of action. It is also used for sedation or as a component of a balanced anaesthetic or total intravenous anaesthetic. Bolus dose recommendations for non-obese patients are made on the basis on TBW. However, in obese patients, fat mass and lean body mass do not increase proportionally. Additionally, blood flow to fat is much less than to lean tissue so that a bolus of propofol based on TBW would result in an increased propofol concentration in blood perfusing lean tissues and could lead to adverse cardiovascular events such as hypotension and myocardial depression [45]. When propofol is given by continuous infusion, the volume of distribution and clearance in obese and non-obese patients is correlated with TBW [16]. There is no difference in elimination half-time between obese and non-obese subjects. The dose of propofol for maintenance infusions in obese patients should be based on TBW. Conversely, propofol

Table 4.3 Intravenous drug dosing in obesity

Drug	Dosing	Comments
Propofol	Induction: LBW Maintenance: TBW	Very lipophilic, high affinity for well-perfused organs, fast onset, short duration of action. Total clearance and Vd at steady state correlate with TBW
Thiopental	LBW	Obese patients have increased Vd and longer elimination half-life, but total clearance normalized for TBW is similar to the non-obese
Etomidate	LBW	Similar pharmacokinetics to propofol/thiopental. Can cause adrenal dysfunction; conflicting studies regarding increased risk of mortality
Dexmedetomidine	LBW	Ideally suited as an analgesic adjuvant in morbidly obese subjects due to minimal respiratory effects. Dosing based on TBW can increase adverse side effects
Midazolam	Single dose: TBW (titrate to effect) Maintenance: LBW	Increased Vd and elimination half-life. Duration of action depends on extent of distribution, not clearance. Start with low dose and titrate to effect to avoid oversedation
Vecuronium, rocuronium	IBW	Pharmacokinetics and pharmacodynamics unaltered with obesity. Prolonged duration of action when dosed based on TBW
Cisatracurium	IBW	Organ-independent Hofmann elimination may make it the non-depolarizing neuromuscular blocker of choice in morbidly obese patients. Duration of action prolonged if given based on TBW
Pancuronium	IBW	Long-acting neuromuscular blocker generally not indicated in obese patients. Dose to maintain constant twitch depression is significantly increased in obese patients
Succinylcholine	TBW	Increased TBW in obesity is associated with increased pseudocholinesterase activity
Sugammadex	TBW	Dose should be based on depth of blockade, generally 2–16 mg/kg. Time to reversal is faster when dose is based on TBW vs IBW or LBW
Fentanyl	LBW	Dosing based on a derived 'pharmacokinetic mass' correlates better with clearance. Dosing based on TBW overestimates dose requirements in the obese
Sufentanil	LBW	Increased Vd and prolonged elimination half-life that correlates with degree of obesity. Clearance is similar in obese and non-obese patients. Start low and titrate to effect
Remifentanil	LBW	Hydrolysis by plasma and tissue esterases results in short context-sensitive half-time. Pharmacokinetics similar in obese and non-obese subjects

IBW, ideal body weight; LBW, lean body weight; TBW, total body weight; Vd, volume of distribution.

given for induction of general anaesthesia as a bolus should be dosed according to the LBW. Morbidly obese patients who were administered a rapid propofol infusion based on LBW had similar times to loss of consciousness as lean control subjects who were administered propofol based on TBW [45]. Some authors have suggested administration of propofol for both maintenance and induction of anaesthesia in obese patients based on TBW [46,47]. However, administration of propofol to obese patients, particularly morbidly obese patients, according to TBW may result in an overdose and the associated haemodynamic consequences (e.g. myocardial depression and hypotension).

Thiopental

Thiopental is a barbiturate used for induction of general anaesthesia. After a single pass, 76% of thiopental distributes to highly perfused tissues such as the brain, lung, kidney, heart, and gut. Two minutes after administration, it redistributes to muscles, resulting in a significant drop in brain concentration, and thus termination of its anaesthetic effect. Thiopental has a very high oil/water partition coefficient, resulting in fast penetration through tissue barriers. The volume of distribution of thiopental is significantly larger in obese versus non-obese patients [48]. As a result of this increase in the volume of distribution, the elimination half-life of thiopental is significantly longer in obese (27.8 hours) versus non-obese patients (6.33 hours). However, total clearance, when normalized to TBW, is not significantly different between obese and non-obese subjects [48]. Computer simulation has been used to show that thiopental induction doses adjusted to LBW result in the same peak plasma concentrations as doses adjusted to cardiac output, suggesting that administering thiopental based on LBW is appropriate [49]. Obese patients have an increased lean body mass and increased cardiac output, which can result in a more rapid redistribution of thiopental after administration. Since the termination of thiopental's effect is due to redistribution, obese patients may have a more rapid awakening after a single bolus dose [9].

Etomidate

Etomidate is an induction agent that causes minimal changes in blood pressure or heart rate. It is the induction agent of choice in haemodynamically unstable patients or those with cardiovascular pathology such as coronary artery disease or obesity cardiomyopathy [50]. Side effects of etomidate include pain on injection, myoclonus, and postoperative nausea and vomiting. Etomidate also inhibits 11-beta-hydroxylase, an enzyme involved in steroid synthesis. This can result in an increased risk of adrenal gland dysfunction and multiorgan system dysfunction [51]. The literature contains conflicting evidence on whether the use of etomidate increases mortality [52–54]. One study specifically evaluating the pharmacodynamics of etomidate in morbidly obese patients suggests dosing based on IBW [55]. Previous authors have suggested dosing etomidate based on TBW but cite inadequate literature to support this practice [56]. Other authors have suggested that because etomidate has similar pharmacokinetics to thiopental and propofol, it should be dosed based on LBW [2].

Dexmedetomidine

Dexmedetomidine is a highly selective alpha-2 agonist with anxiolytic, analgesic, and sedative effects. Dexmedetomidine decreases the release of norepinephrine from presynaptic stores and has a sympatholytic effect, which can result in a decrease in heart rate and blood pressure. It is most commonly given by continuous infusion and has been advocated by many as an adjunct to general anaesthesia in morbidly obese patients due to its ability to avoid respiratory depression [57]. In morbidly obese patients undergoing laparoscopic gastric bypass, a bolus of dexmedetomidine 0.8 mcg/kg followed by an infusion at 0.4 mcg/kg/h has been shown to decrease postoperative pain and the amount of morphine necessary, leading to an improved recovery profile compared with placebo [58]. The addition of dexmedetomidine to a balanced anaesthetic may allow anaesthesiologists to decrease opioid use postoperatively, which may lead to decreased respiratory depression. Clearance of dexmedetomidine is impaired in obese patients [59]. During laparoscopic bariatric surgery, a lower infusion rate of 0.2 mcg/kg/h has been recommended to reduce the risk of bradycardia and hypotension [57]. A prudent approach may be to begin the infusion dosed according to LBW and titrate to effect.

Benzodiazepines

Benzodiazepines are very lipophilic drugs that are used for premedication, sedation, induction, and maintenance of general anaesthesia. After a single dose of midazolam, the intensity and duration of action are dependent on the extent of drug distribution rather than on the rate of elimination and clearance. Total volume of distribution in obese subjects is almost threefold larger than in non-obese subjects, which increases elimination half-life about threefold [60]. The total clearance between obese and non-obese subjects, however, is not different. Some authors advocate that when benzodiazepines are used as a single intravenous dose, the dose should be increased in proportion to TBW to account for the increase in volume of distribution [61,62]. Other authors have recommended giving 'mini loading doses' rather than a large dose based on TBW [63]. If a continuous infusion is used, the dose should be according to IBW since total clearance is not significantly changed in obese subjects [60]. When given as a premedication, the initial dose should be low and titrated to effect to avoid oversedation. Use of longer-acting benzodiazepines should be avoided due to the increased risk of postoperative respiratory depression in obese patients.

Neuromuscular blocking drugs and reversal agents

Neuromuscular blocking drugs are hydrophilic polar compounds and are distributed to a limited extent in excess body fat. The pharmacokinetic and pharmacodynamic profiles of vecuronium in obese and non-obese subjects calculated on the basis of IBW, total volume of distribution, plasma clearance, and elimination half-life are not different [64]. Vecuronium should be dosed according to IBW rather than TBW. When vecuronium is dosed according to TBW, there is a relative overdose, resulting in a prolonged duration of action [65]. This could lead to respiratory difficulties upon emergence and extubation, especially because obese patients have altered respiratory dynamics and a propensity for obstructive sleep apnoea [66].

Rocuronium is a non-depolarizing muscle relaxant that is minimally lipophilic due to its quaternary ammonium group. The pharmacokinetics and pharmacodynamics of rocuronium are not changed in obese versus non-obese patients [67]. However, when rocuronium is administered to morbidly obese patients based on TBW versus IBW, the duration of action is twice as long when TBW is used [68]. Subsequently, concerns arose that dosing based on IBW could lead to a prolonged onset time or poor conditions for tracheal intubation. However, Meyhoff et al. [69] demonstrated that in obese patients undergoing gastric banding or gastric bypass, rocuronium dosed according to IBW versus IBW plus 20% excess weight and IBW plus 40% excess weight did not significantly prolong onset time or provide inferior conditions for tracheal intubation. Thus, it is recommended that rocuronium be dosed on the basis of IBW and that the degree of neuromuscular blockade is carefully monitored [68].

Pancuronium is a long-acting amino steroid neuromuscular blocker. Significantly more pancuronium is necessary to maintain constant twitch depression in obese versus non-obese patients. This increased requirement may be due to the increased extracellular fluid volume in obese individuals [70]. However, dosing of pancuronium should be based on IBW to avoid prolonged neuromuscular blockade. Additionally, unless there is a specific indication for long-term paralysis, neuromuscular blockade with shorter-acting agents such as vecuronium, rocuronium, or cisatracurium is recommended [9].

Cisatracurium is a benzylisoquinoline neuromuscular blocker that is unique in its metabolism by organ-independent Hofmann elimination. Because of this, it is commonly used in patients with end-stage renal or hepatic disease. Some clinicians have deemed it the neuromuscular blocking drug of choice in obese patients [71]. Studies have shown that the duration of cisatracurium is prolonged in obese patients when given based on TBW, and thus it is recommended that it be based on IBW [72].

Succinylcholine is the only depolarizing neuromuscular blocker used clinically. It has a rapid onset and short duration of action. As obese patients have an increased incidence of gastro-oesophageal reflux and a decreased tolerance for apnoea, succinylcholine may be favourable due to its rapid onset of action allowing for rapid tracheal intubation [73]. Its short duration of action may also be advantageous if difficulty securing the airway is encountered and resumption of spontaneous ventilation is necessary [74]. Increasing TBW is associated with increased pseudo-cholinesterase activity and thus succinylcholine should be dosed based on TBW rather than IBW [75]. Potency estimates of succinylcholine in obese patients have been shown to be comparable to non-obese patients when dosed on total body mas [76]. Furthermore, studies have shown that succinylcholine administration based on 1 mg/kg TBW resulted in a more profound block and better tracheal intubating conditions with clinically insignificant postoperative myalgia when compared to 1 mg/kg IBW or LBW [77].

Neostigmine, an anticholinesterase, is the most frequently used drug to reverse neuromuscular blockade and is given with glycopyrrolate or atropine to counteract the cardiovascular effects. When vecuronium is administered based on TBW and reversed with neostigmine 0.04 mg/kg at 25% recovery of twitch height, recovery to a train-of-four ratio of 0.9 was four times longer in obese patients than in non-obese patients [65]. Since obese patients are predisposed to respiratory complications postoperatively, complete reversal of neuromuscular blockade is imperative. Sugammadex falls under the class of drugs known as selective relaxant binding agents. Sugammadex is a modified gamma-cyclodextrin compound with a lipophilic core and hydrophilic exterior that encapsulates steroid-based neuromuscular blocking agents and is renally excreted [78]. Its advantages are that unlike anticholinesterases, it can reverse deep levels of neuromuscular blockade, has no adverse cardiovascular effects, and does not necessitate co-administration of another drug. Dosing recommendations are based on the depth of blockade and range from 2 mg/kg to 16 mg/kg for moderate to profound blockade, respectively [79]. There is no significant effect of bodyweight on the pharmacokinetics of sugammadex [80]. Van Lancker et al. studied sugammadex reversal in obese patients dosed according to IBW, IBW plus 20%, IBW plus 40%, and TBW and concluded that IBW plus 40% was the optimal dose [81]. However, other authors have advocated for dosing based on TBW to ensure adequate reversal of neuromuscular blockade and prevent recurarization [82–84]. The time to reversal of neuromuscular blockade is faster when sugammadex is dosed based on TBW than when it is based on IBW or LBW [81]. Given the high potential for adverse respiratory events with inadequate reversal of neuromuscular blockade and the low incidence of side effects of sugammadex, dosing of sugammadex according to TBW is recommended [82].

Opioids

Obese patients have anatomical, cardiovascular, and respiratory derangements that make them more susceptible to opioid-induced upper airway obstruction and respiratory depression. The incidence of upper airway obstruction and obstructive sleep apnoea are significantly increased in the obese population [39]. The newer synthetic opioids such as fentanyl, sufentanil, and alfentanil are highly lipophilic drugs. In theory, obese patients should have a lower plasma concentration after a single dose due to a larger volume of distribution. However, it has been shown that the lower plasma concentration is due more to the higher cardiac output of obese patients, not from an increased volume of distribution [85]. The increased cardiac output in obese patients lowers plasma fentanyl concentrations during the early distribution phase. Cardiac output is highly correlated with LBW and clearance increases linearly with a 'pharmacokinetic mass,' which is highly correlated to LBW [86]. Fentanyl administration in obese patients should be based on LBW and carefully titrated to effect. Alfentanil is less lipid-soluble than fentanyl and has a smaller volume of distribution. Like fentanyl, the higher cardiac output in obese patients results in a lower alfentanil concentration during the early distribution phase [85]. Studies indicate a slower elimination of sufentanil and alfentanil in obese patients [87]. A study evaluating the accuracy of target-controlled infusions of sufentanil in morbidly obese patients found that a pharmacokinetic model usually applied to normal-weight patients accurately predicted plasma sufentanil concentrations [88]. Dosing regimens for sufentanil and alfentanil should be based on LBW rather than actual body weight to prevent overdosing.

Remifentanil is a very potent opioid that is unique in its hydrolysis by plasma and tissue esterases, resulting in organ-independent clearance and a short context-sensitive half-time, regardless of the duration of infusion. Its fast onset time and high clearance make it suitable for administration by continuous infusion. Remifentanil's pharmacokinetics is more closely related to lean body mass than TBW and thus remifentanil should be dosed according to LBW [89]. Dosing remifentanil in obese patients based on TBW could result in supratherapeutic plasma concentrations and could increase the risk of side effects such as bradycardia and hypotension. Some studies have found that use of remifentanil compared to sufentanil in bariatric patients increased the amount of postoperative opioids necessary in the immediate postoperative period [90].

Inhaled anaesthetics

The newer inhalational agents such as desflurane and sevoflurane have much lower lipid solubility than older agents such as isoflurane. This has led some anaesthesiologists to disfavour isoflurane in obese patients. However, after administration of 0.6 minimum alveolar concentration of isoflurane for surgery lasting 2–4 hours, obese and non-obese subjects had similar times to following commands [91]. The authors proposed that part of the reason might be that the time constants (time to reach 63% of equilibrium) of isoflurane and desflurane are very long (2110 and 1350 minutes, respectively). Furthermore, blood flow to adipose tissue decreases with increasing obesity. These two reasons led the authors to conclude that when isoflurane is used in routine clinical practice, the effect of BMI on isoflurane uptake is clinically insignificant [91]. Sevoflurane is less lipophilic and results in a slightly more rapid uptake and elimination in obese patients compared with isoflurane. Some authors have found that in obese subjects undergoing gastric banding, sevoflurane resulted in a significantly faster recovery and faster discharge from the post-anaesthesia care unit when compared to isoflurane [92]. Desflurane has a blood gas partition coefficient of 0.45 and thus is the least soluble inhaled anaesthetic and theoretically has limited distribution into adipose tissue. Both obese and non-obese patients have faster emergence and recovery with desflurane compared to isoflurane [91]. Comparisons of desflurane with sevoflurane have yielded conflicting results. Some authors found that morbidly obese subjects have faster emergence with desflurane versus sevoflurane [93–95] whereas others did not find significant differences in time to emergence between desflurane and sevoflurane [96,97]. Having a higher BMI is associated with prolonged recovery of protective airway reflexes after general anaesthesia, an effect that is more pronounced when sevoflurane versus desflurane is administered [98]. This effect was even more pronounced than the different blood to gas solubilities would suggest—the slope for time to recovery of protective airway reflexes versus BMI for sevoflurane was fourfold larger than that of desflurane [98].

Local anaesthetics

Regional anaesthesia is frequently favoured in obese patients to reduce the respiratory depression that can accompany general anaesthesia and opioid use. However, obesity can make both neuraxial anaesthesia and peripheral nerve blockade more challenging due to increased adipose tissue and difficulties in identifying anatomical landmarks [99]. Elimination half-life of lidocaine is prolonged in obese subjects compared to non-obese subjects. However, when the volume of distribution is corrected for TBW, there is no difference between obese and non-obese subjects [100]. Obese patients may require less local anaesthetic with neuraxial techniques than their non-obese counterparts [101]. This may be due to fatty infiltration and an increased abdominal pressure and lower volumes of cerebrospinal fluid in obese subjects [102]. Blocks extending above T5 should be avoided, as they may result in respiratory compromise and cardiovascular collapse from autonomic blockade.

REFERENCES

1. Ogden CL, Carroll MD, Kit BK, Flegal KM. Prevalence of childhood and adult obesity in the United States, 2011–2012. JAMA. 2014;**311**(8):806–14.

2. Lemmens HJ. Perioperative pharmacology in morbid obesity. Curr Opin Anaesthesiol. 2010;**23**(4):485–91.

3. Flegal KM, Kit BK, Orpana H, Graubard BI. Association of all-cause mortality with overweight and obesity using standard body mass index categories: a systematic review and meta-analysis. JAMA. 2013;**309**(1):71–82.

4. Duren DL, Sherwood RJ, Czerwinski SA, Lee M, Choh AC, Siervogel RM, et al. Body composition methods: comparisons and interpretation. J Diabetes Sci Technol. 2008;**2**(6):1139–46.

5. Chumlea WC, Schubert CM, Sun SS, Demerath E, Towne B, Siervogel RM. A review of body water status and the effects of age and body fatness in children and adults. J Nutr Health Aging. 2007;**11**(2):111–18.

6. Ellis KJ. Human body composition: in vivo methods. Physiol Rev. 2000;**80**(2):649–80.

7. Williams JE, Wells JC, Wilson CM, Haroun D, Lucas A, Fewtrell MS. Evaluation of Lunar Prodigy dual-energy X-ray absorptiometry for assessing body composition in healthy persons and patients by comparison with the criterion 4-component model. Am J Clin Nutr. 2006;**83**(5):1047–54.

8. Cameron AJ, Magliano DJ, Söderberg S. A systematic review of the impact of including both waist and hip circumference in risk models for cardiovascular diseases, diabetes and mortality. Obes Rev. 2013;**14**(1):86–94.

9. Ingrande J, Lemmens HJ. Dose adjustment of anaesthetics in the morbidly obese. Br J Anaesth. 2010;**105**(Suppl 1):i16–23.

10. Lesser GT, Deutsch S. Measurement of adipose tissue blood flow and perfusion in man by uptake of 85Kr. J Appl Physiol. 1967;**23**(5):621–30.

11. Pai MP, Paloucek FP. The origin of the 'ideal' body weight equations. Ann Pharmacother. 2000;**34**(9):1066–69.

12. Mosteller RD. Simplified calculation of body-surface area. N Engl J Med. 1987;**317**(17):1098.

13. Janmahasatian S, Duffull SB, Ash S, Ward LC, Byrne NM, Green B. Quantification of lean bodyweight. Clin Pharmacokinet. 2005;**44**(10):1051–65.

14. Collis T, Devereux RB, Roman MJ, de Simone G, Yeh J, Howard BV, et al. Relations of stroke volume and cardiac output to body composition: the strong heart study. Circulation. 2001;**103**(6):820–25.

15. James W. Research on Obesity. London: Her Majesty's Stationery Office; 1976.

16. Servin F, Farinotti R, Haberer JP, Desmonts JM. Propofol infusion for maintenance of anesthesia in morbidly obese patients receiving nitrous oxide. A clinical and pharmacokinetic study. Anesthesiology. 1993;**78**(4):657–65.

17. Green B, Duffull SB. What is the best size descriptor to use for pharmacokinetic studies in the obese? Br J Clin Pharmacol. 2004;**58**(2):119–33.

18. Backman L, Freyschuss U, Hallberg D, Melcher A. Cardiovascular function in extreme obesity. Acta Med Scand. 1973;**193**(5):437–46.

19. Lemmens HJ, Bernstein DP, Brodsky JB. Estimating blood volume in obese and morbidly obese patients. Obes Surg. 2006;**16**(6):773–76.

20. Cheymol G. Effects of obesity on pharmacokinetics implications for drug therapy. Clin Pharmacokinet. 2000;**39**(3):215–31.

21. Wasan KM, Lopez-Berestein G. The influence of serum lipoproteins on the pharmacokinetics and pharmacodynamics of lipophilic drugs and drug carriers. Arch Med Res. 1993;**24**(4):395–401.

22. Derry CL, Kroboth PD, Pittenger AL, Kroboth FJ, Corey SE, Smith RB. Pharmacokinetics and pharmacodynamics of triazolam after two intermittent doses in obese and normal-weight men. J Clin Psychopharmacol. 1995;**15**(3):197–205.

23. Barbeau P, Litaker MS, Woods KF, Lemmon CR, Humphries MC, Owens S, Gutin B. Hemostatic and inflammatory markers in obese youths: effects of exercise and adiposity. J Pediatr. 2002;**141**(3):415–20.

24. Nelson CL, Elkassabany NM, Kamath AF, Liu J. Low albumin levels, more than morbid obesity, are associated with complications after TKA. Clin Orthop Relat Res. 2015;**473**(10):3163–72.

25. Brill MJ, Diepstraten J, van Rongen A, van Kralingen S, van den Anker JN, Knibbe CA. Impact of obesity on drug metabolism and elimination in adults and children. Clin Pharmacokinet. 2012;**51**(5):277–304.

26. Emery MG, Fisher JM, Chien JY, Kharasch ED, Dellinger EP, Kowdley KV, et al. CYP2E1 activity before and after weight loss in morbidly obese subjects with nonalcoholic fatty liver disease. Hepatology. 2003;**38**(2):428–35.

27. Ahmed A, Wong RJ, Harrison SA. Nonalcoholic fatty liver disease review: diagnosis, treatment, and outcomes. Clin Gastroenterol Hepatol. 2015;**13**(12):2062–70.

28. Guzzaloni G, Grugni G, Minocci A, Moro D, Morabito F. Liver steatosis in juvenile obesity: correlations with lipid profile, hepatic biochemical parameters and glycemic and insulinemic responses to an oral glucose tolerance test. Int J Obes Relat Metab Disord. 2000;**24**(6):772–76.

29. Michaut A, Moreau C, Robin MA, Fromenty B. Acetaminophen-induced liver injury in obesity and nonalcoholic fatty liver disease. Liver Int. 2014;**34**(7):e171–79.

30. Henegar JR, Bigler SA, Henegar LK, Tyagi SC, Hall JE. Functional and structural changes in the kidney in the early stages of obesity. J Am Soc Nephrol. 2001;**12**(6):1211–17.

31. Hall JE, Crook ED, Jones DW, Wofford MR, Dubbert PM. Mechanisms of obesity-associated cardiovascular and renal disease. Am J Med Sci. 2002;**324**(3):127–37.

32. Demirovic JA, Pai AB, Pai MP. Estimation of creatinine clearance in morbidly obese patients. Am J Health Syst Pharm. 2009;**66**(7):642–48.

33. Díaz ME. Hypertension and obesity. J Hum Hypertens. 2002;**16**(Suppl 1):S18–22.

34. Adams JP, Murphy PG. Obesity in anaesthesia and intensive care. Br J Anaesth. 2000;**85**(1):91–108.

35. Benumof JL. Obesity, sleep apnea, the airway and anesthesia. Curr Opin Anaesthesiol. 2004;**17**(1):21–30.

36. Schumann R. Pulmonary physiology of the morbidly obese and the effects of anesthesia. Int Anesthesiol Clin. 2013;**51**(3):41–51.

37. Auler JOC Jr, Miyoshi E, Fernandes CR, Benseñor FE, Elias L, Bonassa J. The effects of abdominal opening on respiratory mechanics during general anesthesia in normal and morbidly obese patients: a comparative study. Anesth Analg. 2002;**94**(3):741–48.

38. Eichenberger A, Proietti S, Wicky S, Frascarolo P, Suter M, Spahn DR, Magnusson L. Morbid obesity and postoperative pulmonary atelectasis: an underestimated problem. Anesth Analg. 2002;**95**(6):1788–92.

39. Lopez PP, Stefan B, Schulman CI, Byers PM. Prevalence of sleep apnea in morbidly obese patients who presented for weight loss surgery evaluation: more evidence for routine screening for obstructive sleep apnea before weight loss surgery. Am Surg. 2008;74(9):834–38.

40. Katzung BG. Basic & Clinical Pharmacology. 9th ed. Vol. xiv. New York: Lange Medical Books/McGraw-Hill; 2004.

41. Hanley MJ, Abernethy DR, Greenblatt DJ. Effect of obesity on the pharmacokinetics of drugs in humans. Clin Pharmacokinet. 2010;49(2):71–87.

42. Roubenoff R, Kehayias JJ. The meaning and measurement of lean body mass. Nutr Rev. 1991;49(6):163–75.

43. Han T, Harmatz JS, Greenblatt DJ, Martyn JA. Fentanyl clearance and volume of distribution are increased in patients with major burns. J Clin Pharmacol. 2007;47(6):674–80.

44. Eger EI 2nd, Sonner JM. Anaesthesia defined (gentlemen, this is no humbug). Best Pract Res Clin Anaesthesiol. 2006;20(1):23–29.

45. Ingrande J, Brodsky JB, Lemmens HJ. Lean body weight scalar for the anesthetic induction dose of propofol in morbidly obese subjects. Anesth Analg. 2011;113(1):57–62.

46. Casati A, Putzu M. Anesthesia in the obese patient: pharmacokinetic considerations. J Clin Anesth. 2005;17(2):134–45.

47. Leykin Y, Miotto L, Pellis T. Pharmacokinetic considerations in the obese. Best Pract Res Clin Anaesthesiol. 2011;25(1):27–36.

48. Jung D, Mayersohn M, Perrier D, Calkins J, Saunders R. Thiopental disposition in lean and obese patients undergoing surgery. Anesthesiology. 1982;56(4):269–74.

49. Wada DR, Björkman S, Ebling WF, Harashima H, Harapat SR, Stanski DR. Computer simulation of the effects of alterations in blood flows and body composition on thiopental pharmacokinetics in humans. Anesthesiology. 1997;87(4):884–99.

50. Budde AO, Mets B. Pro: etomidate is the ideal induction agent for a cardiac anesthetic. J Cardiothorac Vasc Anesth. 2013;27(1):180–83.

51. Bruder EA, Ball IM, Ridi S, Pickett W, Hohl C. Single induction dose of etomidate versus other induction agents for endotracheal intubation in critically ill patients. Cochrane Database Syst Rev. 2015;1:CD010225.

52. Gu WJ, Wang F, Tang L, Liu JC. Single-dose etomidate does not increase mortality in patients with sepsis: a systematic review and meta-analysis of randomized controlled trials and observational studies. Chest. 2015;147(2):335–46.

53. Chan CM, Mitchell AL, Shorr AF. Etomidate is associated with mortality and adrenal insufficiency in sepsis: a meta-analysis. Crit Care Med. 2012;40(11):2945–53.

54. van den Heuvel I, Wurmb TE, Böttiger BW, Bernhard M. Pros and cons of etomidate—more discussion than evidence? Curr Opin Anaesthesiol. 2013;26(4):404–408.

55. Gaszynski TM, Jakubiak J, Szewczyk T. Etomidate can be dosed according to ideal body weight in morbidly obese patients. Eur J Anaesthesiol. 2014;31(12):713–14.

56. Dargin J, Medzon R. Emergency department management of the airway in obese adults. Ann Emerg Med. 2010;56(2):95–104.

57. Tufanogullari B, White PF, Peixoto MP, Kianpour D, Lacour T, Griffin J, et al. Dexmedetomidine infusion during laparoscopic bariatric surgery: the effect on recovery outcome variables. Anesth Analg. 2008;106(6):1741–48.

58. Bakhamees HS, El-Halafawy YM, El-Kerdawy HM, Gouda NM, Altemyatt S. Effects of dexmedetomidine in morbidly obese patients undergoing laparoscopic gastric bypass. Middle East J Anesthesiol. 2007;19(3):537–51.

59. Cortínez LI, Anderson BJ, Holford NH, Puga V, de la Fuente N, Auad H, et al. Dexmedetomidine pharmacokinetics in the obese. Eur J Clin Pharmacol. 2015;71(12):1501–508.

60. Greenblatt DJ, Abernethy DR, Locniskar A, Harmatz JS, Limjuco RA, Shader RI. Effect of age, gender, and obesity on midazolam kinetics. Anesthesiology. 1984;61(1):27–35.

61. Pieracci FM, Barie PS, Pomp A. Critical care of the bariatric patient. Crit Care Med. 2006;34(6):1796–804.

62. Ogunnaike BO, Jones SB, Jones DB, Provost D, Whitten CW. Anesthetic considerations for bariatric surgery. Anesth Analg. 2002;95(6):1793–805.

63. Erstad BL. Dosing of medications in morbidly obese patients in the intensive care unit setting. Intensive Care Med. 2004;30(1):18–32.

64. Schwartz AE, Matteo RS, Ornstein E, Halevy JD, Diaz J. Pharmacokinetics and pharmacodynamics of vecuronium in the obese surgical patient. Anesth Analg. 1992;74(4):515–18.

65. Suzuki T, Masaki G, Ogawa S. Neostigmine-induced reversal of vecuronium in normal weight, overweight and obese female patients. Br J Anaesth. 2006;97(2):160–63.

66. Memtsoudis SG, Besculides MC, Mazumdar M. A rude awakening—the perioperative sleep apnea epidemic. N Engl J Med. 2013;368(25):2352–53.

67. Pühringer FK, Keller C, Kleinsasser A, Giesinger S, Benzer A. Pharmacokinetics of rocuronium bromide in obese female patients. Eur J Anaesthesiol. 1999;16(8):507–10.

68. Leykin Y, Pellis T, Lucca M, Lomangino G, Marzano B, Gullo A. The pharmacodynamic effects of rocuronium when dosed according to real body weight or ideal body weight in morbidly obese patients. Anesth Analg. 2004;99(4):1086–89.

69. Meyhoff CS, Lund J, Jenstrup MT, Claudius C, Sørensen AM, Viby-Mogensen J, et al. Should dosing of rocuronium in obese patients be based on ideal or corrected body weight? Anesth Analg. 2009;109(3):787–92.

70. Tsueda K, Warren JE, McCafferty LA, Nagle JP. Pancuronium bromide requirement during anesthesia for the morbidly obese. Anesthesiology. 1978;48(6):438–39.

71. Kisor DF, Schmith VD. Clinical pharmacokinetics of cisatracurium besilate. Clin Pharmacokinet. 1999;36(1):27–40.

72. Leykin Y, Pellis T, Lucca M, Lomangino G, Marzano B, Gullo A. The effects of cisatracurium on morbidly obese women. Anesth Analg. 2004;99(4):1090–94.

73. Aceto P, Perilli V, Modesti C, Ciocchetti P, Vitale F, Sollazzi L. Airway management in obese patients. Surg Obes Relat Dis. 2013;9(5):809–15.

74. Loder WA. Airway management in the obese patient. Crit Care Clin. 2010;26(4):641–46.

75. Bentley JB, Borel JD, Vaughan RW, Gandolfi AJ. Weight, pseudocholinesterase activity, and succinylcholine requirement. Anesthesiology. 1982;57(1):48–49.

76. Rose JB, Theroux MC, Katz MS. The potency of succinylcholine in obese adolescents. Anesth Analg. 2000;90(3):576–78.

77. Lemmens HJ, Brodsky JB. The dose of succinylcholine in morbid obesity. Anesth Analg. 2006;102(2):438–42.

78. Partownavid P, Romito BT, Ching W, Berry AA, Barkulis CT, Nguyen KP, et al. Sugammadex: a comprehensive review of the published human science, including renal studies. Am J Ther. 2015;22(4):298–317.

79. Mirakhur RK. Sugammadex in clinical practice. Anaesthesia. 2009;64(Suppl):45–54.

80. Kleijn HJ, Zollinger DP, van den Heuvel MW, Kerbusch T. Population pharmacokinetic-pharmacodynamic analysis for sugammadex-mediated reversal of rocuronium-induced neuromuscular blockade. Br J Clin Pharmacol. 2011;**72**(3):415–33.

81. Van Lancker P, Dillemans B, Bogaert T, Mulier JP, De Kock M, Haspeslagh M. Ideal versus corrected body weight for dosage of sugammadex in morbidly obese patients. Anaesthesia. 2011;**66**(8):721–25.

82. Carron M, Freo U, Parotto E, Ori C. The correct dosing regimen for sugammadex in morbidly obese patients. Anaesthesia. 2012;**67**(3):298–99.

83. Llauradó S, Sabaté A, Ferreres E, Camprubí I, Cabrera A. Sugammadex ideal body weight dose adjusted by level of neuromuscular blockade in laparoscopic bariatric surgery. Anesthesiology. 2012;**117**(1):93–98.

84. Monk TG, Rietbergen H, Woo T, Fennema H. Use of sugammadex in patients with obesity: a pooled analysis. Am J Ther. 2017;**24**(5):e507–16.

85. Björkman S, Wada DR, Stanski DR. Application of physiologic models to predict the influence of changes in body composition and blood flows on the pharmacokinetics of fentanyl and alfentanil in patients. Anesthesiology. 1998;**88**(3):657–67.

86. Shibutani K, Inchiosa MA, Sawada K, Bairamian M. Accuracy of pharmacokinetic models for predicting plasma fentanyl concentrations in lean and obese surgical patients: derivation of dosing weight ('pharmacokinetic mass'). Anesthesiology. 2004;**101**(3):603–13.

87. Scholz J, Steinfath M, Schulz M. Clinical pharmacokinetics of alfentanil, fentanyl and sufentanil. An update. Clin Pharmacokinet. 1996;**31**(4):275–92.

88. Slepchenko G, Simon N, Goubaux B, Levron JC, Le Moing JP, Raucoules-Aimé M. Performance of target-controlled sufentanil infusion in obese patients. Anesthesiology. 2003;**98**(1):65–73.

89. Egan TD, Huizinga B, Gupta SK, Jaarsma RL, Sperry RJ, Yee JB, et al. Remifentanil pharmacokinetics in obese versus lean patients. Anesthesiology. 1998;**89**(3):562–73.

90. De Baerdemaeker LE, Jacobs S, Pattyn P, Mortier EP, Struys MM. Influence of intraoperative opioid on postoperative pain and pulmonary function after laparoscopic gastric banding: remifentanil TCI vs sufentanil TCI in morbid obesity. Br J Anaesth. 2007;**99**(3):404–11.

91. Lemmens HJ, Saidman LJ, Eger EI, Laster MJ. Obesity modestly affects inhaled anesthetic kinetics in humans. Anesth Analg. 2008;**107**(6):1864–70.

92. Torri G, Casati A, Comotti L, Bignami E, Santorsola R, Scarioni M. Wash-in and wash-out curves of sevoflurane and isoflurane in morbidly obese patients. Minerva Anestesiol. 2002;**68**(6):523–27.

93. Strum EM, Szenohradszki J, Kaufman WA, Anthone GJ, Manz IL, Lumb PD. Emergence and recovery characteristics of desflurane versus sevoflurane in morbidly obese adult surgical patients: a prospective, randomized study. Anesth Analg. 2004;**99**(6):1848–53.

94. Gupta A, Stierer T, Zuckerman R, Sakima N, Parker SD, Fleisher LA. Comparison of recovery profile after ambulatory anesthesia with propofol, isoflurane, sevoflurane and desflurane: a systematic review. Anesth Analg. 2004;**98**(3):632–41.

95. La Colla L, Albertin A, La Colla G, Mangano A. Faster wash-out and recovery for desflurane vs sevoflurane in morbidly obese patients when no premedication is used. Br J Anaesth. 2007;**99**(3):353–58.

96. Arain SR, Barth CD, Shankar H, Ebert TJ. Choice of volatile anesthetic for the morbidly obese patient: sevoflurane or desflurane. J Clin Anesth. 2005;**17**(6):413–19.

97. Vallejo MC, Sah N, Phelps AL, O'Donnell J, Romeo RC. Desflurane versus sevoflurane for laparoscopic gastroplasty in morbidly obese patients. J Clin Anesth. 2007;**19**(1):3–8.

98. McKay RE, Malhotra A, Cakmakkaya OS, Hall KT, McKay WR, Apfel CC. Effect of increased body mass index and anaesthetic duration on recovery of protective airway reflexes after sevoflurane vs desflurane. Br J Anaesth. 2010;**104**(2):175–82.

99. Cullen A, Ferguson A. Perioperative management of the severely obese patient: a selective pathophysiological review. Can J Anesth. 2012;**59**(10):974–96.

100. Abernethy DR, Greenblatt DJ. Lidocaine disposition in obesity. Am J Cardiol. 1984;**53**(8):1183–86.

101. Taivainen T, Tuominen M, Rosenberg PH. Influence of obesity on the spread of spinal analgesia after injection of plain 0.5% bupivacaine at the L3–4 or L4–5 interspace. Br J Anaesth. 1990;**64**(5):542–46.

102. Hogan QH, Prost R, Kulier A, Taylor ML, Liu S, Mark L. Magnetic resonance imaging of cerebrospinal fluid volume and the influence of body habitus and abdominal pressure. Anesthesiology. 1996;**84**(6):1341–49.

Opioid pharmacology in obese patients

Jan P. Mulier and Ruben Wouters

Introduction

A primary goal in the care of surgery patients is adequate treatment of their perioperative pain. The guidelines from The Joint Commission (formerly the Joint Commission on Accreditation of Hospital Organizations) in the United States described the measurement of pain as the 'fifth vital signal' [1]. Consequently, pain alleviation is a top priority in postoperative management [2].

Most anaesthesiologists worldwide use opioids as one of the primary components of general anaesthesia for achieving haemodynamic stability intraoperatively and for pain relief postoperatively. There are medical conditions associated with obesity that must be considered when using postoperative opioids to avoid deleterious effects in these patients. The intraoperative use of opioids is less dangerous but induces rapid tolerance [3] and hyperalgesia [4], requiring higher postoperative opioid dosages.

Opioids, however, are not sufficient to treat every postoperative pain and the adverse events and complications induced by opioids cause a real problem for obese patients who frequently have obstructive sleep apnoea (OSA) syndrome and obesity hypoventilation syndrome [5].

The relationship between pain and obesity

Obesity is caused by a combination of environmental, behavioural, and genetic factors. The genotype can provide a background with which the environmental and behavioural factors lead to the phenotypic expression of obesity [6]. Some genetic polymorphisms may lead to obesity, resulting in differences in pharmacodynamics regarding safety and efficacy of drug treatments. The G allele of the OPRM1 gene, which encodes the mu receptor, is frequently involved in obesity rather than in normal-weight patients. This polymorphism has been associated with a decrease in mechanical pain sensitivity, morphine pain relief, and an increase in the requirement for morphine and fentanyl for pain relief [7]. Endogenous opioids and their receptors were used many years ago for pain relief. Subsequently, this system has been linked to eating behaviours. Naltrexone, an opioid antagonist, leads to early satiety and eventual weight loss [8]. Furthermore, genetically engineered obese mice appear to have higher basal endogenous opioid levels [9]. The relationship between opioid analgesic responses and endogenous opioid activity has been studied in animals. One study found evidence that lower endogenous opioid function was associated with higher analgesic responsiveness to morphine [10]. In contrast to this finding, a similar relationship between endogenous opioid function and morphine-related side effects could not be established [11]. A relationship between obesity, endogenous opioid levels, and pain sensation is apparent, but further research is needed to identify the components and mechanisms in order to achieve a more complete understanding of these interactions.

Opioids and adverse events in obese patients

Opioids are by far the most used analgesics in postoperative pain treatment because of their efficacy for pain relief after surgery. Nevertheless, opioid use can also lead to adverse drug events. In another report of The Joint Commission, 21% of medication error-related events involved opioid administration [12]. Opioid-related adverse drug events are common in hospitalized patients, leading to an increase in the length of hospital stay and total hospital costs [13].

When discussing the adverse events of opioids, some remarks concerning OSA and the obese population are necessary.

The prevalence of OSA is very high in obese individuals and tends to be underdiagnosed in this group of patients. A retrospective analysis of 290 patients that received an evaluation for weight loss surgery showed that the incidence of OSA disorder was greater than 70% and tended to increase in incidence as the body mass index increased [14]. More recently, the same prevalence was also reported by other groups [15,16].

OSA is linked to many cardiovascular health problems and other conditions. Several studies showed an association between sleep-disordered breathing and postoperative adverse events [17–19]. Many diseases are linked to OSA and could explain the increased postoperative adverse events.

If and how opioids influence sleep-disordered breathing remains a critical question, but there are few published reports. An observational study investigated the association between postoperative exacerbations of sleep-disordered breathing and several clinical factors, including opioid dose [20]. The 72-hour dosage of opioids was positively associated with the postoperative apnoea–hypopnea index

[19]. Bariatric patients undergoing an opioid anaesthesia have more obstructive breathing (13% vs 0%) and require more oxygen (50% vs 8%) postoperatively in the recovery room in comparison with those undergoing an opioid-free anaesthesia (OFA) [21]. Opioids increase obstructive breathing and should therefore be reduced or better totally avoided in these patients at risk for obstructive breathing [5]. A recent meta-analysis by Gupta et al. found that opioid-induced respiratory depression happens most frequently in the first 24 hours with a higher incidence in patients with OSA syndrome, cardiac or respiratory disease, and receiving a high dose of opioids [22].

It is known that the mu-2 and kappa receptors are very important for respiratory depression and lower motoric tonus after opioid administration. There is some evidence that the tonus genioglossus muscle is heavily affected. This is the most important upper airway dilatator. The mu-opioid receptor mechanism operating at the hypoglossus motor pool causes a suppression of the drive to the genioglossus muscle of the tongue. This could be an explanation for the adverse upper airway function observed during the perioperative period in patients with OSA [23].

In an experimental trial in 2013, an association between nocturnal hypoxaemia in patients at high risk for OSA, and an increased potency of opioid analgesia was reported [24]. The nocturnal hypoxaemia was inversely proportional to the elevation of the cold pain threshold under remifentanil infusion. Nocturnal hypoxaemia potentiated the analgesic effect of mu-opioid agonists. *In vivo* evidence suggested that there was an upregulation of the mu-opioid receptors that might be responsible for the increased potency of these agents [25–27].

We conclude that obese patients are more sensitive to the adverse effects of opioids. The higher incidence of OSA within this population in combination with the increased potency of opioids and the positive association between opioid dose and apnoea–hypopnea index, makes it necessary to lower or, even better, avoid the use of opioids. Nevertheless, adequate perioperative analgesia is imperative but can be achieved by non-opioids and locoregional infiltration. Patients need to breathe deeply to avoid atelectasis and all preventive measures should be taken to avoid perioperative aspiration and pneumonia.

Opioid-induced tolerance and opioid-induced hyperalgesia

Opioid-induced hyperalgesia and acute opioid-induced tolerance are often confused, because they have similar characteristics. When there is an increase in the dose needed to maintain adequate analgesia in patients who already use opioids for the treatment of their pain, opioid-induced tolerance is suspected [28,29].

Tolerance for analgesia starts in rats at 2 hours when a continuous morphine infusion is given, with loss of analgesia after an 8-hour infusion [30]. Similar results were reported for humans receiving a continuous remifentanil infusion where tolerance began at 90 minutes and loss of analgesia was observed after 180 minutes [31]. Tolerance for respiratory depression is, however, very slow [32], increasing the risk of respiratory problems when higher opioid doses are needed.

Opioid-induced hyperalgesia is broadly defined as a state of nociceptive sensitization caused by the exposure to opioids. It can be noted days to weeks after anaesthesia and requires frequent chronic pain therapy. Opioid-induced hyperalgesia is characterized by a paradoxical response whereby a patient receiving opioids for the treatment of pain may actually become more sensitive to certain painful stimuli. This type of pain is not necessarily the same as the underlying pain.

Opioid-induced hyperalgesia is observed when administering a bolus dose of fentanyl to rats, then following their pain levels for the next 2 weeks. If opioids are combined with inflammation, as in surgery, the tolerance and hyperalgesia become even worse. A low dose of fentanyl after 2 weeks caused a paradoxical anti-analgesic effect [33]. The addition of a low dose of ketamine, an *N*-methyl-D-aspartate (NMDA) blocker, reduced the tolerance and hyperalgesia in both severity and in time [34]. Studies have revealed an increased cold pressor test pain threshold and tolerance after fentanyl infusion in human volunteers [4].

In a study using remifentanil during major abdominal surgery, higher postoperative pain scores were observed. The increased morphine demands extended for many postoperative hours. The study described this phenomenon as a combination of acute opioid tolerance and the development of sustained hyperalgesia [3,4]. The same result was found when using high doses of fentanyl. The preoperative administration of 15 mcg/kg fentanyl followed by intraoperative administration of 100 mcg/h fentanyl induced a greater consumption of fentanyl and higher pain intensity after surgery than did the preoperative administration of 1 mcg/kg fentanyl [35]. Other reports found no significant differences [36–38]. A comparison among these studies was not possible because of the different total intraoperative opioid administration procedures. Further investigations are necessary in order to establish a causal relationship.

Morbidly obese: total body weight, lean body weight, and ideal body weight

Individual characteristics need to be considered when determining drug dosages. Particularly in morbidly obese patients, it is necessary to consider the differences in body composition and physiological changes compared to those of normal body weight.

In normal-weight subjects, the total body weight is used to determine the drug dosages. Using this approach in morbidly obese subjects could lead to overdosing because lean body mass and fat mass are not proportional [39]. As fat tissue is poorly vascularized, drug overdosing could therefore occur. Opioids, however, also distribute in the fat compartment after some time, making long-acting opioids dangerous. Very short-acting opioids like remifentanil seem to be safer but induce more tolerance and hyperalgesia. Given this difficulty in using short- and long-acting opioids in obese patients, avoiding all opioids intraoperatively becomes more important in the obese patient.

Opioid-free general anaesthesia

Avoiding opioids during anaesthesia is possible without haemodynamic instability. It is necessary to stabilize the sympathetic system and avoid cardiovascular instability. Opioids at high dosages were the ideal agents to achieve this stability.

The initial use of opioids was often necessary because the drugs used in the past were strong cardiovascular depressant agents and many patients had unknown and untreated cardiovascular coronary diseases. The use of high doses of opioids allowed a reduction in dosages of these drugs and muscle relaxants. Today, safer hypnotics and neuromuscular blocking agents are used to achieve a sufficient depth of anaesthesia and muscle relaxation, and most patients have undergone treatments for their cardiovascular problems.

Drugs that stabilize the sympathetic system are currently in use and are given together in a multitarget approach to avoid the use of opioids.

A sympathetic preoperative blockade with non-opioids allows the reduction of intraoperative and postoperative opioids to almost zero. The opioid paradox is characterized by the observation that the more opioids you give intraoperatively, the more opioids you need postoperatively, or a higher pain score will be noted [21].

The best indications for OFA today are for obese patients, patients with OSA syndrome, opioid addiction, hyperalgesia problems, and chronic pain syndromes better known as complex regional pain syndromes. Due to the reduced side effects such as postoperative nausea and vomiting, OFA is also indicated for most surgical patients with an increased risk for postoperative nausea and vomiting. Vomiting after bariatric surgery increases the risk of high transmural pressures on the fundus of the stomach at the moment of herniation during the vomiting process. A pressure difference of 100–200 mmHg can be achieved and no staple line is able to resist this [40], giving a possible explanation for having most leaks at the last stapler of a sleeve or gastric bypass.

Possible relative contraindications are nodal block and the disorders of autonomic failure better known as orthostatic hypotension (i.e. multiple system atrophy). Patients with a known critical coronary stenosis or an acute coronary ischaemia should not receive OFA. OFA should also be avoided in non-stabilized hypovolaemic shock and poly-trauma patients as peripheral vasodilation can limit the perfusion of critical central organs while opioids induce peripheral vasoconstriction and maintain cardio-cerebral perfusion.

Beginning in 2012, dexmedetomidine became available in Europe, thus making OFA easier by using dexmedetomidine instead of opioids during surgery. If dexmedetomidine is given alone, a 1 mcg/kg loading dose followed by an infusion of 1 mcg/kg/h is needed. Patients will be deep sedated and might have bradycardia and postoperative hypotension. Therefore, a multitarget approach was introduced allowing the reduction of dexmedetomidine to less than 0.3 mcg/kg (ideal body weight) loading followed by less than 0.2 mcg/kg/h infusion over an hour. Lidocaine at 1.5 mg/kg ideal body weight and magnesium at 40 mg/kg ideal body weight at induction and by infusion (lidocaine or procaine at 1–3 mg/kg/hour and magnesium at 5–15 mg/kg/hour) further improved the sympathetic block. If ketamine is added to block nociceptive reactions, the best approach is to give 25 or 50 mg just prior to incision. No hallucinations are possible postoperatively at this dose, even when continued at 0.1 mg/kg/h.

The use of 0.8–1 minimum alveolar concentration of inhalation anaesthetics or propofol is added to achieve hypnosis without awareness verified by a bispectral index monitor. These hypnotics are easier to use than relying on the sedative effects of high doses of dexmedetomidine, lidocaine, or ketamine. Gabapentin at 300 mg or clonidine at 75 mcg can be given as a premedication orally and can be continued the next day postoperatively. A loading dose of ketorolac (0.5 mg/kg lean body weight) or diclofenac (2 mg/kg lean body weight) and dexamethasone (0.1 mg/kg lean body weight) can be added before surgery to reduce inflammation of the peritoneum during laparoscopy. Paracetamol can be added at awakening to achieve an optimal postoperative pain treatment without opioids or epidurals. A low dose of ketamine can be added as an analgesic in a single dose of 10–20 mg or at 50 mg given over the first 12 hours. Ketamine is an NMDA blocker and will prevent hyperalgesia in cases when an opioid is postoperatively required. Using propofol combined with a sympathetic block is also possible but always requires measuring the depth of hypnosis. Opioids are still used only as analgesics postoperatively if non-opioids are not sufficient.

The morphine requirement after general aesthesia without opioids for bariatric surgery in a randomized study using postoperative patient-controlled morphine infusion [21] was reduced on the day of the operation from 15 mg to 5 mg with a significant lower visual analogue scale score (4.7 vs 1.7). The quality of recovery measured by the QoR-40 score on the next day increased, showing an improved quality of recovery after anaesthesia.

Mulier and Dillemans found in a large observational study of 9000 bariatric patients that OFA patients independently required less opioids postoperatively and had less complications after bariatric surgery [41], making this the first outcome study in OFA. OFA was also associated with significantly less healthcare resource utilization, measured as hospital length of stay, admission to a high dependency care unit, surgical reoperation during the first week after surgery, and frequency of readmission to the hospital within 1 month after surgery.

Conclusion

Obese patients require higher doses of opioids but are more sensitive and have more risk for respiratory depression and obstructive breathing. Obese patients should therefore strongly reduce their postoperative opioid consumption. This is more easily achieved by giving an OFA that allows an opioid-free or low-opioid analgesia with enhanced recovery.

REFERENCES

1. Philips DM. JCAHO pain management standards are unveiled. JAMA. 2000;**284**(4):428–29.
2. Huang N, Cunningham F, Laurito CE, Chen C. Can we do better with postoperative pain management? Am J Surg. 2011;**182**(5):440–48.
3. Guignard B, Bossard A. Acute opioid tolerance: intraoperative remifentanil increases postoperative pain and morphine requirement. Anesthesiology. 2000;**93**(2):409–19.
4. Mauermann E, Flitz J, Dolder P, Rentsch K M, Bandschapp O, Ruppen W. Does fentanyl lead to opioid-induced hyperalgesia in healthy volunteers? Anesthesiology. 2016;**124**(2):453–63.
5. Mulier J. Perioperative opioids aggravate obstructive breathing in sleep apnea syndrome: mechanisms and alternative anesthesia strategies. Curr Opin Anesthesiol. 2016;**29**(1):129–33.
6. Lloret-Linares C, Lopes A, Declèves X, Serrie A, Mouly S, Bergmann JF, et al. Challenges in the optimisation of postoperative pain management with opioids in obese patients: a literature review. Obes Surg. 2013;**23**(9):1458–75.

7. Lloret-Linares C, Hajj A, Poitou C, Simoneau G, Clement K, Laplanche JL, et al. Pilot study examining the frequency of several gene polymorphisms involved in morphine pharmacodynamics and pharmacokinetics in a morbidly obese population. Obes Surg. 2011;**21**(8):1257–64.

8. Yeomans MR, Gray RW. Selective effects of naltrexone on food pleasantness and intake. Physiol Behav. 1996;**60**(2):439–46.

9. Khawaja XZ, Chattopadhyay AK, Green IC. Increased beta-endorphin and dynorphin concentrations in discrete hypothalamic regions of genetically obese (ob/ob) mice. Brain Res. 1991;**555**(1):164–68.

10. Bruehl S, Burns JW, Gupta R, Buvanendran A, Chont M, Kinner E, et al. Endogenous opioid function mediates the association between laboratory- evoked pain sensitivity and morphine analgesic responses. Pain. 2010;**151**(9):1856–64.

11. Gupta R, Bruehl S, Burns JW, Buvanendran A, Chont M, Schuster E, et al. Relationship between endogenous opioid function and opioid analgesic side effects. Reg Anesth Pain Med. 2014;**39**(3):219–24.

12. Gordon DB, Dahl J, Phillips P, Frandsen J, Cowley C, Foster RL, et al. The use of "as needed" range orders for opioid analgesics in the management of acute pain; a consensus statement of the American Society for Pain Management Nursing and the American Pain Society. Pain Manag Nurs. 2004;**5**(2):53–58.

13. Oderda G, Evans S, Lloyd J, Lipman A, Chen C, Ashburn M, et al. Cost of opioid-related adverse drug events in surgical patients. J Pain Symptom Manag. 2003;**25**(3):276–83.

14. Lopez PP, Stefan B, Schulman CI, Byers PM. Prevalence of sleep apnea in morbidly obese patients who presented for weight loss surgery evaluation: more evidence for routine screening for obstructive sleep apnea before weight loss surgery. Am Surg. 2008;**74**(9):834–38.

15. Serali AE, Cantor CR, Williams NN, Korus G, Raper SE, Pien G, et al. Obstructive sleep apnea in patients undergoing bariatric surgery: a tertiary center experience. Obes Surg. 2011;**21**(3):316–27.

16. Rao A, Tey BH, Ramalingam G, Poh AG. Obstructive sleep apnea (OSA) in bariatric surgical practice and response of OSA to weight loss after laparoscopic adjustable gastric banding (LAGB). Ann Acad Med Singapore. 2009;**38**(7):587.

17. Chung F, Yegneswaran B, Liao P, Chung SA, Vairavanathan S, Islam S, et al. Validation of the Berlin questionnaire and American Society of Anesthesiologists checklist as screening tools for obstructive sleep apnea in surgical patients. Anesthesiology. 2008;**108**(5):822–30.

18. Kaw R, Chunf F, Pasupuleti V, Mehta J, Gay PC, Hernandez AV. Meta-analysis of the association between obstructive sleep apnoea and postoperative outcome. Br. J Anaesth. 2012;**109**(6):897–96.

19. Kaw R, Paspuleti V, Walker E, Ramaswamy A, Foldvary-Schafer N. Postoperative complications in patients with obstructive sleep apnea. Chest. 2012;**141**(2):436–41.

20. Chung F, Liao P, Elsaid H, Shapiro CM, Kang W. Factors associated with postoperative exacerbation of sleep-disordered breathing. Anesthesiology. 2014;**120**(2):299–311.

21. Mulier J, Wouters R, Dillemans B, De Kock M. A randomized controlled, double-blind trial evaluating the effect of opioid-free versus opioid general anaesthesia on post-operative pain and discomfort measured by the QoR-40. J Clin Anesth Pain Med. 2018;**2**:015.

22. Gupta K, Nagappa M, Prasad A, Abrahamyan L, Wong J, Weingarten TN, et al. Risk factors for opioid-induced respiratory depression in surgical patients: a systematic review and meta-analyses. BMJ Open. 2018;**8**(12):e024086.

23. Hajiha M, DuBord MA, Liu H, Horner RL. Opioid receptor mechanisms at the hypoglossal motor pool and effects on tongue muscle activity in vivo. J Physiol. 2009;**587**(11):2677–92.

24. Doufas AG, Tian L, Padrez KA, Suwanprathes P, Cardell JA, Maecker HT, et al. Experimental pain and opioid analgesia in volunteers at high risk for obstructive sleep apnea. PLoS One. 2013;**8**(1):e54807.

25. Brown KA. Intermittent hypoxia and the practice of anethesia. Anesthesiology. 2009;**110**(4):922–27.

26. Laferriere A, Liu JK, Moss IR. Neurokinin-1 versus mu-opioid receptor binding in rat nucleus tractus solitarius after single and recurrent intermittent hypoxia. Brain Res Bull. 2003;**59**(4):307–13.

27. Lerman J. Unraveling the mysteries of sleep-disordered breathing in children. Anesthesiology. 2006;**105**(4):645–47.

28. Angst MS, Clark JD. Opioid induced hyperalgesia: a qualitative systematic review. Anesthesiology. 2006;**104**(3):570–87.

29. Chu LF, Angst MS. Opioid-induced hyperalgesia in humans: molecular mechanisms and clinical considerations. Clin J Pain. 2004;**24**(6):479–96.

30. Cox BM, Ginsburg M, Osman OH. Acute tolerance to narcotic analgesic drugs in rats. Br J Pharmacol Chemother. 1968;**33**(2):245–56.

31. Vinik HR, Kissin I. Rapid development of tolerance to analgesia during remifentanil infusion in humans. Anesth Analg. 19998;**86**(6):1307–11.

32. Paronis CA, Woods JH. Ventilation in morphine-maintained rhesus monkeys. II Tolerance to the nociceptive but not the ventilatory effects of morphine. J Pharmacol Exp Ther. 1997;**282**(1):355–62.

33. Rivat C, Laboureyras E, Laulin JP, Le Roy C, Richebé P, Simonnet G. Non-nociceptive environmental stress induces hyperalgesia, not analgesia, in pain and opioid-experienced rats. Neuropsychopharmacology. 2007;**32**(10):2217–28.

34. Rivat C, Laulin JP, Corcuff JB, Celerier E, Pain L, Simonnet G. Fentanyl enhancement of carrageenan-induced long-lasting hyperalgesia in rats Anesthesiology. 2002;**96**(2):381–91.

35. Chia YY, Liu K, Wang JJ, Kuo MC, Ho ST. Intraoperative high dose fentanyl induces postoperative fentanyl tolerance. Can J Anesth. 1999;**46**(9):872–7.

36. Lee LH, Irwin MG, Lui SK. Intraoperative remifentanil infusion does not increase postoperative opioid consumption compared with 70% nitrous oxide. Anesthesiology. 2005;**102**(2):398–402.

37. Cortinez LI, Brandes V, Muñoz HR, Guerrero ME, Mur M. No clinical evidence of acute opioid tolerance after remifentanil-based anaesthesia. Br J Anaesth. 2001;**87**(6):866–69.

38. Hansen EG, Duedahl TH, Rømsing J, Hilsted KL, Dahl JB. Intra-operative remifentanil might influence pain levels in the immediate postoperative period after major abdominal surgery. Acta Anaesthesiol Scand. 2005;**49**(10):1464–70.

39. Janmahasatian S, Duffull SB, Ash S, Ward LC, Byrne NM, Green B. Quantification of lean body weight. Clin Pharmacokinet. 2005;**44**(10):1051–65.

40. Rached AA, Basile M, Masri HE. Gastric leaks post sleeve gastrectomy: review of its prevention and management World J Gastroenterol. 2014;**20**(38):13904–10.

41. Mulier J, Dillemans B. Anaesthetic factors affecting outcome after bariatric surgery, a retrospective levelled regression analysis. Obes Surg. 2019;**29**(6):1841–50.

Inhaled anaesthetics and morbid obesity

Luc De Baerdemaeker, Jan Hendrickx, and Andre M. De Wolf

Introduction: intravenous versus inhaled anaesthetics

Obesity affects the pharmacokinetic and pharmacodynamic properties of most intravenous anaesthetics in a complex manner (see Chapter 4). As dose recommendations of intravenous drugs are usually derived from a non-obese population, some sort of dose adjustment has to be made to avoid over- or underdosing, for example, by using dosing scalars. The plethora of dosing scalars available to the clinician reflects our inadequate knowledge. Indeed, the use of these dosing scalars is often illogical because they do not take body composition into account and are unpractical because they require the use of complex formulae such as lean body mass [1] and the pharmacokinetic mass of fentanyl [2]. In this chapter, we will examine to what extent morbid obesity affects the pharmacodynamics and pharmacokinetics of inhaled anaesthetics.

Pharmacodynamics—minimum alveolar concentration and drug interactions

Whether obesity alters the sensitivity of the central nervous system to inhaled anaesthetics remains poorly studied. The few existing studies suggest little or no effect of obesity. Obesity did not affect minimum alveolar concentration $(MAC)_{awake}$ of isoflurane or sevoflurane administered at 1, 1.5, or 2 MAC in 50% nitrous oxide (N_2O) [3]. When Cortínez [4] modelled the hysteresis between the end-expired partial pressure (F_A) of sevoflurane and the bispectral index (BIS) over a 30–60 range with an E-max model, the median effect site partial pressure (Ce) that caused this BIS change (1.52% sevoflurane) did not differ between obese and non-obese patients, indicating that obesity did not alter sensitivity to sevoflurane.

In the non-obese, opioids synergistically interact with inhaled anaesthetics. Opioid concentrations equipotent to 2 ng/mL remifentanil reduce the F_A of inhaled anaesthetics required to ensure loss of response to verbal command, movement on incision, and absence of tachycardia and hypertension by 15%, 50%, and 74%, respectively [5–8]. While it is not known whether obesity affects this pharmacodynamic interaction, obesity does alter the pharmacokinetics of opioids, thus making it difficult to predict the opioid concentration. The lack of data (effect of obesity on pharmacokinetics of intravenous agents) currently precludes model-based approaches towards drug titration using tools like the Smart Pilot (Dräger, Lübeck, Germany): no software is available for a body mass index (BMI) greater than 35 kg/m^2. As in non-obese patients, dexmedetomidine reduces desflurane requirements. During open gastric bypass surgery, a 0.5 mcg/kg bolus followed by a 0.4 mcg/kg/h infusion reduced the F_A of desflurane that maintained BIS at 45–50 by 20% [9]. In patients undergoing laparoscopic bariatric surgery, a dexmedetomidine infusion of 0.2, 0.4, and 0.8 mcg/kg/h reduced the average F_A desflurane concentration by 19%, 20%, and 22%, respectively. However, it did not result in a significantly faster emergence from anaesthesia [10].

Pharmacokinetics—induction and maintenance

When administered in oxygen (O_2)/air, uptake of inhaled anaesthetics is governed by three factors: alveolar minute ventilation (lung wash-in), uptake across the alveolocapillary membrane, and—to a very small extent—metabolism [11]. All of these factors can be affected by obesity.

Alveolar minute ventilation

Assuming no agent is taken up from the alveoli into the blood during initial wash-in (an oversimplification for didactic reasons), the wash-in rate of the lungs depends on the size of the lungs (functional residual capacity (FRC)) and alveolar minute ventilation (V_A). The exponential wash-in process can be described by the time constant tau (τ): $\tau = FRC/V_A$. An exponential process is 95% complete after 3 τ, respectively. This equation, $\tau = FRC/V_A$, mathematically describes what is intuitively obvious: a smaller FRC and larger V_A will hasten lung wash-in. For example, with a 2 L FRC and 4 L/min V_A, τ equals 0.5 minutes, so it will take 3 τ or 1.5 minutes to raise the F_A towards 95% of the inspired partial pressure (F_I).

Obesity reduces FRC by 3–5% per unit of BMI increase in the 20–30 kg/m^2 BMI range, and by an additional 1% per increase above BMI 30 kg/m^2. Even though it is tempting to theoretically speculate how this affects the rate of rise of F_A towards F_I, the clinical implications may be small since anaesthesia is most often induced intravenously anyhow. In addition, some form of mechanical ventilatory support is likely to be used, eliminating hypoventilation as a factor delaying the rise of F_A towards F_I. Even though mask inductions with an inhaled agent are feasible in selected patients, properly fitting a mask in this patient population may be challenging [12]. Reports on larger series are lacking.

Uptake

Uptake of an agent can be discussed by considering mass balances at the Y-piece of the circle breathing system (the difference between the amount entering and leaving the lungs) or by considering the amount being removed across the alveolocapillary membrane. The former includes wash-in of the lungs and uptake by lung tissue, the latter does not.

Uptake expressed as the difference between the amount entering and leaving the lung

Wash-in and uptake is usually graphically represented by the F_A/F_I over time curve, that is, the manner in which F_A rises towards F_I. The F_A/F_I curve can be used to explain what factors impact uptake, but does not really represent uptake itself. If we ignore dead-space (40–50% of tidal volume in real life), incomplete gas mixing, and differences between in- and expired tidal volumes, uptake can be presented by the area *above* the F_A/F_I curve, or $1 - F_A/F_I$ (**Fig. 6.1**). This can be deducted by considering uptake per breath as the amount

of agent going into the lung (F_I × tidal volume) minus the amount leaving the lung (F_A × tidal volume), or ($F_I - F_A$) × tidal volume. After rearranging this mathematically (**Fig. 6.1**), it can be readily appreciated that uptake in the classic F_A/F_I versus time curve is approximated by the area *above* the curve, $1 - F_A/F_I$.

Consequently, uptake across the Y-piece can be represented as the sum of wash-in of the lungs and uptake by the body's different tissue groups. The F_A/F_I versus time curve can now be seen to be a composite of lung wash-in and uptake by the vessel-rich group (VRG), muscle group (MG), and the fat group (FG)—see later for more detail on tissue groups.

Uptake expressed as the amount being removed across the alveolocapillary membrane

Anaesthetic agent uptake across the alveolocapillary membrane opposes the effect of wash-in by V_A. Uptake into the blood can be expressed as the product of the blood/gas partition coefficient ($l_{B/G}$), cardiac output (CO), and the alveolar-to-mixed venous blood partial pressure difference ($F_A - F_v$): uptake = $\lambda_{B/G}$ × CO × ($F_A - F_v$). These three factors are discussed in the following paragraphs, both in general terms and—where information is available and applicable—in terms of how obesity might affect them. The section ends by examining the end-expired–arterial partial pressure gradient and by considering quantitative aspects of uptake.

The blood/gas partition coefficient

Different inhaled anaesthetics have different $\lambda_{B/G}$ values, and this confers them different clinical properties. Reported $\lambda_{B/G}$ values differ slightly between authors (**Table 6.1**). Many factors affect $\lambda_{B/G}$, but BMI is not one of them [13]. Age [14], hypothermia [15], haemodilution [16], and serum cholesterol and triglyceride levels [16, 17], conversely, do affect $\lambda_{B/G}$. Patients with coronary artery disease, for example, have higher triglycerides levels with correspondingly higher $\lambda_{B/G}$ of desflurane, isoflurane, and halothane [18].

Cardiac output

Obesity may increase or decrease CO. In the obese patient without accompanying diseases, the absolute values of CO and blood volume are more related to the fat-free mass and are higher compared to non-obese patients: each 1 kg/m² of BMI increases CO by 0.08 L/min and stroke volume by 1.35 mL [19]. The effect of obesity on CO and stroke volume disappears when indexation to body surface is used [20]. In the obese patient with obesity-related cardiomyopathy, CO is likely to be lower [21].

Even though the above-mentioned obesity-induced changes in CO have been well described, no clinical information is available on the relationship between morbid obesity, CO, and uptake of inhaled anaesthetics. The overall effect of changes in CO on kinetics should match those in the non-obese patient: an increased CO will increase uptake, thus slowing the rate of rise of F_A, and this will slow an inhalational induction (which, as mentioned, is not frequently employed in the obese). When the F_A is target controlled, F_A will no longer be affected by CO (because the anaesthesia machine will adjust agent delivery to maintain the target F_A) and the partial pressure in the central nervous (F_{CNS}) system will rise faster with a higher CO because agent transfer to the CNS will be faster (assuming that cerebral blood flow increases with an increase in CO) [22].

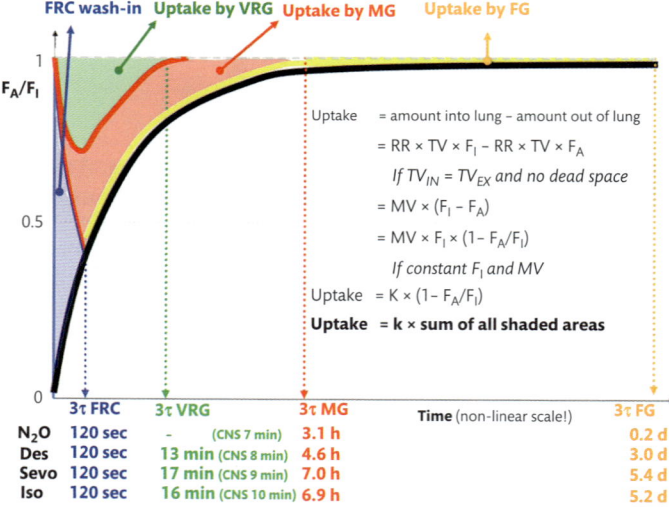

Fig. 6.1 Quantitative interpretation of the F_A/F_I curve. The F_A/F_I curve (thick black line) needs to be interpreted properly—it does not present uptake at all. Uptake can be considered to be proportional to $1 - F_A/F_I$, which is the area above the F_A/F_I curve (see formula in the figure). FRC wash-in and uptake by the VRG, MG, and FG can then schematically be presented as the separate coloured areas above the curve. Uptake across the alveolocapillary membrane is represented by uptake by VRG, MG, and FG (does not include FRC wash-in). Times to 95% saturation of each modern inhaled anaesthetics are displayed at the bottom of the figure. Note that the time axis is not linear in order to allow saturation of the different groups to be schematically displayed. 95% saturation of the CNS (part of the VRG) is displayed separately between brackets. The derivation assumes that the inspired tidal volume (TVIN) is equal to the expired tidal volume (TVEX) and that there is no dead-space ventilation (RR, respiratory rate; K, proportioning constant). Uptake also depends on the absolute value of F_I and minute ventilation (MV).

Table 6.1 Blood/gas partition coefficients ($\lambda_{B/G}$) for desflurane, sevoflurane, and isoflurane

Blood/gas partition coefficient	Desflurane	Sevoflurane	Isoflurane
Eger et al. [11] mean (range)	0.45 (0.42–0.52)	0.65 (0.62–0.69)	1.4 (1.38–1.46)
Esper et al. [13] mean (range)	0.57 (0.56–0.59)	0.74 (0.72–0.77)	1.45 (1.4–1.5)

Source: Data from Eger, E.I., Saidman, L.J., Eger, E.I, Saidman, L.J. Illustrations of inhaled anesthetic uptake, including intertissue diffusion to and from fat. *Anesthesia & Analgesia*, 100(4):1020–33, 2005; Data from Esper, T., Wehner, M., Meinecke, C.D., Rueffert, H. Blood/gas partition coefficients for isoflurane, sevoflurane, and desflurane in a clinically relevant patient population. *Anesthesia & Analgesia*, 120(1): 45–50, 2015.

Tissue saturation, reflected by the $F_A - F_v$ difference

The difference between F_A and F_v (partial pressure in mixed-venous blood) will become smaller when the tissues have taken up more and more anaesthetic agent and become gradually more saturated. This is associated with a reduction in uptake by these tissues. When discussing 'uptake', it is important to distinguish the *amount* of agent a tissue takes up from the *speed* with which tissues saturate. The total *amount* of inert gas a tissue (or organ) can take up (or store) from the blood, depends on the partial pressure of the agent in the arterial blood (F_a) and the capacity of the tissue to store inhaled anaesthetic: total tissue uptake (= tissue capacity) = F_a × volume tissue × $\lambda_{tissue/blood}$. The *speed* with which a tissue saturates towards F_a does not depend on F_a itself, but on the tissue's blood flow: a smaller tissue with low tissue solubility and high tissue blood flow will saturate faster. Mathematically, this can be expressed by its time constant (τ): τ_{tissue} = (volume tissue × $\lambda_{tissue/blood}$)/tissue blood flow.

Eger et al. grouped different organs into different tissues based upon their perfusion: the VRG (consisting of the brain, lungs, kidneys, heart, and liver), the MG, and the FG (Table 6.2). The *capacity* to hold anaesthetic equals the volume of the tissue multiplied by the $\lambda_{tissue/gas}$, and is largest for the FG, followed by the MG, and smallest for the VRG. The *rate* at which they saturate depends both on this capacity (higher capacity = slower equilibration) and the proportion of CO a tissue receives: VRG 75%, MG 20%, and FG 2–5% (2% in the obese (see following paragraph) [23]). The VRG has a small capacity to hold anaesthetic agent and a high tissue blood flow, and thus saturates fast for desflurane (10 minutes) and sevoflurane (15 minutes). The MG has a relatively large capacity and moderate blood flow, and

Table 6.2 Time constants of sevoflurane, desflurane, and isoflurane in non-obese versus obese with a BMI greater than 35 kg/m^2 using combined data on tissue volumes and tissue blood flow

Variable	Normal weight				Obese (BMI >35 kg/m^2)			
	VRG	MG	FG	ITDG	VRG	MG	FG	ITDG
Volume (L)	6	33	14.5	2.9	6	33	45.4	11.3
Tissue/blood partition coefficient = (tissue/gas partition)/(blood/gas partition coefficient)								
Desflurane	1.02	1.37	22.8	22.8	1.02	1.37	22.8	22.8
Sevoflurane	1.49	2.30	45.9	45.9	1.49	2.30	45.9	45.9
Isoflurane	1.54	2.41	48.3	48.3	1.54	2.41	48.3	48.3
Tissue/gas partition coefficient								
Desflurane	0.58	0.78	13	13	0.58	0.78	13	13
Sevoflurane	1.10	1.70	34	34	1.10	1.70	34	34
Isoflurane	2.24	3.50	70	70	2.24	3.50	70	70
Capacity to hold anaesthetic (L) = tissue volume × tissue/gas partition coefficient								
Desflurane	3.48	25.74	188.5	37.7	3.48	25.74	590	147
Sevoflurane	6.6	56.1	493	98.6	6.6	56.1	1544	384
Isoflurane	13.44	115.5	1015	203	13.44	115.5	3178	791
Time constants (min) = 100 × (tissue/blood partition coefficient)/tissue blood flow								
Desflurane	3.39	30.2	962	181	3.39	30.2	1452	211
Sevoflurane	4.95	50.7	1937	364	4.95	50.7	2924	425
Isoflurane	5.12	53.1	2038	383	5.12	53.1	3076	447
Blood flow mL/100 mL tissue/min	30.1	4.54	2.37	12.6	30.1	4.54	1.57	10.8

Source: Data from Eger, E.I., Saidman, L.J., Eger, E.I, Saidman, L.J. Illustrations of inhaled anesthetic uptake, including intertissue diffusion to and from fat. *Anesthesia & Analgesia*, 100(4):1020–33, 2005; Data from Esper, T., Wehner, M., Meinecke, C.D., Rueffert, H. Blood/gas partition coefficients for isoflurane, sevoflurane, and desflurane in a clinically relevant patient population. *Anesthesia & Analgesia*, 120(1): 45–50, 2015; data from Levitt, D.G. Heterogeneity of human adipose blood flow. *BMC Clin Pharmacol*, 7(1), 2007; data from Wang, J., Gallagher, D., Thornton, J.C., Yu, W., Weil, R., Kovac, B., et al. Regional Body Volumes, BMI, Waist Circumference, and Percentage Fat in Severely Obese Adults. *Obesity*,15(11): 2688–98, 2007.

thus saturates after 90–150 minutes with desflurane and sevoflurane, respectively. The FG has a very large capacity to hold anaesthetic agent, but only receives a small proportion of CO, causing the FG to take 3 and 6 days to saturate for 95% with desflurane and sevoflurane, respectively. A fourth compartment, the vessel-poor group, consists of tissues with very low blood flow and low capacity to hold anaesthetic (e.g. tendons). This compartment is ignored because it is unlikely to affect the kinetics.

The fat should be considered as a heterogeneous group, that is, not all fat in the 'FG' is the same. First, adipose tissue blood flow differs between the non-obese (2.8–5 mL/100 g/min) and the obese (1.57 mL/100 g/min), [24], constituting 5% and 2% of CO, respectively. Second, not all of this fat is equally well perfused in the obese patient: 80% or 45.4 L is low-perfused bulk fat, and 20% or 11.3 L constitutes well-perfused fat. The latter has been extrapolated from data suggesting that patients with a BMI of 35–60 kg/m^2 have 51 kg or 56.7 L of fat (assuming a fat density of 0.9 kg/L) [25]. The latter has been referred to by Eger et al. as the inter-tissue diffusion group (ITDG). The existence of this group was postulated while modelling wash-out data of inhaled anaesthetics after a 30-minute anaesthetic [26,27]. The ITDG is thought to represent fat adjacent to highly perfused tissue, for example, peri-renal and mesenteric fat, subcutaneous fat, pericardial fat, fat intercalated between the muscle fibres, and even white matter in the CNS. Anaesthetic agent is thought to diffuse from organs into the fat. The ITDG represents 30% of the body's capacity to store inhaled agent and has a time constant of 200–400 minutes depending on the agent. Levitt et al. expanded on these data to develop a physiologically based pharmacokinetic model. One fat compartment with a blood flow of 3.96 mL/100 mL/min described uptake data well during the first 3 hours. After 3 hours (and up to 6 days), the data were better described by two fat compartments, a slow one with a blood flow of 1.26 mL/100 mL/min and a fast one with a blood flow of 6.66 mL/100 mL/min [28]. Eger et al. [11] suggested that the upper range of the high-flow adipose tissue (10.8 mL/100 mL/min) was due to inter-tissue diffusion of agent from well-perfused tissues to the surrounding fat.

End-expired–arterial gradients

For didactic purposes, discussions on kinetics of inhaled anaesthetics often ignore pulmonary ventilation/perfusion (V/Q) inhomogeneity and assume that the arterial partial pressure (F_a) equals the end-expired partial pressure (F_A). In the obese patient, A–a gradients have been well documented for O_2 and carbon dioxide (CO_2), especially during anaesthesia [29]. They have been well described for potent inhaled anaesthetics—actually, inhaled anaesthetics are used to *study* V/Q scatter: they are an inherent element of the multiple inert gas elimination technique (MIGET) used to study V/Q scatter! Few data exist on inhaled anaesthetics in the obese, and it is unclear whether these gradients are more pronounced in the obese. Cortínez [4] claimed the effect of any V/Q mismatching to be small because they did not find a difference in hysteresis in the sevoflurane F_A and BIS with or without positive-end expiratory pressure, a finding corroborated by Sprung et al. who found that alveolar recruitment failed to increase desflurane F_A in morbidly obese patients, even though the O_2 partial pressure increased [30]. Modern technology (e.g. automated target control delivery, visual drug display systems) might spur a renewed interest in the study of these gradients.

Quantitative aspects

Even though the largest part of this chapter is devoted to uptake, no quantitative uptake data (expressed in mL/min) are provided to the reader, simply because there are none. Closed-circuit anaesthesia with liquid agent injection into the inspiratory limb of the circle breathing system as well as Fick's method have been used to quantify uptake in the non-obese patient, but such data do not exist for the obese patient. Even simpler quantitative data such as O_2 consumption, CO_2 production, and N_2O uptake in the obese during anaesthesia are unknown. With the availability of gas analysers, the clinical relevance of the actual amounts of gas uptake has faded.

Metabolism

The pharmacokinetic effect of metabolism of the modern inhaled agents sevoflurane and desflurane is quite small and can be mostly ignored. Although 20% of the inhaled halothane is metabolized, hepatotoxicity is still relatively rare, but occurs more often in obese women having more than one exposure to the drug within a short time interval. The only reported case of desflurane-related hepatitis [31] is thought to be related to its metabolite trifluoroacetyl chloride (even though desflurane has the lowest metabolism of the inhaled anaesthetics). Sevoflurane metabolism is 2.5%, the highest of the less soluble agents. Even though this theoretically carries a risk of fluoride nephrotoxicity, no renal dysfunction has been reported in obese and non-obese patients anesthetized with sevoflurane [32,33].

Pharmacokinetics–recovery

Many of the factors affecting wash-in and maintenance also affect recovery, but it is not an exact mirror image. This section focuses on recovery after sevoflurane and desflurane administration because these are the most commonly used agents in modern anaesthesia practice, and because considering these two will suffice to highlight the concepts that are clinically relevant to emergence. The combination of a high fat solubility of inhaled anaesthetics and increased fat stores is often invoked to explain delayed emergence in the obese patient. Because sevoflurane's $\lambda_{blood/gas}$ (0.65) and $\lambda_{fat/gas}$ (45.9–60.8) are larger than those of desflurane (0.45 and 22.8–27.7, respectively), desflurane might be expected to be the agent ensuring the more rapid recovery. Things are, however, more complex. We will introduce the reader to the concept of decrement times, compare recovery between the obese and non-obese after desflurane and sevoflurane administration, compare open versus closed systems during emergence, and discuss the risk of rehypnotization.

Decrement times

Decrement times are for inhaled anaesthetics what context-sensitive half-times are for intravenous anaesthetics [34]—they describe how long it takes for F_A to decrease by a certain proportion or 'decrement' (0–100%) after their administration. For intravenous anaesthetics, the 'context' refers to the duration of anaesthesia: the longer the duration of administration, the more drug elimination (via metabolism) rather than redistribution will become responsible for terminating a drug's effect. For inhaled anaesthetics, a longer duration of administration will cause the MG to be more saturated, causing more agent to be released from these tissues groups (and for a longer time) after discontinuing their administration, potentially sustaining a higher F_v for a longer time, and thus delaying emergence. Release of inhaled anaesthetic from the FG has virtually no effect on Fv (except after very long anaesthetics—see later). Gas Man® software (Med Man Simulations, Inc., Boston, MA, USA)-generated decrement times are a great tool to theoretically probe the effect of obesity on the kinetics of inhaled anaesthetics. The next paragraph describes the concept in greater detail.

Fig. 6.2 illustrates how decrements times can help steer drug titration to ensure a swift emergence. **Fig. 6.2a** depicts the dose–response relationship for inhaled anaesthetics, with the x-axis representing the F_A of the inhaled anaesthetic (expressed in MAC equivalents) and the y-axis the probability of not responding to a verbal command (left curve) or of not moving after surgical incision (right curve), expressed as a fraction between 0 and 1. The relationship is sigmoidal and steep, with a median effect partial pressure of 0.35

MAC for hypnosis (= MAC_{awake}) and 1 MAC for immobility [35]. The vertical line parallel to the y-axis that intersects the x-axis at 0.2 MAC is the F_A at which more than 95% of the patients will be awake (assuming 'steady state', meaning F_A has equilibrated with F_{CNS}). Besides hysteresis and drug interactions, two factors will affect the speed with which the patient will regain consciousness. First, the higher F_A has been maintained during the procedure, the more it will have to decrease to reach 0.2 MAC (both in absolute value and in proportion to the maintenance value). The other factor is the context-sensitive half-time. Generally speaking, the more soluble an agent is, the more likely it is that decrement times increase with time. However, the different decrement times are differently affected by the duration of administration (**Fig. 6.2b**). After 4 hours of anaesthesia, 80% decrement times between sevoflurane and desflurane do not differ, but 90% decrement times do. It is important to take this into account when selecting a maintenance F_A—even after 4 hours

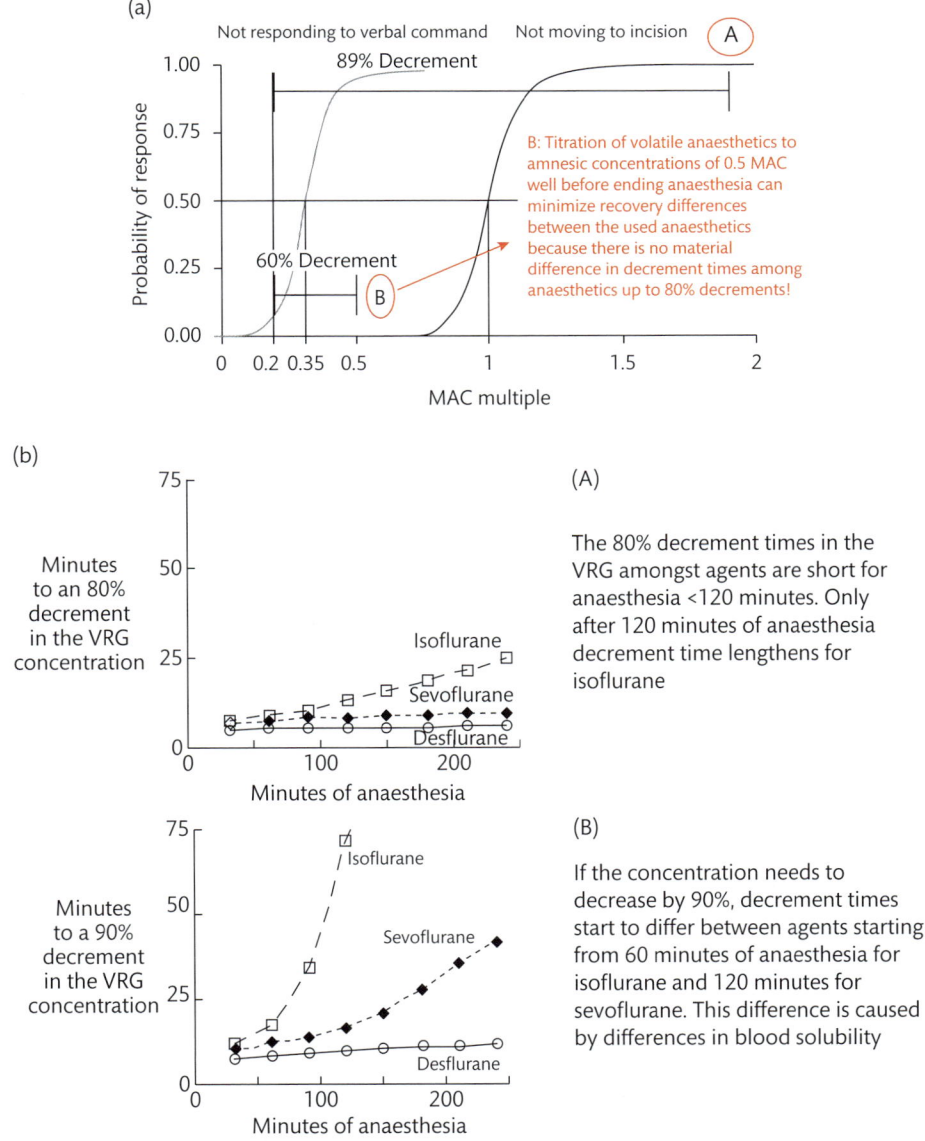

Fig. 6.2 (a) The link between anaesthetic duration and time needed to reach 0.2 MAC and (b) context-sensitive decrement times.

(a) Adapted with permission from Eger, E. I., Shafer, S. The complexity of recovery from anesthesia, *Journal of Clinical Anesthesia*, 17(6): 411–412. Copyright © 2005 Elsevier. DOI: 10.1016/j.jclinane.2005.05.001

(b) Adapted with permission from Eger, E. and Shafer, S. Tutorial: Context-Sensitive Decrement Times for Inhaled Anesthetics, *Anesthesia & Analgesia*, 101(3):688–696, Copyright © 2005 Wolters Kluwer Health, Inc. doi: 10.1213/01.ANE.0000158611.15820.3D

of anaesthesia, emergence times between sevoflurane and desflurane will not differ as long as the maintenance partial pressure has been low enough to ensure that an 80% decrement continues to suffice to ensure the F_A drops below 0.2 MAC.

Recovery in the non-obese

In non-obese patients undergoing ambulatory surgery, the time to eye opening and obeying commands is faster after desflurane than after sevoflurane anaesthesia, but the effects are small and there is a lot of variability among the studies [36]. Time to post-anaesthesia care unit discharge was faster with sevoflurane, and there were no differences between desflurane and sevoflurane in time to home readiness and discharge. These results had been predicted theoretically by Bailey using decrement times: he found no differences in decrement times between sevoflurane and desflurane for decrements up to 80% (i.e. the time for the partial pressure to decrease to 20% of the partial pressure used to maintain anaesthesia) after procedures lasting up to 250 minutes (**Fig. 6.2b**) [34]. Only for 90% decrements did decrement times between these two drugs start to differ after procedures lasting 2 hours or more [37] (**Fig. 6.2b**).

Recovery after desflurane and sevoflurane administration in the obese

Recovery characteristics in the morbidly obese patient after sevoflurane and desflurane anaesthesia were reviewed by Liu et al. [38]. Overall, the results mirror those in the non-obese patient: early recovery characteristics are obtained faster after desflurane anaesthesia, but the effects are modest, of the same magnitude as in the non-obese patients, and vary widely, likely a reflection of the significant heterogeneity in methodology, that is, studies differed in their use of concomitantly administered drugs (midazolam, remifentanil/fentanyl/morphine, N_2O, epidural local anaesthetics), the manner in which the inhaled anaesthetic was titrated (BIS versus F_A), and the manner in which the inhaled anaesthetic was tapered towards the end of the anaesthetic. Overall, after procedures lasting 2–4.2 hours, selecting desflurane instead of sevoflurane saves an average of 3 minutes 25 seconds to eye opening and 4 minutes 17 seconds to extubation (average weighed according to the number of study participants).

The manner in which the anaesthetic is tapered towards the end of an anaesthetic attenuates differences in emergence times between anaesthetics with different solubilities. If decrement times are taken into consideration so that the inhaled anaesthetic is washed out slowly at the end of the anaesthetic while carefully titrating anaesthesia towards BIS levels of 60 or MAC values of 0.5 at the end of surgery ('amnestic levels'), no differences in emergence and recovery profiles could be detected between desflurane and sevoflurane [39,40].

Why do we only detect relatively small differences in emergence time between sevoflurane and desflurane in the obese patient, and why are these differences not more pronounced than in the non-obese? In the obese patient, the large volume of fat combined with the high fat solubility of potent inhaled anaesthetics turns the fat compartment into a huge sink that can absorb large amounts of anaesthetic. Combined with its low perfusion, this causes fat to have very long τ: it takes days for the *partial pressure* of sevoflurane and desflurane in fat to 95% equilibrate (3 τ) with that in the arterial blood, actually 7 days for sevoflurane and 3–4 days for desflurane.

After 6 hours, the fat has been saturated for only 13% and 22% for sevoflurane and desflurane, respectively, and even after a day for only 43% and 63%, respectively. The *amounts* stored in the fat are largely irrelevant for early recovery as long as the partial pressure in the fat remains well below MAC_{awake}.

The following theoretical example illustrates the above-mentioned point very well. Let us assume anaesthesia has been maintained with an F_A of 15 mmHg sevoflurane or 46 mmHg desflurane (2% and 6% of 1 atm, respectively, equipotent doses). After 6 hours, a duration of anaesthesia well beyond the duration of many anaesthetics, the F_{fat} will be 2 mmHg for sevoflurane (= 13% of 15 mmHg) and 10 mmHg for desflurane (= 22% of 6 mmHg). Because this is still well below the MAC_{awake} of sevoflurane (5 mmHg or 0.7% of 1 atm) and desflurane (15 mmHg or 2.0% of 1 atm), it is unlikely that fat can sustain a partial pressure sufficient to keep the patient unconscious—on the contrary, the fat can be expected to continue to take up anaesthetic agent during the initial emergence phase. The take-home message here is that it is not the *amount* of agent taken up by the fat that is clinically relevant, but rather the partial pressure. As long as F_{fat} has not reached that partial pressure responsible for suppression of a certain clinical response, it can be considered clinically irrelevant for that particular clinical end point.

The relationship between partial pressure and concentration (= amount of agent per volume of tissue) is described by Henry's law: concentration = solubility × partial pressure. Applying this principle to the fat in the clinical example described previously allows one to understand why the claim that more sevoflurane than desflurane is stored in fat after, for example, 6 hours of anaesthesia is not only a misconception but flat-out wrong: after 6 hours of anaesthesia with 15 mmHg (2%) sevoflurane or 46 mmHg (6%) desflurane, the fat will contain more desflurane (14.7 mL vapour/100 mL fat) than sevoflurane (8.0 mL vapour/100 mL fat) because the MAC of desflurane is higher than that of sevoflurane. To the best of our knowledge, nobody has ever taken fat tissue samples to confirm these claims.

Theoretically, the ITDG could delay recovery because it has both a shorter time constant than fat but the same ability to hold anaesthetic: a partial pressure equivalent to MAC_{awake} can be attained after 6 hours of 1 MAC administration (**Table 6.3**). However, as mentioned earlier, clinical studies have not been able to tease out clinically relevant differences in emergence times between desflurane and sevoflurane [41,42] and even isoflurane [43] between obese and non-obese patients.

Even if fat would be fully saturated with 1 MAC of anaesthetic agent, it could not significantly contribute to sustain an end-expired partial pressure above MAC_{awake} (0.35 MAC) because it only receives a small part of CO (2% in the morbidly obese—see earlier). Fat can theoretically only delay awakening if it would receive a larger proportion of CO. A Gas Man® simulation supports this notion: even in the more obese model up to 150 kg, sevoflurane and isoflurane decrement times 'do not degrade' for the first 7 and 9 hours of anaesthesia, respectively [44].

Some authors have argued clinical end points other than regaining consciousness might be more important. For example, morbidly obese patients are considered at higher risk of aspiration, not only during induction of anaesthesia but also during emergence. Airway reflexes returned slower with a larger BMI and after the use of sevoflurane rather than desflurane [45].

Table 6.3 Effect of duration of 1 MAC administration on partial pressure in the fat group and the inter-tissue diffusion group of a theoretical patient

Duration (h) of anaesthesia with % end-tidal of 1 MAC	Partial pressure (% of 1 atm)					
	Sevoflurane		Desflurane		Isoflurane	
	FG	ITDG	FG	IDTG	FG	ITDG
1	0.04	0.26	0.24	1.5	0.02	0.14
2	0.08	0.5	0.48	2.6	0.04	0.26
3	0.12	0.7	0.7	3.4	0.06	0.37
6	0.23	1.14	1.32	4.9	0.12	0.62
MAC$_{awake}$ (% of 1 atm)	0.7	0.7	2.0	2.0	0.4	0.4

FG, fat group; ITDG, inter-tissue diffusion group.

Note: % of 1 atm in tissue at time t = MAC.$(1 - e^{-t/\tau})$, with tau values from Table 6.2 are used.

Ventilation and emergence

If fresh gas flow exceeds minute ventilation after discontinuing agent delivery, F_I will be zero and F_A will decrease rapidly if normoventilation is maintained. However, the F_A displayed by the gas analyser will underestimate F_{CNS} due the transport delay of agent from the CNS to the lungs. MAC$_{awake}$ will be a poor tool to guide emergence unless this delay is taken into account. The difficult art of trying to determine the degree of hysteresis in the individual patient can be complemented by tools that calculate the effect site concentration, such as the Smart Pilot® (Dräger, Lübeck, Germany) or MAC Brain® (Getinge, Solna, Sweden), but is not yet available for the obese due a lack of pharmacokinetic/pharmacodynamic models.

Hyperventilation should speed up clearance, and some have recommended to even add CO_2 to the inspired mixture (so-called isocapnic hyperventilation) to minimize hyperventilation-induced cerebral vasoconstriction and to keep the arterial CO_2 partial pressure above the apnoeic threshold. This technique shortened immediate recovery after isoflurane anaesthesia by about 33% in an obese population but had no effect on post-anaesthesia care unit discharge times [46].

Severe hypoventilation (= 0.1–0.3 L/min), for example, induced by opioids or partial airway obstruction, may cause rehypnotization [47]. If the muscle group has been saturated sufficiently to result in F_v above 1–2 MAC$_{awake}$ (e.g. after >4 hours of anaesthesia), rehypnotization will occur. This effect of hypoventilation has not been studied in obese patients or models. The degree of hypoventilation that is likely to cause rehypnotization depends on the solubility of the agent: the same degree of hypoventilation is more likely to cause rehypnotization with the more soluble agent [48]. It is unlikely that release of inhaled anaesthetic from the FG can contribute to this rehypnotization phenomenon, because it cannot release enough inhaled anaesthetic due to its poor perfusion.

Nitrous oxide

N_2O, the shortest-acting agent available to anaesthesia providers, also continues to be used in this challenging population. Even in the non-obese patient, clinical opinion on the use of N_2O differs widely and is shrouded in belief and mystery rather than science. Let us give a few examples of these unsubstantiated claims. Bowel distension during relatively short bariatric procedures is unsupported [49].

The Enigma II trial proved N_2O to be safe during non-cardiac surgery: there was no increase in mortality or wound infections [50]. It also demonstrated that nausea and vomiting can be controlled with antiemetic prophylaxis, and consumption of potent inhaled anaesthetics is reduced [50,51]. The impact of the second gas effect during induction and reverse second gas effect during emergence have been underestimated because researchers have long failed to consider F_a rather than F_A of the concomitantly administered potent inhaled agent [52,53]. In the non-obese patient, the second gas effect improves oxygenation compared to the use of O_2/air mixtures used at the same F_IO_2 [54], but data in the obese patient are lacking. N_2O did not aggravate the haemodynamic consequences of a CO_2 embolism in pigs during laparoscopic surgery [55]. The reverse second gas effect of N_2O [53], higher MAC$_{awake}$ [56], and antagonistic effect on MAC$_{awake}$ [57,58] may all help shorten wake-up times. Still, surprisingly little information is available on the use of N_2O in the obese patient.

Conclusion

MAC does not differ between obese and non-obese patients. Contrary to its effect on intravenous anaesthetics, obesity only modestly affects kinetics of inhaled anaesthetics. These counterintuitive findings underscore the fact that clinical studies rather than belief and intuition should guide the clinician in the choice of drugs and techniques. As clinical differences between desflurane and sevoflurane are small and long-term outcome data are lacking, there is currently no clear evidence to support one agent or technique over another. A proper understanding of decrement times, hysteresis, and isoboles (drug interactions) are particularly useful to help titrate inhaled agents. The manner in which we use these drugs may be more important than the choice of agent.

REFERENCES

1. Janmahasatian S, Duffull SB, Ash S, Ward LC, Byrne NM, Green B. Quantification of lean bodyweight. Clin Pharmacokinet. 2005;44(10):1051–65.
2. Shibutani K, Inchiosa Jr MA, Sawada K, Bairamian M. Accuracy of pharmacokinetic models for predicting plasma fentanyl

concentrations in lean and obese surgical patients: derivation of dosing weight ('pharmacokinetic mass'). Anesthesiology. 2004;**101**(3):603–13.

3. Tabo E, Ohkuma Y, Sakuragi Y, Arai T. [MAC-awake and wake-up time of isoflurane and sevoflurane with reference to the concentration of gas, duration of inhalation and patient's age and obesity]. Masui. 1995;**44**(2):188–92.

4. Cortínez LI, Gambús P, Trocóniz IF, Echevarría G, Muñoz HR. Obesity does not influence the onset and offset of sevoflurane effect as measured by the hysteresis between sevoflurane concentration and bispectral index. Anesth Analg. 2011;**113**(1):70–76.

5. Katoh T, Ikeda K. The effects of fentanyl on sevoflurane requirements for loss of consciousness and skin incision. Anesthesiology. 1998;**88**(1):18–24.

6. Katoh T, Kobayashi S, Suzuki A, Iwamoto T, Bito H, Ikeda K. The effect of fentanyl on sevoflurane requirements for somatic and sympathetic responses to surgical incision. Anesthesiology. 1999;**90**(2):398–405.

7. Katoh T, Nakajima Y, Moriwaki G, Kobayashi S, Suzuki A, Iwamoto T, et al. Sevoflurane requirements for tracheal intubation with and without fentanyl. Br J Anaesth. 1999;**82**(4):561–65.

8. Katoh T, Uchiyama T, Ikeda K. Effect of fentanyl on awakening concentration of sevoflurane. Br J Anaesth. 1994;**73**(3):322–25.

9. Feld JM, Hoffman WE, Stechert MM, Hoffman IW, Ananda RC. Fentanyl or dexmedetomidine combined with desflurane for bariatric surgery. J Clin Anesth. 2006;**18**(1):24–28.

10. Tufanogullari B, White PF, Peixoto MP, Kianpour D, Lacour T, Griffin J, et al. Dexmedetomidine infusion during laparoscopic bariatric surgery: the effect on recovery outcome variables. Anesth Analg. 2008;**106**(6):1741–48.

11. Eger EI, Saidman LJ. Illustrations of inhaled anesthetic uptake, including intertissue diffusion to and from fat. Anesth Analg. 2005;**100**(4):1020–33.

12. Wakamatsu T, Hiromi R, Kato S. [Anesthetic management of morbidly obese patients using inhalation induction with high concentrations of sevoflurane]. Masui. 2005;**54**(7):791–93.

13. Esper T, Wehner M, Meinecke CD, Rueffert H. Blood/gas partition coefficients for isoflurane, sevoflurane, and desflurane in a clinically relevant patient population. Anesth Analg. 2015;**120**(1):45–50.

14. Eger RR, Eger 2nd EI. Effect of temperature and age on the solubility of enflurane, halothane, isoflurane, and methoxyflurane in human blood. Anesth Analg. 1985;**64**(6):640–42.

15. Lockwood GG, Sapsed-Byrne SM, Smith MA. Effect of temperature on the solubility of desflurane, sevoflurane, enflurane and halothane in blood. Br J Anaesth. 1997;**79**(4):517–20.

16. Lerman J, Gregory GA, Willis MM, Eger 2nd EI. Age and solubility of volatile anesthetics in blood. Anesthesiology. 1984;**61**(2):139–43.

17. Malviya S, Lerman J. The blood/gas solubilities of sevoflurane, isoflurane, halothane, and serum constituent concentrations in neonates and adults. Anesthesiology. 1990;**72**(5):793–96.

18. Hu P, Zhou JX, Liu J. Blood solubilities of volatile anesthetics in cardiac patients. J Cardiothorac Vasc Anesth. 2001;**15**(5):560–62.

19. Stelfox HT, Ahmed SB, Ribeiro RA, Gettings EM, Pomerantsev E, Schmidt U. Hemodynamic monitoring in obese patients: the impact of body mass index on cardiac output and stroke volume. Crit Care Med. 2006;**34**(4):1243–46.

20. Collis T, Devereux RB, Roman MJ, de Simone G, Yeh J, Howard BV, et al. Relations of stroke volume and cardiac output to body composition: the strong heart study. Circulation. 2001;**103**(6):820–25.

21. Alpert MA. Obesity cardiomyopathy: pathophysiology and evolution of the clinical syndrome. Am J Med Sci. 2001;**321**(4):225–36.

22. Van Zundert T, Hendrickx J, Brebels A, De Cooman S, Gatt S, De Wolf A. Effect of the mode of administration of inhaled anaesthetics on the interpretation of the F(A)/F(I) curve—a GasMan simulation. Anaesth Intensive Care. 2010;**38**(1):76–81.

23. Lesser GT, Deutsch S. Measurement of adipose tissue blood flow and perfusion in man by uptake of 85Kr. J Appl Physiol. 1967;**23**(5):621–30.

24. Summers LK, Samra JS, Humphreys SM, Morris RJ, Frayn KN. Subcutaneous abdominal adipose tissue blood flow: variation within and between subjects and relationship to obesity. Clin Sci (Lond). 1996;**91**(6):679–83.

25. Wang J, Gallagher D, Thornton JC, Yu W, Weil R, Kovac B, et al. Regional body volumes, BMI, waist circumference, and percentage fat in severely obese adults. Obesity (Silver Spring). 2007;**15**(11):2688–98.

26. Yasuda N, Lockhart SH, Eger EI, Weiskopf RB, Johnson BH, Freire BA, et al. Kinetics of desflurane, isoflurane, and halothane in humans. Anesthesiology. 1991;**74**(3):489–98.

27. Yasuda N, Lockhart SH, Eger EI, Weiskopf RB, Liu J, Laster M, et al. Comparison of kinetics of sevoflurane and isoflurane in humans. Anesth Analg. 1991;**72**(3):316–24.

28. Levitt DG. Heterogeneity of human adipose blood flow. BMC Clin Pharmacol. 2007;**7**(1):1.

29. Porhomayon J, Papadakos P, Singh A, Nader ND. Alteration in respiratory physiology in obesity for anesthesia-critical care physician. HSR Proc Intensive Care Cardiovasc Anesth. 2011;**3**(2):109–18.

30. Sprung J, Whalen FX, Comfere T, Bosnjak ZJ, Bajzer Z, Gajic O, et al. Alveolar recruitment and arterial desflurane concentration during bariatric surgery. Anesth Analg. 2009;**108**(1):120–27.

31. Martin JL, Plevak DJ, Flannery KD, Charlton M, Poterucha JJ, Humphreys CE, et al. Hepatotoxicity after desflurane anesthesia. Anesthesiology. 1995;**83**(5):1125–29.

32. Behne M, Wilke HJ, Harder S. Clinical pharmacokinetics of sevoflurane. Clin Pharmacokinet. 1999;**36**(1):13–26.

33. Higuchi H, Satoh T, Arimura S, Kanno M, Endoh R. Serum inorganic fluoride levels in mildly obese patients during and after sevoflurane anesthesia. Anesth Analg. 1993;**77**(5):1018–21.

34. Bailey JM. Context-sensitive half-times and other decrement times of inhaled anesthetics. Anesth Analg. 1997;**85**(3):681–86.

35. Eger EI, Shafer S. The complexity of recovery from anesthesia. J Clin Anesth. 2005;**17**(6):411–12.

36. Macario A, Dexter F, Lubarsky D. Meta-analysis of trials comparing postoperative recovery after anesthesia with sevoflurane or desflurane. Am J Health Syst Pharm. 2005;**62**(1):63–68.

37. Eger 2nd EI, Shafer SL. Tutorial: context-sensitive decrement times for inhaled anesthetics. Anesth Analg. 2005;**101**(3):688–96.

38. Liu F-L, Cherng Y-G, Chen S-Y, Su Y-H, Huang S-Y, Lo P-H, et al. Postoperative recovery after anesthesia in morbidly obese patients: a systematic review and meta-analysis of randomized controlled trials. Can J Anaesth. 2015;**62**(8):907–17.

39. Arain SR, Barth CD, Shankar H, Ebert TJ. Choice of volatile anesthetic for the morbidly obese patient: sevoflurane or desflurane. J Clin Anesth. 2005;**17**(6):413–19.

40. Vallejo MC, Sah N, Phelps AL, O'Donnell J, Romeo RC. Desflurane versus sevoflurane for laparoscopic gastroplasty in morbidly obese patients. J Clin Anesth. 2007;**19**(1):3–8.

41. La Colla G, La Colla L, Turi S, Poli D, Albertin A, Pasculli N, et al. Effect of morbid obesity on kinetic of desflurane wash-in wash-out curves and recovery times. Minerva Anestesiol. 2007;**73**(5):275–79.

42. Casati A, Marchetti C, Spreafico E, Mamo D. Effects of obesity on wash-in and wash-out kinetics of sevoflurane. Eur J Anaesthesiol. 2004;**21**(3):243–45.

43. Lemmens HJM, Saidman LJ, Eger EI, Laster MJ. Obesity modestly affects inhaled anesthetic kinetics in humans. Anesth Analg. 2008;**107**(6):1864–70.

44. Weber J, Eberhart L, Philip JH. Context-sensitive decrement times for inhaled anesthetics in obese patients. ESA 2016 Annual Meeting abstract 01AP13-5. 2016. http://journals.lww.com/ejanaesthesiology/Documents/ESA2016_LOW.pdf

45. McKay RE, Malhotra A, Cakmakkaya OS, Hall KT, McKay WR, Apfel CC. Effect of increased body mass index and anaesthetic duration on recovery of protective airway reflexes after sevoflurane vs desflurane. Br J Anaesth. 2010;**104**(2):175–82.

46. Katznelson R, Naughton F, Friedman Z, Lei D, Duppin J, Fedorko L, et al. Increased lung clearance of isoflurane shortens emergence in obesity: a prospective randomized-controlled trial. Acta Anaesthesiol Scand. 2011;**55**(8):995–1001.

47. Leeson S, Roberson RS, Philip JH. Hypoventilation after inhaled anesthesia results in reanesthetization. Anesth Analg. 2014;**119**(4):829–35.

48. De Wolf AM, Van Zundert TC, De Cooman S, Hendrickx JF. Theoretical effect of hyperventilation on speed of recovery and risk of rehypnotization following recovery—a GasMan® simulation. BMC Anesthesiol. 2012;**12**(1):22.

49. Brodsky JB, Lemmens HJ, Collins JS, Morton JM, Curet MJ, Brock-Utne JG, et al. Nitrous oxide and laparoscopic bariatric surgery. Obes Surg. 2005;**15**(4):494–96.

50. Myles PS, Leslie K, Chan MT V, Forbes A, Peyton PJ, Paech MJ, et al. The safety of addition of nitrous oxide to general anaesthesia in at-risk patients having major non-cardiac surgery (ENIGMA-II): a randomised, single-blind trial. Lancet. 2014;**384**(9952):1446–54.

51. Myles PS, Chan MT, Kasza J, Paech MJ, Leslie K, Peyton PJ, et al. Severe nausea and vomiting in the Evaluation of Nitrous Oxide in the Gas Mixture for Anesthesia II Trial. Anesthesiology. 2016;**124**(5):1032–40.

52. Peyton PJ, Chao I, Weinberg L, Robinson GJB, Thompson BR. Nitrous oxide diffusion and the second gas effect on emergence from anesthesia. Anesthesiology. 2011;**114**(3):596–602.

53. Peyton PJ, Horriat M, Robinson GJ, Pierce R, Thompson BR. Magnitude of the second gas effect on arterial sevoflurane partial pressure. Anesthesiology. 2008;**108**(3):381–87.

54. Peyton PJ, Stuart-Andrews C, Deo K, Strahan F, Robinson GJB, Thompson BR, et al. Persisting concentrating and second gas effects on oxygenation during N2O anaesthesia. Anaesthesia. 2006;**61**(4):322–29.

55. Diemunsch PA, Noll E, Pottecher J, Diana M, Geny B, Joshi GP. Impact of nitrous oxide on the haemodynamic consequences of venous carbon dioxide embolism: An experimental study. Eur J Anaesthesiol. 2016;**33**(5):356–60.

56. Eger EI II. Age, minimum alveolar anesthetic concentration, and minimum alveolar anesthetic concentration-awake. Anesth Analg. 2001;**93**(4):947–53.

57. Katoh T, Ikeda K, Bito H. Does nitrous oxide antagonize sevoflurane-induced hypnosis? Br J Anaesth. 1997;**79**(4):465–68.

58. Chortkoff BS, Bennett HL, Eger EI 2nd. Does nitrous oxide antagonize isoflurane-induced suppression of learning? Anesthesiology 1993;**79**(4):724–32.

7

Neuromuscular blocking agents in obesity

Ajintha Pathmanathan and Paul Stewart

Introduction

In the early 1500s, Spanish Conquistadors observed the effects of the arrow poison used in hunting by the South Americans Indians. However, it was not until the 1800s that the poison was identified as curare and research commenced into its use in animals and humans to cause temporary paralysis. In 1942, Griffith and Johnson reported the use of extract of curare to improve surgical conditions in 25 patients. It was also the first paper recording the use of neuromuscular blockade in obese patients to obtain satisfactory surgical conditions. They concluded it was a potentially dangerous poison that should be used only by experienced anaesthesiologists in well-equipped operating rooms [1,2].

Today, we have an extensive understanding of neuromuscular transmission, neuromuscular diseases, pharmacological blocking agents, and reversal of these agents. However, there is still a relative paucity of data in the obese patient cohort, an area of medicine which is receiving increased attention due to the high prevalence of obesity.

Mechanism of neuromuscular transmission

Muscle contraction occurs in response to the high-frequency transmission of electrical signals from the motor cortex and spinal cord down the axon and motor nerve to the nerve end plate (Fig. 7.1). Depolarization allows influx of calcium through voltage-gated calcium channels on the presynaptic surface. The calcium released triggers the fusion of the several hundred acetylcholine vesicles to the presynaptic membrane and release of acetylcholine (approximately 5000 molecules) into the synaptic cleft [3].

The acetylcholine diffuses across the synaptic cleft to bind to the post-junctional pentameric transmembrane nicotinic receptor. Simultaneous occupation of the two alpha subunits of the acetylcholine receptor by acetylcholine molecules results in conformational change and transient (1 ms) opening of the ion channel in the core of the receptor. Predominantly sodium and some calcium ions flow through the activated core of the receptor resulting in a rise in the end-plate potential. A potential that cumulatively exceeds the threshold eventually results in an action potential. The sodium-gated voltage channels propagate the action potential along the muscle membrane via a T-tubule system. Calcium ions released from the sarcoplasmic reticulum diffuse into the myofibril resulting in contraction of the muscle fibre.

The concomitant efflux of potassium ions via a separate potassium channel results in end-plate repolarization and detachment of the acetylcholine molecules. These molecules are rapidly hydrolysed into acetyl and choline by the acetylcholinesterase enzyme in the synaptic clefts.

Pre-junctional modulation of acetylcholine release occurs via muscarinic, M_1 (facilitatory) and M_2 (inhibitory) receptors via calcium influx modulation. The pre-junctional nicotinic receptors act via a positive feedback mechanism to increase mobilization of acetylcholine prior to release.

Neuromuscular blocking agents

The commonly used neuromuscular blocking used in anaesthesia practice inhibits acetylcholine action by either agonistic (depolarizing) or antagonistic (non-depolarizing) effects at the post-junctional receptors, preventing muscle contraction (Table 7.1).

Clinical use of paralysis and neuromuscular blocking agents

The modern concept of balanced anaesthesia was first described by Gray and Halton in 1946 as the triad of narcosis, analgesia, and muscle relaxation—the Liverpool technique [4]. Although introduction of the laryngeal mask airway in 1988 by Dr A Brain from the United Kingdom has reduced the need for endotracheal intubation, in many cases paralysis is fundamental to the current practice of anaesthesia.

Paralysis can improve ventilation characteristics and the oxygen balance in patients with high oxygen consumption such as the obese and critically ill patients. Appropriate depth of blockade also minimizes the haemodynamic effects by a reduction in the dose of general anaesthetic agents [5].

Neuromuscular blockade is also used to facilitate intubation and optimize the surgical operating conditions.

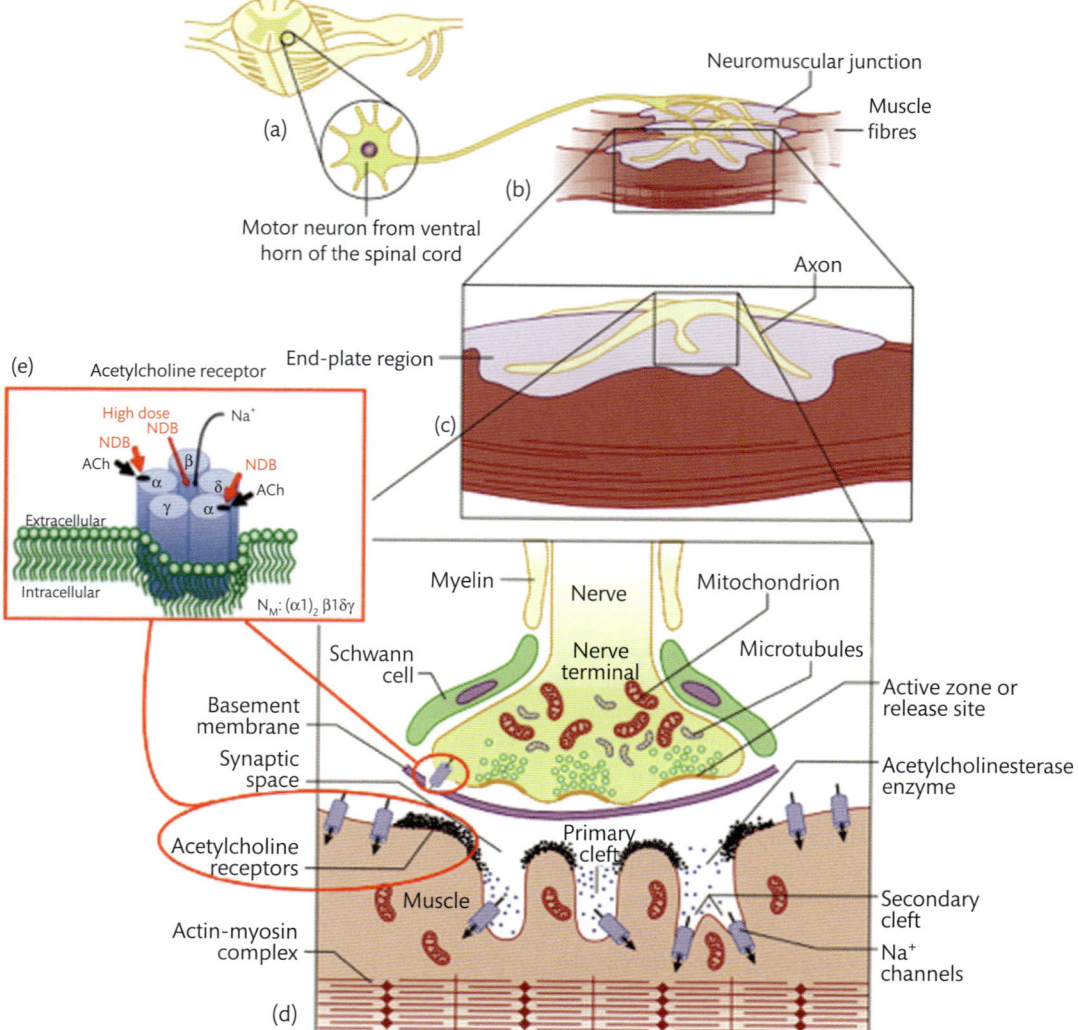

Fig. 7.1 The structure of the adult neuromuscular junction shows three cells that constitute the synapse: the motor neuron (nerve terminal), muscle fibre. (a) The motor nerve arises from the ventral horn of the spinal cord or brainstem. (b) As the nerve divides into branches that innervate individual muscle fibres, (c) each muscle fibre receives only one synapse. The motor nerve further subdivides into numerous presynaptic boutons to terminate on the surface of the muscle fibre. (d) The nerve terminals have vesicles containing acetylcholine clustered in the active zone. The synaptic cleft separates the nerve terminal from the corrugated muscle surface. Dense areas on the shoulders of each fold contain the nicotinic acetylcholine receptors. Sodium (Na^+) channels are present at the bottom of the clefts and throughout the muscle membrane. (e) The acetylcholine receptor is a nicotinic receptor with five subunits. Acetylcholine attaches simultaneously on the two alpha subunits to allow conformational change and influx of cations (Na^+ and Ca^{++}). Non-depolarising blockers prevent acetylcholine from acting at the receptor.

Facilitation of intubation

The use of neuromuscular blockade has been shown to decrease the incidence of difficult intubation by 12–20% [6,7]. Neuromuscular block has been widely recognized to facilitate face mask ventilation, increase chest compliance, abolish laryngeal reflexes, improve visualization of the vocal cords, limit resistance to the laryngoscope, and decrease the frequency of adverse events after intubation such as postoperative hoarseness and laryngeal haematomas [8,9].

Rapid sequence intubation

Since 1961, the rapid sequence technique defined by Sellick using succinylcholine remains in use to prevent gastric aspiration during intubation. A dose of 1–1.5 mg/kg total body weight (TBW) as opposed to ideal body weight (IBW) has been shown to result in more profound and reliable neuromuscular blockade [10].

The advent of rocuronium in the late 1990s saw a number of comparative studies due to its rapid onset and cleaner side effect profile. Succinylcholine has been shown to consistently provide excellent intubating conditions when compared to a standard dose of rocuronium (0.6 mg/kg). There may not be a significant difference with use of high-dose rocuronium (1.2 mg/kg) [11–13].

The introduction of sugammadex enabled rapid reversal of any depth of rocuronium-induced neuromuscular blockade [14,15]. As seen in **Fig. 7.2**, 16 mg/kg of sugammadex can reverse intense neuromuscular blockade 3 minutes after paralysis is induced by rocuronium 1.2 mg/kg more rapidly than with the spontaneous recovery of suxamethonium.

Table 7.1 Commonly used neuromuscular blocks

Name	Compound and properties	Elimination	Onset/duration/dose	Adverse effects
Depolarizing				
Succinylcholine	Dicholine ester of succinic acid (two acetylcholine molecules joined together)	Plasma cholinesterase	Rapid onset: 30–60 s Ultra-short duration: 5–10 min Adult dose: 1–2 mg/kg IV (TBW)	Myalgia Anaphylaxis Hyperkalaemia Sinoatrial nodal block (bradycardia) Malignant Hyperthermia ↑ intragastric, ↑ intracranial, and ↑ intraocular pressure Prolonged paralysis
Non-depolarizing				
Mivacurium	Benzylisoquinoline	Plasma cholinesterase	Slow/short Dose: 0.2–0.25 mg/kg IV (IBW)	Histamine release
Rocuronium	Aminosteroid. Analogue of vecuronium and 6–8× less potent	No metabolism. Hepatic/renal	Rapid/intermediate Adult dose: 0.6 mg/kg IV (IBW) Rapid sequence induction: 1.2 mg/kg IV *Reversal = sugammadex*	Anaphylaxis
Vecuronium	Aminosteroid similar to pancuronium but minus a quaternary methyl group	Hepatic/renal Active metabolite	Slow/intermediate duration Adult dose: 0.08–0.12 mg/kg IV (IBW) *Reversal = sugammadex*	Bradycardia
Cisatracurium	Benzylisoquinoline Stereoisomer of atracurium. Four times as potent	Hofmann elimination. Inactive metabolites	Slow/intermediate Adult dose: 0.1–0.15 mg/kg IV (IBW) for intubation, maintenance infusion 1–2 mcg/kg/min	Laudanosine-related seizure (less than atracurium) No significant histamine release Cardiovascular stability
Atracurium	Benzylisoquinoline	Non-specific esterases and Hofmann degradation	Slow onset. Intermediate duration Dose: 0.3–0.6 mg/kg IV (IBW)	Dose-dependent histamine release. Hypotension and tachycardia. Bronchospasm. Laudanosine-related seizure
Pancuronium	Aminosteroid	Hepatic/renal	Slow/long Dose: 0.1 mg/kg IV (IBW)	Catecholamine release causing hypertension, tachycardia, ventricular arrhythmias, vagal blockade. Allergic reaction if hypersensitive to bromides

IV, intravenous.

Deep or intense neuromuscular blockade

As seen in **Fig. 7.3**, the depth of blockade is defined by the response to either train-of-four (TOF) stimulation or post-tetanic count (PTC) [16].

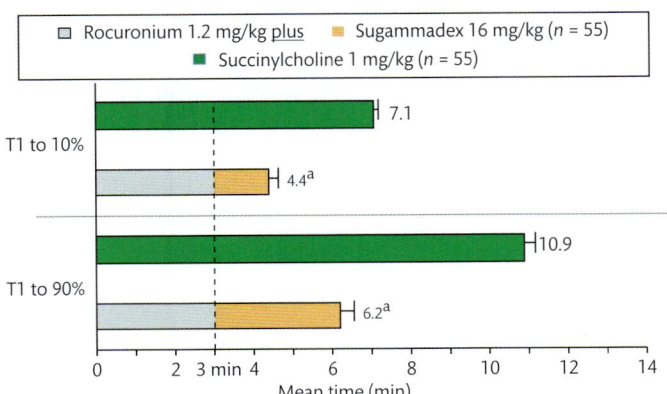

a P<0.001 vs succinylcholine treatment group; results based on intent-to-treat population.

Fig. 7.2 Time to reverse intense blockade induced by rocuronium with sugammadex compared to the spontaneous recovery from blockade induced with succinylcholine.

Source: Data from Lee, C., Jahr, J. S., Candiotti, K. A. et al. Reversal of profound neuromuscular block by sugammadex administered three minutes after rocuronium: a comparison with spontaneous recovery from succinylcholine. *Anesthesiology*, 110:1020–5, 2009.

Use of deep neuromuscular blockade in certain laparoscopic procedures may improve surgical conditions. In open abdominal surgery, neuromuscular blockade will improve surgical conditions [17]. The debate as to whether deep neuromuscular blockade decreases length of stay and improves patient or surgical outcomes continues [18,19]. There is some evidence in laparoscopic surgery that lower peritoneal pressures may decrease postoperative pain, including shoulder tip pain [20,21].

Dosing of neuromuscular blockers and reversal agents in obese patients

It is well known, however, that pharmacokinetic and pharmacodynamic features differ in obese patients. Obese individuals have increased cardiac output, increased volume of central and peripheral compartments, increased adiposity, increased lean body weight, liver and kidney abnormalities, increased splanchnic blood flow, and changes in plasma protein concentration and functional binding.

The suggested scalar for dosing of succinylcholine in morbidly obese patients is TBW for rapid sequence induction as plasma cholinesterase concentrations and volume of extracellular fluid are increased in obese patients [22]. The current evidence suggests IBW be used as a scalar for appropriate dosing of all non-depolarizing neuromuscular blockers and reversal agents. Use of TBW has been shown

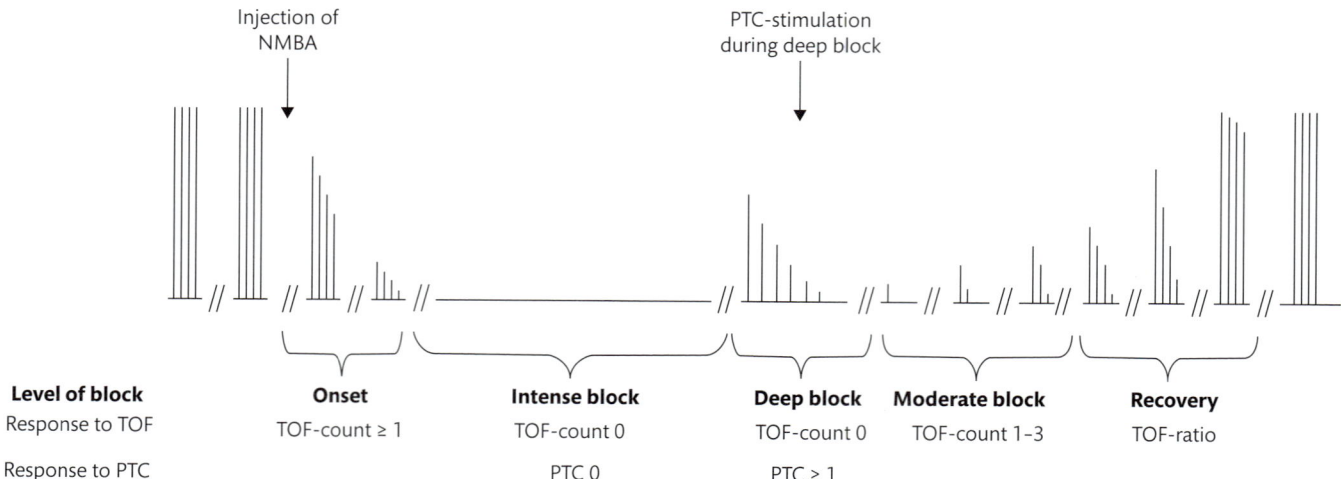

Levels of block after a normal intubating dose of a non-depolarizing neuromuscular blocking agent (NMBA), as classified using post-tetanic count (PTC) and train-of-four (TOF) stimulation. During intense (profound) block, there are no responses to either TOF or PTC stimulation. During deep block, there is response to PTC, but not to TOF stimulation. Intense (profound) block and deep block together constitutes the 'Period of no response to TOF stimulation'. The reappearance of the response to TOF stimulation heralds the start of moderate block. Finally, when all four responses to TOF stimulation are present and a TOF ratio can be measured, the recovery period has started.

Fig. 7.3 Classification of the depth of neuromuscular blockade.

Adapted with permission from Viby-Mogensen, J., Mirakhur, R.K., Eriksson, L. I., et al. Good clinical research practice in pharmacodynamic studies of neuromuscular blocking agents II: the Stockholm revision. *Acta Anaesthesiologica Scandinavica*, 51(7): 789–808. Copyright © 2007 John Wiley and Sons. DOI: 10.1111/j.1399-6576.1996.tb04389.x

to significantly increase the duration of action of non-depolarizing blockers [23–26].

However, with the use of quantitative neuromuscular monitoring and availability of sugammadex as a reversal agent, the dose of rocuronium and vecuronium can be titrated to required depth, as rapid and complete reversal is now possible.

The other non-depolarizing neuromuscular agents need to be used with additional caution as neostigmine cannot reverse deep neuromuscular blockade. Neostigmine has a ceiling effect due to maximal inhibition of acetylcholinesterase at doses of 70 mcg/kg, not exceeding a total dose of 5 mg [22]. Specifically, in obese patients, neostigmine has been shown to have a fourfold increase in time to achieve a TOF of 0.9 compared with normal-weight individuals [27].

Monitoring neuromuscular blockade

Neuromuscular monitoring provides key information in order to refine all stages of the management of neuromuscular blockade. This is essential in obese patients who have varying pharmacokinetics, pharmacodynamics, increased incidence of obstructive sleep apnoea, and higher risk of upper airway obstruction.

Guidelines published by anaesthesia societies from the Czech Republic, the United Kingdom, France, and Australia, recommend routine and preferably quantitative neuromuscular function monitoring [28–30]. The Association of Anaesthetists of Great Britain and Ireland introduced guidelines in 2016 stating that quantification of neuromuscular blockade 'is essential for all stages of anaesthesia when neuromuscular blockade drugs are administered. This is best monitored using an objective, quantitative peripheral nerve stimulator' [29]. Monitoring can be divided into five specific

phases. On induction prior to administration of neuromuscular blocking agents, prior to intubation, maintenance of blockade, assessment of blockade prior to reversal, and confirmation of adequacy of recovery (**Fig. 7.4**).

1. *Prior to induction of neuromuscular blockade*. Calibration should be performed during the induction of anaesthesia but prior to the administration of the muscle relaxant. This is important to establish the current required to produce a supramaximal stimulation and to confirm that the equipment is functioning.

2. *Assessment prior to intubation*. Adequate depth of neuromuscular blockade will reduce the incidence of difficult intubations [7]. Due to interindividual variability of onset of blockade, confirmation of depth of neuromuscular blockade should be confirmed prior to an attempt at intubation.

3. *Monitoring during maintenance of blockade*. Monitoring of blockade during this period will allow titration of the muscle relaxant bolus' or infusions to provide constant levels of blockade and consistent surgical conditions. Madsen et al. performed a systematic review and found support for deep blockade improves surgical conditions when compared to moderate blockade [16,17].

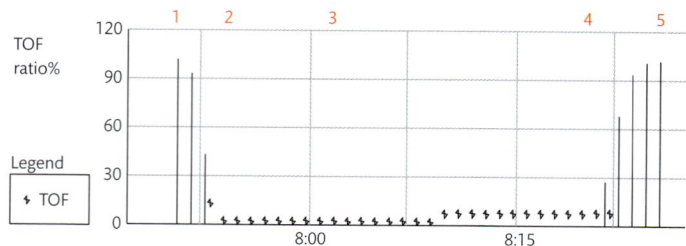

Fig. 7.4 Phases of monitoring neuromuscular blockade.

4. *Assessment of blockade prior to reversal.* It is essential to assess the depth of blockade to select the appropriate reversal agent and the dosage.

5. *Confirmation of adequacy of reversal.* Confirmation of a TOF ratio (TOFR) of greater than 0.9 can only be performed with a quantitative neuromuscular function monitor to exclude the adverse effects of residual neuromuscular blockade.

Neostigmine may cause muscle weakness if administered after full recovery from neuromuscular blockade [31]. It has been suggested that 20 mcg/kg rather than 60–70 mcg/kg of neostigmine can be administered if four twitches are present with no fade on TOF monitoring to reduce the potential of neostigmine-induced muscle weakness.

Clinical signs

Traditional teaching led anaesthesiologists to use clinical signs to time extubation and exclude residual neuromuscular blockade. However, signs such as sustained eye opening, 5-second head lift, protrusion of the tongue, arm lift to the opposite shoulder, sustained tongue depressor test, sustained handgrip for 5 seconds, sustained leg lift for 5 seconds, normal tidal volume, and vital capacity are insensitive and cannot exclude residual neuromuscular blockade [32].

Many of these signs require an awake, cooperative, and, in some cases, an already extubated patient. The limitations of solely using clinical signs is not only the impracticality but evidence suggesting this practice would place patients at risk of upper airway obstruction, aspiration, postoperative pulmonary complications, and increased morbidity and mortality [33,34].

Furthermore, it may be possible to perform all these tests in a poorly reversed patient with a TOFR of less than 0.9 and in some individuals at a TOFR of 0.4 [35]. A reason why this occurs is because the pharyngeal and upper airway muscles responsible for maintenance of the opening of the airway and coordination of swallowing are particularly sensitive to the effects of neuromuscular blocking agents and are the last to recover [36,37]. Therefore, a patient may be able to breath, because the diaphragm is the most resistant muscle to relaxants and the first to recover but experience upper airway obstruction due to weakness of the pharyngeal muscles. Evidence suggests that respiratory and upper airway function do not return to normal unless the TOFR, measured by quantitative monitors (mechanomyography or electromyography) at the adductor pollicis, is at least 0.9.

Therefore, clinical signs are not a useful indicator of adequate recovery of neuromuscular function.

Which muscles to monitor?

Commonly, the ulnar nerve is stimulated and the response is assessed by the evoked response at the first dorsal interosseous muscle, abductor digiti minimi, or the adductor pollicis. These muscle groups may recover up to 30 minutes after the recovery of the diaphragm but are slower to recover than the pharyngeal muscle (**Fig. 7.5**) [38]. Therefore, this is a relatively safe muscle to monitor and easily accessible.

Stimulation of the facial nerve and monitoring of the facial muscles (the orbicularis oculi and corrugator supercilii) can lead to overdosing of the muscle relaxant or even to premature extubation

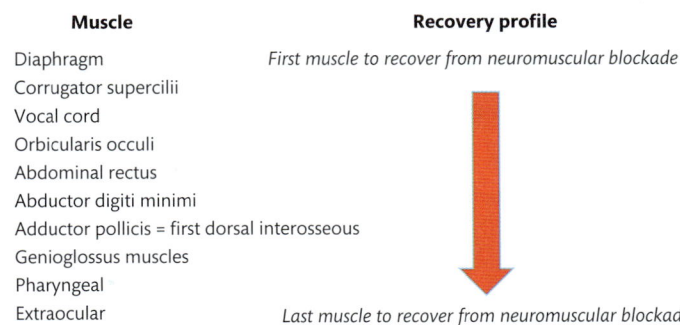

Muscle	Recovery profile
Diaphragm	*First muscle to recover from neuromuscular blockade*
Corrugator supercilii	
Vocal cord	
Orbicularis occuli	
Abdominal rectus	
Abductor digiti minimi	
Adductor pollicis = first dorsal interosseous	
Genioglossus muscles	
Pharyngeal	
Extraocular	*Last muscle to recover from neuromuscular blockade*

Fig. 7.5 Recovery profile of different muscle groups.

Adapted from Phillips, S., Stewart, P.A., Freelander, N., Heller, G., Comparison of evoked electromyography in three muscles of the hand during recovery from non-depolarising neuromuscular blockade. *Anaesthesia and Intensive Care*, 40(4): 690–696. Copyright © 2012 SAGE. https://doi.org/10.1177/0310057X1204000416

because these muscles, like the diaphragm, are more resistant and recover earlier than the pharyngeal muscles [39]. Unfortunately, the facial muscles may also be stimulated directly and result in inaccurate assessment of the depth of neuromuscular blockade [40].

Neuromuscular monitoring

Neuromuscular monitors can be classified into subjective/qualitative stimulators or objective/quantitative monitors. Subjective monitors are the conventional peripheral nerve stimulators where the response to stimulation is evaluated by visual or tactile means. The quantitative monitors are mechanomyography, kinemyography, electromyography, or acceleromyography (AMG), providing a numeric output of the TOFR and twitch height.

The most useful modes of stimulation used are listed in **Table 7.2** [41–43]. The depth of blockade can be assessed using TOF stimuli and the PTC.

Quantitative neuromuscular monitoring

Mechanomyography

In response to stimulation of the ulnar nerve, a force transducer is used to measure the response at the adductor pollicis. It has been used for research and is not available commercially.

Electromyography

This monitor (**Fig. 7.6**) is viewed by some as an alternative gold standard to mechanomyography. When the supramaximal stimulus at any muscle group is determined, a characteristic biphasic waveform can be confirmed on the monitor. This biphasic waveform disappears with the onset of the muscle relaxant.

Acceleromyography

AMG is available for use in clinical practice. A small piezoelectric crystal generates a voltage related to the acceleration of the muscle being stimulated. Based on Newton's law (force = mass × acceleration), the force can be calculated. AMG TOFRs recover earlier than those ratios determined by electromyography and mechanomyography. Therefore, residual neuromuscular blockade may not be excluded until sometime after the TOFR reaches 1.0.

Table 7.2 The most useful modes of stimulation

Type of stimulus	Acceptable outcome	Comments
Single-twitch stimulus	Quantitative baseline assessment	Single twitch each second (1 Hz) is used when determining the supramaximal stimulation current and also to determine the PTC after the application of a tetanic stimulus
Double-burst stimulation (DBS) 2–3 short bursts of 50 Hz tetanic stimuli of 2–3 impulses (separated by 750 ms interval)	Visual or tactile. No palpable fade	An experienced anaesthesiologist is unable to detect fade with DBS at TOFR of >0.6. Not suitable to exclude residual neuromuscular blockade
Train of four (TOF) 4 stimuli at 2 Hz (every 2 s) at intervals of >12 s	Visual or tactile. Measurement of fade—qualitative (visual) or quantitative (TOF ratio)	Qualitative fade by experienced anaesthesiologists cannot be determined at TOFR >0.4. Useful as a gauge for depth of blockade. Not suitable to exclude residual neuromuscular blockade. Quantitative measurement confirming TOFR >0.9 is required to exclude residual neuromuscular blockade prior to extubation
PTC Counting the number of responses when a sequence of ST stimulation at 1 Hz is applied for 20 s following a 5 s, 50 Hz tetanus	Visual or tactile. Quantitative count	Extremely painful (patients need to be anaesthetized). TOF or additional PTC cannot be used for another 3–5 min due to increased acetylcholine (false positive). This may result in early extubation or administration of excessive amounts of muscle relaxant [40–42]

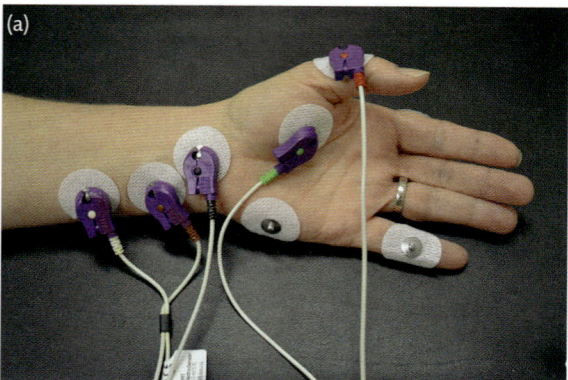

Adductor pollicis (EMG-AP)

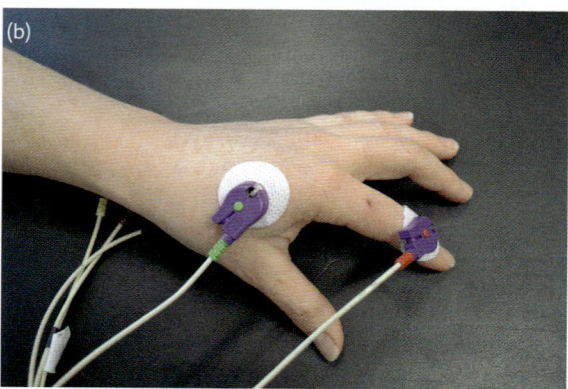

First dorsal interosseous (EMG-FDI)

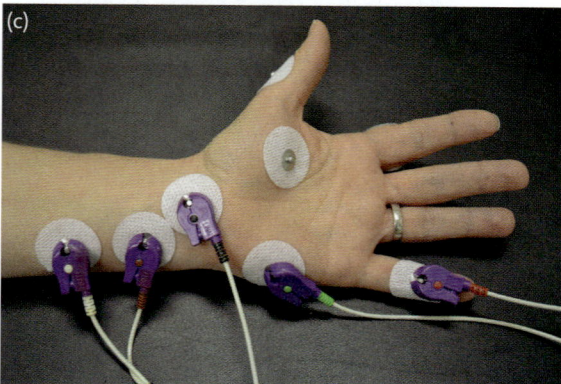

Abductor digiti minimi (EMG-ADM)

Fig. 7.6 Electromyography at (a) adductor pollicis, (b) first dorsal interosseous muscle, and (c) abductor digiti minimi.

Adapted from Phillips, S., Stewart, P.A., Freelander, N., Heller, G., Comparison of evoked electromyography in three muscles of the hand during recovery from non-depolarising neuromuscular blockade. *Anaesthesia and Intensive Care*, 40(4): 690–696. Copyright © 2012 SAGE. https://doi.org/10.1177/0310057X1204000416

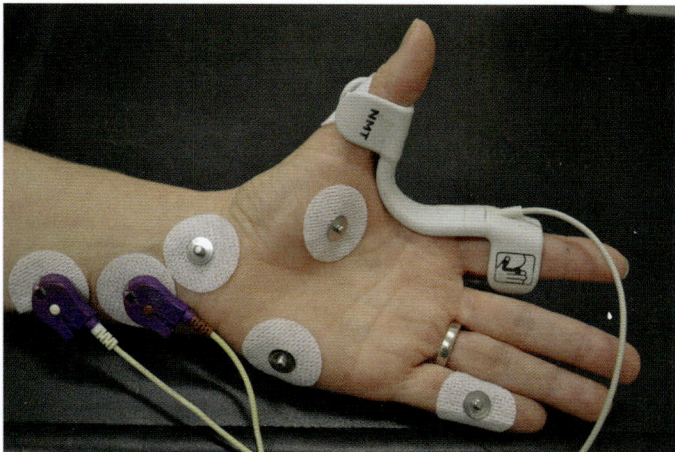

Fig. 7.7 Kinemyographic measurement of muscle contraction following stimulation of the ulnar nerve.

There are a number of devices used to record AMG and each has different characteristics. The TOF-Watch SX® (Organon, Ireland) and the Stimpod™ (Xavant Technology, Pretoria, South Africa) may provide a baseline recording of 150% or more in the absence of neuromuscular blocking agents. Therefore, with these devices it is essential to assess the baseline prior to neuromuscular blockade so that this level can be used as the target to confirm recovery. The application of a preload with a hand adapter may improve the accuracy of the readings. The thumb must be allowed to move freely to obtain reliable readings so this form of monitoring may not be suitable if the arms are placed by the sides under the drapes.

Kinemyography

For the measurement with kinemyography (Fig. 7.7), a piezoelectric strip is placed between the thumb and the second finger. When the ulnar nerve is stimulated, an electrical signal proportional to the degree of bending is generated. Again, the thumb must be allowed to move freely to obtain accurate recordings. Kinemyography is very precise and is simple to use in clinical practice.

Practical tips to improve quality of monitoring

These steps include preparation of the skin (removing hair and oil), ensuring moist electrodes, placing the stimulating electrodes in the correct anatomical position over the nerve selected for stimulation, placing the negative stimulating electrode distally, ensuring 3–6 cm between the stimulating electrodes, use of supramaximal stimulation, calibration of the device before neuromuscular blocking agent is administered, and maintaining the skin surface temperature above 32°C.

In the cold operating theatre with infusions of cold solutions into the arm, recordings made may result in inaccurate readings. Lower core temperature will also prolong the duration of action of the muscle relaxants and reversal may be incomplete.

If AMG or kinemyography monitoring is used, the hand must be allowed unimpeded movement to provide accurate results. If the baseline TOF recordings of AMG devices are greater than 100% then the target for adequate reversals should be that obtained before administration of muscle relaxant.

Reversal agents

Neostigmine

Up until the relatively recent entry of sugammadex to the market, neostigmine has been the mainstay of neuromuscular blockade reversal. Due to costs and restricted access, neostigmine is still commonly used.

The main drawback to neostigmine use has been its slow and unpredictable onset of action and its lack of efficacy in reversing deep blockade. It exhibits a ceiling effect at doses of 70 mcg/kg.

Furthermore, neostigmine also has a high side effect profile secondary to its unwanted muscarinic effects such as bradycardia, bronchospasm, increased secretions, nausea and vomiting, increased peristalsis, increased urination, muscle cramps, visual disturbances, and, in some cases, convulsions [43]. As a result, antimuscarinic drugs such as atropine or glycopyrrolate are given concomitantly. These have their own side effects including dry mouth, mydriasis, confusion, urinary retention, constipation, nausea and vomiting, severe allergic reactions, cardiac arrhythmias, tachycardia, and prolonged QT [44].

If neostigmine is selected as a reversal agent, it is essential to use quantitative neuromuscular function monitoring to confirm adequacy of reversal. A number of studies show increased respiratory complications when neostigmine is administered or when administration is unwarranted at doses of greater than 60 mcg/kg or without the guidance of neuromuscular function monitoring [45–48]. Kirkegaard et al. identified that some individuals who receive neostigmine to reverse moderate neuromuscular blockade may require more than 90 minutes to reach a TOF of greater than 0.9 [49]. Even today studies demonstrate that greater than 30% of patients reversed with neostigmine experience residual neuromuscular blockade [50,51].

There is now evidence to suggest that upper airway dysfunction (e.g. dysphagia or partial upper airway obstruction) may occur even with a recovery of an acceleromyographic TOFR of 0.9 [52,53]. Thus, an acceleromyographic TOFR threshold of 1.0 for at least 15 minutes or more is now recommended [54].

Inhalational agents will also affect the recovery times when neostigmine is used as a reversal agent. Kim et al. identified that time of reversal of neuromuscular blockade in patients undergoing sevoflurane anaesthesia was three times longer than under propofol anaesthesia. In contrast to this, sugammadex reversal times were unchanged [55].

Sugammadex

Sugammadex has been a game-changing innovation in anaesthesia practice since its introduction in 2006. It is relatively fast acting, safe, and side effect free in comparison to acetylcholinesterase inhibitors. Sugammadex is a modified gamma-cyclodextrin molecule which acts as a reversal agent by encapsulating in a tight one-to-one complex inactivating both rocuronium and vecuronium [56].

The molecule is highly hydrophilic, distributing into the central compartment [56,57]. To provide a greater safety margin and more rapid reversal times, TBW dosing is recommended in

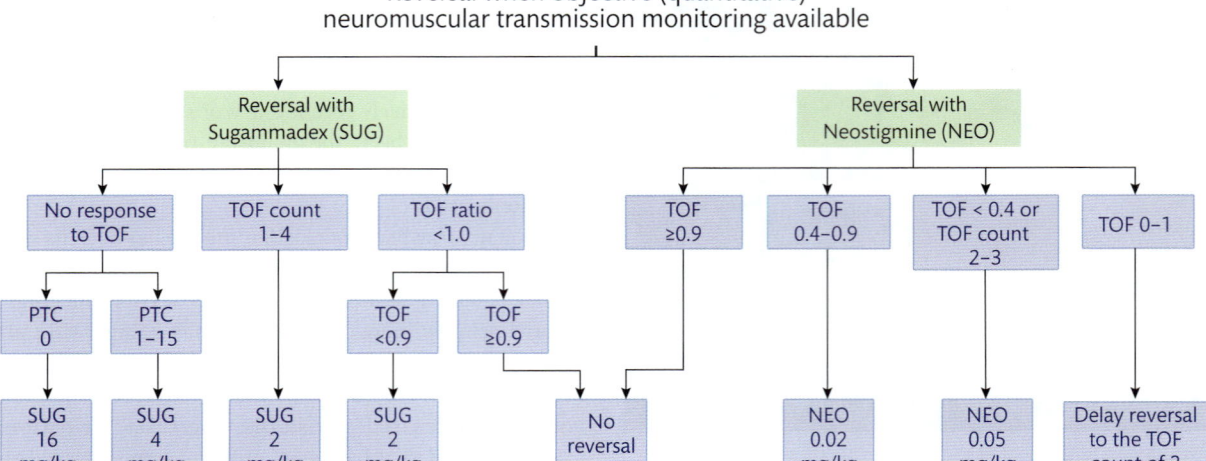

Fig. 7.8 Algorithmic approach to the use of sugammadex and neostigmine with the benefit of quantitative neuromuscular transmission monitoring (NMT).

Reproduced with permission from Miller, R., Eriksson, L, Fleischer, L, et al. *Miller's Anaesthesia*, 1060. Copyright © 2009 Elsevier. Adapted with permission from Eikermann, M., Kopman, A. F., Antagonism of non-depolarising neuromuscular block: current practice, *Anaesthesia*, 64(s1):22–30. Copyright © 2009 John Wiley and Sons.

the prescribing information. The dose for reversal of intense, deep, or moderate blockade is 16 mg/kg, 4 mg/kg, or 2 mg/kg respectively.

The requirement for rapid and complete reversal of neuromuscular blockade in obese patients is evident because of their increased risk of respiratory complications. In 2015, Brueckmann et al. reported a zero incidence of residual neuromuscular blockade in a post-anaesthesia care unit (PACU) by reversing rocuronium with sugammadex, using the correct dose, guided by neuromuscular function monitoring [50]. Sugammadex is an important milestone in the reduction of residual curarization and adverse PACU events, shortening time to discharge from the operating and recovery rooms, and resulting in increased safety for all, especially obese patients [49].

Fig. 7.8 provides an algorithmic approach to the use of sugammadex and neostigmine with the benefit of quantitative neuromuscular monitoring. Note the response to sugammadex in patients paralysed with vecuronium is slower than with rocuronium. Patients receiving sugammadex recover faster in comparison to those receiving neostigmine [56].

Residual neuromuscular blockade

Residual neuromuscular blockade in PACU settings is common (with an incidence of 30–40%) yet the prevalence is under-reported and thereby under-recognized by anaesthetists and PACU staff. Residual neuromuscular blockade is defined as a TOFR of less than 0.9 measured with mechanomyography or electromyography at the adductor pollicis.

The outcomes of residual neuromuscular paralysis include pharyngeal dysfunction, upper airway obstruction, increased risk of gastric content aspiration, impaired hypoxic ventilatory drive, unpleasant symptoms of muscle weakness, postoperative pulmonary complications, delayed discharge from recovery, and associations with major morbidity and mortality [58]. Given the oxygen demands and impaired respiratory mechanics of obese patients, the risks are more profound.

It is essential for safe care and early recovery after surgery in every obese patient requiring neuromuscular blockade to have quantitative neuromuscular function monitoring. The requirement for monitoring and adequate reversal of neuromuscular blocking agents is important in reducing morbidity and mortality in the recovery period and improving efficiency of surgical and ambulatory care centres [59].

Conclusion

Neuromuscular blockers are an essential component to balanced anaesthesia techniques for surgery requiring intubation and muscle relaxation or paralysis. Neuromuscular blockade should be considered in obese patients to facilitate intubation, reduce the risk of difficult intubation, and optimize surgical conditions. There is no specific agent of choice; however, rocuronium, vecuronium, atracurium, and cisatracurium are the most commonly used agents in the obese population.

The pharmacokinetics and pharmacodynamics of neuromuscular blocker and reversal agents is known to vary in obese patients. Although guidance is available suggesting the use of IBW as the scalar for dosing non-depolarizing blocker agents, the utilization of monitoring to guide dosing is recommended.

For rapid sequence induction and deep neuromuscular blockade, the combination of high-dose rocuronium and sugammadex for reversal is recommended. Neostigmine is not a suitable reversal agent for deep neuromuscular blockade. Furthermore, it is not recommended particularly in obese patients at risk of upper airway obstruction due to slower reversal times and high interindividual variability.

The risk of complications due to inadequate blockade and residual neuromuscular blockade are likely to be more significant in the obese population, therefore quantitative neuromuscular monitoring is very strongly recommended to confirm adequacy of reversal with a TOFR of greater than 0.9. A number of international guidelines now recommend the use of quantitative neuromuscular monitoring for all phases of surgery including induction, maintenance, and confirmation of recovery for every patient receiving neuromuscular blocking agents.

CASE REPORT

Mrs A was a 92 kg (body mass index = 39 kg/m²) obese patient having a revision laparoscopic sleeve gastrectomy. She had no prior history of obstructive sleep apnoea but had hypertension, diabetes, reflux, and asthma. Intraoperatively she was induced with fentanyl 100 mcg, propofol and Precedex® (dexmedetomidine) infusion, and rocuronium 50 mg. The procedure took 1.5 hours and the patient had deep neuromuscular blockade using qualitative neuromuscular monitoring (peripheral nerve stimulator). The anaesthesia chart records the TOF count to be 0/4 prior to reversal. The patient was extubated deep and the endotracheal tube replaced with a laryngeal mask airway. The patient was administered sugammadex 200 mg (2 mg/kg) and the TOF count obtained was 4/4 with no documented fade.

On return to PACU, the laryngeal mask airway appears to have been removed as the patient became agitated. The bariatric anaesthetist was phoned in theatre and notified of the following symptom—hypertension (blood pressure 254/105 mmHg) and oxygen saturation 94% on 15 L oxygen by Hudson mask. Clonidine and naloxone were ordered over the phone and administered intravenously. Additional clonidine for hypertension and naloxone for desaturation were administered assuming the patient had opioid overdosage. A second anaesthetist also reviewed the patient in PACU and the patient received further doses of clonidine and naloxone.

On further review by the bariatric anaesthetist, the diagnosis of residual neuromuscular blockade (possibly due to recurarization or inadequate dosage of sugammadex for reversal) was made. A second dose of sugammadex 200 mg (2 mg/kg) was administered resulting in immediate recovery and normalization of blood pressure and oxygen saturation. The patient was sent to the intensive care unit postoperatively due to persistent hypercapnia and potentially undiagnosed obstructive sleep apnoea.

Key learning points

'Faced with a patient who is hypoxaemic, has airway obstruction, or is not comfortable in the PACU, most anaesthesiologists and recovery staff do not spontaneously think of residual neuromuscular blockade as a likely cause. Residual neuromuscular blockade may be particularly difficult to identify in the obese patient' [60].

1. Patients can appear to breathe adequately due to early return of diaphragmatic muscle function but can obstruct due to upper airway muscle paralysis. The upper airway muscles are the last to recover from neuromuscular blockade.

2. Quantitative neuromuscular transmission monitoring is required from induction to recovery. Only quantitative neuromuscular transmission monitoring can confirm the adequate reversal with a TOFR of greater than 0.9.

3. Dosage of sugammadex is based on depth of blockade—in deep blockade the dose of sugammadex is 4 mg/kg. The recommended dosage for reversal of intense blockade with sugammadex is 16 mg/kg.

4. In using subjective peripheral nerve stimulator and interpreting TOF count 4/4 without fade it should be noted that patients can still have residual nerve blockade. PTC would have identified deep blockade or intense blockade.

5. There is significant interindividual variability in duration of neuromuscular blockade. Even a small dose of rocuronium can last hours in some patients. Quantitative neuromuscular monitoring is required to identify this occurrence [61].

6. Always consider residual neuromuscular blockade for a distressed patient in PACU.

7. Performing extubation only when the patient is awake and responsive will reduce the risk of critical respiratory events in the post-anaesthetic care unit [61].

REFERENCES

1. Dale H. Chemical transmission of the effects of nerve impulses. Br Med J. 1934;**1**(3827):835–41.
2. Griffith HR, Enid Johnson G. The use of curare in general anesthesia. Anesthesiology. 1942;**3**(4):418–20.
3. Martyn JAJ. Neuromuscular physiology and pharmacology. In: Miller RD, ed. Miller's Anesthesia. Philadelphia, PA: Churchill Livingstone; 2010:341–60.
4. Gray TC, Halton J. Curarine with balanced anaesthesia. Br Med J. 1946;**2**(4469):293–95.
5. Leslie K, Myles PS, Forbes A, Chan MTV. The effect of bispectral index monitoring on long-term survival in the B-aware trial. Anesth Analg. 2010;**110**(3):816–22.
6. Schlaich N, Mertzlufft F, Soltesz S, Fuchs-Buder T. Remifentanil and propofol without muscle relaxants or with different doses of rocuronium for tracheal intubation in outpatient anaesthesia. Acta Anaesthesiol Scand. 2000;**44**(6):720–26.
7. Combes X, Andriamifidy L, Dufresne E, Suen P, Sauvat S, Scherrer E, et al. Comparison of two induction regimens using or not using muscle relaxant: impact on postoperative upper airway discomfort. Br J Anaesth. 2007;**99**(2):276–81.
8. Mencke T, Echternach M, Kleinschmidt S, Lux P, Barth V, Plinkert PK, et al. Laryngeal morbidity and quality of tracheal intubation: a randomized controlled trial. Anesthesiology. 2003;**98**(5):1049–56.
9. Frerk C, Mitchell VS, McNarry AF, Mendonca C, Bhagrath R, Patel A, et al. Difficult Airway Society 2015 guidelines for management of unanticipated difficult intubation in adults. Br J Anaesth. 2015;**115**(6):827–48.
10. Lemmens HJM, Brodsky JB. The dose of succinylcholine in morbid obesity. Anesth Analg. 2006;**102**(2):438–42.
11. Hunter JM. Rocuronium: the newest aminosteroid neuromuscular blocking drug. Br J Anaesth. 1996;**76**(4):481–83.
12. Furyk J. How does rocuronium compare with succinylcholine in people undergoing rapid sequence induction intubation? Cochrane Clinical Answers. March 2017. https://www.cochranelibrary.com/cca/doi/10.1002/cca.1513/full
13. Tran DTT, Newton EK, Mount VAH, Lee JS, Wells GA, Perry JJ. Rocuronium versus succinylcholine for rapid sequence induction intubation. Cochrane Database Syst Rev. 2015;**10**:CD002788.
14. Magorian T, Flannery KB, Miller RD. Comparison of rocuronium, succinylcholine, and vecuronium for rapid-sequence induction of anesthesia in adult patients. Anesthesiology. 1993;**79**(5):913–18.
15. Tang L, Li S, Huang S, Ma H, Wang Z. Desaturation following rapid sequence induction using succinylcholine vs. rocuronium in overweight patients. Acta Anaesthesiol Scand. 2011;**55**(2):203–208.
16. Fuchs-Buder T, Claudius C, Skovgaard LT, Eriksson LI, Mirakhur RK, Viby-Mogensen J, et al. Good clinical research practice in pharmacodynamic studies of neuromuscular blocking

agents II: the Stockholm revision. Acta Anaesthesiol Scand. 2007;**51**(7):789–808.

17. Madsen MV, Staehr-Rye AK, Gätke MR, Claudius C. Neuromuscular blockade for optimising surgical conditions during abdominal and gynaecological surgery: a systematic review. Acta Anaesthesiol Scand. 2015;**59**(1):1–16.

18. Kopman AF, Naguib M. Laparoscopic surgery and muscle relaxants: is deep block helpful? Anesth Analg. 2015;**120**(1):51–58.

19. Martini CH, Boon M, Bevers RF, Aarts LP, Dahan A. Evaluation of surgical conditions during laparoscopic surgery in patients with moderate vs deep neuromuscular block. Br J Anaesth. 2014;**112**(3):498–505.

20. Kopman AF, Naguib M. Laparoscopic surgery and muscle relaxants: is deep block helpful? Anesth Analg. 2015;**120**(1):51–58.

21. Torensma B, Martini CH, Boon M, Olofsen E, In 't Veld B, Liem RSL, et al. Deep neuromuscular block improves surgical conditions during bariatric surgery and reduces postoperative pain: a randomized double blind controlled trial. PLoS One. 2016;**11**(12):e0167907.

22. Ingrande J, Lemmens HJM. Dose adjustment of anaesthetics in the morbidly obese. Br J Anaesth. 2010;**105** Suppl 1:i16–23.

23. Tsueda K, Warren JE, McCafferty LA, Nagle JP. Pancuronium bromide requirement during anesthesia for the morbidly obese. Anesthesiology. 1978;**48**(6):438–39.

24. Schwartz AE, Matteo RS, Ornstein E, Halevy JD, Diaz J. Pharmacokinetics and pharmacodynamics of vecuronium in the obese surgical patient. Anesth Analg. 1992;**74**(4):515–18.

25. Leykin Y, Pellis T, Lucca M, Lomangino G, Marzano B, Gullo A. The effects of cisatracurium on morbidly obese women. Anesth Analg. 2004;**99**(4):1090–94.

26. Kirkegaard-Nielsen H, Helbo-Hansen HS, Lindholm P, Severinsen IK, Pedersen HS. Anthropometric variables as predictors for duration of action of atracurium-induced neuromuscular block. Anesth Analg. 1996;**83**(5):1076–80.

27. Suzuki T, Masaki G, Ogawa S. Neostigmine-induced reversal of vecuronium in normal weight, overweight and obese female patients. Br J Anaesth. 2006;**97**(2):160–63.

28. Czech Society of Anaesthesiology and Intensive Care Medicine. Practice parameters for the safe and effective use of neuromuscular blocking drugs in anaesthesia. 2010. https://www.akutne.cz/index.php?pg=vyukove-materialy--guidelines-old

29. Checketts MR, Alladi R, Ferguson K, Gemmell L, Handy JM, Klein AA, et al. Recommendations for standards of monitoring during anaesthesia and recovery 2015: Association of Anaesthetists of Great Britain and Ireland. Anaesthesia. 2016;**71**(1):85–93.

30. Anon. Indications of neuromuscular blockade in anaesthesia. Short text. Ann Fr Anesth Reanim. 2000;**19** Suppl 2:352s–355s.

31. Kent N, Liang S, Phillips S, Smith N, Khandkar C, Eikermann M, Stewart P. Therapeutic doses of neostigmine, depolarising neuromuscular blockade and muscle weakness in awake volunteers: a double-blind, placebo-controlled, randomised volunteer study. Anaesthesia. 2018;**73**(9):1079–89.

32. Stanec A, Heyduk J, Stanec G, Orkin LR. Tetanic fade and post-tetanic tension in the absence of neuromuscular blocking agents in anesthetized man. Anesth Analg. 1978;**57**(1):102–107.

33. Heier T, Caldwell JE, Feiner JR, Liu L, Ward T, Wright PMC. Relationship between normalized adductor pollicis train-of-four ratio and manifestations of residual neuromuscular block: a study using acceleromyography during near steady-state concentrations of mivacurium. Anesthesiology. 2010;**113**(4):825–32.

34. Cammu G, De Witte J, De Veylder J, Byttebier G, Vandeput D, Foubert L, et al. Postoperative residual paralysis in outpatients versus inpatients. Anesth Analg. 2006;**102**(2):426–29.

35. Heier T, Caldwell JE, Feiner JR, Liu L, Ward T, Wright PMC. Relationship between normalized adductor pollicis train-of-four ratio and manifestations of residual neuromuscular block: a study using acceleromyography during near steady-state concentrations of mivacurium. Anesthesiology. 2010;**113**(4):825–32.

36. Smith CE, Donati F, Bevan DR. Potency of succinylcholine at the diaphragm and at the adductor pollicis muscle. Anesth Analg. 1988;**67**(7):625–30.

37. Laycock JR, Donati F, Smith CE, Bevan DR. Potency of atracurium and vecuronium at the diaphragm and the adductor pollicis muscle. Br J Anaesth. 1988;**61**(3):286–91.

38. Phillips S, Stewart PA, Freelander N, Heller G. Comparison of evoked electromyography in three muscles of the hand during recovery from non-depolarising neuromuscular blockade. Anaesth Intensive Care. 2012;**40**(4):690–96.

39. Ungureanu D, Meistelman C, Frossard J, Donati F. The orbicularis oculi and the adductor pollicis muscles as monitors of atracurium block of laryngeal muscles. Anesth Analg. 1993;**77**(4):775–79.

40. Naguib M, Brull SJ, Johnson KB. Conceptual and technical insights into the basis of neuromuscular monitoring. Anaesthesia. 2017;72 Suppl 1:16–37.

41. Brull SJ, Silverman DG. Tetanus-induced changes in apparent recovery after bolus doses of atracurium or vecuronium. Anesthesiology. 1992;**77**(4):642–45.

42. Dupuis JY, Martin R, Tessonnier JM, Tétrault JP. Clinical assessment of the muscular response to tetanic nerve stimulation. Can J Anaesth. 1990;**37**(4 Pt 1):397–400.

43. Capron F, Fortier L-P, Racine S, Donati F. Tactile fade detection with hand or wrist stimulation using train-of-four, double-burst stimulation, 50-hertz tetanus, 100-hertz tetanus, and acceleromyography. Anesth Analg. 2006;**102**(5):1578–84.

44. Welliver M, McDonough J, Kalynych N, Redfern R. Discovery, development, and clinical application of sugammadex sodium, a selective relaxant binding agent. Drug Des Devel Ther. 2009;2:49–59.

45. Grosse-Sundrup M, Henneman JP, Sandberg WS, Bateman BT, Uribe JV, Nguyen NT, et al. Intermediate acting non-depolarizing neuromuscular blocking agents and risk of postoperative respiratory complications: prospective propensity score matched cohort study. BMJ. 2012;**345**:e6329.

46. Meyer MJ, Bateman BT, Kurth T, Eikermann M. Neostigmine reversal doesn't improve postoperative respiratory safety. BMJ. 2013;**346**:f1460.

47. Sasaki N, Meyer MJ, Malviya SA, Stanislaus AB, MacDonald T, Doran ME, et al. Effects of neostigmine reversal of nondepolarizing neuromuscular blocking agents on postoperative respiratory outcomes: a prospective study. Anesthesiology. 2014;**121**(5):959–68.

48. McLean DJ, Diaz-Gil D, Farhan HN, Ladha KS, Kurth T, Eikermann M. Dose-dependent association between intermediate-acting neuromuscular-blocking agents and postoperative respiratory complications. Anesthesiology. 2015;**122**(6):1201–13.

49. Kirkegaard H, Heier T, Caldwell JE. Efficacy of tactile-guided reversal from cisatracurium-induced neuromuscular block. Anesthesiology. 2002;**96**(1):45–50.

50. Brueckmann B, Sasaki N, Grobara P, Li MK, Woo T, de Bie J, et al. Effects of sugammadex on incidence of postoperative residual neuromuscular blockade: a randomized, controlled study. Br J Anaesth. 2015;**115**(5):743–51.

51. Stewart PA, Liang SS, Li QS, Huang ML, Bilgin AB, Kim D, et al. The impact of residual neuromuscular blockade,

oversedation, and hypothermia on adverse respiratory events in a postanesthetic care unit. Anesth Analg. 2016;**123**(4):859–68.

52. Eikermann M, Blobner M, Groeben H, Rex C, Grote T, Neuhäuser M, et al. Postoperative upper airway obstruction after recovery of the train of four ratio of the adductor pollicis muscle from neuromuscular blockade. Anesth Analg. 2006;**102**(3):937–42.

53. Eikermann M, Vogt FM, Herbstreit F, Vahid-Dastgerdi M, Zenge MO, Ochterbeck C, et al. The predisposition to inspiratory upper airway collapse during partial neuromuscular blockade. Am J Respir Crit Care Med. 2007;**175**(1):9–15.

54. Carron M, Freo U, Parotto E, Ori C. The correct dosing regimen for sugammadex in morbidly obese patients. Anaesthesia. 2012;**67**(3):298–99.

55. Kim KS, Cheong MA, Lee HJ, Lee JM. Tactile assessment for the reversibility of rocuronium-induced neuromuscular blockade during propofol or sevoflurane anesthesia. Anesth Analg. 2004;**99**(4):1080–85.

56. Mirakhur RK. Sugammadex in clinical practice. Anaesthesia. 2009;**64**:45–54.

57. Van Lancker P, Dillemans B, Bogaert T, Mulier JP, De Kock M, Haspeslagh M. Ideal versus corrected body weight for dosage of sugammadex in morbidly obese patients. Anaesthesia. 2011;**66**(8):721–25.

58. Berg H, Roed J, Viby-Mogensen J, Mortensen CR, Engbaek J, Skovgaard LT, et al. Residual neuromuscular block is a risk factor for postoperative pulmonary complications. A prospective, randomised, and blinded study of postoperative pulmonary complications after atracurium, vecuronium and pancuronium. Acta Anaesthesiol Scand. 1997;**41**(9):1095–103.

59. Butterly A, Bittner EA, George E, Sandberg WS, Eikermann M, Schmidt U. Postoperative residual curarization from intermediate-acting neuromuscular blocking agents delays recovery room discharge. Br J Anaesth. 2010;**105**(3):304–309.

60. Donati F. Neuromuscular monitoring: what evidence do we need to be convinced? Anesth Analg. 2010;**111**(1):6–8.

61. Debaene B, Plaud B, Dilly M-P, Donati F. Residual paralysis in the PACU after a single intubating dose of nondepolarizing muscle relaxant with an intermediate duration of action. Anesthesiology. 2003;**98**(5):1042–48.

SECTION 2
Obesity and physiology

Metabolic syndrome

Patrick J. Neligan

Introduction

Two patients are scheduled for major surgery. They are both 58 years old and are obese: they have identical body mass indices (BMIs) of 38 kg/m². Neither smoke. One patient has significant underlying cardiovascular disease (CVD), consequent of obesity, the other does not. One is at elevated risk for perioperative complications, the other is not. The reason for the disorientating difference in risk profile results not from the patient's weight and BMI, but from fat distribution and the metabolic activity of adipose tissue.

Fat distribution

Not all obese individuals are created equally. This is the major problem associated with using BMI as a predictor of future ill health. The distribution of body fat has a significant impact on the development of metabolic disease. Individuals are divided into roughly two groups—those with peripheral (pear shaped—gluteofemoral obesity) fat distribution, the majority of whom are female, and those with central (apple shaped—abdominal obesity) fat distribution, the majority of whom are male. Abdominal girth reflects visceral obesity and this can be recorded as waist circumference or waist-to-hip (WTH) ratio. A WTH ratio of greater than 1.0 in males, and greater than 0.85 in females, suggests central obesity [1].

Visceral fat distribution plays a key role in the pathogenesis of metabolic disease and CVD and waist circumference is a better predictor of the development of metabolic disease and CVD and death than BMI [2–5]. For example, in a study of 27,098 participants in 52 countries, WHR showed a graded and highly significant association with myocardial infarction and was a superior predictor of cardiac events than BMI [4]. The European Prospective Investigation into Cancer and Nutrition (EPIC) study examined the association of BMI, waist circumference, and WHR with the risk of death among 359,387 participants from nine European countries [5]. The participants were followed up for almost 10 years; 14,723 died. Waist circumference and WHR, and hence visceral adiposity, were strongly associated with the risk of death. BMI was also associated with the risk of death but in a J-shaped distribution, with higher risks of death observed in the lower and upper BMI categories than in the middle categories. Abdominal obesity increased the risk of death irrespective of the BMI.

Non-alcoholic fatty liver disease

In obese patients, the liver becomes overloaded with carbohydrate and fat. This results in a significant increase in insulin production, with progressively reducing effectiveness. Fat accumulates within the liver. Fatty liver (hepatic steatosis) is resistant to the action of insulin and hepatic glucose production increases, inducing further hyperinsulinaemia and worsening steatosis. Insulin levels remain high between meals. More than 30% of American adults have hepatic steatosis [6]. With weight loss the liver shrinks in size, consequent of reduced fat content. Hepatic insulin sensitivity improves, leading to a reduction in blood glucose.

Type 2 diabetes (T2D) is characterized by both hepatic steatosis and dysregulated glucose metabolism [7]. Fatty liver precedes the onset and diagnosis of T2D [8]. There appears to be an inflection point where endogenous insulin fails to suppress glucose production and facilitate muscular storage. The islet cells decompensate and the patient develops T2D. In the short term, reversal of hepatic steatosis appears to result in reversal of T2D. However, in the long term (>2 or 3 years), irreversible islet cell damage occurs and diabetes persists. Non-alcoholic fatty liver disease (NAFLD) is almost universal among diabetic people who are morbidly obese [9]. It is associated with coronary arterial disease [10,11] and should be considered a risk indicator.

Non-alcoholic steatohepatitis (NASH) is an inflammatory disease that results from hepatic steatosis. It is characterized by macrovesicular steatosis, lobular inflammation, and hepatocellular ballooning [12]. NASH is reversible, in its early stages, with weight loss. However, sustained liver injury leads to fibrosis and cirrhosis in 10–25% of affected individuals [13]. It is estimated that 12–20% of patients with hepatic steatosis will go on to develop NASH [14]. Of these, roughly one in eight will develop cirrhosis over the next 5 years.

From insulin resistance to type 2 diabetes

Insulin resistance is a clinical condition where there is reduced biological activity in response to circulating insulin. Insulin is secreted mainly in response to plasma glucose, and obese patients tend to consume very large quantities of refined carbohydrates. Consequently, in obesity, circulating insulin levels rise and this results in a series of metabolic abnormalities. These include the various components of the metabolic syndrome (MetS) and, as previously mentioned, NAFLD. Patients who develop insulin resistance may be genetically susceptible, but a number of environmental factors may also trigger this problem—including lifestyle, diet, stress, and smoking [15–19].

The metabolic consequences of insulin resistance result in a progressive cycle of hyperglycaemia, dyslipidaemia, endothelial dysfunction, inflammation, and atherosclerosis [20]. Simultaneously, as the pancreatic beta cells increase output to maintain normoglycemia, fatty deposition around these cells progressively reduces synthetic reserve [15]. Patients may initially manifest impaired glucose tolerance, but physiological reserve depletes over time, beta cells burn out and diabetes ensues [21].

Metabolic syndrome

The term MetS refers to a collection of clinical findings that, when clustered together, are believed to be associated with elevated long-term risk for morbidity and mortality compared with the sum of the individual components alone. These include central obesity, hypertension, dyslipidaemia, and insulin resistance or impaired glucose tolerance.

The International Diabetes Federation (IDF; https://idf.org/) has described a syndrome as 'a recognizable complex of symptoms and physical or biochemical findings for which a direct cause is not understood … the components coexist more frequently than would be expected by chance alone. When causal mechanisms are identified, the syndrome becomes a disease.'

In 1988, Gerald Reaven referred to this cluster of symptoms as 'Syndrome X' and believed that insulin resistance and hyperinsulinaemia caused metabolic dysfunction that led eventually to T2D and CVD [22–24]. Over the past quarter of a century, the understanding of these processes has been refined, and insulin resistance has been marginalized in favour of central obesity.

Three major definitions of MetS currently exist: the World Health Organization (WHO) (**Box 8.1**) definition [25], the National Cholesterol Education Program (NCEP)—Adult Treatment Panel III definition (**Box 8.2**) [26–28], and the IDF definition (**Box 8.3**) [29]. The major difference between the IDF and the NCEP is the emphasis on waist circumference (as a marker of central obesity) and ethnicity-specific adjustments in this to ensure generalizability.

The NCEP and the IDF definitions have a lower threshold for blood pressure (130/85 versus 140/90 mmHg) than the WHO. The NCEP does not require waist circumference to be elevated in all patients, whereas the WHO and the IDF do. The NCEP does not require frank glucose intolerance or diabetes, whereas the WHO and the IDF do. And finally, the NCEP and the IDF do not require microalbuminuria, whereas the WHO does [26,30].

Depending on which definition is used, between 25.1% (NCEP definition) [31] and 27% (WHO definition) [32] of the population have MetS. African American females and Mexican Americans of both sexes are at particular risk. Among Finnish males, the prevalence of MetS ranged from 8.8% (WHO definition) to 14.3% (NCEP definition) [29].

Although obesity is not an essential component of MetS, there is a strong correlation between visceral fat deposits and MetS. The

---

> **Box 8.1** Metabolic syndrome—World Health Organization criteria (1999)
>
> 1. Must have abnormal glucose metabolism:
>   a. diabetes mellitus
>   b. impaired glucose tolerance
>   c. impaired fasting glucose insulin resistance;
>
> *And* two of the following:
> 1. Blood pressure: ≥140/90 mmHg.
> 2. Dyslipidaemia:
>   a. triglycerides: ≥1.695 mmol/L.
>   b. high-density lipoprotein cholesterol ≤0.9 mmol/L (male), ≤1.0 mmol/L (female).
> 3. Central obesity: waist:hip ratio >0.90 (male); >0.85 (female), and/or body mass index >30 kg/m²
> 4. Microalbuminuria: urinary albumin excretion ratio ≥20 mg/min or albumin:creatinine ratio ≥30 mg/g.
>
> Source: Data from Alberti, K.G., Zimmet, P.Z. Definition, diagnosis and classification of diabetes mellitus and its complications. Part 1: diagnosis and classification of diabetes mellitus provisional report of a WHO consultation. *Diabetic Medicine*, 15(7):539–53, 1998 John Wiley & Sons.

presence of MetS, not elevated BMI, predicts future CVD in women [33]. Consequently, definitions of MetS emphasize waist circumference rather than BMI. It is possible to be obese without MetS; sometimes referred to as the metabolically 'healthy' obese [34].

> **Box 8.2** Metabolic syndrome—National Cholesterol Education Program (American Heart Association) definitions
>
> **NCEP I 2001**
> The US NCEP—Adult Treatment Panel III (2001) requires at least three of the following:
> 1. Central obesity defined by waist circumference:
>   a. ≥102 cm or 40 inches (male).
>   b. ≥88 cm or 36 inches (female).
> 2. Dyslipidaemia: triglycerides ≥1.695 mmol/L (150 mg/dL).
> 3. Dyslipidaemia:
>   a. HDL <40 mg/dL (male).
>   b. HDL <50 mg/dL (female).
> 4. Blood pressure ≥130/85 mmHg.
> 5. Fasting plasma glucose ≥6.1 mmol/L (110 mg/dl).
>
> **NCEP II–ATP III/American Heart Association 2005 (updated definitions)**
> 1. Central obesity:
>   a. waist circumference: men ≥40 inches (102 cm).
>   b. waist circumference: women—≥35 inches (88 cm).
> 2. Dyslipidaemia: triglycerides: ≥150 mg/dL.
> 3. Dyslipidaemia: reduced HDL:
>   a. Men ≤40 mg/dL.
>   b. Women ≤50 mg/dL.
> 4. Hypertension: ≥130/85 mmHg or use of antihypertensives.
> 5. Elevated fasting glucose: ≥100 mg/dL (5.6 mmol/L) or use of medication for hyperglycaemia.
>
> Adapted with permission from Third Report of the National Cholesterol Education Program (NCEP) Expert Panel on Detection, Evaluation, and Treatment of High Blood Cholesterol in Adults (Adult Treatment Panel III) Final Report, *Circulation*, 106(25):3143. Copyright © 2002 Wolters Kluwer Health, Inc.; and Adapted with permission from Grundy, S. M., Brewer, H. B., Cleeman, J. I., et al, Definition of Metabolic Syndrome, *Circulation*, 109(3):433–438. Copyright © 2004 Wolters Kluwer Health, Inc.; and Adapted with permission from Grundy, S. M., Cleeman, J. I., Daniels, S. R., et al, Diagnosis and Management of the Metabolic Syndrome, *Circulation*, 112(17):2735–2752. Copyright © 2005 Wolters Kluwer Health, Inc.

Box 8.3 Metabolic syndrome—International Diabetes Federation 2006 definitions

For a person to be defined as having MetS they must have:
1. Central obesity:
   a. waist circumference ≥94 cm for Europid men.
   b. waist circumference ≥80 cm for Europid women.
   c. (ethnicity-specific values for other groups).

Plus *any two* of the following four factors:
1. Dyslipidaemia, elevated triglycerides ≥150 mg/dL (1.7 mmol/L), or specific treatment for dyslipidaemia.
2. Dyslipidaemia, reduced HDL:
   a. <40 mg/dL (1.03 mmol/L) in males.
   b. <50 mg/dL (1.29 mmol/L) in females.
   c. or specific treatment for dyslipidaemia.
3. Hypertension: systolic blood pressure ≥130 or diastolic blood pressure ≥85 mm Hg, or treatment of previously diagnosed hypertension.
4. Elevated fasting plasma glucose ≥100 mg/dL (5.6 mmol/L), or previously diagnosed type 2 diabetes.

If above 5.6 mmol/L or 100 mg/dL, an oral glucose tolerance test is strongly recommended but is not necessary to define presence of the syndrome.

Source: Data from Alberti, K. G. M. M., Zimmet, P., Shaw, J., Metabolic syndrome—a new world-wide definition. A Consensus Statement from the International Diabetes Federation, *Diabetic Medicine*, 23(5):469–480, 2006 John Wiley & Sons.

Box 8.4 Adipocytokines associated with the metabolic syndrome

Acute phase reactants
↑ C-reactive protein.
↑ SAA.

Adipokines
↓ Adiponectin.
↑ Leptin.
↑ Resistin.

Macrophage-derived factors
↑ Resistin.
↑ IL-1β.

Proinflammatory cytokines and chemokines
↑ TNFα.
↑ IL-1, IL-6, IL-8, IL-10, IL-18.
↑ CCL2.

Prothrombotic factors
↑ PAI-1.
↑ Fibrinogen.
↑ Factor VII.

CCL, chemotactic cytokine 2; IL, interleukin; PAI, plasminogen activator inhibitor 1; SSA, serum amyloid A.

Metabolic syndrome and inflammation

Visceral fat is an endocrine, paracrine, and immunological organ. Various pro- and anti-inflammatory cytokines are produced. As adipose tissue mass increases with obesity, the balance tilts towards more inflammatory and less anti-inflammatory activity [35]. Obesity is thus a state of chronic inflammation [36].

Insulin is an anti-inflammatory hormone. As we have seen, increased circulating free fatty acids, derived from highly metabolic visceral fat, can reduce insulin activity and promote hepatic steatosis. There is a strong relationship between NAFLD and the development of MetS [37]. Increased secretion of interleukin (IL)-6 and tumour necrosis factor-alpha (TNFα) are associated with increased turnover of adipose tissue triglyceride stores, insulin resistance, and increased circulating free fatty acids. There is enhanced production of glucose and very-low-density lipoprotein by the liver. Triglyceride levels are increased and this reduces high-density lipoprotein (HDL) size. Smaller HDLs are more easily filtered by the kidney, increasing excretion and lowering plasma HDL levels. Low-density lipoprotein size is reduced: these smaller, less dense particles are more atherogenic.

With visceral obesity, tissue macrophages invade adipose tissue and release TNFα. This, in turn, causes the release of IL-1, IL-6, and other cytokines. There is an alteration in the relative concentrations of adipose-derived hormones, collectively known as 'adiopkines' (**Box 8.4**). Leptin is involved in the control of satiety and is markedly proinflammatory. Adiponectin, which is thought to be anti-inflammatory and enhances insulin sensitivity, is reduced in visceral obesity. Resistin, an adipokine that antagonizes insulin, is elevated. There are elevated levels of plasminogen activator inhibitor-1 (PAI-1), and increased C-reactive protein levels, consistent with activation of inflammation. Cytokines and free fatty acids increase the production of fibrinogen and PAI-1 by the liver and adipose tissue. This results in a prothrombotic state [38]. This adipocytokine profile, which is characteristic of MetS and NAFLD, is associated with increased risk for myocardial ischaemia and infarction [39–41].

Metabolic syndrome and cardiovascular risk

MetS increases the risk of cardiovascular and coronary heart disease by 1.5–3 times [42,43]. This results, presumably, from a combination of active inflammation, hypercoagulability, atherogenesis, hyperglycaemia, insulin resistance, and increased circulating lipids. In a post hoc analysis of two cardiovascular trials, the Scandinavian Simvastatin Survival Study (4S) and the Air Force/Texas Coronary Atherosclerosis Prevention Study, patients with MetS were 1.5 times more likely to have major coronary events versus those without [44].

In an 11-year study of 3585 elderly subjects without diabetes or coronary heart disease, patients who had MetS, according to the 2005 NCEP definition, were 20–30% more likely to experience a cardiovascular event than subjects without MetS [45].

Sundström et al. followed a cohort of 2322 men, between the age of 50 and 70 years, for 32.7 years, and looked at cardiovascular morbidity using NCEP definitions [46]. The presence of MetS predicted total and cardiovascular mortality in individuals with and without known CVD and diabetes.

A 10-year Dutch study of 1364 subjects, without pre-existing CVD or diabetes, found that MetS was associated with about a twofold increase in age-adjusted risk of fatal CVD in men and non-fatal CVD in woman [47].

Huang and colleagues enrolled 124,513 participants, aged 20–94 years, in Taiwan, and followed them over 8 years [48]. The baseline prevalence of MetS was 22.4% by the NCEP II (2005) definitions and 13.9% by the IDF definition. Both systems identified an elevated risk of overall mortality and cardiovascular mortality with the NCEP II definition being more robust: the hazard ratios of all-cause and CVD mortality were 1.21 (95% confidence interval (CI) 1.09–1.34) and 1.77 (95% CI 1.40–2.24), respectively, in men and 1.30 (95% CI 1.12–1.49) and 1.69 (95% CI 1.19–2.42), respectively, in women.

Wilson and colleagues [49] followed a cohort of 3323 middle-aged adults without known CVD or T2D for 8 years. Baseline prevalence of the MetS was 26.8% in men and 16.6% in women. MetS predicted the development of CVD and T2D in men and women. In men, the hazard ratio for CVD was 2.88 (95% CI 1.99–4.16) and 6.92 (95% CI 4.47–10.81) for T2D.

A study that followed 4258 elderly subjects without pre-existing CVD, for, on average, 15 years found that subjects with MetS had a 22% higher mortality (relative risk (RR) 1.22; 95% CI 1.11–1.34), than those without [50]. However, mortality was better predicted by the presence of hyperglycaemia and hypertension than by the diagnosis of MetS. Subjects having both hypertension and elevated fasting glucose had 82% higher mortality (RR 1.82; 95% CI 1.58–109).

A study in Finland looked at the relationship between cerebrovascular disease and MetS in 1131 men with no history of CVD or DM, over an average of 14.3 years [51]. There was a 2.05-fold increase in the risk of stroke of all causes and a 2.41-fold increase in the risk for ischaemic stroke.

Metabolic syndrome in the perioperative period

MetS is associated with long-term complications such as T2D, CVD, and cerebrovascular disease, but does this translate to elevated perioperative risk?

Wei Pan and colleagues performed a retrospective analysis of nearly 10,000 patients that had attended the Texas Heart Institute over a 10-year period [52]. Patients were subdivided on the basis of BMI into obese with diabetes or without. The combination of elevated BMI and diabetes was associated with an elevated risk of postoperative respiratory failure, atrial and ventricular arrhythmias, renal insufficiency, and leg wound infections. These data suggest that diabetes and obesity, as seen in MetS, have synergistic risk.

In a study of almost 1200 patients who underwent coronary artery bypass grafting (CABG) over 10 years, preoperative MetS (46.6%) was associated with long-term poor prognosis in terms of all-cause death (hazard ratio (HR) 1.34; 95% CI 1.03–1.74; $P = 0.028$) and cardiac death (HR 2.31; 95% CI 1.36–3.92; $P = 0.002$) [53]. Patients with MetS had HRs of 2.47 (95% CI 1.22–4.99; $P = 0.012$) for postoperative stroke and 3.81 (95% CI 1.42–10.3; $P = 0.008$) for postoperative acute kidney injury [54].

In a study of 5304 patients who had undergone CABG, 2411 (46%) patients had MetS. The operative mortality after CABG surgery was 2.4% in patients with MetS and 0.9% in patients without MetS ($P < 0.0001$). After adjustment for other risk factors: MetS plus diabetes increased mortality by 2.7 times ($P = 0.007$), MetS without DM increased mortality by 2.36 times ($P = 0.007$); diabetes alone did not increase risk [55]. A similar study of 1133 non-diabetic patients who underwent revascularization demonstrated that patients with both MetS and hypertension had a HR of 3.91 ($P = 0.001$) for cardiac mortality and 2.09 for stroke ($P = 0.03$) [56].

Adverse outcomes are not limited to patients undergoing cardiovascular surgery. A study of 114 patients undergoing colorectal surgery demonstrated that MetS was associated with a higher rate of complications (40.5% vs 11.1%; $P < 0.001$) and a longer length of hospital stay (11.2 vs 8.1 days; $P = 0.006$) [57]. A very large cohort study of patients undergoing spinal fusion showed that patients with MetS had significantly longer length of stay, higher hospital costs, higher rates of non-routine discharges, and increased rates of major life-threatening complications [58]. Similarly, patients undergoing major joint arthroplasty were at elevated perioperative risk, particularly where one or more element of the MetS definition was uncontrolled [59]. A study of 430 consecutive patients undergoing percutaneous nephrolithotomy revealed a HR of 2.7 ($P < 0.05$) for major complications associated with MetS [60].

A very large cohort study of more than 300,000 patients in the American College of Surgeons database looked at adverse outcomes in patients over a range of BMIs and whether or not they had MetS [61]. For patients with elevated BMI, without MetS, mortality was lower or equal to that of normal-weight patients, up to a BMI of 40 kg/m^2. For all obese patients with MetS there was an increase in perioperative mortality. For example, patients with MetS and BMI greater than 40 kg/m^2 had a twofold increased risk of death (odds ratio (OR) 1.99; 95% CI 1.41–2.80). The same cohort had an elevated risk of cardiac events (OR 2.66; 95% CI 1.68–4.19) and acute kidney injury (OR 7.29; 95% CI 5.27–10.1). For patients with BMI greater than 30 kg/m^2 and MetS there was an elevated risk of cardiac events, acute kidney injury, central nervous system events, wound infections, and sepsis, compared with obese patients without MetS. Only pulmonary complications were more frequent in the metabolically normal obese population, compared with normal-weight controls. This tendency for obese patients to have equal or fewer complications in perioperative medicine and critical illness, has been termed the 'obesity paradox'.

Obesity paradox

To date, multiple studies have failed to link increased BMI with adverse outcomes in patients undergoing surgery or becoming critically ill. For example, a series of studies that looked at obesity and cardiac surgery failed to show any increase in risk [62–65], with only one large cohort study, in patients with higher BMIs, reporting increased perioperative risk [66].

A prospective study from Pennsylvania looked at the impact of obesity over 4 years in 2800 medical intensive care unit (ICU) patients [67]. BMI had no impact on outcomes, such as length of stay, mechanical ventilation, ventilation free days, costs, and so on. It is noteworthy, however, that obese patients were more likely younger and female, suggesting age-related bias and under-representation of patients with metabolic disease. A larger study of 41,000 critically ill patients confirmed that low BMI, as seen in the perioperative study [61], rather than high BMI, was associated with worse outcomes [68]. A 5-year study of 10,000 surgical ICU patients revealed no difference in ICU outcomes with regard to BMI [69]. The 60-day mortality was lower in overweight and obese patients (BMI 25–39.9 kg/m^2) (OR 0.83; 95% CI 0.69–0.99; P 0.047). Again, the worst outcomes were in patients with BMI less than 20 (17.8% vs 11.1%; $P = 0.006$) and BMI greater than 40 kg/m^2.

Two meta-analyses looked at obesity outcomes in ICUs in 2008 [70] and 2009 [71]. Hogue and colleagues demonstrated that there was lower hospital mortality for obese and morbidly obese subjects (RR 0.76; 95% CI 0.59–0.92; and RR 0.83; 95% CI 0.66–1.04, respectively) compared with normal weight controls [71]. Oliveros and colleagues found similar results, but longer duration of stay for patients with BMI greater than 40 kg/m^2 [70].

The obesity paradox, whereby lower-BMI patients have worse outcomes, and higher-BMI patients (up to 40 kg/m²) have better outcomes, has been demonstrated in a variety of setting outside of perioperative medicine and critical care. This includes patients with acute coronary syndromes [72], in chronic heart failure [73], following coronary revascularization [74], in pneumonia [75], in end-stage kidney disease [76], and in many other settings.

It is important to understand that, on a population basis, long-term outcomes from obesity, whether patients are metabolically healthy or unhealthy, may be worse than for 'normal-weight' individuals [77]. Nonetheless, it is clear that BMI as a tool for predicting risk, in perioperative medicine and critical illness, is no longer fit for purpose. This probably relates to the fact that, as overall nutrition improves, lean body mass increases in proportion to fat body mass up to an inflection point BMI for about 35 kg/m². This likely increases physiological reserve and may be responsible for improved outcomes in critical illness. What is clear then, in anaesthesia practice, is that for obese and morbidly obese patients, determining whether they are metabolically healthy or have MetS, may radically change their perioperative risk profile.

Perioperative screening and therapeutics

Once diagnosed, MetS requires significant lifestyle modification that emphasizes reduced calorie intake, particularly refined carbohydrates, leading to weight loss. Patients should be treated with interventions that target individual components of MetS, that include tight control of hypertension, dyslipidaemia, and diabetes. However, for the clinician who encounters a patient with MetS at the preoperative assessment centre, is it appropriate to commence such therapy and do these interventions modulate perioperative risk?

On the surface, the preoperative diagnosis of MetS should increase our ability to delineate risk. The presence of coronary arterial disease is known to increase perioperative risk [78]. In a large cohort of patients, the prevalence of coronary arterial disease was 19.2% in patients with MetS and T2D, 13.9% with MetS alone, and 7.5% with diabetes alone [79]. So, one would think that identifying patients with MetS, preoperatively, should ensure that patients with elevated cardiac risk are accounted for and therapeutic interventions made to modulate risk. Unfortunately, to date, no large epidemiological studies have been performed to support this hypothesis. Moreover, the results of trials of perioperative pharmacotherapy to reduce risk have been disappointing.

Two problems derive from this. The first is the diagnosis of MetS: should all perioperative patients that have central obesity be screened? Using the current definitions, this would require fasting blood glucose and fasting lipid profiles. Is this cost-effective?

The second problem is that once MetS has been diagnosed, what intervention is likely to reduce perioperative morbidity? Accumulated data on preoperative pharmacotherapy has yielded disappointing results. Early enthusiasm for perioperative beta blockade has been tempered by data arising from the POISE trial [80]. This was a large, prospective, randomized control trial of 8351 patients in 190 hospitals in 23 countries. Patients with, or at risk of, atherosclerotic disease who were undergoing non-cardiac surgery were randomized to receive extended-release metoprolol (n = 4174) or placebo (n = 4177) started 2–4 hours before surgery

and continued for 30 days. Administration of metoprolol was associated with a lower incidence of myocardial infarction (absolute risk reduction 1.2%; P <0.001), but a higher mortality rate (absolute risk increase of 0.8%; P <0.04) and an increase in the risk of stroke (absolute risk increase 0.5%; P <0.01). The POISE investigators undertook a series of meta-analyses of published trials of perioperative beta blockers, including their own. Although beta blockade appeared to reduce the perioperative risk of myocardial infarction, it did so at elevated risk for mortality and stroke [80].

Perioperative beta blockade can only be recommended for patients already receiving this therapy, and it should not be stopped in the perioperative period.

Dyslipidaemia is a core component of MetS. Statin therapy is well established for prevention of CVD [81]. To date, no randomized controlled trial has satisfactorily proven the effectiveness of statin therapy in the perioperative period, and although retrospective analyses have suggested a benefit, this is likely overestimated [82].

It seems that the major benefit of statins in the perioperative period arise from *not stopping* these drugs when previously prescribed. Studies have demonstrated that acute statin withdrawal increases markers of inflammation and oxidative stress, and that statin withdrawal during unstable periods is associated with an increased risk of adverse cardiac events [83–85].

In the clinical arena there is accumulating data that hyperglycaemia, and poor control of diabetes, results in worse outcomes from myocardial ischaemia and stroke [86–89]. Insulin appears to be cardioprotective in the presence of ischaemia [90,91]. In cardiac surgery, meticulous control of blood glucose significantly reduces the incidence of deep sternal wound infections [92,93], and mortality (in diabetic patients) [94]. Van den Berghe and colleagues demonstrated a significant mortality benefit from tight glycaemic control, using insulin infusions, in surgical critical care patients, predominantly those who had undergone cardiothoracic surgery [95]. A follow-up study in medical intensive care failed to confirm efficacy [96]. Subsequent trials found that 'tight glycaemic control' was associated with an excess of morbidity and mortality consequent, principally, of hypoglycaemia [97,98].

Currently, there are insufficient data to support tight glycaemic control for the majority of perioperative patients, perhaps with the exception of those undergoing cardiac or neurosurgery.

Key points

1. Obesity is a metabolic disease that arises from excessive energy consumption.
2. Obesity increases the risk for cardiovascular, cerebrovascular, and neoplastic disease.
3. NAFLD appears to be an early indicator of escalating endocrine and metabolic dysfunction; it precedes T2D and MetS and may progress to NASH or cirrhosis.
4. Central obesity closely correlates with cardiovascular risk. It is believed that this results from metabolically active visceral fat: there is a persistent proinflammatory, prothrombotic, and atherogenic state.
5. MetS involves central obesity, dyslipidaemia, hypertension, and insulin resistance.

6. Compared with elevated BMI, patients with MetS are more likely to develop CVD and cerebrovascular disease.

7. Patients with elevated BMI (up to a BMI of 40 kg/m²) should not be considered to have elevated perioperative risk or increased mortality in the ICU. In fact, many studies have demonstrated lower risk than with 'normal-weight' patients: this is known as the 'obesity paradox'.

8. Obesity plus MetS or diabetes does increase perioperative risk.

9. It is unclear whether or not patients should be screened for MetS preoperatively as minimal data are currently available regarding therapeutic interventions or modifications that may reduce risk.

REFERENCES

1. Björntorp P. Aging and body composition. Nutrition. 1997;**13**(6):572–73.
2. Wang Y, Rimm EB, Stampfer MJ, Willett WC, Hu FB. Comparison of abdominal adiposity and overall obesity in predicting risk of type 2 diabetes among men. Am J Clin Nutr. 2005;**81**(3):555–63.
3. Folsom AR, Kaye SA, Sellers TA, Hong CP, Cerhan JR, Potter JD, et al. Body fat distribution and 5-year risk of death in older women. JAMA. 1993;**269**(4):483–87.
4. Yusuf S, Hawken S, Èunpuu S, Bautista L, Franzosi MG, Commerford P, et al. Obesity and the risk of myocardial infarction in 27,000 participants from 52 countries: a case-control study. Lancet. 2005;**366**(9497):1640–49.
5. Pischon T, Boeing H, Hoffmann K, Bergmann M, Schulze MB, Overvad K, et al. General and abdominal adiposity and risk of death in Europe. N Engl J Med. 2008;**359**(20):2105–20.
6. Browning JD, Szczepaniak LS, Dobbins R, Nuremberg P, Horton JD, Cohen JC, et al. Prevalence of hepatic steatosis in an urban population in the United States: impact of ethnicity. Hepatology. 2004;**40**(6):1387–95.
7. Taylor R. Pathogenesis of type 2 diabetes: tracing the reverse route from cure to cause. Diabetologia. 2008;**51**(10):1781–89.
8. Kotronen A, Yki-Jarvinen H. Fatty liver: a novel component of the metabolic syndrome. Arterioscler Thromb Vasc Biol. 2008;**28**(1):27–38.
9. Adams LA, Angulo P, Lindor KD. Nonalcoholic fatty liver disease. CMAJ. 2005;**172**(7):899–905.
10. Schindhelm RK, Dekker JM, Nijpels G, Heine RJ, Diamant M. No independent association of alanine aminotransferase with risk of future type 2 diabetes in the Hoorn study. Diabetes Care. 2005;**28**(11):2812.
11. Ekstedt M, Franzen LE, Mathiesen UL, Thorelius L, Holmqvist M, Bodemar G, et al. Long-term follow-up of patients with NAFLD and elevated liver enzymes. Hepatology. 2006;**44**(4):865–73.
12. Neuschwander-Tetri BA, Caldwell SH. Nonalcoholic steatohepatitis: summary of an AASLD Single Topic Conference. Hepatology. 2003;**37**(5):1202–19.
13. Moller DE, Kaufman KD. Metabolic syndrome: a clinical and molecular perspective. Annu Rev Med. 2005;**56**(1):45–62.
14. Day CP. Non-alcoholic fatty liver disease: current concepts and management strategies. Clin Med. 2006;**6**(1):19–25.
15. Boden G. Role of fatty acids in the pathogenesis of insulin resistance and NIDDM. Diabetes. 1997;**461**(1):3–10.
16. Bouchard C. Genetic factors in the regulation of adipose tissue distribution. Acta Med Scand Suppl. 1988;**732**:135–41.
17. Colditz G, Willett W, Rotnitzky A, Manson J. Weight gain as a risk factor for clinical diabetes mellitus in women. Ann Intern Med. 1995;**122**(7):481–6.
18. Ginsberg H. Insulin resistance and cardiovascular disease. J Clin Invest. 2000;**106**(4):453–8.
19. Hsueh W, Quinones M. Role of endothelial dysfunction in insulin resistance. Am J Cardiol. 2003;**92**(4A):10–17J.
20. DeFronzo RA, Ferrannini E. Insulin resistance: a multifaceted syndrome responsible for NIDDM, obesity, hypertension, dyslipidemia, and atherosclerotic cardiovascular disease. Diabetes Care. 1991;**14**(3):173–94.
21. Martyn JA, Kaneki M, Yasuhara S. Obesity-induced insulin resistance and hyperglycemia: etiologic factors and molecular mechanisms. Anesthesiology. 2008;**109**(1):137–48.
22. Reaven GM. Banting lecture 1988. Role of insulin resistance in human disease. Diabetes. 1988;**37**(12):1595–607.
23. Haffner S, Valdez R, Hazuda H. Prospective analysis of the insulin-resistance syndrome (syndrome X). Diabetes. 1992;**41**(6):715–22.
24. Björntorp P. Metabolic implications of body fat distribution. Diabetes Care. 1991;**14**(12):1132–43.
25. Alberti KG, Zimmet PZ. Definition, diagnosis and classification of diabetes mellitus and its complications. Part 1: diagnosis and classification of diabetes mellitus provisional report of a WHO consultation. Diabet Med. 1998;**15**(7):539–53.
26. Third report of the National Cholesterol Education Program (NCEP) expert panel on detection, evaluation, and treatment of high blood pressure in adults (Adult Treatment Panel III): final report. Circulation. 2002;**106**(25):3143–421.
27. Grundy SM, Brewer HB, Cleeman JI, Smith SC, Lenfant C. Definition of metabolic syndrome: Report of the National Heart, Lung, and Blood Institute/American Heart Association. Circulation. 2004;**109**(3):433–38.
28. Grundy SM, Cleeman JI, Daniels SR, Donato KA, Eckel RH, Franklin BA, et al. Diagnosis and management of the metabolic syndrome: an American Heart Association/National Heart, Lung, and Blood Institute Scientific Statement. Circulation. 2005;**112**(17):2735–52.
29. Alberti KGMM, Zimmet P, Shaw J. Metabolic syndrome—a new world-wide definition. A consensus statement from the International Diabetes Federation. Diabet Med. 2006;**23**(5):469–80.
30. Grundy S, Hansen B, Smith S. AHA/NHLBI/ADA conference proceedings: clinical management of metabolic syndrome. Report of the American Heart Association/National Heart, Lung, and Blood Institute/American Diabetes Association Conference on Scientific Issues Related to Management. Circulation. 2004;**109**(4):551–56.
31. Ford E, Giles W. A comparison of the prevalence of the metabolic syndrome using two proposed definitions. Diabetes Care. 2003;**26**(3):575–81.
32. Ford ES, Giles WH, Mokdad AH. Increasing prevalence of the metabolic syndrome among U.S. Adults. Diabetes Care. 2004;**27**(10):2444–49.
33. Kip KE, Marroquin OC, Kelley DE, Johnson BD, Kelsey SF, Shaw LJ, et al. Clinical importance of obesity versus the metabolic syndrome in cardiovascular risk in women: a report from the Women's Ischemia Syndrome Evaluation (WISE) Study. Circulation. 2004;**109**(6):706–13.
34. Karelis AD, St Pierre DH, Conus F, Rabasa-Lhoret R, Poehlman ET. Metabolic and body composition factors in subgroups

of obesity: what do we know? J Clin Endocrinol Metab. 2004;**89**(6):2569–75.

35. Matsuzawa Y, Funahashi T, Kihara S, Shimomura I. Adiponectin and metabolic syndrome. Arterioscler Thromb Vasc Biol. 2004;**24**(1):29–33.

36. Wisse BE. The inflammatory syndrome: the role of adipose tissue cytokines in metabolic disorders linked to obesity. J Am Soc Nephrol. 2004;**15**(11):2792–800.

37. Hamaguchi M, Kojima T, Takeda N, Nakagawa T, Taniguchi H, Fujii K, et al. The metabolic syndrome as a predictor of nonalcoholic fatty liver disease. Ann Intern Med. 2005;**143**(10):722–8.

38. Cornier MA, Dabelea D, Hernandez TL, Lindstrom RC, Steig AJ, Stob NR, et al. The metabolic syndrome. Endocr Rev. 2008;**29**(7):777–822.

39. Pischon T, Girman CJ, Hotamisligil GS, Rifai N, Hu FB, Rimm EB. Plasma adiponectin levels and risk of myocardial infarction in men. JAMA. 2004;**291**(14):1730–7.

40. Pai JK, Pischon T, Ma J, Manson JE, Hankinson SE, Joshipura K, et al. Inflammatory markers and the risk of coronary heart disease in men and women. N Engl J Med. 2004;**351**(25):2599–610.

41. Ridker PM, Rifai N, Pfeffer M, Sacks F, Lepage S, Braunwald E. Elevation of tumor necrosis factor-alpha and increased risk of recurrent coronary events after myocardial infarction. Circulation. 2000;**101**(18):2149–53.

42. Dandona P, Aljada A, Chaudhuri A. The potential influence of inflammation and insulin resistance on the pathogenesis and treatment of atherosclerosis-related complications in type 2 diabetes. J Clin Endocrinol Metab. 2003;**88**(6):2422–29.

43. Meigs J, Mittleman M, Nathan D. Hyperinsulinemia, hyperglycemia, and impaired hemostasis: the Framingham Offspring Study. JAMA. 2000;**283**(2):221–28.

44. Girman C, Rhodes T, Mercuri M. The metabolic syndrome and risk of major coronary events in the Scandinavian Simvastatin Survival Study (4S) and the Air Force/Texas Coronary Atherosclerosis Prevention Study (AFCAPS/TexCAPS). Am J Cardiol. 2004;**93**(2):136–41.

45. McNeill AM, Katz R, Girman CJ, Rosamond WD, Wagenknecht LE, Barzilay JI, et al. Metabolic syndrome and cardiovascular disease in older people: The Cardiovascular Health Study. J Am Geriatr Soc. 2006;**54**(9):1317–24.

46. Sundstrom J, Riserus U, Byberg L, Zethelius B, Lithell H, Lind L. Clinical value of the metabolic syndrome for long term prediction of total and cardiovascular mortality: prospective, population based cohort study. BMJ. 2006;**332**(7546):878–82.

47. Dekker JM, Girman C, Rhodes T, Nijpels G, Stehouwer CD, Bouter LM, et al. Metabolic syndrome and 10-year cardiovascular disease risk in the Hoorn Study. Circulation. 2005;**112**(5):666–73.

48. Huang KC, Lee LT, Chen CY, Sung PK. All-cause and cardiovascular disease mortality increased with metabolic syndrome in Taiwanese. Obesity (Silver Spring). 2008;**16**(3):684–89.

49. Wilson PW, D'Agostino RB, Parise H, Sullivan L, Meigs JB. Metabolic syndrome as a precursor of cardiovascular disease and type 2 diabetes mellitus. Circulation. 2005;**112**(20):3066–72.

50. Mozaffarian D, Kamineni A, Prineas RJ, Siscovick DS. Metabolic syndrome and mortality in older adults: the Cardiovascular Health Study. Arch Intern Med. 2008;**168**(9):969–78.

51. Kurl S, Laukkanen JA, Niskanen L, Laaksonen D, Sivenius J, Nyyssonen K, et al. Metabolic syndrome and the risk of stroke in middle-aged men. Stroke. 2006;**37**(3):806–11.

52. Pan W, Hindler K, Lee VV, Vaughn WK, Collard CD. Obesity in diabetic patients undergoing coronary artery bypass graft surgery is associated with increased postoperative morbidity. Anesthesiology. 2006;**104**(3):441–47.

53. Kajimoto K, Kasai T, Miyauchi K, Hirose H, Yanagisawa N, Yamamoto T, et al. Metabolic syndrome predicts 10-year mortality in non-diabetic patients following coronary artery bypass surgery. Circ J. 2008;**72**(9):1481–86.

54. Kajimoto K, Miyauchi K, Kasai T, Yanagisawa N, Yamamoto T, Kikuchi K, et al. Metabolic syndrome is an independent risk factor for stroke and acute renal failure after coronary artery bypass grafting. J Thorac Cardiovasc Surg. 2009;**137**(3):658–63.

55. Echahidi N, Pibarot P, Després JP, Daigle JM, Mohty D, Voisine P, et al. Metabolic syndrome increases operative mortality in patients undergoing coronary artery bypass grafting surgery. J Am Coll Cardiol. 2007;**50**(9):843–51.

56. Kasai T, Miyauchi K, Kajimoto K, Kubota N, Dohi T, Kurata T, et al. The adverse prognostic significance of the metabolic syndrome with and without hypertension in patients who underwent complete coronary revascularization. J Hypertens. 2009;**27**(5):1017–24.

57. Lohsiriwat V, Pongsanguansuk W, Lertakyamanee N, Lohsiriwat D. Impact of metabolic syndrome on the short-term outcomes of colorectal cancer surgery. Dis Colon Rectum. 2010;**53**(2):186–91.

58. Memtsoudis SG, Kirksey M, Ma Y, Chiu YL, Mazumdar M, Pumberger M, et al. Metabolic syndrome and lumbar spine fusion surgery: epidemiology and perioperative outcomes. Spine (Phila Pa 1976). 2012;**37**(11):989–95.

59. Zmistowski B, Dizdarevic I, Jacovides CL, Radcliff KE, Mraovic B, Parvizi J. Patients with uncontrolled components of metabolic syndrome have increased risk of complications following total joint arthroplasty. J Arthroplasty. 2013;**28**(6):904–907.

60. Tefekli A, Kurtoglu H, Tepeler K, Karadag MA, Kandirali E, Sari E, et al. Does the metabolic syndrome or its components affect the outcome of percutaneous nephrolithotomy? J Endourol. 2007;**22**(1):35–40.

61. Glance MD, Wissler MD, Mukamel P, Li P, Diachun MD, Salloum MD, et al. Perioperative outcomes among patients with the modified metabolic syndrome who are undergoing noncardiac surgery. Anesthesiology. 2010;**113**(4):859–72.

62. Birkmeyer NJ, Charlesworth DC, Hernandez F, Leavitt BJ, Marrin CA, Morton JR, et al. Obesity and risk of adverse outcomes associated with coronary artery bypass surgery. Northern New England Cardiovascular Disease Study Group. Circulation. 1998;**97**(17):1689–94.

63. Jin R, Grunkemeier GL, Furnary AP, Handy JR, Jr Is obesity a risk factor for mortality in coronary artery bypass surgery? Circulation. 2005;**111**(25):3359–65.

64. Kim J, Hammar N, Jakobsson K, Luepker RV, McGovern PG, Ivert T. Obesity and the risk of early and late mortality after coronary artery bypass graft surgery. Am Heart J. 2003;**146**(3):555–60.

65. Reeves BC, Ascione R, Chamberlain MH, Angelini GD. Effect of body mass index on early outcomes in patients undergoing coronary artery bypass surgery. J Am Coll Cardiol. 2003;**42**(4):668–76.

66. Prabhakar G, Haan CK, Peterson ED, Coombs LP, Cruzzavala JL, Murray GF. The risks of moderate and extreme obesity for coronary artery bypass grafting outcomes: a study from the Society of Thoracic Surgeons' database. Ann Thorac Surg. 2002;**74**(4):1125–30.

67. Ray DE, Matchett SC, Baker K, Wasser T, Young MJ. The effect of body mass index on patient outcomes in a medical ICU. Chest. 2005;**127**(6):2125–31.

68. Tremblay A, Bandi V. Impact of body mass index on outcomes following critical care. Chest. 2003 Apr;**123**(4):1202–1207.

69. Hutagalung R, Marques J, Kobylka K, Zeidan M, Kabisch B, Brunkhorst F, et al. The obesity paradox in surgical intensive care unit patients. Intensive Care Med. 2011;**37**(11):1793–99.

70. Oliveros H, Villamor E. Obesity and mortality in critically ill adults: a systematic review and meta-analysis. Obesity. 2008;**16**(3):515–21.

71. Hogue CW, Stearns JD, Colantuoni E, Robinson KA, Stierer T, Mitter N, et al. The impact of obesity on outcomes after critical illness: a meta-analysis. Intensive Care Med. 2009;**35**(7):1152–70.

72. Niedziela J, Hudzik B, Niedziela N, G-àsior M, Gierlotka M, Wasilewski J, et al. The obesity paradox in acute coronary syndrome: a meta-analysis. Eur J Epidemiol. 2014;**29**(11):801–12.

73. Sharma A, Lavie CJ, Borer JS, Vallakati A, Goel S, Lopez-Jimenez F, et al. Meta-analysis of the relation of body mass index to all-cause and cardiovascular mortality and hospitalization in patients with chronic heart failure. Am J Cardiol. 2015;**115**(10):1428–34.

74. Sharma A, Vallakati A, Einstein AJ, Lavie CJ, Arbab-Zadeh A, Lopez-Jimenez F, et al. Relationship of body mass index with total mortality, cardiovascular mortality, and myocardial infarction after coronary revascularization: evidence from a meta-analysis. Mayo Clin Proc. 2014;**89**(8):1080–100.

75. Nie W, Zhang Y, Jee SH, Jung KJ, Li B, Xiu Q. Obesity survival paradox in pneumonia: a meta-analysis. BMC Med. 2014;**12**:61.

76. Park J, Ahmadi SF, Streja E, Molnar MZ, Flegal KM, Gillen D, et al. Obesity paradox in end-stage kidney disease patients. Prog Cardiovasc Dis. 2014;**56**(4):415–25.

77. Kramer CK, Zinman B, Retnakaran R. Are metabolically healthy overweight and obesity benign conditions? A systematic review and meta-analysis. Ann Intern Med. 2013;**159**(11):758–69.

78. Eagle KA, Berger PB, Calkins H, Chaitman BR, Ewy GA, Fleischmann KE, et al. ACC/AHA guideline update for perioperative cardiovascular evaluation for noncardiac surgery—executive summary: a report of the American College of Cardiology/American Heart Association Task Force on Practice Guidelines (Committee to Update the 1996 Guidelines on Perioperative Cardiovascular Evaluation for Noncardiac Surgery). J Am Coll Cardiol. 2002;**39**(3):542–53.

79. Alexander CM, Landsman PB, Teutsch SM, Haffner SM. NCEP-defined metabolic syndrome, diabetes, and prevalence of coronary heart disease among NHANES III participants age 50 years and older. Diabetes. 2003;**52**(5):1210–14.

80. Devereaux PJ, Yang H, Yusuf S, Guyatt G, Leslie K, Villar JC, et al. Effects of extended-release metoprolol succinate in patients undergoing non-cardiac surgery (POISE trial): a randomised controlled trial. Lancet. 2008;**371**(9627):1839–47.

81. Colhoun HM, Betteridge DJ, Durrington PN, Hitman GA, Neil HA, Livingstone SJ, et al. Primary prevention of cardiovascular disease with atorvastatin in type 2 diabetes in the Collaborative Atorvastatin Diabetes Study (CARDS): multicentre randomised placebo-controlled trial. Lancet. 2004;**364**(9435):685–96.

82. Biccard BM. A peri-operative statin update for non-cardiac surgery. Part II: statin therapy for vascular surgery and peri-operative statin trial design. Anaesthesia. 2008;**63**(2):162–71.

83. Heeschen C, Hamm CW, Laufs U, Snapinn S, Bohm M, White HD. Withdrawal of statins increases event rates in patients with acute coronary syndromes. Circulation. 2002;**105**(12):1446–52.

84. Le MY, Godet G, Coriat P, Martinon C, Bertrand M, Fleron MH, et al. The impact of postoperative discontinuation or continuation of chronic statin therapy on cardiac outcome after major vascular surgery. Anesth Analg. 2007;**104**(6):1326–33.

85. Schouten O, Hoeks SE, Welten GM, Davignon J, Kastelein JJ, Vidakovic R, et al. Effect of statin withdrawal on frequency of cardiac events after vascular surgery. Am J Cardiol. 2007;**100**(2):316–20.

86. Capes SE, Hunt D, Malmberg K, Gerstein HC. Stress hyperglycaemia and increased risk of death after myocardial infarction in patients with and without diabetes: a systematic overview. Lancet. 2000;**355**(9206):773–78.

87. Wahab NN, Cowden EA, Pearce NJ, Gardner MJ, Merry H, Cox JL. Is blood glucose an independent predictor of mortality in acute myocardial infarction in the thrombolytic era? J Am Coll Cardiol. 2002;**40**(10):1748–54.

88. Iwakura K, Ito H, Ikushima M, Kawano S, Okamura A, Asano K, et al. Association between hyperglycemia and the no-reflow phenomenon in patients with acute myocardial infarction. J Am Coll Cardiol. 2003;**41**(1):1–7.

89. O'Neill PA, Davies I, Fullerton KJ, Bennett D. Stress hormone and blood glucose response following acute stroke in the elderly. Stroke. 1991;**22**(7):842–47.

90. Jonassen AK, Sack MN, Mjos OD, Yellon DM. Myocardial protection by insulin at reperfusion requires early administration and is mediated via Akt and p70s6 kinase cell-survival signaling. Circ Res. 2001;**89**(12):1191–98.

91. Lazar HL, Chipkin SR, Fitzgerald CA, Bao Y, Cabral H, Apstein CS. Tight glycemic control in diabetic coronary artery bypass graft patients improves perioperative outcomes and decreases recurrent ischemic events. Circulation. 2004;**109**(12):1497–502.

92. Zerr KJ, Furnary AP, Grunkemeier GL, Bookin S, Kanhere V, Starr A. Glucose control lowers the risk of wound infection in diabetics after open heart operations. Ann Thorac Surg. 1997;**63**(2):356–61.

93. Furnary AP, Zerr KJ, Grunkemeier GL, Starr A. Continuous intravenous insulin infusion reduces the incidence of deep sternal wound infection in diabetic patients after cardiac surgical procedures. Ann Thorac Surg. 1999;**67**(2):352–60.

94. Furnary AP, Gao G, Grunkemeier GL, Wu Y, Zerr KJ, Bookin SO, et al. Continuous insulin infusion reduces mortality in patients with diabetes undergoing coronary artery bypass grafting. J Thorac Cardiovasc Surg. 2003;**125**(5):1007–21.

95. van den Berghe G, Wouters P, Weekers F, Verwaest C, Bruyninckx F, Schetz M, et al. Intensive insulin therapy in the critically ill patients. N Engl J Med. 2001;**345**(19):1359–67.

96. van den Berghe G, Wilmer A, Hermans G, Meersseman W, Wouters PJ, Milants I, et al. Intensive insulin therapy in the medical ICU. N Engl J Med. 2006;**354**(5):449–61.

97. Brunkhorst FM, Engel C, Bloos F, Meier-Hellmann A, Ragaller M, Weiler N, et al. Intensive insulin therapy and pentastarch resuscitation in severe sepsis. N Engl J Med. 2008;**358**(2):125–39.

98. NICE-SUGAR Study Investigators. Intensive versus conventional glucose control in critically ill patients. N Engl J Med. 2009;**360**(13):1283–97.

Cardiorespiratory physiology including airway changes in obesity

Jahan Porhomayon and Peter J. Papadakos

Introduction

Obesity is a serious disorder resulting in major health consequences. Obese adults are at increased risk for acute and chronic medical conditions. The rise in the rate of obesity in school-aged children, adolescents, and young adults in the last 30 years is a clear healthcare crisis that needs to be addressed. Despite recent national reports in the United States highlighting positive downward trends in the rate of obesity in younger children, we are still faced with approximately 12.7 million children struggling with obesity [1,2].

The prevalence of clinically severe obesity is increasing at a much faster rate among adults in the United States than is the prevalence of moderate obesity. This is consistent with the public health idea that the population weight distribution is shifting, which disproportionately increases extreme weight categories. Because comorbidities and resulting medical service use are much higher among severely obese individuals, the widely published trends for overweight/obesity underestimate the consequences for population health. The aggressive and costly expansion of bariatric surgery in recent years has had no visible effect on containing morbid obesity rates in the United States [3]. The increasing obesity prevalence encompassed all segments of the population across sex, race, educational status, and socioeconomic status.

Airway-related obesity disorder

Previous studies have determined that neck circumference and obesity were predictors of difficult intubation in morbidly obese surgical patients [4]. It has been reported that even tracheostomy tube placement could fail because of anatomical changes due to obesity and a short neck [5]. Obesity and anatomical variations, such as retrognathia, increase the likelihood of upper airway collapse by altering the passive mechanical behaviour of the upper airway. Fat deposits were observed anterior to the laryngopharyngeal airspace, in submental regions, in all obese subjects [6]. This characteristic depends on the mechanical properties of each upper airway tissue in isolation, their geometrical arrangements, and their physiological interactions. Recent measurements of respiratory-related deformation of the airway wall have shown that there are different patterns of airway soft tissue movement during the respiratory cycle. In obese patients with obstructive sleep apnoea (OSA), airway dilation appears less coordinated compared with that in healthy subjects (matched for body mass index). Intrinsic mechanical properties of airway tissues are altered in obese OSA patients, but the factors underlying these changes have yet to be elucidated. How neural drive to the airway dilators relates to the biomechanical behaviour of the upper airway (movement and stiffness) is still poorly understood [7]. Additionally, increased neck circumference has been associated with increased upper airway collapsibility in adolescents in the hypotonic but not the activated state [8]. Although obesity with enlargement of soft tissue structures is considered the predominant mechanism leading to upper airway narrowing, abnormal craniofacial development on a genetic or developmental basis also plays an important contributory role [9].

Obesity and the respiratory system

The prevalence of obesity has increased considerably during the past 30 years. Possible consequences of obesity on respiratory physiology include a restrictive disorder, changes in ventilatory mechanics, and an alteration of respiratory drive. Apart from the well-established relation between obesity and OSA–hypopnea syndrome, obesity is associated with other respiratory disorders as well. On the one hand, epidemiological and animal data suggest a causal relationship between obesity and asthma. On the other hand, morbid obesity is associated, through an alteration of the respiratory drive involving leptin, with a diurnal and nocturnal alveolar hypoventilation defining the obesity–hypoventilation syndrome [10].

Obesity, along with its pathophysiological changes, increases the risk of intraoperative and perioperative respiratory complications. Obesity affects every organ system and causes significant chronic medical comorbidities. In particular, perioperative hypoxaemia is quite common due to a decrease in expiratory reserve volume, and the change increases in direct proportion with increasing body mass index. To avoid hypoxaemia during induction of general an-aesthesia, evaluation of the difficult airway is very important. In morbid obesity, there is an increased hindrance to breathing caused by the effects of the increased mass on the chest wall and abdomen. Subjects with morbid obesity can maintain normal concentrations of carbon dioxide by increasing inspiratory neuromuscular drive and/or by altering central breath timing [11]. Obesity decreases total respiratory compliance by as much as two-thirds of the normal value as measured in non-obese individuals [12,13]. The decrease in com-pliance was thought to result primarily from a reduced chest wall compliance associated with the deposition of fat in and around the ribs, the diaphragm, and the abdomen. Subsequent investigations in healthy obese subjects revealed higher total respiratory system and chest wall elastance during voluntary muscle relaxation than during paralysis [14], suggesting that incomplete relaxation may have contributed to lower chest wall compliance reported in total lung capacity (TLC) and vital capacity (VC) [14,15] which decrease linearly with a rising body mass index [16]; however, the changes are small, and TLC is usually maintained above the lower limit of normal. A marked abnormality of lung volumes in mild to mod-erate obesity should raise suspicion of an underlying intrinsic lung disease or neuromuscular pathology except in those with morbid obesity or those with excessive central adiposity (waist-to-hip ratio ≥0.95) [14].

Spirometry is normal in mild obesity. As body mass index in-creases, there is a reduction in expiratory flow and a decrease in forced expiratory volume in 1 second (FEV_1) and forced vital cap-acity (FVC) [15]. The ratio of FEV_1 to FVC is preserved and even increased, which is attributed to peripheral airway closure and gas trapping, hence reducing the VC. However, the reduction in FEV_1 and FVC is strongly correlated with abdominal obesity. FVC, FEV_1, and TLC were found to be significantly lower in subjects with upper body fat distribution or central obesity earlier studies.

Obesity and sleep disorders

Obesity is an important risk factor for OSA syndrome and pa-tients using a nasal continuous positive airway pressure or bi-level positive airway pressure device at home should be treated in a post-anaesthesia care unit [17]. OSA–hypopnea syndrome in-volves recurring episodes of total obstruction (apnoea) or partial obstruction (hypopnea) of airways during sleep. OSA–hypopnea syndrome affects mainly obese individuals and it is defined by an apnoea–hypopnea index of five or more episodes per hour associ-ated with daytime somnolence [18]. In addition to anatomical fac-tors and neuromuscular and genetic factors, sleep disorders are also involved in the pathogenesis of sleep apnoea. Obesity affects upper airway anatomy because of fat deposition and metabolic activity of adipose tissue. OSA–hypopnea syndrome and metabolic syndrome have several characteristics such as visceral obesity, hypertension, and insulin resistance. Inflammatory cytokines might be related to the pathogenesis of sleep apnoea and metabolic syndrome. Sleep ap-noea treatment includes obesity treatment, use of equipment such as continuous positive airway pressure machines, drug therapy, and even surgical procedures in selected patients. Currently, there is no specific drug therapy available with proven efficacy for the treatment of OSA–hypopnea syndrome. Body weight reduction results in

improvement of sleep apnoea and obesity treatment must be empha-sized, including lifestyle changes, anti-obesity drugs, and bariatric surgery [19]. The use of magnetic resonance imaging has revealed that spontaneous sleep caused significant obstruction and nar-rowing of various sites of the pharyngeal airway in the OSA patients, but not in the non-OSA subjects. During wakefulness, the non-OSA subjects showed no marked narrowing of the pharyngeal airways, whereas a transient but significant narrowing was observed in the OSA patients. The mean values of both the cross-sectional area and the anterior–posterior diameter at the soft palate were significantly reduced by spontaneous sleep in the OSA patients [20]. Investigators have determined that a diagnosis of OSA imparts an increased risk of postoperative respiratory failure, cardiac events, and intensive care unit transfer than patients with a non-OSA diagnosis [21,22].

Anaesthetic management

The presence of coexisting disease, difficulty with airway manage-ment, and respiratory compromise, as well as alterations in drug metabolism in obese patients, combine to make understanding this particular disorder vital for the clinical anaesthesiologist [23,24]. Obese patients show a markedly increased perioperative morbidity and mortality [25–27]. Due to the severe impairment of the cardiopulmonary system, the extremely obese patient is at high risk for cardiac and pulmonary complications. It is now recom-mended that a multidisciplinary approach for surgery on obese patients involving an anaesthesiologist early in their care improves outcome [28] (Fig. 9.1).

Among the abundant pathophysiological disorders are reduc-tions in functional residual capacity and total compliance as well as oxygen costs of breathing that are increased by a factor of 4–16 [29]. Changes in static and dynamic respiratory mechanics, upper

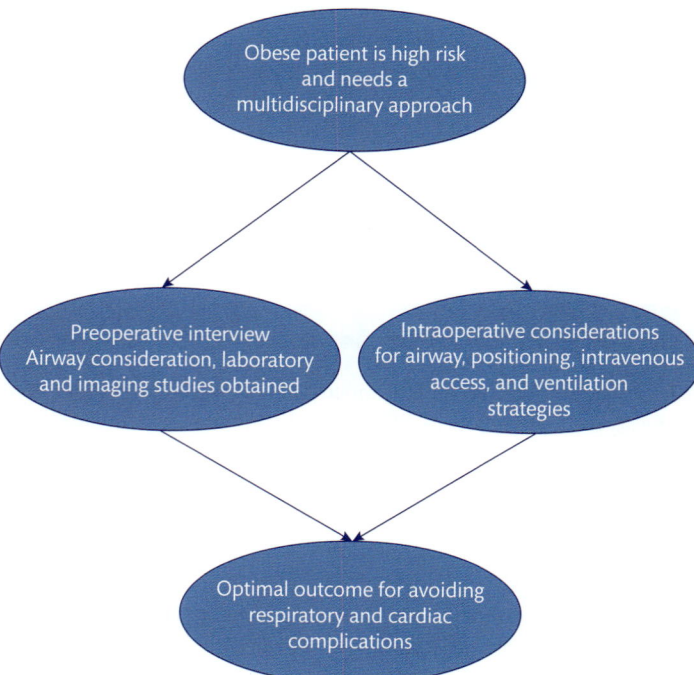

Fig. 9.1 Suggested outline for approaching an obese surgical patient.

airway anatomy, as well as multiple preoperative comorbidities and altered drug metabolism characterize obese patients and will impact the anaesthetic plan at multiple levels [30]. During the preoperative evaluation, patients should be assessed to identify who is at risk for difficult ventilation and intubation [31] and postoperative complications. Benzodiazepine loading doses should be adjusted on actual weight, and maintenance doses should be adjusted on ideal body weight. Propofol dosages are calculated on total body weight. The loading dose of lipophilic opioids is based on total body weight, whereas maintenance dosages should be cautiously reduced because of the higher sensitivity of the obese patient to their depressant effects. Pharmacokinetic parameters of muscle relaxants are minimally affected by obesity, and their dosage is based on ideal rather than total body weight. Inhalation anaesthetics with very low lipid solubility, such as sevoflurane and desflurane, allow for quick modification of the anaesthetic plan during surgery and rapid emergence at the end of surgery, hence representing very flexible anaesthetic drugs for use in this patient population. Drug dosing is generally based on the volume of distribution for the loading dose and on the clearance for maintenance. In the obese patient, the volume of distribution is increased if the drug is distributed both in lean and fat tissues whereas the anaesthetic drug clearance is usually normal or increased [32].

An effective strategy to minimize intubation and extubation airway complications should include pre-emptive optimization of patients' conditions, careful timing of extubation [33], the presence of experienced personnel trained in advanced airway management, and the availability of the necessary equipment and appropriate airway monitoring [34]. Even after weight loss, patients with post-gastric surgery are still at increased risk of pulmonary aspiration during induction of general anaesthesia [35]. The analgesic plan should be executed starting in the preoperative area, to increase the success of ventilation at the end of the case and prevent reintubation. Intraoperative ventilatory settings should be customized to the changes in respiratory mechanics for the specific patient and procedure [36], to minimize the risk of lung damage. Several non-invasive ventilatory modalities are available [33] to increase the success rate of extubation at the end of the case and to prevent reintubation [37]. Detailed preoperative examination and discussion should take place with an emphasis on comorbidities and their impact on anaesthesia. Particular laboratory studies, such as arterial blood gases, electrocardiogram, selected pulmonary function tests, and serum hepatic profile, can be quite useful. Intraoperative concerns encompass the choice of airway (awake versus sedation or anaesthesia) [38], patient positioning [39], availability of a difficult airway cart in the operating room or post-anaesthesia recovery room [40], regional versus general anaesthesia [41], anaesthetic biotransformation, and variables influencing intraoperative oxygenation [30]. Obesity and snorers are the high-risk groups of perioperative desaturation [42,43]. Postoperative concerns are directed towards minimizing postoperative hypoxaemia, peripheral intravenous access, and fluid imbalances. Specific choices of anaesthetic agents and techniques await further clinical and laboratory investigations in this unique subset of the population [44]. Patients with sleep-disordered breathing must be managed according to institutional protocols [45–47].

In summary, the management of obese or super-obese patients undergoing surgery and anaesthesia requires a team approach to prevent complications. A thorough understanding of the pathophysiology of the obese patient is necessary in order to make appropriate adjustments to anaesthesia and the surgical plan.

REFERENCES

1. Karp SM, Gesell SB. Obesity prevention and treatment in school-aged children, adolescents, and young adults—where do we go from here? Prim Prev Insights. 2015;5:1–4.
2. Anandam A, Akinnusi M, Kufel T, Porhomayon J, El-Solh AA. Effects of dietary weight loss on obstructive sleep apnea: a meta-analysis. Sleep Breath. 2013;17(1):227–34.
3. Sturm R. Increases in morbid obesity in the USA: 2000–2005. Public Health. 2007;121(7):492–96.
4. Riad W, Vaez MN, Raveendran R, Tam AD, Quereshy FA, Chung F, et al. Neck circumference as a predictor of difficult intubation and difficult mask ventilation in morbidly obese patients: a prospective observational study. Eur J Anaesthesiol. 2016;33(4):244–49.
5. Hwang SM, Jang JS, Yoo JI, Kwon HK, Lee SK, Lee JJ, et al. Difficult tracheostomy tube placement in an obese patient with a short neck – a case report. Korean J Anesthesiol. 2011;60(6):434–36.
6. Horner RL, Mohiaddin RH, Lowell DG, Shea SA, Burman ED, Longmore DB, et al. Sites and sizes of fat deposits around the pharynx in obese patients with obstructive sleep apnoea and weight matched controls. Eur Respir J. 1989;2(7):613–22.
7. Bilston LE, Gandevia SC. Biomechanical properties of the human upper airway and their effect on its behavior during breathing and in obstructive sleep apnea. J Appl Physiol. 2014;116(3):314–24.
8. Yuan H, Schwab RJ, Kim C, He J, Shults J, Bradford R, et al. Relationship between body fat distribution and upper airway dynamic function during sleep in adolescents. Sleep. 2013;36(8):1199–207.
9. Shepard JW, Jr, Gefter WB, Guilleminault C, Hoffman EA, Hoffstein V, Hudgel DW, et al. Evaluation of the upper airway in patients with obstructive sleep apnea. Sleep. 1991;14(4):361–71.
10. Réthoret-Lacatis C, Janssens JP. Obesity and respiratory disorders. Rev Med Suisse. 2008;4(180):2512–14, 2516–17.
11. Burki NK, Baker RW. Ventilatory regulation in eucapnic morbid obesity. Am Rev Respir Dis. 1984;129(4):538–43.
12. von Ungern-Sternberg BS, et al. Comparison of perioperative spirometric data following spinal or general anaesthesia in normal-weight and overweight gynaecological patients. Acta Anaesthesiol Scand. 2005;49(7):940–48.
13. Naimark A, Cherniack RM. Compliance of the respiratory system and its components in health and obesity. J Appl Physiol. 1960;15:377–82.
14. Rubinstein I, Zamel N, DuBarry L, Hoffstein V. Airflow limitation in morbidly obese, nonsmoking men. Ann Intern Med. 1990;112(11):828–32.
15. von Ungern-Sternberg BS, Regli A, Schneider MC, Kunz F, Reber A. Effect of obesity and site of surgery on perioperative lung volumes. Br J Anaesth. 2004;92(2):202–207.
16. Söderberg M, Thomson D, White T. Respiration, circulation and anaesthetic management in obesity. Investigation before and after jejunoileal bypass. Acta Anaesthesiol Scand. 1977;21(1):55–61.
17. Takeda K. Preoperative assessment of obese patients. Masui. 2010;59(7):874–78.
18. Munish M, et al. The use of practice guidelines by the American Society of Anesthesiologists for the identification of surgical

patients at high risk of sleep apnea. Chron Respir Dis. 2012;**9**(4):221–30.

19. de Sousa AG, Cercato C, Mancini MC, Halpern A. Obesity and obstructive sleep apnea-hypopnea syndrome. Obes Rev. 2008;**9**(4):340–54.

20. Ikeda K, Ogura M, Oshima T, Suzuki H, Higano S, Takahashi S, et al. Quantitative assessment of the pharyngeal airway by dynamic magnetic resonance imaging in obstructive sleep apnea syndrome. Ann Otol Rhinol Laryngol. 2001;**110**(2):183–89.

21. Hai F, Porhomayon J, Vermont L, Frydrych L, Jaoude P, El-Solh AA. Postoperative complications in patients with obstructive sleep apnea: a meta-analysis. J Clin Anesth. 2014;**26**(8):591–600.

22. Reddy R, Adamo D, Kufel T, Porhomayon J, El-Solh AA. Treatment of opioid-related central sleep apnea with positive airway pressure: a systematic review. J Opioid Manag. 2014;**10**(1):57–62.

23. Richards TA, Kaye AD, Fields AM. Morbid obesity—a review. Middle East J Anesthesiol. 2005;**18**(1):93–105.

24. Ortiz VE, Kwo J. Obesity: physiologic changes and implications for preoperative management. BMC Anesthesiol. 2015;**15**:97.

25. Wilson AT, Reilly CS. Anaesthesia and the obese patient. Int J Obes Relat Metab Disord. 1993;**17**(8):427–35.

26. Waisath TC, et al. Body mass index and the risk of postoperative complications with dentoalveolar surgery: a prospective study. Oral Surg Oral Med Oral Pathol Oral Radiol Endod. 2009;**108**(2):169–73.

27. Joshi GP, Ahmad S, Riad W, Eckert S, Chung F. Selection of obese patients undergoing ambulatory surgery: a systematic review of the literature. Anesth Analg. 2013;**117**(5):1082–91.

28. Lindauer B, Steurer MP, Müller MK, Dullenkopf A. Anesthetic management of patients undergoing bariatric surgery: two year experience in a single institution in Switzerland. BMC Anesthesiol. 2014;**14**:125.

29. Peters J, Steinhoff H. Anesthesia problems in extreme obesity. Anaesthesist. 1983;**32**(8):374–81.

30. Porhomayon J, et al. Strategies in postoperative analgesia in the obese obstructive sleep apnea patient. Clin J Pain. 2013;**29**(11):998–1005.

31. Weinberg L, Tay S, Lai CF, Barnes M. Perioperative risk stratification for a patient with severe obstructive sleep apnoea undergoing laparoscopic banding surgery. BMJ Case Rep. 2013;**2013**:bcr2012008336.

32. Casati A, Putzu M. Anesthesia in the obese patient: pharmacokinetic considerations. J Clin Anesth. 2005;**17**(2):134–45.

33. Nicholson A, Cook TM, Smith AF, Lewis SR, Reed SS. Supraglottic airway devices versus tracheal intubation for airway management during general anaesthesia in obese patients. Cochrane Database Syst Rev. 2013;**9**:CD010105.

34. Cavallone LF, Vannucci A. Review article: extubation of the difficult airway and extubation failure. Anesth Analg. 2013;**116**(2):368–83.

35. Koolwijk J, Schors M, el Bouazati S, Noordergraaf GJ. Airway management concerns in patient with gastric banding procedures. BMJ Case Rep. 2013;**2013**: bcr2013201009.

36. Watson RA, Pride NB. Postural changes in lung volumes and respiratory resistance in subjects with obesity. J Appl Physiol (1985). 2005;**98**(2):512–17.

37. Pedoto A. Lung physiology and obesity: anesthetic implications for thoracic procedures. Anesthesiol Res Pract. 2012;**2012**:154208.

38. Uakritdathikarn T, Asampinawat T, Wanasuwannakul T, Yoosamran B. Awake intubation with Airtraq laryngoscope in a morbidly obese patient. J Med Assoc Thai. 2008;**91**(4):564–67.

39. Ebert TJ, Shankar H, Haake RM. Perioperative considerations for patients with morbid obesity. Anesthesiol Clin. 2006;**24**(3):621–36.

40. Porhomayon J, El-Solh AA, Nader ND. National survey to assess the content and availability of difficult-airway carts in critical-care units in the United States. J Anesth. 2010;**24**(5):811–14.

41. Kim HJ, Kim WH, Lim HW, Kim JA, Kim DK, Shin BS, et al. Obesity is independently associated with spinal anesthesia outcomes: a prospective observational study. PLoS One. 2015;10(4):e0124264.

42. Uakritdathikarn T, Chongsuvivatwong V, Geater AF, Vasinanukorn M, Thinchana S, Klayna S. Perioperative desaturation and risk factors in general anesthesia. J Med Assoc Thai. 2008;**91**(7):1020–29.

43. Mendonca J, et al. Obese patients: respiratory complications in the post-anesthesia care unit. Rev Port Pneumol. 2014;**20**(1):12–19.

44. Vaughan RW. Anesthetic management of the morbidly obese patient. Contemp Anesth Pract. 1982;**5**:71–94.

45. Unetani H, et al. Perioperative management of a morbidly obese patient with sleep apnea syndrome. Masui. 2003;**52**(6):646–49.

46. Porhomayon J, et al. Respiratory perioperative management of patients with obstructive sleep apnea. J Intensive Care Med. 2014;**29**(3):145–53.

47. Porhomayon J, El-Solh A, Chhangani S, Nader ND. The management of surgical patients with obstructive sleep apnea. Lung. 2011;**189**(5):359–67.

Obstructive sleep apnoea
Incidence, physiology, and management

Raviraj Raveendran and Frances Chung

Introduction

Obstructive sleep apnoea (OSA) is the most common breathing disorder of sleep, characterized by recurrent episodes of upper airway obstruction with recurrent cycles of desaturation and reoxygenation, leading to fragmentation of sleep associated with daytime fatigue and sleepiness. The incidence of OSA is increasing in proportion to the increase in obesity incidence. A significant number of OSA patients are not diagnosed when they present for elective surgery [1], and up to 24% of surgical patients are found to be at high risk based on screening, of whom 81% have not been previously diagnosed with OSA [2,3]. Recent outcome studies on surgical populations have shown the importance of diagnosis and optimizing these patients before surgery [4,5]. Since OSA is an important risk factor for other comorbid conditions such as hypertension, ischaemic heart disease, cardiac arrhythmias, pulmonary hypertension, and stroke, identification and management of OSA has been given more importance in recent years. Recent understanding of sleep physiology, pathogenesis of OSA, and anaesthetic effects on OSA has resulted in significant changes in the perioperative management of OSA patients [6,7]. In this chapter, we review the epidemiology, pathophysiology, and management of OSA in morbidly obese patients.

Definition of obstructive sleep apnoea

The gold standard for the diagnosis of OSA requires an overnight polysomnography or sleep study. The severity of OSA is determined by the apnoea–hypopnea index (AHI), which is defined as the average number of abnormal breathing events per hour of sleep. Apnoea refers to cessation of airflow for 10 seconds, while hypopnea occurs with reduced airflow with desaturation of at least 4% [8]. The American Academy of Sleep Medicine diagnostic criteria for OSA requires either an AHI of 15 or greater, or an AHI of at least 5 with symptoms, such as daytime sleepiness, loud snoring, or observed obstruction during sleep [9]. The Canadian Thoracic Society guidelines for diagnosing OSA require the presence of an AHI of at least 5 on polysomnography, and either of (1) daytime sleepiness or (2) two other symptoms of OSA (e.g. choking or gasping during sleep, unrefreshing sleep, recurrent awakenings, daytime fatigue) [10]. Severity of OSA is mild for an AHI of at least 5 to less than 15, moderate for an AHI 15–30, and severe for an AHI greater than 30 events/hour [9].

Epidemiology and risk factors for obstructive sleep apnoea

The prevalence of OSA is increasing in parallel with obesity. The actual incidence varies according to the variation in the definition of OSA. In the Wisconsin Sleep Cohort study, by defining OSA as an AHI of at least 5 events/hour the prevalence was 24% in men and 9% in women aged 30–60 years [11]. According to a North American study, the reported incidence was 13% of men and 6% in women, in which OSA was defined with an AHI greater than 15 events/hour [12]. The prevalence of OSA was as high as 78% in morbidly obese patients scheduled for bariatric surgery [13]. More recent data from Europe had an alarming level of OSA incidence of 23.4% and 49% for female and male subjects, respectively [14]. In addition, the incidence varies with race and ethnicity of the study population. The prevalence of OSA is higher in black compared to white populations, but the incidence of non-obese OSA is highest in Chinese people [15]. Since it is difficult to have a rigid cut-off point with definition, OSA should be considered as a spectrum of disease similar to hypertension and diabetes mellitus.

The incidence of OSA increases with age and males are three time more prone to OSA [16]. Obesity is the most important risk factor for OSA. A 10% increase in body mass index increases the OSA incidence up to six times [17]. In a 2015 retrospective study on obese patients with hypoxaemia, the incidence of OSA was 80% [18]. Males with central or android obesity are more prone to have OSA than the gynaecoid type of obesity. Craniofacial abnormalities including abnormal maxillary or short mandibular size, a wide craniofacial base, and adenoid and tonsillar hypertrophy increase the risk of OSA [19]. Smokers have a three times higher risk of OSA than non-smokers [20]. The incidence of OSA during pregnancy in the first and third trimesters was 10.5% and 26.7%, respectively, in one study [21]. Other medical conditions precipitate OSA, including congestive heart failure, chronic obstructive pulmonary disease, acromegaly, hypothyroidism, and end-stage renal disease.

Pathophysiology of obstructive sleep apnoea

In general, sleep reduces tonic activation of upper airway dilator musculature leading to increased airway compliance and an enhanced collapsibility, which is more pronounced during rapid eye movement sleep. In the awake state, the upper airway stability and patency is maintained by increased genioglossus muscle tone by pulling the tongue forward [22]. This normal physiological change is exaggerated in OSA patients, whose airway is narrower, longer, and more collapsible, and it mainly depends on compensatory activation of airway dilator muscles to maintain patency during wakefulness. There are anatomical and non-anatomical factors contributing to the pathogenesis of OSA. The non-anatomical factors include neuromuscular mechanism, lung volume, ventilator control, arousal threshold, and rostral fluid shift [23].

Considering the anatomical factors, OSA patients have smaller pharyngeal airways in comparison with non-OSA controls, with a narrower cross-sectional area of the airway lumen, which is more vulnerable to collapse [24]. Also, they have bigger tongues, greater lateral pharyngeal wall width, and longer soft palates than controls [25]. Obesity is one of the major risk factors for OSA, which contributes by increases in parapharyngeal fat and fat deposition in the tongue [26]. Other craniofacial abnormalities including smaller cranial base, smaller maxilla, and mandibular retrognathia are likely to encroach on upper airway soft tissues and result in a smaller airway space [27]. The box model describes an excess soft tissue with the normal skeletal frame (obesity) or normal soft tissue with the restricted skeletal frame (craniofacial abnormality). Both increase the closing pressure in the upper airway [28]. This anatomical imbalance contributes to OSA [29], which is further influenced by sex and ethnicity. The upper airway is more collapsible in the supine compared to the lateral position and this may be related to upper airway dilator muscle responsiveness and reduction in lung volume in supine position.

Considering the non-anatomical factors, upper airway pharyngeal muscle tone is maintained by input from chemoreceptor and mechanoreceptor output from the brainstem respiratory centre, which is influenced by sleep and the awake state. In comparison with non-OSA patients, OSA patients have an increase in pharyngeal muscle activity during the awake state. During sleep, the activity of the dilator muscle in OSA patients reduces more than in non-OSA patients [30,31]. This loss of neuromuscular compensation contributes to the pharyngeal muscle collapse during sleep. Lung volumes are important to maintain the upper airway patency. An increase in lung volume results in caudal traction on the trachea, which increases the pharyngeal lumen size and reduces pharyngeal extraluminal tissue pressure [32]. Lung volumes are markedly reduced by a combination of increased abdominal

fat mass and recumbent posture. Reduction of lung volume may decrease longitudinal tracheal traction forces and pharyngeal wall tension, which predisposes to narrowing of the airway. In addition, obesity-related leptin resistance may impair the neuroanatomical interactions necessary for stable breathing, thereby contributing to the pathogenesis of OSA [33].

Though anatomical changes and deficiencies in compensatory mechanisms by pharyngeal muscle activity are key factors for the upper airway collapse in OSA, the ventilatory control system plays an important role [34]. Neuronal output from the central respiratory generator controls breathing to maintain the optimal levels of oxygen and carbon dioxide. OSA patients are likely to have instability of this control system which leads to periods of cyclic breathing and an obstructed airway [35]. This instability is called loop gain. A high loop gain causes an excessive response to hypoxia, which leads to hyperventilation and potentiation of apnoea. It has been shown that there is a strong correlation between high loop gain and OSA with a non-collapsible upper airway [36].

Arousal is a protective reflex to avoid hypoxia after an obstruction event during sleep. This terminates apnoea and resumes breathing. At the same time, this leads to hyperventilation and further potentiates the apnoea. Some OSA patients have a low arousal threshold which allows them to wake from sleep before the compensatory mechanisms become activated. OSA patients with a high arousal threshold may be more prone to respiratory depression with opioids. Understanding the phenotype of OSA is essential in the management of these patients [37].

There is a high prevalence of OSA among patients with heart and renal failure due to nocturnal rostral fluid shift. At night in the supine position, gravity moves the accumulated leg fluid rostrally and increases fluid volume in the neck region; this increases tissue pressure and collapsibility of the pharyngeal [38].

Comorbid conditions associated with obstructive sleep apnoea

Repeat episodes of upper airway obstruction with OSA causes marked changes in intrathoracic pressure and fluctuations in cardiac preload and afterload, which precipitate to cardiac remodelling and reduction in cardiac function. Hypoxaemia due to OSA also boosts the release of acute phase proteins and reactive oxygen species, causing secondary release of mediators and an augmented prothrombotic and proinflammatory state, which accelerate the atherosclerosis [39].

OSA is an independent risk factor for hypertension. Sleep disturbances and recurrent hypoxaemia cause sympathetic overactivity, acute blood pressure swings during sleep, endothelial damage, and nocturnal as well as daytime hypertension. The increase in right ventricular cavity size and wall thickness is related to OSA. OSA is one of the common reasons for resistance hypertension [40]. OSA is also an important risk factor for coronary artery disease. In general, the incidence of OSA is 30% among patients with coronary artery disease [41] and the incidence of coronary artery disease is up to 57% in untreated OSA patients compared to 6.6% in treated OSA patients [42]. Also, the frequency of apnoea and hypopnea is an independent risk factor for mortality among coronary artery disease patients. A 2014 study shows the severity of OSA is associated with myocardial injury [43].

A large prospective study on 700 patients with heart failure showed that 76% of patients had sleep-disordered breathing, of whom 40% had central sleep apnoea and 36% had OSA [44]. In heart failure patients with preserved ejection fraction, 48% had an AHI of 15 events/hour and 25% had clinical OSA [45]. Rostral neck oedema is an important factor in both obstructive and central apnoea generation in heart failure [38]. The Sleep Heart Health Study showed an incidence of 58% for heart failure in patients with severe OSA (AHI >30 events/hour) [46]. In the same study, the risk of atrial fibrillation among patients with OSA was about four times higher than in those with no sleep-disordered breathing [47]. The pathophysiological mechanisms including cardiac remodelling, structural changes such as left atrial dilation and electrical remodelling, and autonomic dysregulation have been implicated as predisposing factors in OSA patients to atrial fibrillation. The prevalence of pulmonary hypertension in severe OSA patients is up to 20% [48].

A systematic review in 2015 shows that OSA is associated with an increase in prothrombotic markers and the incidence of thromboembolic complications is two to three times higher in OSA patients [49]. OSA is a risk factor for beta-cell dysfunction and insulin resistance, which is independent of obesity. OSA is associated with glycated haemoglobin and vascular complications in patients with type 2 diabetes. Continuous positive airway pressure (CPAP) might improve insulin resistance and glycaemic measures [50]. One study showed a 30% higher risk of diabetes in severe OSA patients [51]. There is emerging evidence of the association of OSA with the presence and severity of non-alcoholic fatty liver disease [52].

There is evidence showing the relationship between OSA and chronic obstructive pulmonary disease, also called the overlap syndrome. A study showed that 57% of patients with moderate to severe chronic obstructive pulmonary disease have OSA [53]. This group of OSA patients have an increased risk of cardiac mortality and CPAP use was shown to be associated with reduction of mortality [54]. There is a strong association between ischaemic stroke and AHI in men with mild to moderate sleep apnoea [55].

The increased incidence of OSA during pregnancy is related to weight gain, increase in blood volume, which promotes rostral spread of fluid causing oedema of upper airway, and change in sensitivity of the respiratory centre due to hormonal changes [56]. OSA is associated with preeclampsia or gestational hypertension, eclampsia [57], and gestational diabetes [58].

Obesity hypoventilation syndrome is a triad of obesity, daytime hypoventilation, and sleep-disordered breathing without a neuromuscular, mechanical, or metabolic cause of hypoventilation. The prevalence of obesity hypoventilation syndrome is 10–20% in obese patients with OSA and 0.15–0.3% in the general adult population. Compared to eucapnic obese patients, patients with obesity hypoventilation syndrome present with severe upper airway obstruction, restrictive chest physiology, blunted central respiratory drive, pulmonary hypertension, and increased mortality. The mainstay of therapy is non-invasive positive airway pressure [59] (Fig. 10.1). Malignant obesity hypoventilation syndrome is defined as a patient with a body mass index greater than 40 kg/m² with awake hypercapnia ($PaCO_2$ >45 mmHg), the metabolic syndrome, and multiorgan dysfunction related to obesity [60].

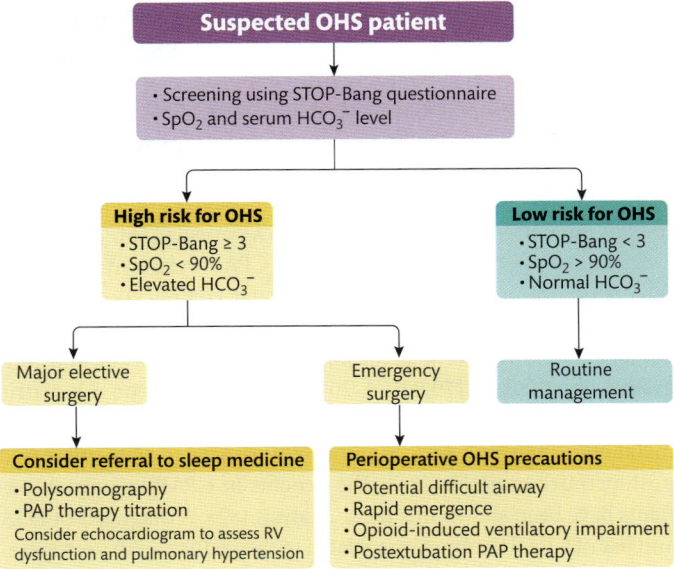

Fig. 10.1 Mechanisms by which obesity and OSA result in chronic hypercapnia. HCO_3^-, serum bicarbonate; OHS, obesity hypoventilation syndrome; PAP, positive airway pressure; RV, right ventricular; SpO_2, pulse oximeter oxygen saturation.

Reproduced with permission from Chau, E.H.L., Lam, D., et al. Obesity Hypoventilation Syndrome: A Review of Epidemiology, Pathophysiology, and Perioperative Considerations, Anaesthesia, 117(1):118–205. Copyright © 2012 Wolters Kluwer Health, Inc. doi: 10.1097/ALN.0b013e31825add60.

Obstructive sleep apnoea and anaesthesia

Anaesthetic agents, including sedative-hypnotics, opioids, and muscle relaxants, exaggerate OSA-related airway instability and worsen the apnoea. Surgical stress responses during the postoperative period significantly alter the sleep architecture [61]. In recent years, the impact of anaesthesia on OSA patients has come to light due to the evidence from major outcome studies. The American Society of Anesthesiologists [62,63], the Society for Ambulatory Anesthesia [64], and the Society of Anesthesia and Sleep Medicine [65,66] have published guidelines to emphasize the importance of patient selection and management of OSA patients.

Chronic untreated OSA is an independent risk factor for increased mortality in the general population [67,68]. Patients with OSA have a two times higher risk of pulmonary complications after non-cardiac surgery [69]. In bariatric surgical patients, OSA was found to be an independent risk factor for adverse postoperative events [70]. Flink et al. reported a 53% incidence of postoperative delirium in OSA patients versus 20% in non-OSA patients and initiation of CPAP may reduce the incidence [71,72].

A meta-analysis by Kaw et al. showed that the presence of OSA increased the odds of postoperative cardiac events including myocardial infarction, cardiac arrest, and arrhythmias (odds ratio (OR) 2.1), respiratory failure (OR 2.4), desaturation (OR 2.3), intensive care unit transfers (OR 2.8), and reintubations (OR 2.1) [73]. Mokhlesi et al. examined large nationally representative cohorts in elective orthopaedic, prostate, abdominal, and cardiovascular surgery in 1 million patients [4] and 90,000 patients undergoing bariatric surgery [74]. Both studies showed increased complications but not an increase in mortality. A large population study showed

OSA patients are more likely to receive ventilatory support, more intensive care unit, stepdown, and telemetry services, consume more economic resources, and have longer lengths of hospitalization [5]. Patients with a STOP-Bang score of 3 or more are at greater risk of postoperative adverse events and longer length of stay [75]. A recent meta-analysis on a cardiac surgery population showed that the incidence of major adverse cardiac or cerebrovascular events was 33.3% in OSA patients versus 18.1% in non-OSA patients [76].

Diagnosis of OSA and prescription of CPAP were associated with a reduction of postoperative cardiovascular complications [77,78]. Metabolic syndrome is a risk factor for postoperative pulmonary complications, deep venous thrombosis, atrial fibrillation, and congestive heart failure [79,80]. A 2015 outcome study on a bariatric surgical population showed that pulmonary complications and metabolic syndrome were significantly associated with increased postoperative mortality [81]. The benefits of CPAP in surgical patients have been shown in a meta-analysis [82]. A diagnosis of OSA and use of CPAP therapy were related with a reduction in postoperative complications, especially cardiac arrest and shock [83]. Another study of 2000 OSA patients in 50 hospitals in the United States found that OSA patients with CPAP treatment have less cardiorespiratory complications than OSA patients without CPAP therapy [84]. Compared to OSA alone, patients with obesity hypoventilation syndrome are more likely to have perioperative complications. A recent study showed patients with obesity hypoventilation syndrome are more likely to develop postoperative respiratory failure (OR 10.9), postoperative heart failure ($P < 0.0001$), prolonged intubation (OR 5.4), postoperative intensive care unit transfer (OR 3.8), and prolonged hospital stay [85].

Diagnostic tools for obstructive sleep apnoea

The gold standard for diagnosing OSA is overnight polysomnography. Since polysomnography is a time-consuming and expensive test, various screening tools such as the STOP-Bang questionnaire, sleep apnoea clinical score, Berlin questionnaire, and Epworth sleepiness score are available [86]. Among these tools, the STOP-Bang questionnaire (Fig. 10.2) [87] has the highest methodological validity in predicting a diagnosis of OSA [88–90] and a STOP-Bang score of 5–8 identified patients with a high probability of moderate to severe OSA [91,92]. The addition of serum HCO_3^- level of at least 28 mmol/L to a STOP-Bang score of 3 or greater improves the specificity [93]. For obese or morbidly obese patients, a STOP-Bang score of 4 or more can be used as a cut-off [94]. A recent meta-analysis shows the high performance of STOP-Bang in surgical population and sleep clinic [95]. Patients with a positive STOP-Bang score are more likely to have increased postoperative complications [96, 97].

The oxygen desaturation index (ODI) from a high-resolution nocturnal oximeter is a sensitive and specific screening tool to identify sleep-disordered breathing in surgical patients [98]. The ODI is a good predictor of the AHI. An ODI greater than 10 events/hour demonstrates high sensitivity (93%) and reasonable specificity (75%) to detect moderate and severe OSA. Patients with preoperative mean overnight SpO_2 less than 93%, or ODI greater than 29 events/hour have been shown to be at higher risk for postoperative adverse

events [99]. These screening tests do not differentiate OSA from other sleep disorders, such as central sleep apnoea and obesity hypoventilation syndrome, and therefore a polysomnography and blood gas test are indicated to diagnose hypercarbia and effortless apnoea, respectively. A functional algorithm could help to guide screening and the management of the obese patients with OSA [100].

Treatment modalities for obstructive sleep apnoea

The goal of the treatment is to improve the symptoms of OSA and quality of sleep by normalizing the AHI. CPAP is the gold standard treatment for OSA. Though CPAP is a 'one-size-fits-all' solution by preventing upper airway collapse, recent understanding of the pathophysiology of OSA has widened the treatment options [101]. General measures are patient education on the benefits of weight loss and exercise, avoiding the supine position during sleep, and avoiding alcohol and sedative medications such as benzodiazepines. CPAP works by creating a positive pharyngeal transmural pressure and increasing the end-expiratory lung volume. CPAP is the most common mode and other modes are bi-level positive airway pressure, and autotitrating positive airway pressure. Non-adherence to CPAP therapy is high, 20–40% of patients are unable to tolerate and initiate CPAP treatment. These patients may benefit from alternate methods such as oral appliances and upper airway surgery. Uvulopalatopharyngoplasty is one of the most common surgical procedures which involves resection of the uvula, redundant retrolingual soft tissue, and palatine tonsillar tissue. Other surgical treatment options are radiofrequency ablation, maxillomandibular advancement, septoplasty, rhinoplasty, nasal turbinate reduction, nasal polypectomy, palatal advancement pharyngoplasty, tonsillectomy, adenoidectomy, palatal implants, tongue reduction (partial glossectomy, lingual tonsillectomy), and genioglossus advancement. In 2010, the American Academy of Sleep Medicine published a guideline for surgical treatment for OSA [102]. Hypoglossal nerve stimulation with an implantable neurostimulator device is a new treatment that may be suitable for selected patients with moderate to severe OSA who are non-compliant with positive airway pressure therapy [103].

Perioperative management of obstructive sleep apnoea patients

Perioperative management includes identification of OSA patients, optimization, intraoperative risk mitigation, and postoperative monitoring. The Society of Anesthesia and Sleep Medicine has published recent guidelines on preoperative and intraoperative management of OSA patients [65,66]. The American Society of Anesthesiologists published guidelines on the perioperative management of OSA patients [62,63] based on the severity of sleep apnoea, invasiveness of surgery, type of anaesthesia, and the need for postoperative opioids. Based on a systematic review of recent evidence, the Society for Ambulatory Anesthesia has recommended a consensus statement on the preoperative selection of patients with OSA for ambulatory surgery [64]. It recommends the STOP-Bang questionnaire as a screening tool.

Yes   No
☐   ☐   **Snoring?**
          Do you **Snore Loudly** (loud enough to be heard through closed doors or your bed-partner elbows you for snoring at night)?

Yes   No
☐   ☐   **Tired?**
          Do you often feel **Tired, Fatigued, or Sleepy** during the daytime (such as falling asleep during driving)?

Yes   No
☐   ☐   **Observed?**
          Has anyone **Observed** you **Stop Breathing** or **Choking/Gasping** during your sleep?

Yes   No
☐   ☐   **Pressure?**
          Do you have or are being treated for **High Blood Pressure?**

Yes   No
☐   ☐   **Body Mass Index more than 35 kg/m2?**

Yes   No
☐   ☐   **Age older than 50 years?**

Yes   No
☐   ☐   **Neck size large? (Measured around Adams apple)**
          For male, is your shirt collar 17 inches or larger?
          For female, is your shirt collar 16 inches or larger?

Yes   No
☐   ☐   **Gender = Male?**

Scoring Criteria

For general population

Low risk of OSA: Yes to 0–2 questions

Intermediate risk of OSA: Yes to 3–4 questions

High risk of OSA: Yes to 5–8 questions

Yes to 2 of 4 STOP questions + individual's gender is male

Yes to 2 of 4 STOP questions + BMI >35 kg/m^2

Yes to 2 of 4 STOP questions + neck circumference: male 17 inches

female 16 inches

Fig. 10.2 The STOP-Bang questionnaire.

Reproduced courtesy of Dr Frances Chung and UHN. Copyright of University Health Network. Accurate at time of press. For up-to-date information and permission licensing, please access www.stopbang.ca.

General anaesthesia in OSA patients is challenging as the administration of sedatives, anaesthetics, and analgesics could further worsen pharyngeal obstruction in a pre-existing dysfunctional airway. A recent meta-analysis showed that OSA patients had a 3.5-fold higher chance of difficult intubation and a 3.4-fold chance of difficult mask ventilation [104]. Perioperatively, various methods can be used to mitigate the risks and adverse outcomes in OSA patients (Table 10.1). While planning general anaesthesia, anticipation of difficult intubation, use of short-acting opioids, propofol, and desflurane or sevoflurane will minimize airway-related complications [100]. Since OSA is one of the predisposing factors for opioid-induced ventilator impairment [105,106], intraoperative use of opioid-sparing agents such as non-steroidal anti-inflammatory drugs, paracetamol, tramadol, cyclooxygenase-2 inhibitors, and adjuvants such as the anticonvulsants pregabalin and gabapentin are useful in reducing postoperative opioid requirements. During

Table 10.1 Perioperative precautions and risk mitigation for patients with sleep disordered breathing

Anaesthetic concern	Principles of management
Preoperative Screening	• OSA screening recommended to be a part of standard pre-anaesthetic evaluation • Additional evaluation for hypoventilation syndrome, severe pulmonary hypertension, and resting hypoxaemia in the absence of other cardiopulmonary disease
SASM Guidelines [65]	• Continue PAP therapy, advise patients to bring PAP equipment to the surgical facility
Ambulatory surgery criteria, SAMBA Guideline [64]	• OSA patients with optimized comorbid conditions • Patient using PAP therapy • Postoperative pain mainly managed mainly with non-opioid analgesia
Intraoperative Airway management (difficult mask ventilation and tracheal intubation)	• HELP positioning (Head Elevated Laryngoscopy Position) • Pre-oxygenation with 25-degree head-up position and CPAP • Nasal oxygen insufflation or THRIVE technique • Anticipated difficult airway—difficult airway equipment • Rapid sequence induction with cricoid pressure for patients with GORD
Ventilation	• Recruitment manoeuvre + PEEP to avoid atelectasis • Protective ventilation—low TV and plateau pressure • Second-generation supraglottic device for better seal
Opioid-related respiratory depression	• Minimize opioid use • Use of short-acting agents (e.g. remifentanil) • Multimodal approach to analgesia (NSAIDs, acetaminophen, tramadol, ketamine, gabapentin, pregabalin, dexmedetomidine, clonidine, dexamethasone) • Consider local and regional anaesthesia where appropriate
Extubation	• Extubate wide-awake in the sitting position if possible • Consider sugammadex to prevent inadequate reversal
Monitored anaesthetic care	• Avoid deep sedation with unsecured airway • Intraoperative capnography for monitoring of ventilation
Postoperative	• Resume PAP therapy to avoid postoperative atelectasis • Monitored bed for OSA patients with recurrent respiratory events, OHS and overlap syndrome patient • Avoid long-acting opioid prescription for ambulatory surgical patient

CPAP, continuous positive airway pressure; GORD, gastro-oesophageal reflux disease; NSAIDs, non-steroidal anti-inflammatory drugs; OHS, obesity hypoventilation syndrome; OSA, obstructive sleep apnoea; PAP therapy, positive airway pressure therapy; PEEP, positive end-expiratory pressure; SAMBA, Society for Ambulatory Anesthesia; SASM, Society of Anesthesia and Sleep Medicine; THRIVE, transnasal humidified rapid-insufflation ventilatory exchange; TV, tidal volume;

emergence, extubating awake with adequate reversal of neuromuscular block in a semi-upright posture reduces the incidences of oxygen desaturation in the immediate postoperative period. A recent meta-analysis on the use of intraoperative neuromuscular blocking agents showed that OSA patients had more postoperative hypoxemias, respiratory failure, and residual neuromuscular blockade compared to non-OSA patients [107]. Local and regional anaesthesia techniques may be preferable to general anaesthesia to avoid manipulation of the airway and reduce postoperative requirement for analgesia [100]. A secured airway is preferred to an unprotected one for procedures requiring deep level of sedation.

All patients with known or suspected OSA who have received general anaesthesia should stay an additional 60 minutes in the post-anaesthesia care unit (PACU) after meeting the modified Aldrete discharge criteria [100,108]. The occurrence of recurrent respiratory events in the PACU (episodes of apnoea ≥10 seconds, bradypnea <8 breaths/min, repeated oxygen desaturation <90%, or pain-sedation mismatch) is an indication for continuous postoperative monitoring (**Fig. 10.3**) [99]. Any of the above-mentioned events occurring repeatedly in separate 30-minute intervals are considered recurrent PACU respiratory events. Patients with suspected OSA and who develop recurrent respiratory events in the PACU are at increased risk of postoperative respiratory complications [109,110]. These patients may require postoperative CPAP therapy with a monitoring facility [111]. Monitoring with continuous oximetry is recommended for patients who needs parenteral opioids due to possible drug-induced respiratory depression [112]. Continuing CPAP therapy in the postoperative period reduces the risk of postoperative complications [82]. Other than oral or systemic administration of opioid-sparing agents, other alternative techniques include local anaesthetic wound infiltration, peripheral nerve block catheters, and neuraxial infusions of local anaesthetic agents. Postoperative parenteral opioids should be managed by the use of patient-controlled analgesia with no basal infusion and a strict hourly dose limit.

A PACU order-based approach facilitates postoperative decision-making for patients with sleep apnoea. The orders prompt anaesthesiologists to consider the factors and events associated with a higher risk of complications from OSA, diagnostic follow-up, and possible sleep medicine consult [113]. One study found that patients had no increase in postoperative complications if managed on the OSA risk management protocol [114]. The disturbances in sleep architecture were greatest on the first postoperative night and breathing disturbances during sleep were greatest on the third postoperative night [61]. Preoperative AHI, male sex, and 72-hour opioid dose were positively associated with postoperative AHI [115]. A recent study showed that postoperative oxygen therapy improved the oxygenation without increases in AHI and hypercapnia among most of the OSA patients [116]. It is necessary to have appropriate monitoring based on the OSA risk.

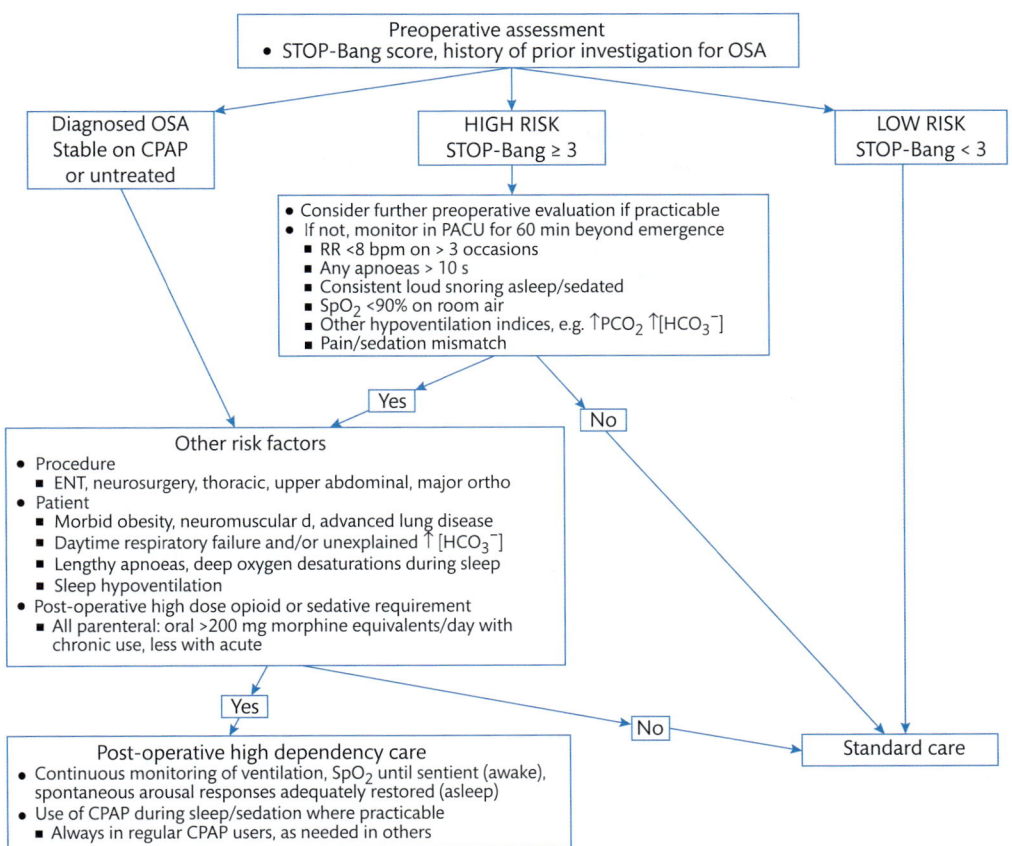

Fig. 10.3 Postoperative management of the diagnosed or suspected OSA patient after general anaesthesia. ENT, ear, nose, and throat; HCO$_3^-$, serum bicarbonate; PACU, post-anaesthesia care unit; PCO$_2$, partial pressure of carbon dioxide; RR, respiratory rate; SpO$_2$, pulse oximeter oxygen saturation. Reproduced with permission from Chung, F., Hillman, D. R., Anaesthetic management of sleep-disordered breathing in adults, *Respirology*, 22(2):230–239. Copyright © 2016 John Wiley and Sons. https://doi.org/10.1111/resp.12967

Conclusion

OSA is a growing problem for both developed and developing countries. The understanding of pathophysiology of OSA in recent years has resulted in significant changes in the treatment pathways, especially in perioperative care. Although patients with OSA are shown to have significant perioperative morbidity, algorithm-based management and the use of CPAP show promising results in perioperative outcomes. Anaesthesiologists have a vital role in managing OSA patients by identifying OSA and associated comorbid conditions, ensuring preoperative optimization, and providing protocol-based perioperative care.

REFERENCES

1. Singh M, Liao P, Kobah S, Wijeysundera DN, Shapiro C, Chung F. Proportion of surgical patients with undiagnosed obstructive sleep apnoea. Br J Anaesth. 2013;**110**(4):629–36.
2. Finkel KJ, Searleman AC, Tymkew H, Tanaka CY, Saager L, Safer-Zadeh E, et al. Prevalence of undiagnosed obstructive sleep apnea among adult surgical patients in an academic medical center. Sleep Med. 2009;**10**(7):753–58.
3. Stierer TL, Wright C, George A, Thompson RE, Wu CL, Collop N. Risk assessment of obstructive sleep apnea in a population of patients undergoing ambulatory surgery. J Clin Sleep Med. 2010;**6**(5):467–72.
4. Mokhlesi B, Hovda MD, Vekhter B, Arora VM, Chung F, Meltzer DO. Sleep-disordered breathing and postoperative outcomes after elective surgery: analysis of the nationwide inpatient sample. Chest. 2013;**144**(3):903–14.
5. Memtsoudis SG, Stundner O, Rasul R, Chiu YL, Sun X, Ramachandran SK, et al. The impact of sleep apnea on postoperative utilization of resources and adverse outcomes. Anesth Analg. 2014;**118**(2):407–18.
6. Malhotra A, Orr JE, Owens RL. On the cutting edge of obstructive sleep apnoea: where next? Lancet Respir Med; 2015;**3**(5):397–403.
7. Pham L V, Schwartz AR. The pathogenesis of obstructive sleep apnea. J Thorac Dis.2015;**7**(8):1358–72.
8. Berry RB, Budhiraja R, Gottlieb DJ, et al. Rules for scoring respiratory events in sleep: update of the 2007 AASM manual for the scoring of sleep and associated events. J Clin Sleep Med. 2012;**8**(5):597–619.
9. Epstein LJ, Kristo D, Strollo PJ, Friedman N, Malhotra A, Patil SP, et al. Clinical guideline for the evaluation, management and long-term care of obstructive sleep apnea in adults. J Cinical Sleep Med. 2009;**5**(3):263–76.
10. Fleetham J, Ayas N, Bradley D, Fitzpatrick M, Oliver TK, Morrison D, et al. Canadian Thoracic Society 2011 guideline update: diagnosis and treatment of sleep disordered breathing. Can Respir J. 2011;**18**(1):25–47.

11. Young T, Palta M, Dempsey J, Skatrud J. The occurrence of sleep-disordered breathing among middle-aged adults. N Engl J Med. 1993;**328**(17):1230–35.

12. Peppard PE, Young T, Barnet JH, Palta M, Hagen EW, Hla KM. Increased prevalence of sleep-disordered breathing in adults. Am J Epidemiol. 2013;**177**(9):1006–14.

13. Lopez PP, Stefan B, Schulman CI, Byers PM. Prevalence of sleep apnea in morbidly obese patients who presented for weight loss surgery evaluation: more evidence for routine screening for obstructive sleep apnea before weight loss surgery. Am Surg. 2008;**74**(9):834–38.

14. Haba-Rubio J, Marques-Vidal P, Andries D, Tobback N, Preisig M, Vollenweider P, et al. Objective sleep structure and cardiovascular risk factors in the general population: the HypnoLaus Study. Sleep. 2015;**38**(3):391–400.

15. Chen X, Wang R, Zee P, Lutsey PL, Javaheri S, Alcántara C, et al. Racial/ethnic differences in sleep disturbances: the Multi-Ethnic Study of Atherosclerosis (MESA). Sleep. 2015;**38**(6):877–88.

16. Quintana-Gallego E, Carmona-Bernal C, Capote F, Sánchez-Armengol Á, Botebol-Benhamou G, Polo-Padillo J, et al. Gender differences in obstructive sleep apnea syndrome: a clinical study of 1166 patients. Respir Med. 2004;**98**(10):984–89.

17. Peppard PE, Young T, Palta M, Dempsey J, Skatrud J. Longitudinal study of moderate weight change and sleep-disordered breathing. JAMA. 2000;**284**(23):3015–21.

18. Povitz M, James MT, Pendharkar SR, Raneri J, Hanly PJ, Tsai WH. Prevalence of sleep-disordered breathing in obese patients with chronic hypoxemia. A cross-sectional study. Ann Am Thorac Soc. 2015;**12**(6):921–27.

19. Young T, Skatrud J, Peppard PE. Risk factors for obstructive sleep apnea in adults. JAMA. 2004;**291**(16):2013–16.

20. Wetter DW, Young TB, Bidwell TR, Badr MS, Palta M. Smoking as a risk factor for sleep-disordered breathing. Arch Intern Med. 1994;**154**(19):2219–24.

21. Pien GW, Pack AI, Jackson N, Maislin G, Macones GA, Schwab RJ. Risk factors for sleep-disordered breathing in pregnancy. Thorax. 2014;**69**(4):371–77.

22. Eckert DJ, White DP, Jordan AS, Malhotra A, Wellman A. Defining phenotypic causes of obstructive sleep apnea. Identification of novel therapeutic targets. Am J Respir Crit Care Med. 2013;**188**(8):996–1004.

23. Dempsey JA, Xie A, Patz DS, Wang D. Physiology in Medicine: obstructive sleep apnea pathogenesis and treatment—considerations beyond airway anatomy. J Appl Physiol. 2014;**116**(1):3–12.

24. Haponik EF, Smith PL, Bohlman ME, Allen RP, Goldman SM, Bleecker ER. Computerized tomography in obstructive sleep apnea. Correlation of airway size with physiology during sleep and wakefulness. Am Rev Respir Dis. 1983;**127**(2):221–26.

25. Schwab RJ, Pasirstein M, Pierson R, Mackley A, Hachadoorian R, Arens R, et al. Identification of upper airway anatomic risk factors for obstructive sleep apnea with volumetric magnetic resonance imaging. Am J Respir Crit Care Med. 2003;**168**(5):522–30.

26. Pahkala R, Seppä J, Ikonen A, Smirnov G, Tuomilehto H. The impact of pharyngeal fat tissue on the pathogenesis of obstructive sleep apnea. Sleep Breath. 2014;**18**(2):275–82.

27. Lee RW, Sutherland K, Cistulli P. Craniofacial morphology in obstructive sleep apnea: a review. Clin Pulm Med. 2010;**17**(4):189–95.

28. Watanabe T, Isono S, Tanaka A, Tanzawa H, Nishino T. Contribution of body habitus and craniofacial characteristics to segmental closing pressures of the passive pharynx in patients with sleep-disordered breathing. Am J Respir Crit Care Med. 2002;**165**(2):260–65.

29. Tsuiki S, Isono S, Ishikawa T, Yamashiro Y, Tatsumi K, Nishino T. Anatomical balance of the upper airway and obstructive sleep apnea. Anesthesiology. 2008;**108**(6):1009–15.

30. Mezzanotte WS, Tangel DJ, White DP. Influence of sleep onset on upper-airway muscle activity in apnea patients versus normal controls. Am J Respir Crit Care Med. 1996;**153**(6 Pt 1):1880–87.

31. Worsnop C, Kay A, Pierce R, Kim Y, Trinder J. Activity of respiratory pump and upper airway muscles during sleep onset. J Appl Physiol. 1998;**85**(3):908–20.

32. Amatoury J, Kairaitis K, Wheatley JR, Bilston LE, Amis TC. Peripharyngeal tissue deformation and stress distributions in response to caudal tracheal displacement: pivotal influence of the hyoid bone? J Appl Physiol. 2014;**116**(7):746–56.

33. Drager LF, Togeiro SM, Polotsky VY, Lorenzi-Filho G. Obstructive sleep apnea: a cardiometabolic risk in obesity and the metabolic syndrome. J Am Coll Cardiol. 2013;**62**(7):569–76.

34. Younes M. Role of respiratory control mechanisms in the pathogenesis of obstructive sleep disorders. J Appl Physiol. 2008;**105**(5):1389–405.

35. Dempsey JA, Veasey SC, Morgan BJ, O'Donnell CP. Pathophysiology of sleep apnea. Physiol Rev. 2010;**90**(1):47–112.

36. Wellman A, Jordan AS, Malhotra A, Fogel RB, Katz ES, Schory K, et al. Ventilatory control and airway anatomy in obstructive sleep apnea. Am J Respir Crit Care Med. 2004;**170**(11):1225–32.

37. Subramani Y, Singh M, Wong J, Kushida CA, Malhotra A, Chung F. Understanding phenotypes of obstructive sleep apnea: applications in anesthesia, surgery, and perioperative medicine. Anesth Analg. 2017;**124**(1):179–91.

38. White LH, Bradley TD. Role of nocturnal rostral fluid shift in the pathogenesis of obstructive and central sleep apnoea. J Physiol. 2013;**591**(Pt 5):1179–93.

39. Badran M, Golbidi S, Ayas N, Laher I. Nitric oxide bioavailability in obstructive sleep apnea: interplay of asymmetric dimethylarginine and free radicals. Sleep Disord. 2015;**2015**:1–10.

40. Khan A, Patel NK, O'Hearn DJ, Khan S. Resistant hypertension and obstructive sleep apnea. Int J Hypertens. 2013;**2013**:193010.

41. Schäfer H, Koehler U, Ewig S, Hasper E, Tasci S, Lüderitz B. Obstructive sleep apnea as a risk marker in coronary artery disease. Cardiology. 1999;**92**(2):79–84.

42. Peker Y, Hedner J, Norum J, Kraiczi H, Carlson J. Increased incidence of cardiovascular disease in middle-aged men with obstructive sleep apnea: a 7-year follow-up. Am J Respir Crit Care Med. 2002;**166**(2):159–65.

43. Einvik G, Røsjø H, Randby A, Namtvedt SK, Hrubos-Strøm H, Brynildsen J, et al. Severity of obstructive sleep apnea is associated with cardiac troponin I concentrations in a community-based sample: data from the Akershus Sleep Apnea Project. Sleep. 2014;**37**(6):1111–16.

44. Oldenburg O, Lamp B, Faber L, Teschler H, Horstkotte D, Töpfer V. Sleep-disordered breathing in patients with symptomatic heart failure: a contemporary study of prevalence in and characteristics of 700 patients. Eur J Heart Fail. 2007;**9**(3):251–57.

45. Bitter T, Faber L, Hering D, Langer C, Horstkotte D, Oldenburg O. Sleep-disordered breathing in heart failure with normal left ventricular ejection fraction. Eur J Hear Fail. 2009;**11**(6):602–608.

46. Gottlieb DJ, Yenokyan G, Newman AB, O'Connor GT, Punjabi NM, Quan SF, et al. Prospective study of obstructive sleep apnea and incident coronary heart disease and heart failure: the Sleep Heart Health Study. Circulation. 2010;**122**(4):352–60.

47. Mehra R, Benjamin EJ, Shahar E, Gottlieb DJ, Nawabit R, Kirchner HL, et al. Association of nocturnal arrhythmias with sleep-disordered breathing: the sleep heart health study. Am J Respir Crit Care Med. 2006;**173**(8):910–16.

48. Sajkov D, McEvoy RD. Obstructive sleep apnea and pulmonary hypertension. Prog Cardiovasc Dis. 2009;**51**(5):363–70.

49. Lippi G, Mattiuzzi C, Franchini M. Sleep apnea and venous thromboembolism. A systematic review. Thromb Haemost. 2015;**114**(5):958–63.

50. Tahrani AA, Ali A, Stevens MJ. Obstructive sleep apnoea and diabetes: an update. Curr Opin Pulm Med. 2013;**19**(6):631–38.

51. Kendzerska T, Gershon AS, Hawker G, Tomlinson G, Leung RS. Obstructive sleep apnea and incident diabetes: a historical cohort study. Am J Respir Crit Care Med. 2014;**190**(2):1–43.

52. Musso G, Cassader M, Olivetti C, Rosina F, Carbone G, Gambino R. Association of obstructive sleep apnoea with the presence and severity of non-alcoholic fatty liver disease. A systematic review and meta-analysis. Obes Rev. 2013;**14**(5):417–31.

53. Soler X, Gaio E, Powell FL, Ramsdell JW, Loredo JS, Malhotra A, et al. High prevalence of obstructive sleep apnea in patients with moderate to severe COPD. Ann Am Thorac Soc. 2015;**12**(8):1219–25.

54. Stanchina ML, Welicky LM, Donat W, Lee D, Corrao W, Malhotra A. Impact of CPAP use and age on mortality in patients with combined COPD and obstructive sleep apnea: the overlap syndrome. J Clin Sleep Med. 2013;**9**(8):767–72.

55. Redline S, Yenokyan G, Gottlieb DJ, Shahar E, O'Connor GT, Resnick HE, et al. Obstructive sleep apnea-hypopnea and incident stroke: the sleep heart health study. Am J Respir Crit Care Med. 2010;**182**(2):269–77.

56. Abdullah HR, Nagappa M, Siddiqui N, Chung F. Diagnosis and treatment of obstructive sleep apnea during pregnancy. Curr Opin Anaesthesiol. 2016;**29**(3):317–24.

57. Louis JM, Mogos MF, Salemi JL, Redline S, Salihu HM. Obstructive sleep apnea and severe maternal-infant morbidity/mortality in the United States, 1998–2009. Sleep. 2014;**37**(5):843–49.

58. Reutrakul S, Zaidi N, Wroblewski K, Kay HH, Ismail M, Ehrmann DA,et al. Interactions Between Pregnancy, Obstructive Sleep Apnea, and Gestational Diabetes Mellitus. J Clin Endocrinol Metab. 2013;**98**(10):4195–202.

59. Chau EHL, Lam D, Wong J, Mokhlesi B, Chung F. Obesity hypoventilation syndrome: a review of epidemiology, pathophysiology, and perioperative considerations. Anesthesiology. 2012;**117**(1):188–205.

60. Marik PE, Varon J. The malignant obesity hypoventilation syndrome (MOHS). Curr Respir Med Rev. 2014;**24**:197–205.

61. Chung F, Liao P, Yegneswaran B, Shapiro CM, Kang W. Postoperative changes in sleep-disordered breathing and sleep architecture in patients with obstructive sleep apnea. Anesthesiology. 2014;**120**(2):287–98.

62. Gross JB, Bachenberg KL, Benumof JL, Diego S, Caplan RA, Connis RT, Cote CJ, et al. Practice guidelines for the perioperative management of patients with obstructive sleep apnea. Anesthesiology. 2006;**104**(5):1081–93.

63. American Society of Anesthesiologists Task Force on Perioperative Management of Patients with Obstructive Sleep Apnea. Practice guidelines for the perioperative management of patients with obstructive sleep apnea. An updated report by the American Society of Anesthesiologists Task Force on Perioperative Management of Patients with Obstructive Sleep Apnea. Anesthesiology. 2014;**120**(2):268–86.

64. Joshi GP, Ankichetty SP, Gan TJ, Chung F. Society for Ambulatory Anesthesia consensus statement on preoperative selection of adult patients with obstructive sleep apnea scheduled for ambulatory surgery. Anesth Analg. 2012;**115**(4):1060–68.

65. Chung F, Memtsoudis SG, Ramachandran SK, Nagappa M, Opperer M, Cozowicz C, et al. Society of Anesthesia and Sleep Medicine guidelines on preoperative screening and assessment of adult patients with obstructive sleep apnea. Anesth Analg. 2016;**123**:452–73.

66. Memtsoudis SG, Cozowicz C, Nagappa M, Wong J, Joshi GP, Wong DT, et al. Society of Anesthesia and Sleep Medicine guideline on intraoperative management of adult patients with obstructive sleep apnea. Anesth Analg. 2018;**127**(4):967–87.

67. Young T, Finn L, Peppard PE, Szklo-Coxe M, Austin D, Nieto FJ, et al. Sleep disordered breathing and mortality: eighteen-year follow-up of the Wisconsin sleep cohort. Sleep. 2008;**31**(8):1071–78.

68. Marshall NS, Wong KKH, Liu PY, Cullen SRJ, Knuiman MW, Grunstein RR. Sleep apnea as an independent risk factor for all-cause mortality: the Busselton Health Study. Sleep. 2008;**31**(8):1079–85.

69. Memtsoudis S, Liu SS, Ma Y, Chiu YL, Walz JM, Gaber-Baylis LK, et al. Perioperative pulmonary outcomes in patients with sleep apnea after noncardiac surgery. Anesth Analg. 2011;**112**(1):113–21.

70. Flum DR, Belle SH, King WC, Wahed AS, Berk P, Chapman W, et al. Perioperative safety in the longitudinal assessment of bariatric surgery. N Engl J Med. 2009;**361**(5):445–54.

71. Flink BJ, Rivelli SK, Cox EA, White WD, Falcone G, Vail TP, et al. Obstructive sleep apnea and incidence of postoperative delirium after elective knee replacement in the nondemented elderly. Anesthesiology. 2012;**116**(4):788–96.

72. Lam EWK, Chung F, Wong J. Sleep-disordered breathing, postoperative delirium, and cognitive impairment. Anesth Analg. 2017;**124**(5):1626–35.

73. Kaw R, Chung F, Pasupuleti V, Mehta J, Gay PC, Hernandez AV. Meta-analysis of the association between obstructive sleep apnoea and postoperative outcome. Br J Anaesth. 2012;**109**(6):897–906.

74. Mokhlesi B, Hovda MD, Vekhter B, Arora VM, Chung F, Meltzer DO. Sleep-disordered breathing and postoperative outcomes after bariatric surgery: Analysis of the nationwide inpatient sample. Obes Surg. 2013;**23**(11):1842–51.

75. Nagappa M, Patra J, Wong J, et al. Association of STOP-Bang Questionnaire as a screening tool for sleep apnea and postoperativecomplications:a systematic review and Bayesian meta-analysis of prospective and retrospective cohort studies. Anesth Analg. 2017;**125**(4):1301–308.

76. Nagappa M, Ho G, Patra J, Wong J, Singh M, Kaw R, Cheng D, Chung F. Postoperative outcomes in obstructive sleep apnea patients undergoing cardiac surgery: a systematic review and meta-analysis of comparative studies. Anesth Analg. 2017;**125**(6):2030–37.

77. Mutter TC, Chateau D, Moffatt M, Ramsey C, Roos LL, Kryger M. A matched cohort study of postoperative outcomes in obstructive sleep apnea: could preoperative diagnosis and treatment prevent complications? Anesthesiology. 2014;**121**(4):707–18.

78. Chung F, Nagappa M, Singh M, Mokhlesi B. CPAP in the perioperative setting: evidence of support. Chest 2016;**140**(2):586–97.

79. Tung A. Anaesthetic considerations with the metabolic syndrome. Br J Anaesth. 2010;**105** Suppl:i24–33.

80. Pomares J, Mora-García G, Palomino R, León Y De, Gómez-Alegría C, Gómez-Camargo D. Metabolic syndrome and perioperative complications during scheduled surgeries with spinal anesthesia. Open J Anesthesiol. 2014;**4**(7):167–76.

81. Schumann R, Shikora SA, Sigl JC, Kelley SD. Association of metabolic syndrome and surgical factors with pulmonary adverse events, and longitudinal mortality in bariatric surgery. Br J Anaesth. 2015;**114**(1):83–90.

82. Nagappa M, Mokhlesi B, Wong J, Wong DT, Kaw R, Chung F. The effects of continuous positive airway pressure on postoperative outcomes in obstructive sleep apnea patients undergoing surgery: a systematic review and meta-analysis. Anesthes Analg. 2015;**120**(5):1013–23.

83. Mutter TC, Chateau D, Moffatt M, Ramsey C, Roos LL, Kryger M. A matched cohort study of postoperative outcomes in obstructive sleep apnea: could preoperative diagnosis and treatment prevent complications? Anesthesiology 2014;**121**(4):707–18.

84. Abdelsattar ZM, Hendren S, Wong SL, Campbell DA, Ramachandran SK. The Impact of untreated obstructive sleep apnea on cardiopulmonary complications in general and vascular surgery: a cohort study. Sleep. 2015; **38**(8):1205–10.

85. Kaw R, Bhateja P, Paz Y, Mar H, Hernandez AV, Ramaswamy A, et al. Postoperative complications in patients with unrecognized obesity hypoventilation syndrome undergoing elective non-cardiac surgery. Chest. 2016;**149**(1):11–13.

86. El-Sayed IH. Comparison of four sleep questionnaires for screening obstructive sleep apnea. Egypt J Chest Dis Tuberc. 2012;**61**(4):433–41.

87. Chung F, Yegneswaran B, Liao P, Chung SA, Vairavanathan S, Islam S, et al. STOP questionnaire: a tool to screen patients for obstructive sleep apnea. Anesthesiology. 2008;**108**(5):812–21.

88. Abrishami A, Khajehdehi A, Chung F. A systematic review of screening questionnaires for obstructive sleep apnea. Can J Anesth. 2010;**57**(5):423–38.

89. Ramachandran SK, Josephs LA. A meta-analysis of clinical screening tests for obstructive sleep apnea. Anesthesiology. 2009;**110**(4):928–39.

90. Chung F, Abdullah HR, Liao P. STOP-Bang questionnaire: a practical approach to screen for obstructive sleep apnea. Chest; 2016;**149**(3):1–26.

91. Chung F, Subramanyam R, Liao P, Sasaki E, Shapiro C, Sun Y. High STOP-Bang score indicates a high probability of obstructive sleep apnoea. Br J Anaesth. 2012;**108**(5):768–75.

92. Chung F, Liao P, Farney R. Correlation between the STOP-Bang score and the severity of obstructive sleep apnea. Anesthesiology 2015;**122**(6):1436–37.

93. Chung F, Chau E, Yang Y, Liao P, Hall R, Mokhlesi B. Serum bicarbonate level improves specificity of STOP-bang screening for obstructive sleep apnea. Chest. 2013;**143**(12):1284–93.

94. Chung F, Yang Y, Liao P. Predictive performance of the stop-bang score for identifying obstructive sleep apnea in obese patients. Obes Surg. 2013;**23**(12):2050–57.

95. Nagappa M, Liao P, Wong J, Auckley D, Ramachandran SK, Memtsoudis S, et al. Validation of the STOP-Bang questionnaire as a screening tool for obstructive sleep apnea among different populations: a systematic review and meta-analysis. PLoS One. 2015;**10**(12):e0143697.

96. Vasu TS, Doghramji K, Cavallazzi R, Grewal R, Hirani A, Leiby B, et al. Obstructive sleep apnea syndrome and postoperative complications: clinical use of the STOP-BANG questionnaire. Arch Otolaryngol Head Neck Surg. 2010;**136**(10):1020–24.

97. Nagappa M, Patra J, Wong J, Subramani Y, Singh M, Ho G, Wong DT, Chung F. Association of STOP-Bang questionnaire as a screening tool for sleep apnea and postoperative complications: a systematic review and bayesian meta-analysis of prospective and retrospective cohort studies. Anesth Analg 2017;**125**(4):1301–308.

98. Chung F, Liao P, Elsaid H, Islam S, Shapiro CM, Sun Y. Oxygen desaturation index from nocturnal oximetry: a sensitive and specific tool to detect sleep-disordered breathing in surgical patients. Anesth Analg. 2012;**114**(5):993–1000.

99. Chung F, Zhou L, Liao P. Parameters from preoperative overnight oximetry predict postoperative adverse events. Minerva Anestesiol. 2014;**80**(10):1084–95.

100. Seet E, Chung F. Management of sleep apnea in adults—functional algorithms for the perioperative period: continuing professional development. Can J Anaesth. 2010;**57**(9):849–64.

101. Sutherland K, Cistulli PA. Recent advances in obstructive sleep apnea pathophysiology and treatment. Sleep Biol Rhythm. 2015;**13**(1):26–40.

102. Caples SM, Rowley JA, Prinsell JR, Pallanch JF, Elamin MB, Katz SG, et al. Surgical modifications of the upper airway for obstructive sleep apnea in adults: a systematic review and meta-analysis. Sleep. 2010;**33**(10):1396–407.

103. Certal VF, Zaghi S, Riaz M, Vieira AS, Pinheiro CT, Kushida C, et al. Hypoglossal nerve stimulation in the treatment of obstructive sleep apnea: a systematic review and meta-analysis. Laryngoscope. 2015;**125**(5):1254–64.

104. Nagappa M, Wong DT, Cozowicz C, Ramachandran SK, Memtsoudis SG, Chung F. Is obstructive sleep apnea associated with difficult airway? evidence from a systematic review and meta-analysis of prospective and retrospective cohort studies. PLoS One. 2018:4;**13**(10):e0204904.

105. Lam KK, Kunder S, Wong J, Doufas AG, Chung F. Obstructive sleep apnea, pain, and opioids: is the riddle solved? Curr Opin Anaesthesiol. 2015;**29**(1):134–40.

106. Cozowicz C, Chung F, Doufas AG, Nagappa M, Memtsoudis SG. Opioids for acute pain management in patients with obstructive sleep apnea: a systematic review. Anesth Analg. 2018;**127**(4):988–1001.

107. Hafeez KR, Tuteja A, Singh M, Wong DT, Nagappa M, Chung F, Wong J. Postoperative complications with neuromuscular blocking drugs and/or reversal agents in obstructive sleep apnea patients: a systematic review. BMC Anesthesiol. 2018;**18**(1):91.

108. Seet E, Chung F. Obstructive sleep apnea: preoperative assessment. Anesthesiol Clin. 2010;**28**(2):199–215.

109. Gali B, Whalen FX, Schroeder DR, Gay PC, Plevak DJ. Identification of patients at risk for postoperative respiratory complications using a preoperative obstructive sleep apnea screening tool and postanesthesia care assessment. Anesthesiology. 2009;**110**(4):869–77.

110. Orlov D, Ankichetty S, Chung F, Brull R. Cardiorespiratory complications of neuraxial opioids in patients with obstructive sleep apnea: a systematic review. J Clin Anesth. 2013;**25**(7):591–99.

111. Sundar E, Chang J, Smetana GW. Perioperative screening for and management of patients with obstructive sleep apnea. J Clin Outcomes Manag. 2011;**18**:399–411.

112. Weinger MB, Lee LA. No patient shall be harmed by opioid-induced respiratory depression. APSF Newsl. 2011;**26**(2):21, 26–28. http://www.apsf.org/newsletters/html/2011/fall/01_opioid.htm

113. Swart P, Chung F, Fleetham J. An order-based approach to facilitate postoperative decision-making for patients with sleep apnea. Can J Anesth. 2013;**60**(3):321–24.

114. Chong CT, Tey J, Leow SL, Low W, Kwan KM, Wong YL, et al. Management plan to reduce risks in perioperative care of patients with obstructive sleep apnoea averts the need for presurgical polysomnography. Ann Acad Med Singapore. 2013;**42**(3):110–19.

115. Chung F, Liao P, Elsaid H, Shapiro CM, Kang W. Factors associated with postoperative exacerbation of sleep-disordered breathing. Anesthesiology. 2014;**120**(2):299–311.

116. Liao P, Wong J, Singh M, Wong DT, Islam S, Andrawes M, et al. Postoperative oxygen therapy in patients with OSA: a randomized controlled trial. Chest 2017;**151**(3):597–611.

Continuous positive airway pressure
Physiology and perioperative implications

Rainer Lenhardt and Jerrad R. Businger

Pathophysiology of the respiratory system

The morbidly obese patient has a large body mass consisting mainly of increased body fat with only a minimal increase in lean body mass compared with a non-obese patient. To quantify the amount of tissue mass (muscle, fat, and bone) in an individual, body mass index (BMI) has been used for many years. Patients with a higher BMI have more impairment of respiratory function, particularly when their BMI exceeds 45 kg/m² [1]. In addition, the pattern of fat distribution may play an important role in reduced respiratory function. While peripheral or gluteofemoral fat deposition may not contribute to respiratory decline, android fat deposition has a major impact on respiratory function. Intra-abdominal fat deposition reduces thorax compliance due to increased intra-abdominal pressure. In the obese patient, intra-abdominal pressure is typically between 6 to 12 mmHg compared with an intra-abdominal pressure between 0 to 6 mmHg in non-obese patients [2]. Thoracic fat deposition further negatively affects chest wall compliance. Overall, central fat deposition results in a decrease of static and dynamic lung volumes [3]. As a consequence, functional residual capacity (FRC) and forced vital capacity are reduced [4]. Reduction in FRC and forced vital capacity contribute to an increase in postoperative atelectasis with a concomitant risk of developing hypoxia and hypercapnia.

Obesity has been linked with asthma [5] and chronic obstructive pulmonary disease (COPD) [6]. Both diseases are characterized by an increase in bronchial airway resistance. Bronchoconstriction can increase expiratory flow limitation during tidal breathing, which may enhance postoperative respiratory symptoms. Obese asthma patients are more likely to develop expiratory flow limitation during tidal breathing compared to non-obese asthma patients [7]. Expiratory flow limitation during tidal breathing in combination with reduced lung volume may further increase the severity of symptoms postoperatively.

Morbidly obese patients have an increased metabolic demand resulting in an increase in blood volume, left ventricular stroke work, and left ventricular stroke volume. Stroke volume augments cardiac output, which is increased linearly by body weight. Increased activity of catecholamines and the renin–angiotensin system foster systemic and pulmonary hypertension and left ventricular hypertrophy and, subsequently, left ventricular dysfunction resulting in cardiac failure. Increased stroke work of the left ventricle predisposes patients to elevated left ventricular filling pressures, pulmonary wedge pressures, and may eventually lead to pulmonary hypertension [8].

Pulmonary hypertension results in right ventricular hypertrophy and right ventricular enlargement. As these manifestations persist, eventually right heart failure will occur and occasionally result in sudden death. Another risk factor in morbidly obese patients for the development of pulmonary hypertension is ongoing hypoxaemia and hypercapnia from obstructive sleep apnoea (OSA) and obesity hypoventilation syndrome (OHS).

OSA is a very common comorbidity of morbid obesity that is estimated to affect up to 90% of morbidly obese patients. Excessive deposition of fatty tissue in the pharynx and larynx reduces the physiological airway aperture, particularly during sleep. The subsequent obstruction of the pharyngeal and laryngeal structures causes snoring and reduction in breathing (hypopnea) or even complete cessation of breathing (apnoea). The breathing interruptions occur during sleep secondary to temporary airway closure. As a consequence, patients may become hypoxic and hypercapnic. Moreover, these patients suffer from sleep fragmentation and complain of daytime sleepiness. During the day, OSA patients appear to be eucapnic. The gold standard to diagnose OSA is the apnoea–hypopnea index using polysomnography. However, there is a high incidence of undiagnosed surgical patients suffering from OSA. A simple screening tool, the STOP-Bang questionnaire, has been developed and validated for the diagnosis of OSA in the preoperative environment [9].

OSA can develop into OHS. Obesity hypoventilation syndrome is a combination of daytime hypercapnia and sleep-disordered breathing that is unrelated to any other pulmonary or neuromuscular disorder. OHS has an incidence of about 5% in morbidly obese and super-obese patients. In addition to OSA symptoms, OHS patients suffer from extensive daytime sleepiness and become hypercapnic even during daytime hours. OHS can be diagnosed by means of polysomnography and arterial blood gas analysis. As with OSA, a modified STOP-Bang questionnaire can be used to assess patients preoperatively [10]. Both syndromes, OSA and OHS, carry a significantly increased risk of hypoxaemia and hypercapnia in the perioperative period.

General anaesthesia is induced in the supine position. Consequently, changes in the elastic properties of the respiratory system and cephalad displacement of the diaphragm occurs. The ensuing reduction of the movement of the chest wall and the diaphragm decreases lung volume and results in about a 25% loss of FRC in a 70 kg patient. In contrast, an obese patient in the supine position may have a reduced FRC by as much as 50%. In fact, the increase in BMI has a linear relationship with the reduction of FRC and lung volume [11]. Both effects cause a mismatch in ventilation/perfusion ratio (V/Q mismatch) with the risk of hypoxia and hypercapnia more likely to occur in morbidly obese compared with non-obese patients.

Reduction in lung volume and FRC renders obese patients prone to diminished oxygen reserve during induction, maintenance, and emergence from anaesthesia. This is indicated by formation of atelectasis in the dependent lungs within minutes after induction of general anaesthesia [12]. The greater the BMI, the faster oxygen saturation will decrease after induction [13]. Hence, obese patients are routinely preoxygenated with 100% oxygen before induction and during emergence from general anaesthesia [14]. This results in an elevated fractional inspired oxygen concentration (FiO_2) during anaesthesia, frequently above 0.5 FiO_2. Following extubation, morbidly obese patients exhibit a reduction in lung volume and FRC rendering them susceptible to significant atelectasis.

A high FiO_2 causes reabsorption atelectasis [15], potentially exacerbating atelectasis already caused by supine positioning and general anaesthesia. Perioperative opioid administration can further reduce postoperative ventilation and enhance the V/Q mismatch putting the morbidly obese patient at higher risk for hypoxaemia and hypercapnia immediately after emergence from general anaesthesia and during the immediate recovery period.

In summary, the combination of obesity, surgery, and general anaesthesia contributes to a deterioration of respiratory mechanics during anaesthesia and in the postoperative period. The change in respiratory mechanics mimics a restrictive respiratory pattern and can persist for many days after surgery. Restrictive respiration increases the work of breathing with an increase in oxygen consumption and may further compromise oxygenation and carbon dioxide elimination [16]. Obese patients tend to have a rapid and shallow breathing pattern postoperatively. Faster breathing increases deadspace ventilation and reduces alveolar ventilation. The alveolar–arterial gradient is typically increased [17]. Thus, these patients are more likely to need reintubation or may have to stay on the ventilator for an extended period of time.

Obese patients with or without OSA or OHS have adipose tissue deposition in the pharynx and paralaryngeal tissues. Redundant fat tissue may cause grossly reduced airway patency after emergence from anaesthesia and extubation of the trachea. Airway obstruction is further pronounced in the supine position. The narrowing of the upper airways can compromise breathing efforts and render patients prone to hypoxaemia and hypercapnia.

Non-invasive ventilation

Non-invasive positive pressure ventilation has been shown to improve oxygenation and reduce the rate of reintubations in morbidly obese patients [18]. Non-invasive positive pressure ventilation has been recommended by the American Society of Anesthesiologists for morbidly obese patients with OSA in the postoperative period [19]. Non-invasive ventilation (NIV) has been widely used in patients with exacerbation of COPD, in asthma attacks, and cardiogenic pulmonary oedema. A subset of patients with respiratory failure profit from the use of NIV in the intensive care unit (ICU) including patients with chronic hypercapnic respiratory failure who are being weaned from mechanical ventilation [20,21]. NIV is a mainstay in treating OSA and OHS and its long-term application has been shown to reduce mortality and morbidity in this patient population [22,23].

NIV has entered into the perioperative environment, mainly in patients with postoperative hypoxaemia or hypercapnia with impending respiratory failure and the risk for reintubation. NIV can be used as a therapeutic intervention for postoperative high-risk patients and morbidly obese patients exhibiting respiratory failure. Additionally, NIV can be applied in obese patients with concomitant OSA or OHS perioperatively in a prophylactic way.

NIV is defined as non-invasive delivery of continuous positive pressure throughout the breathing cycle (continuous positive airway pressure (CPAP)) or by two different positive pressure levels, a higher pressure level during inspiration and a lower pressure level during expiration (bi-level positive airway pressure (BiPAP)). NIV is applied by mask to nose only (nasal mask), to mouth and nose together (Fig. 11.1), or by a helmet that covers and seals the whole head. As opposed to tracheal intubation, NIV does not interfere with the upper airway directly. There is no connection to the pharynx or vocal cords and the patient's ability to swallow and speak are preserved, although speaking may interrupt positive airway pressure. Of paramount importance is the fact that patients can cough and protect their airways from overt or silent aspiration. As a result, potential complications of invasive ventilation are less likely to occur. These include the risk of post-intubation tracheal stenosis or ventilator-associated pneumonia or aspiration pneumonia.

As mentioned previously, NIV can be applied in two different ways: CPAP or BiPAP. CPAP describes a ventilation mode that is characterized by an elevated airway pressure during the entire phase of the breathing cycle. Most importantly, positive airway pressures are delivered during expiration allowing restriction of gas flow from

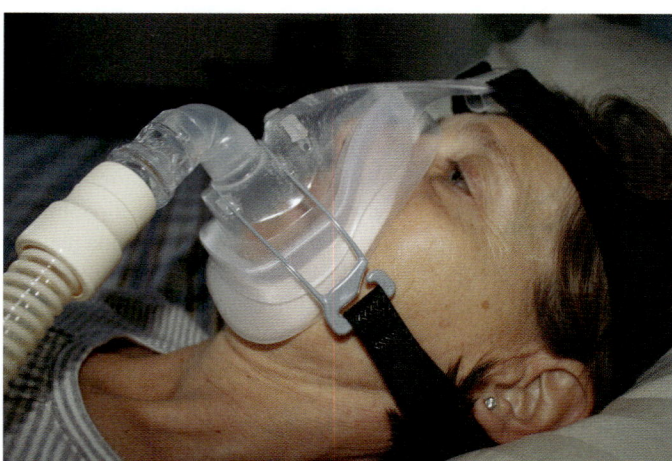

Fig. 11.1 Example of a CPAP mask covering nose and mouth.

the alveoli to the environment thus preventing the formation of atelectasis. Maintaining positive pressure in the upper airways keeps smaller, more distal airways open and prevents dynamic airway collapse in the small bronchi during expiration. Likewise, keeping upper airways open allows for constant gas flow during expiration and reduces the dynamic upper airway obstruction as observed in OSA and OHS. Lastly, CPAP increases the difference between negative pleural pressures and airway pressures during inspiration. This difference in pressures decreases the work of breathing for the patient significantly. Therefore, CPAP appears to be helpful for patients with a weak thoracic pump, including patients with COPD or morbidly obese patients.

CPAP represents the least invasive form of NIV and may not reduce the work of breathing in all patients at risk for respiratory failure. Some patients present with a combination of COPD and morbid obesity or other source of respiratory muscle weakness. For these patients, CPAP will not be sufficient to avert impending respiratory failure after general anaesthesia. In this case, the thoracic pump will be too weak to profit from CPAP alone and a more invasive form of NIV is needed.

CPAP may be combined with inspiratory pressure support. Pressure support further reduces the work of breathing by augmenting each tidal volume. Pressure support is triggered by the patient's breathing efforts (patient triggered). The support is a boost of positive pressure, set by the operator of the NIV device (pressure targeted), and will typically end at 25% of the patient's airflow (flow-cycled). Pressure support is typically set to 5–10 cm H_2O above CPAP with the goal to achieve an augmented tidal volume of about 6 mL/kg of predicted body weight.

When using a combination of CPAP and pressure support, an expiratory positive airway pressure (EPAP) and an inspiratory positive airway pressure (IPAP) will be set. In other words, two different airway pressures are used during the respiratory cycle, which has been referred to as BiPAP. Ventilation with BiPAP is different from bi-level ventilation in intubated patients in the critical care unit. In intubated patients, bi-level ventilation offers a mandatory ventilation pattern with a compulsory change in pressure levels on a set rate; whereas BiPAP ventilation in spontaneously breathing, non-intubated patients is solely triggered by the patent's effort to inhale.

Several different BiPAP ventilators have become available, all with a proprietary algorithm to adjust for different patient needs. For instance, in one device auto-titrating bi-level positive airway pressure, IPAP and EPAP are adjusted automatically and individually to overcome increased airway resistance due to upper airway obstruction or bronchoconstriction. Another device regulates IPAP only with adaptive servo ventilation. This means IPAP is adjusted for each inspiration with the goal to maintain a moving target ventilation set at 90% of the patient's recent average minute ventilation. Yet, another ventilator has a built-in algorithm that uses prior peak flows to target the level of IPAP. In addition, volume-assured and volume-controlled ventilation support are available. Volume-assured pressure support IPAP is adjusted to achieve a target tidal volume set by the healthcare provider. In volume-controlled ventilation, the patient will receive a preset tidal volume irrespective of the underlying lung pathology, similar to volume control used for intubated patients. This method appears to be the most invasive ventilation of all available non-invasive ventilation methods.

> **Box 11.1** Indications for use of non-invasive ventilation
>
> - Treatment of airway obstruction as in OSA.
> - Treatment of postoperative hypoxaemia.
> - Treatment of postoperative hypercarbia.
> - COPD exacerbation.
> - Cardiogenic pulmonary oedema.
> - Prevention of atelectasis in high-risk surgical patients.

Morbidly obese patients may be treated with any of the above-mentioned ventilation support methods. The patients may be in full synchrony and feel an almost immediate improvement and reduction of their breathing workload. At all times, patient comfort must be guaranteed. Hence, close communication with the patient is mandatory to assure adequate comfort and synchrony between the patients' breathing efforts and positive pressure breaths delivered by the NIV ventilator.

In cases where patient discomfort is present though, adjustments can be made based on patient request. Likewise, changes in pressure settings should be made when target tidal volumes are not reached. An alternative to measured tidal volumes is to titrate positive airway pressures to a target partial pressure of carbon dioxide, if an arterial line is available to frequently analyse arterial blood gas.

Non-invasive ventilators are stand-alone devices. These devices are very versatile and can be utilized in every room with oxygen wall outlets, such as a post-anaesthesia care unit, ICU, or on the regular patient ward. Modern hospital-based NIV ventilators are microprocessor driven and have fast responding pressure and flow meters that allow for immediate adjustment of airway flows to target preset airway pressures. Such ventilators have the capacity to detect and measure air leaks that may occur because of ill-fitting face masks or an indwelling nasogastric tube that creates an improper seal. Leak correction is prompt in response to leakage and will increase airflow to maintain the level of preset positive airway pressure both during inspiration and expiration.

Postoperative respiratory failure in the morbidly obese patient may be treated with CPAP or BiPAP alone. However, some obese patients will require additional oxygen to improve hypoxaemia. Modern non-invasive ventilators are equipped to deliver high inspired oxygen with the FiO_2 titrated to the desired oxygen saturation. This is in sharp contrast to simple CPAP or BiPAP ventilators that are used at home in patients with OSA or morbidly obese patients with obesity hypoventilation syndrome (OHS). Indications for NIV are listed in **Box 11.1**.

Contraindications to non-invasive ventilation

Morbidly obese patients can profit from NIV in the postoperative phase as described previously. Specifically, the rate of reintubation may be reduced postoperatively, if NIV is applied in an appropriate manner. The most important preconditions for successful NIV application are that the patient is willing and understands the reason to attach a mask on his/her face tightly. Cooperation of the patient requires the patient to be awake, alert, and breathing spontaneously. If the patient is hypercapnic, mental status changes may initially cause

Box 11.2 Contraindications for use of non-invasive ventilation

- Unconsciousness/inability to protect airway.
- Agitated or uncooperative.
- Inadequate respiratory drive.
- Medically unstable—hypotensive shock, upper gastrointestinal bleed.
- Upper airway or upper gastrointestinal surgery.
- Persistent nausea/vomiting.
- Copious secretions.
- Facial trauma.

the patient to resist a CPAP mask. However, with correction of hypercapnia, the mental status usually improves within minutes.

If the patient is unable to follow instructions from the provider, NIV is contraindicated. This includes any form of coma or reduced alertness, but also agitation and restlessness. This includes patients who are unable to protect their airway or who are suffering from postoperative nausea and vomiting. Obviously, apnoeic patients must be intubated. Whenever NIV is applied, well-trained staff have to be readily available to troubleshoot any potentially dangerous situation such as vomiting into the CPAP mask.

In addition, postoperative application of NIV may be contraindicated after certain surgical procedures such as oesophagus or gastric surgery or in obese patients with pneumothorax. Patients with facial fractures, skull base fractures, or significant facial trauma should not be put on a facial mask postoperatively either.

Patients with massive production of secretions or patients with frequent coughing episodes (e.g. long-time smokers) will frequently open their mouth during NIV treatment. As a consequence, this interferes with NIV in patients wearing a nasal mask or causes a major leak in a face mask, both of which thwart the effect of positive airway pressure ventilation. Contraindications for NIV use are given in **Box 11.2**.

Clinical application

As previously described, induction of general anaesthesia causes a reduction in FRC and ultimately a decrease in oxygen reserve. This phenomenon is accentuated in the obese population causing them to have a higher-risk scenario of hypoxia and hypercapnia. In order to help circumvent this scenario, obese patients are routinely preoxygenated with 100% oxygen. However, this is not without compromise as reabsorption atelectasis can occur. NIV is an alternative to preoxygenating with 100% oxygen. Implementing NIV in obese patients prior to induction of anaesthesia improves preoxygenation and is effective in reducing desaturation compared with standard preoxygenation techniques [24].

The successful application of NIV following surgery in the post-anaesthesia care unit is well accepted. Its utility as a therapeutic intervention for patients with either hypercapnic or non-hypercapnic respiratory failure has been proven to be an effective strategy to decrease invasive ventilation across a variety of settings. Moreover, it is now known that certain surgeries, including upper abdominal, cardiac, thoracic, and bariatric, are prone to higher risks of postoperative pulmonary decompensation. Undertaking these surgeries in an obese patient, who already exhibits altered respiratory function, creates an increased risk of significant postoperative respiratory compromise. As a result, the prophylactic application of NIV aimed at preventing and reversing atelectasis in patients undergoing these high-risk surgeries is worthy of exploration.

Of special note is bariatric surgery where all patients are suffering from some magnitude of obesity. Moreover, the number of bariatric surgical procedures performed worldwide has increased significantly recently. It should be noted that although the complication rates following bariatric surgery are relatively low, the likelihood of postoperative respiratory compromise is much higher given the patient population. Several studies have been performed in bariatric surgical patients in order to evaluate the effectiveness of NIV.

Gaszynski et al. found that CPAP improved oxygenation compared to traditional oxygen delivery via nasal cannula in 19 morbidly obese patients after undergoing gastric bypass surgery [25]. Similar results were exhibited by another study using NIV in postoperative patients after undergoing Roux-en-Y gastric bypass surgery. The authors concluded that NIV leads to improved oxygenation, without increasing surgical complications such as anastomotic dehiscence [26].

In another study, Joris et al. examined 30 patients undergoing bariatric surgery and assigned them to either oxygenation via face mask, low-support BiPAP (8/4), or high-support BiPAP (12/4) for the first 24 hours following surgery. Pulmonary function tests and oxygen saturation were then measured at specific time intervals. The results revealed that the patients with the higher support BiPAP postoperatively had improved pulmonary function tests and oxygen saturations. Furthermore, these benefits were maintained at day 2 following discontinuation of NIV and allowed for faster recovery back to baseline pulmonary function [27].

Ebeo et al. also evaluated whether a benefit existed in postoperative pulmonary function in patients utilizing NIV in the first 24 hours following open gastric bypass surgery. The study demonstrated that NIV leads to higher levels of forced vital capacity, forced expiratory volume in 1 second, and percentage of haemoglobin oxygen saturation postoperatively and these benefits persisted for a period of time following discontinuation of NIV. However, despite these benefits the authors noted no difference in length of hospital stay [28].

Although these studies are small in magnitude, they all offer the same take-away message: the prophylactic application of NIV in the postoperative setting for morbidly obese patients undergoing bariatric surgery improves oxygenation. These findings are paramount moving forward given the exponential increase of bariatric surgeries and the increasing number of patients with morbid obesity who are presenting for other surgical procedures.

Whether this link exists for obese patients undergoing different types of surgery and clinical settings is yet to be fully determined. However, it has been shown that successful application of NIV following cardiac, thoracic, and abdominal surgeries in non-obese patients is a viable intervention both prophylactically and therapeutically. It could be surmised then that similar results would be expected in the obese patient population. Ultimately, at this point we are at the juvenile stages of our understanding surrounding the full potential benefits of NIV in the perioperative period. Further studies are required to shed light on the optimal ventilatory settings, timing of application, and length of application of NIV within this patient subgroup who appears to largely benefit from NIV.

Approaching the obese patient in the post-anaesthesia care unit with acute respiratory distress is managed in the same manner as the non-obese patient. However, this must be done in a timely and diligent manner as obese patients can deteriorate to severe hypoxic and hypercapnic states much quicker than a non-obese patient for reasons previously outlined. Postoperatively, there is a wide array of problems that can lead to acute respiratory distress. Potential causes include, but are not limited to, pharmacotherapy, such as residual anaesthetic agents, opiates, benzodiazepines, and neuromuscular blockers.

Pulmonary problems, such as airway obstruction, bronchospasm from asthma or COPD exacerbation, pneumothorax, atelectasis, pulmonary embolism, or mucous plugging may occur, and neurological issues such anxiety, pain, or delirium can worsen respiratory distress. Bedside evaluation of the patient is paramount, paying particular attention to lung auscultation, airway evaluation, and the patient's breathing pattern. Respiratory mechanics should be optimized by positioning the patient in a 30-degree head-up position to help facilitate lung recruitment and FRC. Pulmonary therapy such as incentive spirometry, facilitation of coughing, and mobilization of secretions should be implemented. Supplemental oxygen, if not already available, should be administered. If any reversible causes are identified, then appropriate interventions to reverse the process should be undertaken. In instances where prompt reversal is not attainable and the underlying reason for respiratory distress is deemed temporary, for example, significant atelectasis, then the application of NIV must be considered.

However, in patients that are comatose, agitated, or suffering from a process that will not readily resolve such as aspiration, NIV is contraindicated and prompt securing of the airway with intubation and invasive ventilation should ensue. In addition, in those patients where NIV was initiated and improvement in symptoms, partial pressure of oxygen, or partial pressure of carbon dioxide does not occur within the first hour of intervention, then intubation should be considered.

How to apply non-invasive ventilation to the patient

The obese patient ought to be instructed about the principles of non-invasive ventilation early on. The instruction should take place in the preoperative setting, regardless, if NIV is planned to be applied prophylactically pre-induction or as a therapeutic option postoperatively. Whenever NIV is applied, standard monitoring must be utilized. This includes monitoring of oxygen saturation and respiratory rate along with basic cardiovascular monitoring.

In the recovery room, the morbidly obese patient should be placed in a semi-recumbent position with adequate pain control, allowing for improvement of FRC. The device mask is attached to the patient's face and adjusted to seal properly. Usually, CPAP is started at 5–8 cmH$_2$O at a FiO$_2$ of 0.4. Guided by vital signs and arterial blood gas, if available, CPAP may be titrated up to 10–12 cmH$_2$O with the goal of achieving normoxia and normocapnia.

Apart from the CPAP set point, it is equally important to set the flow trigger to −1 to −2 L/minute. Alternatively, a pressure trigger may be used at 1–2 cmH$_2$O. If autotriggering is induced, higher flow or pressure triggers should be used than those for normal-weight patients.

If normoxia and normocapnia cannot be achieved or if the patient has labouring breathing with marked tachypnoea with the initial settings, pressure support ventilation (PSV) should be added to the CPAP mode. PSV can be started with 3–5 cmH$_2$O and should gradually be increased to 10–15 cmH$_2$O above the CPAP level as tolerated by the patient. CPAP and PSV together constitute the BiPAP mode. Patient synchrony with the ventilator set on CPAP or BiPAP is crucial. If the patient continues to be uncomfortable and the breathing workload of the patient appears to be too high, intubation and positive pressure ventilation should be initiated. See **Fig. 11.2**.

Conversely, if respiratory status improves, CPAP or BiPAP should be continued for 3 hours with a subsequent break from the tightly attached mask. Duration of CPAP or BiPAP should be determined on an individual basis guided by oxygen saturation, breathing rate and pattern of the patient, and arterial blood gas analysis. The morbidly obese patient who does not have significant improvement of respiratory insufficiency in the recovery room should be transferred to a critical care unit for continuation of NIV and close monitoring for potential need of reintubation.

There are many different ventilators for NIV commercially available. All NIV ventilators are very accurate and have the ability to compensate for potential leaks. Ventilator settings are similar to ICU ventilators. FiO$_2$, pressure levels for CPAP/BiPAP, and flow or pressure triggers can be adjusted. There are no data showing superiority of one NIV ventilator over another. However, it should be noted

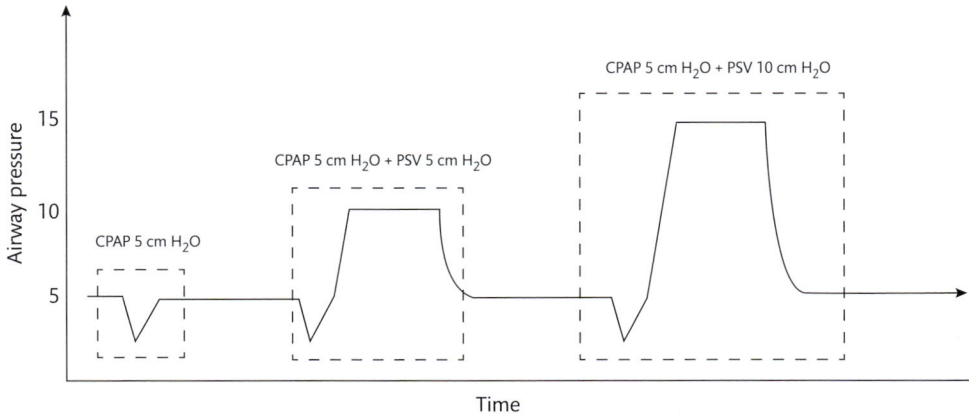

Fig. 11.2 Different modes of CPAP and combination of CPAP plus PSV. Inspiratory trigger at −2 cmH$_2$O with CPAP 5 cmH$_2$O; CPAP 5 cmH$_2$O and PSV 5 cmH$_2$O; and CPAP 5 cmH$_2$O and PSV 10 cmH$_2$O.

> **Box 11.3** Algorithm for non-invasive ventilation
>
> - Set pressure trigger to -2 cmH_2O.
> - Start CPAP at 6 cmH_2O.
> - Increase CPAP by 2 cmH_2O as needed.
> - CPAP maximum at 10 cmH_2O.
> - If hypoxia or hypercarbia persists, start PSV at 5 cmH_2O above CPAP.
> - Gradually increase PSV by 2 cmH_2O up to a maximum of 15 cmH_2O above CPAP.
> - Increase FiO_2 guided by oxygen saturation.
> - Give CPAP/PSV break every 3 hours.

that multifunction hospital ventilators are preferred over simple ventilators in the morbidly obese patient population both in the recovery room and ICU. Factors affecting NIV application are shown in **Box 11.3**.

Conclusion

As morbid obesity continues to increase worldwide, there is an ever-increasing likelihood of routinely giving anaesthetic care for patients afflicted with this disease and its associated comorbidities. Obese patients will present within a variety of clinical settings, from the perioperative arena to the ICU. As outlined previously, one important comorbidity suffered by morbidly obese individuals concerns the respiratory system—spanning the spectrum from baseline respiratory dysfunction to OHS and OSA. The combination of obesity, surgery, and general anaesthesia contributes to a deterioration of respiratory mechanics during anaesthesia and in the postoperative period. Consequently, the anaesthesiologist must be well versed, not only with understanding the underlying pathophysiology of patients suffering from morbid obesity such as the aforementioned respiratory dysfunction, but how best to optimally care for this growing subset of patients to ensure the most favourable outcomes. Application of CPAP and/or BiPAP is one important intervention that has been shown not only to benefit morbidly obese patients as a therapeutic intervention, but also as a potential prophylactic intervention to circumvent unwanted perioperative respiratory complications and ensure optimal delivery of care and patient outcomes.

REFERENCES

1. D'Ávila Melo SM, Melo VA de, Menezes Filho RS de, Santos FA. Effects of progressive increase in body weight on lung function in six groups of body mass index. Rev Assoc Med Bras. 2011;**57**(5):509–15.
2. Wilson A, Longhi J, Goldman C, McNatt S. Intra-abdominal pressure and the morbidly obese patients: the effect of body mass index. J Trauma. 2010;**69**(1):78–83.
3. Jones RL, Nzekwu MM. The effects of body mass index on lung volumes. Chest. 2006;**130**(3):827–33.
4. Mahadev S, Salome CM, Berend N, King GG. The effect of low lung volume on airway function in obesity. Respir Physiol Neurobiol. 2013;**188**(2):192–99.
5. Shore SA, Johnston RA. Obesity and asthma. Pharmacol Ther. 2006;**110**(1):83–102.
6. Behrens G, Matthews CE, Moore SC, Hollenbeck AR, Leitzmann MF. Body size and physical activity in relation to incidence of chronic obstructive pulmonary disease. CMAJ. 2014;**186**(12):E457–69.
7. Mahadev S, Farah CS, King GG, Salome CM. Obesity, expiratory flow limitation and asthma symptoms. Pulm Pharmacol Ther. 2013;**26**(4):438–43.
8. Alpert MA, Lavie CJ, Agrawal H, Kumar A, Kumar SA. Cardiac effects of obesity. J Cardiopulm Rehabil Prev. 2016;**36**(1):1–11.
9. Chung F, Subramanyam R, Liao P, Sasaki E, Shapiro C, Sun Y. High STOP-Bang score indicates a high probability of obstructive sleep apnoea. Br J Anaesth. 2012;**108**(5):768–75.
10. Bingol Z, Pıhtılı A, Kıyan E. Modified STOP-BANG questionnaire to predict obesity hypoventilation syndrome in obese subjects with obstructive sleep apnea. Sleep Breath. 2016; **20**(2):495–500.
11. Neligan PJ. Metabolic syndrome: anesthesia for morbid obesity. Curr Opinion Anaesthesiol. 2010;**23**(3):375–83.
12. Eichenberger AS, Proietti S, Wicky S, Frascarolo P, Suter M, Spahn DR, et al. Morbid obesity and postoperative pulmonary atelectasis: an underestimated problem. Anesth Analg. 2002;**95**(6):1788–92.
13. Jense HG, Dubin SA, Silverstein PI, O'Leary-Escolas U. Effect of obesity on safe duration of apnea in anesthetized humans. Anesth Analg. 1991;**72**(1):89–93.
14. Shah U, Wong J, Wong DT, Chung F. Preoxygenation and intraoperative ventilation strategies in obese patients: a comprehensive review. Curr Opinion Anaesthesiol. 2016;**29**(1):109–18.
15. Rothen HU, Sporre B, Engberg G, Wegenius G, Reber A, Hedenstierna G. Prevention of atelectasis during general anaesthesia. Lancet. 1995;**345**(8962):1387–91.
16. Parameswaran K, Todd DC, Soth M. Altered respiratory physiology in obesity. Can Respir J. 2006;**13**(4):203–10.
17. Salome CM, King GG, Berend N. Physiology of obesity and effects on lung function. J Appl Physiol. 2010;**108**(1):206–11.
18. Gupta RM, Parvizi J, Hanssen AD, Gay PC. Postoperative complications in patients with obstructive sleep apnea syndrome undergoing hip or knee replacement: a case-control study. Mayo Clin Proc. 2001;**76**(9):897–905.
19. American Society of Anesthesiologists Task Force on Perioperative Management of patients with obstructive sleep apnea. Practice guidelines for the perioperative management of patients with obstructive sleep apnea: an updated report by the American Society of Anesthesiologists Task Force on Perioperative Management of patients with obstructive sleep apnea. Anesthesiology. 2014;**120**(2):268–86.
20. Girault C, Bubenheim M, Abroug F, Diehl JL, Elatrous S, Beuret P, et al. Noninvasive ventilation and weaning in patients with chronic hypercapnic respiratory failure: a randomized multicenter trial. Am J Respir Crit Care Med. 2011;**184**(6):672–79.
21. Brochard L, Mancebo J, Elliott MW. Noninvasive ventilation for acute respiratory failure. Eur Respir J. 2002;**19**(4):712–21.
22. Kryger MH, Berry RB, Massie CA. Long-term use of a nasal expiratory positive airway pressure (EPAP) device as a treatment for obstructive sleep apnea (OSA). J Clin Sleep Med. 2011;**7**(5):449–53B.
23. Mokhlesi B, Kryger MH, Grunstein RR. Assessment and management of patients with obesity hypoventilation syndrome. Proc Am Thorac Soc. 2008;**5**(2):218–25.

24. Delay J-M, Sebbane M, Jung B, Nocca D, Verzilli D, Pouzeratte Y, et al. The effectiveness of noninvasive positive pressure ventilation to enhance preoxygenation in morbidly obese patients: a randomized controlled study. 2008;**107**(5):1707–13.

25. Gaszynski T, Tokarz A, Piotrowski D, Machala W. Boussignac CPAP in the postoperative period in morbidly obese patients. Obes Surg. 2007;**17**(4):452–56.

26. Pessoa KC, Araújo GF, Pinheiro AN, Ramos MRS, Maia SC. Noninvasive ventilation in the immediate postoperative of gastrojejunal derivation with Roux-en-Y gastric bypass. Rev Bras Fisioter. 2010;**14**(4):290–95.

27. Joris JL, Sottiaux TM, Chiche JD, Desaive CJ, Lamy ML. Effect of bi-level positive airway pressure (BiPAP) nasal ventilation on the postoperative pulmonary restrictive syndrome in obese patients undergoing gastroplasty. Chest. 1997;**111**(3):665–70.

28. Ebeo CT, Benotti PN, Byrd RP, Elmaghraby Z, Lui J. The effect of bi-level positive airway pressure on postoperative pulmonary function following gastric surgery for obesity. Respir Med. 2002;**96**(9):672–76.

SECTION 3
Non-bariatric surgery

Thoracoabdominal surgeries in obese patients

Deepu S. Ushakumari and Stephanie Rayos Callison

Introduction

The prevalence of obesity has been steadily increasing, and it is now common for anaesthesiologists to care for obese patients in the perioperative setting. In addition, lung cancer is the second most common type of cancer in both males and females and the leading cause of cancer-related deaths [1]. In 2006–2010, 25% of patients with lung cancer who presented for lobectomy were obese [2]. Obesity carries with it significant comorbidities, including hypertension, coronary artery disease, and diabetes, all of which contribute to higher perioperative morbidity and mortality in patients presenting for thoracic surgery.

In this chapter, unique mechanical and physiological changes to the respiratory system conferred by obesity, as well as its effect on the interpretation of studies, will be reviewed. Recommendations are included on clinical examination and evaluation of relevant cardiopulmonary test results; intraoperative challenges encountered in obese patients presenting for thoracic surgery, including intravenous (IV) access, monitoring, lung isolation, positioning, and potential postoperative complications, their risk factors, and ways to mitigate them, are also reviewed.

Pulmonary physiological changes in obesity and its implications in thoracic anaesthesia

Pulmonary function changes

Obese individuals have a restrictive profile in pulmonary function tests with a rapid, shallow breathing pattern. A relative increase in dead-space ventilation (ratio of volume of dead space to tidal volume) causes increased oxygen cost of breathing, and obese individuals perform poorly on pulmonary function tests [3].

Lung volume changes

Both static and dynamic lung volumes are altered in obesity. Functional residual capacity (FRC) is reduced by the obese abdomen displacing the diaphragm into the chest [4]. However, residual volume (RV) is unaltered, resulting in a reduced expiratory reserve volume (ERV) in obesity. A decrease in ERV is the most consistent pulmonary function abnormality in obesity [3]. ERV is further diminished in the supine position due to increased displacement of the diaphragm into the chest cavity. Beyond a certain point, the ERV may decrease to less than the closing volume, leading to closure of smaller airways and air trapping [5]. Since RV is unchanged, the relationship of FRC less than closing capacity is equivalent to ERV less than closing volume.

FRC is linearly related to height, and obese individuals have a decreased FRC compared to lean people of the same height. In a white male adult aged 25–65 years:

$$FRC = (5.95 \times height) + (0.019 \times age) - (0.086 \times BMI) - 5.3$$

where FRC is in litres, height in metres, age in years, and BMI (body mass index) in kg/m² [6].

The proposed relationship between FRC after induction of anaesthesia and anthropometry is:

$$FRC \ (\% \ of \ pre\text{-}anaesthetic \ value) = 137.7 - 164.4 \times (weight \ in \ kg/ height \ in \ cm).$$

Accordingly, FRC decreases significantly after induction of anaesthesia in the obese patient but does not do so in the non-obese individual [7].

Dynamic lung volumes such as vital capacity and total lung capacity are usually normal in obesity [8]. The RV/ total lung capacity ratio is normal or slightly increased [9]. Measurements such as forced expiratory volume in 1 second (FEV_1), forced vital capacity (FVC), forced expiratory flow in 25–75% phase of expiration, and minute volume are decreased in obesity, but these decreases are small and the values often fall within the normal range in otherwise healthy children and adults [10,11]. The FEV_1/FVC ratio is usually normal or even slightly increased in obese patients, sometimes in spite of morbid obesity [12]. Thus, the changes in major spirometric findings in obesity are an effect of obesity on lung volumes and not directly due to airway obstruction [12]. Mid-expiratory flow obstruction is seen in morbidly obese subjects [11].

Spirometry in mild to moderate obesity paints a restrictive picture, and severe and morbid obesity replicates an obstructive picture. The mechanism may be related to decreased lung volumes, small airway collapse, or a combination of both [3].

Lung mechanics, airway resistance, and compliance

Compliance

The total respiratory compliance is reduced up to two-thirds of the normal value in obesity. Both a decrease in lung compliance (caused by increased pulmonary blood volume, increased alveolar surface tension, and closure of dependent airways) and a decrease in chest wall compliance (caused by fat accumulation on the thorax, abdomen, and diaphragm) contribute to this, but the contribution of the latter outweighs the former [14]. The reduction in lung compliance and obesity share an exponential relationship [15]. Interestingly, the chest wall pressure–volume curve of obese patients is similar to that of a normal subject with mass loading of the thorax [16]. Thus, the excess fat acts as an inspiratory threshold load and once it is overcome, the chest wall behaves normally [12].

Resistance

Reduction in FRC affects airway resistance and reactance. Airway resistance is increased in the obese [17]; however, specific airway resistance (resistance adjusted for the lung volumes) is in the normal range. This apparent increased airway resistance is likely due to the reduction in lung volumes [18,19]. However, some studies refute this and suggest there is an additional increase in resistance not attributable to the decreased lung volumes [20–22]. Proposed explanations include exposure to proinflammatory adipokines, continual opening and closing of small airways in dependent lung regions, and lipid deposition in the lungs affecting surfactant function [12,23].

Work of breathing

Both oxygen consumption (VO_2) and carbon dioxide production (VCO_2) are significantly increased in obese individuals. Multiple reports have documented an increased VO_2 even in sedated obese patients [14,24]. The percentage of VO_2 used for spontaneous ventilation is negligible in lean individuals but is significant in the obese, as documented by a study on anaesthetized paralysed individuals [24]. Altered upper airway mechanics, impaired lung mechanics as detailed previously, neurohormonal influences, altered ventilatory drive, impaired gas exchange, and overutilized respiratory muscles are all factors bequeathing the increased work of breathing [25,26].

These changes in respiratory mechanics worsen in the supine position and get progressively worse under general anaesthesia and one-lung ventilation (OLV). After adding on the surgical insult caused by thoracotomy and lung parenchyma resection, respiratory mechanics are significantly altered in the immediate postoperative period, with such changes persisting for 1–2 months [27].

Respiratory muscles

Respiratory muscle endurance, measured by maximal voluntary ventilation, is reduced by 20% in healthy obese people and by 45% in obese people with obesity hypoventilation syndrome (OHS) [28]. Fibre stretching by the additional load puts the diaphragmatic muscles at a length-tension disadvantage and causes diaphragmatic dysfunction [29]. The tidal expiratory flow limitation leads to intrinsic positive end-expiratory pressure (PEEP), which in turn imposes a threshold load on the muscles of inspiration. In addition, inspiratory muscles also experience an increased neural drive in morbidly obese individuals [30]. The oxygen cost of respiratory muscles is also greater in obese individuals [26].

Ventilation/perfusion distribution, gas exchange, and airway closure

Ventilation and perfusion in a healthy non-obese lung are highest in the dependent zones. This regional distribution of alveolar ventilation may be reversed in some obese individuals. In obese individuals with ERV reduction to 20% of predicted, ventilation is preferentially distributed to the upper zones of the lung, leaving the dependent zones underventilated and overperfused [31]. This results in ventilation/perfusion (V/Q) mismatch, the severity of which correlates to the decrease in ERV [3]. These findings have been even observed in the lateral decubitus position [32]. One of the proposed mechanisms responsible is a change in lung configuration (caused by the limitation of chest wall and diaphragm movement) leading to basal air trapping at low lung volumes [5,33]. FRC is decreased so much in some obese individuals that it may drop below the closing capacity, and small airway closure can occur even at tidal breaths [34,35]. The degree of airway closure in tidal breathing correlates to the partial pressure of oxygen (PaO_2) [34].

Increasing obesity increases measures of gas exchange, such as carbon monoxide diffusion capacity (DLCO) and the ratio of DLCO to alveolar volume (DLCO/VA) [8], both of which return to more normal levels with weight loss. Increased DLCO is likely due to increased pulmonary blood volume and flow. A normal or low-normal DLCO and DLCO/VA is suggestive of loss of a pulmonary capillary bed due to some other reason [3]. An increased alveolar–arterial oxygen gradient ($A–aO_2$) and a mild decrease in PaO_2 may be seen even in eucapnic obese individuals and is associated with abdominal obesity in the morbidly obese [12]. However, the effect of weight loss on gas exchange is variable, with conflicting evidence regarding changes in arterial oxygen tension with loss of weight [35,36].

Control of breathing and ventilatory responsiveness

Mildly obese patients compensate for the rising level of CO_2 during exercise and rebreathing by increasing their minute ventilation. However, morbidly obese patients are unable to do this, and some may even be hypercapnic at rest—so-called OHS. The proposed theories for CO_2 accumulation include decreased ventilatory response to CO_2, inefficient respiratory muscles, impaired central respiratory drive, increased work of breathing, increased inspiratory threshold, and abnormal ventilatory load compensation [3,28]. In OHS, hypoxic drive is one-sixth and hypercapnic drive is one-third of that of non-obese subjects [37]. Whether the decreased ventilatory response to CO_2 (40% in simple obesity and 65% in OHS) precedes obesity or is acquired later is an unresolved inquisition [3]. OHS is discussed elsewhere in this textbook (see Chapter 20).

Sleep apnoea syndromes

Both central sleep apnoea syndrome and obstructive sleep apnoea syndrome (OSAS) are observed more frequently in obese individuals [38]. The periodic apnoea or hypopnea episodes lead to pulmonary vasoconstriction and structural alterations in the walls of pulmonary arterioles resulting in permanent daytime pulmonary hypertension [39].

Obesity and exercise lung physiology

Healthy obese individuals demonstrate exertional dyspnoea and shorter 6-minute walking distance [40]. The discomfort from increased load on the feet and joints and skin friction limits exercise capacity [40]. In a eucapnic obese subject at rest, the respiratory rate is approximately 40% higher than a person with a normal BMI. The duration of inspiration (T_i) as a fraction of total breath duration (T_i/T_{tot}) is normal. In obese patients without OHS, the tidal volume is normal even at maximal exercise. However, individuals with OHS have a 25% higher response rate and a 25% lower tidal volume than subjects with simple obesity, whereas T_i/T_{tot} remains normal with exercise [4].

Oxygen uptake (VO_2) at rest is roughly 25% greater and is also increased with exertion in obese subjects [28]. Relative work inefficiency exists, with an increase in VO_2 for a given workload [41]. Peak exercise capacity, peak VO_2, peak oxygen pulse (VO_2/heart rate), and anaerobic threshold are normal in moderately obese subjects [42]. Exercise spirometry suggests that obese individuals have expiratory flow limitation during exercise [43]. This may be due to the abnormally low decrease in end-expiratory lung volumes with exercise in obesity [3]. Dead-space ventilation, which may be increased at rest, decreases towards the normal range with exercise [44].

Dyspnoea in obesity

Dyspnoea at rest may be reported in obese individuals, but it is unclear if this is solely due to obesity [45]. However, dyspnoea on exertion is reported by almost 80% of obese subjects. Comorbidities such as diastolic dysfunction, coronary artery disease, pulmonary hypertension, and gastro-oesophageal reflux disease all contribute to this phenomenon [46]. In a study by Ofir et al., the respiratory mechanics related to obesity did not contribute to the breathlessness in obese individuals [12,47]. Obese individuals have a higher respiratory rate, and oxygen cost of breathing increases parabolically with respiratory rate. This increased oxygen cost of breathing may be contributing to breathlessness with exercise [48]. Flow receptor stimulation caused by airway obstruction at low lung volumes increase the sensation of breathlessness [3,49]. Orthopnoea in morbidly obese subjects correlate to the greater reduction in expiratory flow and ERV in the supine position [50].

Obesity and obstructive airway disease

Obesity has long been considered to be a risk factor for obstructive lung disease, including asthma [51]. Proposed reasons for this include smaller airway calibre at low lung volumes, airway hyper-responsiveness, and absence of the bronchoprotective effect of deep inhalations [3], but a causal relationship has not been definitively established. Asthma may be overdiagnosed in obese individuals and an objective confirmation for the diagnosis is recommended to avoid missing alternate aetiologies for dyspnoea [10]. The association between obesity and chronic obstructive pulmonary disease (COPD) is believed to be paradoxical. Low BMI has been associated with increased mortality in COPD, but when BMI is adjusted for muscle mass, this association is lost [52]. Low maximum exercise capacity is a strong predictor of mortality in COPD. Maximum exercise capacity increases with increasing BMI but declines when BMI enters the obese range. Further studies are required to investigate the belief that obesity is protective in COPD [3]. A combination of increased weight and airway obstruction can substantially decrease the respiratory quality of life in patients with moderate COPD, suggesting that even a modest weight loss may be especially beneficial [53].

Preoperative risk assessment and preparation

During a brief preoperative evaluation, the physician anaesthesiologist has to identify patients at a higher risk, formulate perioperative management, and focus resources to improve outcomes [54]. By virtue of their comorbidities and altered physiological state as discussed previously, many obese individuals stratify into the high-risk category.

Recent advances in anaesthesia, novel minimally invasive and lung-sparing surgical techniques, as well as improved postoperative management have significantly reduced the morbidity and mortality after thoracic surgery. However, these advances have also expanded the group of patients who are considered 'operable' and continue to pose a challenge to the anaesthesiologist. Respiratory complications, such as atelectasis, pneumonia, and respiratory failure, occur in 15–20% of patients and are responsible for the expected 3–4% mortality [55]. The anaesthesiologist also has to consider the risk of postponing or denying a potentially curative surgery in lung cancer patients.

The preoperative assessment begins with a complete history and physical examination and a compendium of information from multiple sources: electronic records, laboratory results, radiological images, consultation notes from other services, and tests designed to evaluate perioperative risk for a particular individual [56].

Patient interview and physical examination

A thorough patient interview to assess functional tolerance, respiratory quality of life, possible aetiologies for dyspnoea, and use of appetite-suppressant drugs is very important in obese patients presenting for surgery. Airway assessment should focus on identifying patients at a higher risk for difficult ventilation or intubation, or both, and include review of previous airway management records. While elevated BMI with or without OSAS is not a predictor of difficult laryngoscopy [57,58], obese patients with OSAS are at risk for difficult mask ventilation [59]. Airway management in obesity is discussed elsewhere in this textbook (see Chapter 21). Clinical examination should look for clinical features of OSAS, OHS, difficult IV access, and difficult regional anaesthesia techniques.

Discussion of smoking history and the benefits of smoking cessation are of particular importance in obese patients. Pulmonary complications are decreased in thoracic surgical patients who cease smoking for longer than 5–8 weeks before surgery [60]. Carboxyhaemoglobin concentrations are decreased in patients who cease smoking more than 12 hours before surgery [61]. Smoking cessation increases the relative oxygen tension and higher wound tissue oxygen concentration correlates with better wound healing and resistance to infection. These are particularly important in the proinflammatory milieu of obesity. Sputum volume, which is higher in smokers who have been abstinent for less than 8 weeks, is an independent risk factor for pulmonary complications [62]. However, there is no paradoxical increase in risk for pulmonary complications conferred by smoking cessation in the weeks immediately prior to lung resection surgery [63].

Cardiovascular disease

The strong association between smoking and cardiovascular disease as well as lung cancer makes it highly likely that thoracic surgery patients are smokers with a higher risk for perioperative cardiac complications [64]. Signs and symptoms of cardiac disease may masquerade as pulmonary symptoms. The American College of Cardiology/American Heart Association guideline for perioperative cardiovascular evaluation for non-cardiac surgery provides an excellent approach for assessment of thoracic surgical patients [65]. Cardiovascular changes in obesity and risk factors for cardiovascular disease are discussed in detail in Chapter 13. Combining coronary artery bypass grafting with lung cancer surgery has been associated with increased morbidity and mortality risk [66]. One study suggests no increased risk when combining off-pump coronary artery bypass grafting with lung cancer surgery, but further studies are required to prove such observations [67]. The incidence of dysrhythmias is 30–50% in the first week after pulmonary resection in non-obese individuals [68]. This is likely to be higher in obese patients who have a naturally higher risk of dysrhythmias due to myocardial hypertrophy and hypoxaemia, coronary artery disease, increased plasma catecholamine secretions, fatty infiltration of conduction systems, OSAS, and pulmonary hypertension [69]. Careful evaluation for such predispositions in obese thoracic surgery patients will help plan strategies to decrease the incidence of postoperative dysrhythmias.

Renal dysfunction

Although obesity was not listed as a risk factor for postoperative renal dysfunction, the increased prevalence of comorbidities (e.g. hypertension and diabetes mellitus) combined with renal structural changes in obese patients confer an increased risk of perioperative acute kidney injury (AKI) [70–72]. There is a positive correlation between high BMI and incidence of chronic kidney disease [73]. In addition, obese patients are more likely to be taking drugs which alter the glomerular pressure, such as renin–angiotensin–aldosterone axis modifiers, increasing the likelihood of renal dysfunction [74].

Chronic obstructive pulmonary disease

COPD is considered a systemic inflammatory process when coexisting with obesity [75]. There are several similarities between the physiological effects of COPD and obesity. Patients with severe COPD retain CO_2 due to their inability to maintain the increased work of breathing required to overcome inefficient pulmonary mechanics—similar to obesity. Oxygen supplementation in these patients is associated with a further rise in $PaCO_2$, as high fractional inspired oxygen (FiO_2) causes a relative decrease in alveolar ventilation, and increased V/Q mismatch [76]. COPD patients desaturate more frequently and to lower oxygen values than normal patients during sleep [54]—similar to OHS, but there is no increased incidence of sleep apnoea syndromes in COPD patients. Moreover, the rapid, shallow breathing pattern seen in obesity worsens during these periodic COPD-associated desaturations. The fall in oxygen saturation during sleep in COPD patients is associated with an increase in pulmonary artery pressure and is worse in subjects with coexisting obesity. Right ventricular dysfunction is noted in up to 50% of COPD patients [54]. When this is added to the right ventricular strain and increased pulmonary vascular resistance in a patient with OSAS/OHS, the dysfunctional right ventricle may not be able to tolerate sudden increases in afterload [77]. COPD patients often have an incomplete expiratory phase due to flow limitation and increased airway resistance termed auto-PEEP (intrinsic PEEP)—similar to obesity. During spontaneous respiration, the auto-PEEP adds an increased inspiratory load to the already increased expiratory load, similar to obesity. All of these similarities in respiratory physiology should be considered when evaluating lung function tests in a morbidly obese thoracic surgical patient with severe COPD.

Assessment of pulmonary function

Suboptimal image quality of chest X-rays in obesity can be due to inadequate penetration of X-rays, insufficient contrast from scatter radiation, patient motion artefacts, or inability to fit the entire area of interest on an image receptor [78]. Chest radiography and ultrasonography are the imaging modalities most affected by obesity [79].

The 'three-legged' stool for pre-thoracotomy respiratory assessment focuses on three areas: respiratory mechanics, lung parenchymal function, and cardiopulmonary interaction [54].

Respiratory mechanics

All pulmonary resection patients should have a preoperative baseline spirometry [54]. Interpretation of the test results on respiratory mechanics should consider the alterations in respiratory physiology with obesity. Baseline spirometry values for obese patients undergoing lung resection have not yet been elucidated. Predicted postoperative FEV_1 (ppoFEV_1) is touted as the most valid single test for predicting post-thoracotomy respiratory complications, where: Risk stratification for complications: ppoFEV_1 greater than 40%—low risk; ppoFEV_1 less than 30%—high risk [55].

These absolute values traditionally used for predicting postoperative complications are not indexed to body weight and consequently are less applicable to the obese thoracic surgical patient. However, it has been demonstrated that ppoFEV_1 and FVC decrease proportionally as BMI increases [80].

Lung parenchymal function

Conventionally, pressures of PaO_2 less than 60 mmHg and $PaCO_2$ greater than 45 mmHg were used as cut-off values for pulmonary resection [54]. However, DLCO has evolved to be the most useful test for gas exchange capacity of the lung, as it measures the total functioning alveolar–capillary interface surface area. Postoperative DLCO is calculated similarly as ppoFEV_1 previously described and values less than 40% have a much higher risk for postoperative respiratory complications [81]. Again, these values are not indexed to body weight and must be interpreted with caution in obese subjects.

The National Emphysema Treatment Trial showed that patients with ppoFEV_1 or DLCO less than 20% had an unacceptably high perioperative mortality rate [82]. Pierce et al. suggested that a product of ppoFEV_1 and postoperative DLCO, termed predicted postoperative product, less than 1650 was the best predictor of surgical mortality [83].

Cardiopulmonary interaction

Cardiopulmonary exercise testing is currently the 'gold standard' for assessment of cardiopulmonary function, while maximal oxygen consumption (VO_2 max) is regarded as the most useful predictor of post-thoracotomy outcome [54]. Simple bedside measures like the 6-minute walk test show an excellent correlation with VO_2 max and can be used in resource-limited settings. A VO_2 max less than 10 mL/kg/min or 40% predicted is considered an absolute contraindication to lung resection. Exercise testing in obesity shows no differences in terms of ST segment abnormalities or effort-induced angina between obese and non-obese individuals but demonstrates a very low functional capacity and complex dysrhythmias in some obese individuals [84]. Obese individuals demonstrate a decreased ability to take in, deliver, and consume additional oxygen needed during aerobic exercise [85]. A degree of right ventricular dysfunction, proportional to the amount of functioning pulmonary vascular bed removed, is seen after pulmonary resections [86]. This may be worsened in obese individuals with pre-existing right ventricular strain and pulmonary hypertension, as in OHS.

Split lung function tests

Radionuclide perfusion scanning and oxygen-enhanced magnetic resonance imaging are newer techniques which have replaced the anatomically calculated estimates of postoperative pulmonary function and are considered more accurate in obese subjects [87,88]. Any patient with a preoperative FEV_1 or DLCO less than 80% should be considered for V/Q lung scanning. Since this test is performed at rest, as opposed to spirometry which is a forced manoeuvre, it may be more reliable in obese individuals with expiratory flow limitation [54].

Patients receiving chemotherapy for lung cancer may demonstrate a reduction in DLCO and improvement in spirometry. However, a decrease in DLCO/VA after chemotherapy is associated with increased risk of pulmonary complications [89]. These measurements may be altered by changes in body weight seen in obese patients receiving chemotherapy.

Final preoperative assessment

This is usually performed immediately before surgery, and important considerations include airway assessment, establishment of monitoring, plan for regional anaesthesia, predicting the technique and equipment for lung isolation, and assessing the risk for hypoxaemia during OLV [54].

Intraoperative considerations

Monitoring

Preoperative preparation of a patient for thoracic surgery includes establishing standard American Society of Anesthesiologists monitors and placing invasive monitors for specific patients or procedures. Obese patients may prove challenging in one or more of these steps.

Thoracic surgical procedures require placement of at least one large-bore peripheral IV catheter and obese patients often have difficult IV access, as their increased subcutaneous tissue mass makes peripheral veins more difficult to palpate or visualize [90,91]. Ultrasonography and vein finders can be a valuable tool in obese paediatric and adult patients [92].

Thoracic surgery sometimes requires central venous cannulation, especially for pneumonectomies and large tumours with significant expected blood loss. The altered anatomy, including a short neck and redundant soft tissue, makes it challenging to place central lines in obese patients [93]. In addition, the standard-length central venous catheters may be too short in obese patients [94]. The use of pulmonary artery catheters may be of value in patients with cor pulmonale, severe pulmonary hypertension, and those presenting for lung transplant.

Invasive arterial pressure monitoring is indicated if prolonged OLV is anticipated. Due to the inaccurate estimation of non-invasive blood pressure by oscillator-cuff methods, obese patients are more likely to require arterial lines. The same considerations discussed previously regarding difficult peripheral IV access apply to potentially difficult arterial line placement. Continuous non-invasive arterial pressure monitoring devices showed initial promise, but the fidelity of these devices is questionable [95].

Increased subcutaneous and epicardial fat may alter the interpretation of electrocardiographic monitoring. Obese patients have high false-positive rates for myocardial infarction [96], repolarization abnormalities, QRS duration, and QT intervals [97].

Regional anaesthesia

Regional anaesthetic techniques such as thoracic epidural analgesia (TEA) and thoracic paravertebral block (TPVB) play a remarkable role in making recovery faster and smoother. Continuous epidural and paravertebral catheters are frequently placed preoperatively for open thoracic surgeries. These techniques are described later in this chapter.

Preoxygenation

The technique of breathing a higher FiO_2 (approximately 1) denitrogenates the FRC and prolongs the apnoea time (delay until the SpO_2 reaches 90%). This is of particular importance in obese patients with anticipated difficult mask ventilation/intubation. An extra layer of complexity is added when lung isolation is required which is most commonly achieved by placement of a double-lumen endotracheal tube (DLT). Relative to non-obese patients, decreased FRC, increased oxygen consumption, and increased DLCO in obese patients predisposes them to rapid desaturation [98]. Preoxygenation in obese patients can be enhanced by positive pressure ventilation and optimal positioning [98,99]. Optimal positioning options include placing the patient upright in a sitting (25 degrees), reverse Trendelenburg, or ramped position [100]. Another technique to increase apnoea time is to passively insufflate oxygen via a 10-French catheter in the nasopharynx at 5 L/min during laryngoscopy attempts [101].

Induction of anaesthesia

The decisions regarding type of induction (standard IV versus rapid sequence induction) and technique for intubation (after induction versus awake fibreoptic) are made on a case-by-case basis [102]. Dosage considerations include altered volume of distribution of drugs, uneven distribution of lean body weight as a part of the total body weight, and oil/water solubility of the drug used [103]. The prudence of a vigilant anaesthesiologist monitoring clinical end points can oftentimes produce better outcomes than empirical drug dosing regimens in obese patients where the pharmacokinetic profile of the same drug may vary at different times [104]. Obese patients are also at increased risk for aspiration due to the higher incidence of gastro-oesophageal reflux disease and higher resting gastric volumes. Despite this, the routine use of rapid sequence induction is not recommended [105].

Intubation and lung isolation

Obese patients with OSAS have smaller pharyngeal areas compared to non-obese cohorts, limiting both effective ventilation and optimal visualization required to secure the airway [106]. Moreover, obese patients have limited neck mobility and mouth opening [107]. Obesity, per se, has not been shown to be a predictor of difficult intubation. However, obese patients with OSAS, higher Mallampati score, large neck circumference, and increased pre-tracheal soft tissue by ultrasonography at the level of the vocal cords are more difficult to intubate [108,109]. Placement of a rigid DLT could be even more challenging, although this has never been studied or documented.

Positioning patients in the 'sniffing position' with elevation of the chest and shoulders on a ramp alleviates some soft tissue compression of airway structures, improves pulmonary reserve, and facilitates intubation [110]. Use of mask straps, oral airways, and alternative airway devices such as video laryngoscopy and fibreoptic bronchoscopy may assist in securing the airway. The management priority should be to safely secure the airway before considering lung isolation techniques. When the placement of a DLT is difficult due to increased bulk of the tube relative to a smaller pharyngeal area or to a misalignment of axis caused by soft tissue, a single-lumen tube should be placed to secure the airway and prevent desaturation [111].

Left-sided DLTs are the most commonly used devices for lung isolation. Appropriate DLT size (largest feasible) is chosen based on anthropometry and radiographic measurements of the anatomy. However, in patients with difficult airways, in patients with tracheostomy tubes, and for single lobar blockade, use of bronchial blockers is recommended [111,112]. An alternative technique is to use an airway exchange catheter (at least 83 cm long) to exchange a single-lumen endotracheal tube for a DLT. DLTs make it easier to suction the non-ventilated lung; however, no clear superiority of DLTs or bronchial blockers has been established in clinical practice [113]. The lung isolation strategy should be customized for each patient depending on ease of intubation, type of surgery, institutional preference, and experience with the device. Regardless of the type of lung isolation technique employed, flexible fibreoptic confirmation of placement is mandatory, in addition to clinical confirmation [114]. X-rays provide a definitive confirmation. A novel point-of-care method to confirm lung isolation is with ultrasonography to look for pleural/lung movement.

Once the airway is secured, any positioning device used to attain a head-elevated position, such as a ramp, is removed prior to positioning the patient for surgery.

Positioning

The lateral decubitus position is required for most thoracic surgeries. Requirements unique to shifting a morbidly obese patient from a supine to a lateral position include additional personnel to shift the patient, proportionally larger rolls just inferior to the axilla, larger bean bags, and operating room tables with more weight-support capability. Bean bags, safety straps to secure the patient to the table, and non-sliding base cushions will all help prevent the inadvertent

fall of a patient from the operating room table. Ensuring neutral positioning of the cervical spine in the lateral position can be difficult in morbidly obese patients with short necks. Brachial plexus injuries are the most common nerve injuries associated with the lateral position; these include stretch injuries of the non-dependent arm and compression injuries of the dependent arm. Pressure sores and nerve injuries are more likely in diabetic obese patients [115]. The arms should not be positioned beyond the 90–90 position; flexion and abduction should be less than 90 degrees. Pulsatile monitors (arterial line and pulse oximetry) on opposite arms will help in early detection of vascular compression. Optimal positioning of the airway device should be confirmed clinically and bronchoscopically after any change in position. Bronchial blockers have a higher chance of displacement than DLTs after positioning the patient and is more likely in obese patients.

Anaesthetic management

Fluid management

Thoracic surgery literature recommends judicious fluid administration to avoid shunting and pulmonary oedema in the dependent lung. Lymphatic disruption plays a role in the 'lower lung syndrome'. Obese patients are more likely to have prolonged surgeries due to difficult surgical exposure. Obese subjects have relatively (compared to normal BMI) less intracellular, extracellular, and absolute total body water content [116]. Indexed blood volume (blood volume in mL/kg total body weight) decreases in a non-linear manner with increasing weight [117]. Recent evidence indicates a higher incidence of kidney dysfunction after restrictive fluid management. Therefore, goal-directed fluid therapy and maintenance of euvolemia is recommended [118]. Goal-directed fluid therapy is possible, despite the use of the lateral position and OLV [119]. This is especially important in obese patients with altered body water composition and vascular permeability [120]. Bariatric surgery literature suggests a high incidence of primary AKI in patients with a higher BMI and intraoperative hypotension [121]. Research is needed to look at the incidence of renal failure in obese thoracic surgery patients.

Temperature management

Temperature management can be arduous in obese patients with higher body surface areas undergoing open thoracotomy, with significant heat loss. Hypothermia inhibits hypoxic pulmonary vasoconstriction and may contribute to hypoxia during OLV [122,123]. Multiple interventions can assist in maintaining normothermia in the obese patient, including increasing ambient operating room temperature, use of multiple forced-air heating devices, and use of fluid and airway circuit warmers. Literature is inconclusive to suggest that obesity increases the chance of perioperative hypothermia if active body surface warming devices are used diligently [124].

One-lung ventilation

A necessary prerequisite for most thoracic surgeries, OLV can be challenging in a patient with abnormal lung function and superimposed restrictive pulmonary physiology of obesity. Relative hypoxaemia is expected due to the reduction in FRC, alterations in the V/Q relationship, and changes to the oxygen–haemoglobin dissociation curve [125]. OLV is recognized as a risk factor for postoperative pulmonary complications and acute lung injury, which has recently been classified as mild acute respiratory distress syndrome [126]. Protective OLV strategies will reduce acute lung injury, intensive care unit (ICU) admissions, and length of hospital stay [127]. Mechanisms known to trigger ventilator-induced lung injury, such as exposure to non-physiological tidal volumes and loss of normal FRC, are almost always present during OLV. When this is superimposed onto OLV-driven oxidative stress, capillary shear stress due to hypoperfusion, and ischaemia-reperfusion injury on re-expanding the operated lung at the end of OLV, thoracic surgery provides a perfect framework for postoperative pulmonary complications [128]. Obese patients are more likely to suffer more than one of these consequences due to their proinflammatory physiological state, altered blood volume distribution, and higher delivered tidal volumes to the ventilated lung. However, studies are required to prove these associations.

Hypoxaemia during one-lung ventilation

OLV should be limited to the minimum duration possible, and protective ventilation strategies such as low FiO_2, optimal tidal volumes, use of PEEP, recruitment manoeuvres, and lower plateau pressures should be used [129]. The incidence of hypoxaemia during OLV has decreased significantly to around 10% [130]. Continuous pulse oximetry can be supplemented with intermittent arterial blood gas analysis to ensure normoxaemia. Hypoxaemia during OLV can be managed by the following:

- Continuous positive airway pressure to the non-ventilated lung (5–10 cmH_2O)—found to be more effective in low-volume ventilation strategies and is recommended as the first measure [131].
- PEEP to the ventilated lung—PEEP to the ventilated lung in OLV may shift it to a point above the lower inflection point of the pressure–volume loop (optimal PEEP); the resulting increase in pulmonary vascular resistance will increase shunt and hypoxaemia [132].
- Periodic re-inflation of the non-ventilated lung in cooperation with the surgeon.

Other methods described include adjusting ventilator settings, continuous insufflation of oxygen to the non-ventilated lung, clearing the ventilated lung of secretions, and repositioning the DLT to ensure correct positioning. Obese patients are more likely to have technically challenging dissections and are at risk for getting a pneumothorax on the dependent side. This differential diagnosis should be considered while troubleshooting rising peak inspiratory pressure on the ventilated lung and hypoxaemia.

Other techniques sometimes used as an alternative to OLV in the thoracic anaesthesia such as apnoeic oxygenation, high-frequency positive pressure ventilation, and high-frequency jet ventilation are not very useful in morbidly obese patients due to a faster rate of rise of $PaCO_2$.

Tracheal extubation

Following lung surgery, spontaneous ventilation is preferable to positive pressure ventilation for improved V/Q matching, pulmonary toilet, and decreased stress on endobronchial suture lines. In a morbidly obese patient, the optimal position for extubation is the reverse Trendelenburg or seated-up position to increase FRC.

Once extubation criteria are met, the bronchial cuff may be deflated and the DLT may then be withdrawn into the trachea, or the DLT may be switched to a single-lumen tube. Both these manoeuvres decrease airflow resistance and facilitate extubation [133].

Obese patients are more likely to require non-invasive positive pressure ventilation in the immediate postoperative period, and this has to be discussed with the surgeon in cases involving upper gastrointestinal anastomoses or in patients with copious secretions.

The intraoperative period concludes with transfer out of the OR to the post-anaesthesia care unit or ICU as needed.

Postoperative considerations

Risk factors identified for postoperative complications and 30-day hospital mortality after pneumonectomy include higher American Society of Anesthesiologists classification score, coronary artery disease, congestive heart failure, prior acute myocardial infarction, diabetes, cerebrovascular disease, chronic renal insufficiency, lower FEV_1, malnutrition, intraoperative blood loss greater than 4 units, right-sided pneumonectomy, and surgery performed at low-volume centres [134]. Although obesity is not identified as an independent risk factor, obese individuals are more likely to have more than one of these independent risk factors. Interestingly, low BMI (<18.5 kg/m²) is clearly associated with increased complications after thoracotomy similar to reports from non-thoracic surgeries [135]. However, we cannot confirm the phenomenon of the 'obesity paradox' which purports lesser complications in obese populations and this has been addressed in Chapter 22.

Emergence

Obese patients are more likely to get higher doses of neuromuscular blocking agents and opioids and have a slower emergence. The use of inhaled anaesthetics with lower blood–gas partition coefficient may aid in a faster recovery, but evidence for this observation is equivocal [136]. Use of short-acting medications in morbidly obese patients will facilitate a shorter immediate recovery time (time from surgical closure to extubation). Morbidly obese patients with higher immediate recovery times have an increased risk of postoperative respiratory complications [137]. Careful consideration is required in calculating the dose of neuromuscular reversal agents and in the use of neuromuscular monitoring equipment. Monitoring devices may not be able to achieve ulnar nerve supramaximal stimulations over 70 mA if the wrist circumference is greater than 18 cm [138]. The novel reversal agent, sugammadex, has been shown to hasten the time needed to achieve 90% train-of-four ratio [139]. However, recurarization after sugammadex has been documented in obese patients [140]. Appropriate dosing guidelines for the use of sugammadex in obese patients are scant, as studies looking at this have recommended different doses [141].

Early hypoxaemia and lung dysfunction

Respiratory failure is the most common cause of morbidity after thoracic surgery. Airway obstruction and reintubation are common in obese patients with COPD in the immediate postoperative period [142]. Early extubation is advocated to prevent the risk of pulmonary barotrauma and infection [143]. There is no evidence that obesity increases risk for rare complications such as pulmonary blowout. Patients are observed for hypoxia (PaO_2 <60 mmHg) and respiratory acidosis ($PaCO_2$ >45 mmHg) either in the post-anaesthesia care unit or in the ICU. It is recommended that obese patients be placed on continuous pulse oximetry, as intermittent clinical observations may fail to detect even significant periods of desaturation [144]. The desaturation episodes may last up to 30 minutes and are not eliminated by the use of supplemental oxygen alone [145,146]. Supplemental oxygen should be administered for at least the first 2–3 days after thoracic surgery, until the normal sleep pattern is re-established [144]. Maintaining a semi-upright position (30–45 degrees) and other measures to decrease atelectasis, such as incentive spirometry, chest physiotherapy, and early ambulation, go hand-in-hand with aggressive pain control to prevent hypoxaemia. Use of thoracic epidural will decrease the pulmonary complications in high-risk patients [147], including the morbidly obese. When comparing video-assisted thoracoscopic surgery (VATS) to open thoracotomy, VATS patients had significantly less postoperative pneumonia, faster chest tube removal, and quicker ICU discharge times [148]. A VATS approach may help decrease postoperative respiratory complications in morbidly obese patients.

Higher BMI confers an increased risk for acute respiratory distress syndrome in critically ill patients with primary graft dysfunction after lung transplantation [149,150]. Animal studies suggest a predisposition to atelectrauma in obesity, because tidal volume ventilation falls very close to the lower inflection point of the pressure–volume curve [151].

Obese patients left intubated after surgery should be placed on mechanical ventilation settings calculated using predicted body weight and Acute Respiratory Distress Syndrome Network recommendations. Obese individuals may have elevated baseline pleural pressures, and this has led to endorsements that obese patients are at lower risk for volutrauma caused by alveolar stretch in a high plateau pressure setting with higher transpulmonary pressure. However, outcome studies are lacking for this observation [152]. Obesity has long been considered an independent risk factor for prolonged mechanical ventilation and extubation failure; nevertheless, this has been disproven in an analysis [153].

Cardiovascular complications

Supraventricular dysrhythmias are common after pneumonectomy, with rates of 4–25% after standard and 27–44% after extrapleural pneumonectomy [134]. The peak incidence is between postoperative days 1 and 4 [134]. Postoperative new-onset atrial fibrillation is more common in obese patients [154]. The risk for atrial fibrillation increases 4% for every 1-unit increase in BMI [155]. Non-cardiac thoracic surgical patients who develop atrial fibrillation have increased lengths of hospital stay, higher mortality rates, and higher hospital charges [156]. Protocols designed to decrease the incidence of atrial fibrillation in morbidly obese patients undergoing thoracic surgery seem justified.

Higher BMI correlates with increased right ventricular mass and modestly lower right ventricular ejection fraction independent of other cardiovascular risk factors and left ventricular function [157]. Alterations in right ventricular structure and function, as well as an increase in pulmonary vascular resistance, are more common in obese patients with OSAS or OHS [158].

Acute cardiac herniation is a rare complication after pneumonectomy or any thoracic surgery which involves opening the pericardium [159,160]. This is a surgical emergency and does not have an increased incidence in obesity.

Postoperative haemorrhage

Thoracic surgical procedures have the potential to cause significant bleeding, particularly those which include extensive dissection and manipulation [161]. Obesity has not been shown to increase the risk for bleeding in cardiac surgery, but thoracic surgical literature pertaining to this is lacking. Obese patients are more likely to be on pharmacological thromboembolic prophylaxis, and the benefits of these drugs should be carefully weighed against the risk of bleeding. Increased chest tube drainage (>200 mL/hour), hypotension, and tachycardia may be signs of post-thoracotomy haemorrhage. An empty hemithorax after a pneumonectomy has the potential to accommodate a huge volume of blood (2–3 L approximately equal to half expected blood volume), and increased blood volume of obese patients creates this potential scenario, where a large blood loss may go undetected.

Pain management

Severe pain is expected after a thoracotomy incision and is worsened by continuous breathing movements. It has major implications: splinting leading to atelectasis and respiratory failure, difficulty in coughing leads to inadequate clearing of secretions and pneumonia, ipsilateral shoulder pain, and it sometimes results in a chronic pain condition called post-thoracotomy pain syndrome [162]. Obese patients are more likely to be converted from a VATS procedure to an open thoracotomy and become a challenge for acute postoperative pain management. Even thoracoscopic incisions can result in significant pain [162]. An opioid-sparing multimodal analgesia regimen is highly recommended in obese individuals, particularly those with OHS.

TEA is considered the gold standard for post-thoracotomy pain management. Continuous epidural analgesia decreases oxygen requirements and left ventricular stroke work in obese subjects after abdominal surgeries [163]. However, such studies in obese thoracic surgical patients are lacking. The 15% failure rate of TEA is likely to be even higher in obese subjects with non-palpable bony landmarks [164]. Cephalad spread of medications instilled into the epidural space has been shown to correlate with BMI in pregnant obese patients [165]. Respiratory benefits of TEA include greater postoperative FEV_1 and FVC, improved coughing and clearing of secretions, and decreased respiratory morbidity [166]. Obese patients with the tenuous FRC– closing capacity relationship can gain very much from these benefits, as recovery of spirometric values are quicker in patients who received TEA [135]. The use of local anaesthetic in TEA decreases the incidence of postoperative dysrhythmia [167]; this can be tremendously beneficial for obese patients, who are more susceptible to development of dysrhythmias. Superior pain control provided by TEA, along with its opioid-sparing effect, can minimize unwanted side effects of IV opioids and improve postoperative patient mobility [168]. Catastrophic complications of TEA such as epidural haematoma and abscess are rare in obesity. TEA is the preferred thoracic pain management technique available at this time and is highly recommended in obese thoracic surgical

Table 12.1 Comparison of thoracic epidural analgesia and thoracic paravertebral block

		TEA	TPVB
Reported failure rate		6%	10–15%
Risk	Dural puncture	Higher	Lower
	Pleural puncture	Lower	Higher
Incidence	Hypotension	Higher	Lower
	Urinary retention	Higher	Lower
	Nausea	Higher	Lower
Other considerations	Efficacy of adding opioids	Improved pain management	No added pain benefit
	Anaesthesiologist's comfort level in placement	Higher	Lower

patients. Some practitioners recommend the use of TEA for VATS lobectomies [169].

TPVBs are steadily gaining popularity with the increasing use of ultrasound guidance in the placement of nerve blocks. Multiple studies have compared TEA to TPVBs and have demonstrated no difference in postoperative pain scores, pulmonary function, or respiratory complications [169,170]. Slight differences exist between the two regional techniques; see Table 12.1 [164]. TPVBs seem more promising for the obese; however, research specifically in this patient population is needed before routine use of this technique can be recommended.

Other pain management techniques include intrathecal opioid analgesia, intercostal analgesia, intrapleural analgesia, cryoanalgesia, and IV pain medications [164]. Studies on these interventions in obese patients are lacking and use of IV opioids in obesity is rife with problems. Use of non-steroidal anti-inflammatory drugs may be complicated in the setting of restrictive fluid management for lung resection surgery in an obese patient who is more susceptible to renal injury. Analgesic adjuncts such as low-dose ketamine, dexmedetomidine, gabapentin, and pregabalin play a significant role in obese post-thoracotomy pain management.

Renal system

Obesity is a well-known risk factor for chronic kidney disease [171] and AKI due to its associated comorbidities and association with increased glomerular filtration rate. Obesity-induced intra-abdominal hypertension contributes to renal dysfunction [172]. Elevated creatinine in the post-thoracotomy period is associated with increased mortality, and obese patients are more likely to have higher creatinine values due to their predisposition for renal dysfunction [173–175]. Creatinine-defined AKI criteria are more applicable than indexed urine output criteria in the obese population [176]. Equations commonly used for glomerular filtration rate estimation may be inaccurate in obese patients [177]; instead, use of the Chronic Kidney Disease Epidemiology Collaboration equation is recommended [178].

Thromboembolic risk and prophylaxis

Obese patients are at increased risk for venous thromboembolism, as many of them have pre-existing lower extremity venous stasis [179,180]. Other factors which may elevate risk in the perioperative period include the possibility of lung cancer, decreased mobility, and increased circulating procoagulants due to the stress response.

Pharmacological prophylaxis may be inadequate, as fixed-dose regimens may underdose patients with higher BMI; weight-based dosing of low-molecular-weight-heparin is recommended [181]. In patients with decreased mobility, pulmonary embolism is a real risk, and all efforts should be made to decrease the period of immobilization [182].

Infection risk

Obesity alone increases the risk for postoperative infections [183]. These infections range from skin and soft tissue infection, wound dehiscence, respiratory infections, and urinary infections, to bloodstream infections [184]. Factors contributing to this include inadequate tissue perfusion, the proinflammatory state of obesity, immunological dysfunction, inadequate antibiotic dosing, and higher prevalence of diabetes [144]. Obese patients are not at an increased risk for pressure ulcers, as the cushioning effect of redundant soft tissue may counteract the pressure exerted by extra weight [185]. A BMI greater than 30kg/m² multiplies the risk for catheter-associated infections and nosocomial pneumonia more than twofold [186].

Nutrition

Nutrition goals in obesity are targeted at maintaining euglycemia, obtaining adequate nutrients to promote wound healing, and enhancing utilization of endogenous fat [144]. Obese individuals may be more receptive to lifestyle and dietary modifications in the postoperative period. High-protein hypocaloric feeds with vitamin and trace element supplementation is recommended for the critically ill obese patient [187].

Early mobilization and physical therapy

Enhanced recovery programmes with early mobilization are being increasingly utilized in thoracic surgery. These should be equally applied to obese patients as faster recovery of the obese patient may occur when the incidences and risks of respiratory complications, lower extremity blood clots, and pressure ulcers are decreased. TEA should not be considered a contraindication for mobilization, and dosing regimens should be titrated to avoid motor blockade [144].

Rhabdomyolysis is recognized to be more common in morbidly obese patients [135]. Risk factors include morbid obesity, male sex, hypertension, diabetes, peripheral vascular disease, and, most importantly, long-duration surgery in a non-physiological position (e.g. left lateral position). Local signs of rhabdomyolysis include pain, swelling, numbness, or weakness, and these may be masked by the presence of TEA. Once rhabdomyolysis is diagnosed, aggressive hydration and diuresis are required to prevent AKI [135].

Protocol-based postoperative management with contributions from various teams are necessary to have optimal outcomes in obese post-thoracotomy individuals.

Key points

- Obese individuals may have a restrictive or obstructive pattern on spirometry, and a reduced FRC due to decreased ERV. This can sometimes make FRC less than closing capacity, even in the supine position, and leads to air trapping.
- Obesity is associated with a decrease in lung compliance and increases in resistance, work of breathing, and V/Q mismatch.
- OHS subjects have a decreased ventilatory response to CO_2, which predisposes them to opioid-induced ventilatory depression.
- VO_2 is increased in obese patients, which makes them likely to have dyspnoea at both rest and exertion without any underlying pulmonary pathology.
- Smoking history and OSAS history are particularly important in obese patients.
- Obese individuals with COPD have a very high risk for postoperative pulmonary complications and should be optimized preoperatively using a well-planned regimen.
- Establishment of invasive monitoring and regional anaesthesia can be challenging in obese individuals.
- Establishment of OLV is not considered to be more difficult in obese patients versus individuals with a normal BMI. However, obese individuals are more likely to have hypoxaemia on OLV.
- During extubation, position the patient head-up and take steps to prevent atelectasis. In addition, many obese patients will benefit from extubation followed by a rapid transfer to a non-invasive positive-pressure ventilation or continuous positive airway pressure.
- Early postoperative hypoxaemia is common in obese post-thoracotomy patients. Excellent pain control using multimodal analgesic regimens, along with TEA or TPVB, will help decrease postoperative morbidity and duration of hospital stay.
- Obese patients are more likely to develop postoperative supraventricular dysrhythmia and will benefit from dysrhythmia prevention protocols.
- Institution-specific protocol-based postoperative management will help attain optimal outcomes after thoracic surgery in obese patients.

CASE REPORT

A 60-year-old, 150 cm tall, 124 kg female (BMI 55 kg/m²), with a 45 pack-year smoking history with COPD, OSAS, and non-small cell lung cancer presents for a right VATS, lobectomy, and possible thoracotomy. Her medications include a phentermine/topiramate combination for seizures and weight loss.

How would you evaluate and prepare this patient for surgery?

A structured preoperative assessment should include respiratory quality of life, objective measurement of functional capacity (e.g. Duke activity status index), airway assessment, severity of OSAS, reinforcement for preoperative smoking cessation, teaching of incentive spirometry, prehabilitation, and medication management (do not abruptly stop appetite-suppressant drugs combined with anticonvulsants). Focused review of lung imaging studies, pulmonary function tests, and cardiac workup should be done. Discussion with the patient about lung isolation techniques, and possible neuraxial and regional anaesthetic techniques will help alleviate anxiety.

What respiratory physiological changes do you anticipate?

COPD with coexistent obesity is considered a systemic inflammatory process. CO_2 retention, increased work of breathing, rapid, shallow breathing pattern, periodic oxygen desaturations causing increased pulmonary vascular resistance, and right ventricular dysfunction may be present. We can expect a decreased FRC and expiratory reserve volume with a high closing volume to FRC ratio. V/Q mismatch, changes in oxygen–haemoglobin dissociation curve, and relative hypoxaemia can be expected in a supine position leading to a decreased apnoea time. Worsening of V/Q mismatch and hypoxaemia with OLV in a lateral position as well as hypercapnia with an increased PaCO2– end-tidal CO_2 gradient are anticipated due to the restrictive lung physiology. In addition, securing and maintaining lung isolation using a DLT or a single-lumen tube with bronchial blocker and fibreoptic confirmation may be challenging.

How will you manage hypoxaemia during one-lung ventilation?

Minimizing duration of OLV, protective ventilation strategies such as low FiO2, optimal tidal volumes, use of PEEP, recruitment manoeuvres, and lower plateau pressures will decrease lung injury. Continuous positive airway pressure to the non-dependent lung, application of optimal PEEP to the dependent lung, and periodic reinflation of the non-dependent lung can help minimize hypoxaemia. If unsuccessful, continuous insufflation of oxygen to the non-ventilated lung, clearing the ventilated lung of secretions, and repositioning the DLT to ensure correct positioning can be tried. Be vigilant for a pneumothorax on the dependent side in challenging dissections.

How will you manage pain during and after the surgery?

An opioid-sparing multimodal analgesia regimen is highly recommended especially in the presence of OHS. This regimen includes the use of regional anaesthesia, continuous local anaesthetic wound infiltration techniques, non-steroidal anti-inflammatory drugs, paracetamol (acetaminophen), and analgesic adjuncts such as ketamine, gabapentin, and dexmedetomidine. If converted to an open thoracotomy, a TEA will be highly beneficial. Superior pain control, opioid-sparing, improved patient mobility, greater postoperative FEV1 and FVC, and improved coughing and clearing of secretions can be expected with TEA, thereby decreasing respiratory morbidity.

What postoperative complications do you anticipate?

Respiratory failure is the most common cause of morbidity after thoracic surgery. Anticipate airway obstruction and possible reintubation in the immediate postoperative period. Continuous pulse oximetry and supplemental oxygen is recommended for at least 24–48 hours. Maintaining a semi-upright position, incentive spirometry, chest physiotherapy, and early ambulation can decrease atelectasis. New-onset atrial fibrillation, right ventricular dysfunction, and pulmonary hypertension can be anticipated. Renal dysfunction and elevated creatinine postoperatively can be prevented by optimizing volume status and avoiding nephrotoxic agents. The patient is at increased risk for venous thromboembolism and postoperative infections. Early mobilization, optimal use of anticoagulants, and rapid discontinuation of tubes and lines will decrease risks of predictable complications and expedite her recovery.

REFERENCES

1. American Cancer Society (US). Key Statistics for Lung Cancer. Atlanta: American Cancer Society (US). http://www.cancer.org/cancer/lungcancer-non-smallcell/detailedguide/non-small-cell-lung-cancer-key-statistics

2. St. Julien JB, Aldrich MC, Sheng S, et al. Obesity increases operating room time for lobectomy in the society of thoracic surgeons database. Annals of Thoracic Surgery. 2012;**94**(6):1841–47.

3. Parameswaran K, Todd DC, Soth M. Altered respiratory physiology in obesity. Canadian Respiratory Journal. 2006;**13**(4):203–10.

4. Pelosi P, Gregoretti C. Perioperative management of obese patients. Best Practice & Research. Clinical Anaesthesiology. 2010;**24**(2):211–25.

5. Caro CG, Butler J, Dubois AB. Some effects of restriction of chest cage expansion on pulmonary function in man: an experimental study. Journal of Clinical Investigation. 1960;**39**:573–83.

6. Cotes JE Chin DJ, Miller MR. Lung Function, Physiology, Measurement and Application in Medicine. Oxford: Blackwell; 2006.

7. Don HF, Wahba M, Cuadrado L, Kelkar K. The effects of anesthesia and 100% oxygen on the functional residual capacity of the lungs. Anesthesiology. 1970;**32**(6):521–29.

8. Ray CS, Sue DY, Bray G, Hansen JE, Wasserman K. Effects of obesity on respiratory function. American Review of Respiratory Disease. 1983;**128**(3):501–506.

9. Jones RL, Nzekwu MM. The effects of body mass index on lung volumes. Chest. 2006;**130**(3):827–33.

10. Sin DD, Jones RL, Man SF. Obesity is a risk factor for dyspnea but not for airflow obstruction. Archives of Internal Medicine. 2002;**162**(13):1477–81.

11. Schachter LM, Salome CM, Peat JK, Woolcock AJ. Obesity is a risk for asthma and wheeze but not airway hyperresponsiveness. Thorax. 2001;**56**(1):4–8.

12. Salome CM, King GG, Berend N. Physiology of obesity and effects on lung function. Journal of Applied Physiology (Bethesda, MD: 1985). 2010;**108**(1):206–11.

13. Biring MS, Lewis MI, Liu JT, Mohsenifar Z. Pulmonary physiologic changes of morbid obesity. American Journal of the Medical Sciences. 1999;**318**(5):293–97.

14. Naimark A, Cherniack RM. Compliance of the respiratory system and its components in health and obesity. Journal of Applied Physiology. 1960;**15**:377–82.

15. Pelosi P, Croci M, Ravagnan I, et al. The effects of body mass on lung volumes, respiratory mechanics, and gas exchange during general anesthesia. Anesthesia and Analgesia. 1998;**87**(3):654–60.

16. Sharp JT, Henry JP, Sweany SK, Meadows WR, Pietras RJ. Effects of mass loading the respiratory system in man. Journal of Applied Physiology. 1964;**19**:959–66.

17. Yap JC, Watson RA, Gilbey S, Pride NB. Effects of posture on respiratory mechanics in obesity. Journal of Applied Physiology (Bethesda, MD: 1985). 1995;**79**(4):1199–205.

18. Zerah F, Harf A, Perlemuter L, Lorino H, Lorino AM, Atlan G. Effects of obesity on respiratory resistance. Chest. 1993;**103**(5):1470–76.

19. Nicolacakis K, Skowronski ME, Coreno AJ, et al. Observations on the physiological interactions between obesity and asthma. Journal of Applied Physiology (Bethesda, MD: 1985). 2008;**105**(5):1533–41.

20. King GG, Brown NJ, Diba C, et al. The effects of body weight on airway calibre. European Respiratory Journal. 2005;**25**(5):896–901.

21. Watson RA, Pride NB. Postural changes in lung volumes and respiratory resistance in subjects with obesity. Journal of Applied Physiology (Bethesda, MD: 1985). 2005;**98**(2):512–17.

22. Inselman LS, Chander A, Spitzer AR. Diminished lung compliance and elevated surfactant lipids and proteins in nutritionally obese young rats. Lung. 2004;**182**(2):101–17.

23. Milic-Emili J, Torchio R, D'Angelo E. Closing volume: a reappraisal (1967+2007). European Journal of Applied Physiology. 2007;**99**(6):567–83.

24. Kress JP, Pohlman AS, Alverdy J, Hall JB. The impact of morbid obesity on oxygen cost of breathing (VO(2RESP)) at rest. American Journal of Respiratory and Critical Care Medicine. 1999;**160**(3):883–86.

25. Sood A. Altered resting and exercise respiratory physiology in obesity. Clinics in Chest Medicine. 2009;**30**(3):445–54, vii.

26. Lin CK, Lin CC. Work of breathing and respiratory drive in obesity. Respirology (Carlton, Vic.). 2012;**17**(3):402–11.

27. Nakata M, Saeki H, Yokoyama N, Kurita A, Takiyama W, Takashima S. Pulmonary function after lobectomy: video-assisted thoracic surgery versus thoracotomy. Annals of Thoracic Surgery. 2000;**70**(3):938–41.

28. Koenig SM. Pulmonary complications of obesity. American Journal of the Medical Sciences. 2001;**321**(4):249–79.

29. Sharp JT, Druz WS, Kondragunta VR. Diaphragmatic responses to body position changes in obese patients with obstructive sleep apnea. American Review of Respiratory Disease. 1986;**133**(1):32–37.

30. Chlif M, Keochkerian D, Choquet D, Vaidie A, Ahmaidi S. Effects of obesity on breathing pattern, ventilatory neural drive and mechanics. Respiratory Physiology & Neurobiology. 2009;**168**(3):198–202.

31. Holley HS, Milic-Emili J, Becklake MR, Bates DV. Regional distribution of pulmonary ventilation and perfusion in obesity. Journal of Clinical Investigation. 1967;**46**(4):475–81.

32. Hurewitz AN, Susskind H, Harold WH. Obesity alters regional ventilation in lateral decubitus position. Journal of Applied Physiology (Bethesda, MD: 1985). 1985;**59**(3):774–83.

33. Demedts M. Regional distribution of lung volumes and of gas inspired at residual volume: influence of age, body weight and posture. Bulletin Europeen de Physiopathologie Respiratoire. 1980;**16**(3):271–85.

34. Hedenstierna G, Santesson J, Norlander O. Airway closure and distribution of inspired gas in the extremely obese, breathing spontaneously and during anaesthesia with intermittent positive pressure ventilation. Acta Anaesthesiologica Scandinavica. 1976;**20**(4):334–42.

35. Hakala K, Mustajoki P, Aittomaki J, Sovijarvi AR. Effect of weight loss and body position on pulmonary function and gas exchange abnormalities in morbid obesity. International Journal of Obesity and Related Metabolic Disorders. 1995;**19**(5):343–46.

36. Thomas PS, Cowen ER, Hulands G, Milledge JS. Respiratory function in the morbidly obese before and after weight loss. Thorax. 1989;**44**(5):382–86.

37. Zwillich CW, Sutton FD, Pierson DJ, Greagh EM, Weil JV. Decreased hypoxic ventilatory drive in the obesity-hypoventilation syndrome. American Journal of Medicine. 1975;**59**(3):343–48.

38. Bady E, Achkar A, Pascal S, Orvoen-Frija E, Laaban JP. Pulmonary arterial hypertension in patients with sleep apnoea syndrome. Thorax. 2000;**55**(11):934–39.

39. Kay JM, Suyama KL, Keane PM. Effect of intermittent normoxia on muscularization of pulmonary arterioles induced by chronic hypoxia in rats. American Review of Respiratory Disease. 1981;**123**(4 Pt 1):454–58.

40. Hulens M, Vansant G, Claessens AL, Lysens R, Muls E. Predictors of 6-minute walk test results in lean, obese and morbidly obese women. Scandinavian Journal of Medicine & Science in Sports. 2003;**13**(2):98–105.

41. Dempsey JA, Reddan W, Balke B, Rankin J. Work capacity determinants and physiologic cost of weight-supported work in obesity. Journal of Applied Physiology. 1966;**21**(6):1815–20.

42. American Thoracic Society; American College of Chest Physicians. ATS/ACCP Statement on cardiopulmonary exercise testing. American Journal of Respiratory and Critical Care Medicine. 2003;**167**(2):211–77.

43. Johnson BD, Weisman IM, Zeballos RJ, Beck KC. Emerging concepts in the evaluation of ventilatory limitation during exercise: the exercise tidal flow-volume loop. Chest. 1999;**116**(2):488–503.

44. Dempsey JA, Reddan W, Rankin J, Balke B. Alveolar-arterial gas exchange during muscular work in obesity. Journal of Applied Physiology. 1966;**21**(6):1807–14.

45. Bai J, Peat JK, Berry G, Marks GB, Woolcock AJ. Questionnaire items that predict asthma and other respiratory conditions in adults. Chest. 1998;**114**(5):1343–48.

46. Bulpitt CJ, Palmer AJ, Battersby C, Fletcher AE. Association of symptoms of type 2 diabetic patients with severity of disease, obesity, and blood pressure. Diabetes Care. 1998;**21**(1):111–15.

47. Ofir D, Laveneziana P, Webb KA, O'Donnell DE. Ventilatory and perceptual responses to cycle exercise in obese women. Journal of Applied Physiology (Bethesda, MD: 1985). 2007;**102**(6):2217–26.

48. Luce JM. Respiratory complications of obesity. Chest. 1980;**78**(4):626–31.

49. Pankow W, Podszus T, Gutheil T, Penzel T, Peter J, Von Wichert P. Expiratory flow limitation and intrinsic positive end-expiratory pressure in obesity. Journal of Applied Physiology (Bethesda, MD: 1985). 1998;**85**(4):1236–43.

50. Ferretti A, Giampiccolo P, Cavalli A, Milic-Emili J, Tantucci C. Expiratory flow limitation and orthopnea in massively obese subjects. Chest. 2001;**119**(5):1401–408.

51. Chinn S. Obesity and asthma: evidence for and against a causal relation. Journal of Asthma. 2003;**40**(1):1–16.

52. Oga T, Nishimura K, Tsukino M, Sato S, Hajiro T. Analysis of the factors related to mortality in chronic obstructive pulmonary disease: role of exercise capacity and health status. American Journal of Respiratory and Critical Care Medicine. 2003;**167**(4):544–49.

53. Swinburn CR, Cooper BG, Mould H, Corris PA, Gibson GJ. Adverse effect of additional weight on exercise against gravity in patients with chronic obstructive airways disease. Thorax. 1989;**44**(9):716–20.

54. Slinger PD, Campos JH. Anesthesia for thoracic surgery. In: Miller RD, ed. Miller's Anesthesia. Vol 2. 7th ed. Philadelphia, PA: Churchill Livingstone; 2010:1819–82.

55. Slinger PD, Johnston MR. Preoperative assessment: an anesthesiologist's perspective. Thoracic Surgery Clinics. 2005;**15**(1):11–25.

56. American Society of Anesthesiologists Task Force on Preanesthesia Evaluation. Practice advisory for preanesthesia evaluation: a report by the American Society of Anesthesiologists Task Force on Preanesthesia Evaluation. Anesthesiology. 2002;**96**(2):485–96.

57. Ezri T, Medalion B, Weisenberg M, Szmuk P, Warters RD, Charuzi I. Increased body mass index per se is not a predictor of difficult laryngoscopy. Canadian Journal of Anaesthesia. 2003;**50**(2):179–83.

58. Neligan PJ, Porter S, Max B, Malhotra G, Greenblatt EP, Ochroch EA. Obstructive sleep apnea is not a risk factor for difficult intubation in morbidly obese patients. Anesthesia and Analgesia. 2009;**109**(4):1182–86.

59. Leoni A, Arlati S, Ghisi D, et al. Difficult mask ventilation in obese patients: analysis of predictive factors. Minerva Anestesiologica. 2014;**80**(2):149–57.

60. Vaporciyan AA, Merriman KW, Ece F, et al. Incidence of major pulmonary morbidity after pneumonectomy: association with timing of smoking cessation. Annals of Thoracic Surgery. 2002;**73**(2):420–25.

61. Akrawi W, Benumof JL. A pathophysiological basis for informed preoperative smoking cessation counseling. Journal of Cardiothoracic and Vascular Anesthesia. 1997;**11**(5):629–40.

62. Yamashita S, Yamaguchi H, Sakaguchi M, et al. Effect of smoking on intraoperative sputum and postoperative pulmonary complication in minor surgical patients. Respiratory Medicine. 2004;**98**(8):760–66.

63. Barrera R, Shi W, Amar D, et al. Smoking and timing of cessation: impact on pulmonary complications after thoracotomy. Chest. 2005;**127**(6):1977–83.

64. Bernstein WK, Deshpande S. Preoperative evaluation for thoracic surgery. Seminars in Cardiothoracic and Vascular Anesthesia. 2008;**12**(2):109–21.

65. Fleisher LA, Fleischmann KE, Auerbach AD, et al. 2014 ACC/AHA guideline on perioperative cardiovascular evaluation and management of patients undergoing noncardiac surgery: executive summary. Journal of Nuclear Cardiology. 2015;**22**(1):162–215.

66. Johnson JA, Landreneau RJ, Boley TM, et al. Should pulmonary lesions be resected at the time of open heart surgery? American Surgeon. 1996;**62**(4):300–303.

67. Dyszkiewicz W, Jemielity MM, Piwkowski CT, Perek B, Kasprzyk M. Simultaneous lung resection for cancer and myocardial revascularization without cardiopulmonary bypass (off-pump coronary artery bypass grafting). Annals of Thoracic Surgery. 2004;**77**(3):1023–27.

68. Ritchie AJ, Bowe P, Gibbons JR. Prophylactic digitalization for thoracotomy: a reassessment. Annals of Thoracic Surgery. 1990;**50**(1):86–88.

69. Shenkman Z, Shir Y, Brodsky JB. Perioperative management of the obese patient. British Journal of Anaesthesia. 1993;**70**(3):349–59.

70. Chagnac A, Weinstein T, Korzets A, Ramadan E, Hirsch J, Gafter U. Glomerular hemodynamics in severe obesity. American Journal of Physiology. Renal Physiology. 2000;**278**(5):F817–22.

71. Amann K, Benz K. Structural renal changes in obesity and diabetes. Seminars in Nephrology. 2013;**33**(1):23–33.

72. Kumar AB, Bridget Zimmerman M, Suneja M. Obesity and post-cardiopulmonary bypass-associated acute kidney injury: a single-center retrospective analysis. Journal of Cardiothoracic and Vascular Anesthesia. 2014;**28**(3):551–56.

73. Kramer HJ, Saranathan A, Luke A, et al. Increasing body mass index and obesity in the incident ESRD population. Journal of the American Society of Nephrology. 2006;**17**(5):1453–59.

74. Arora P, Rajagopalam S, Ranjan R, et al. Preoperative use of angiotensin-converting enzyme inhibitors/angiotensin receptor blockers is associated with increased risk for acute kidney injury after cardiovascular surgery. Clinical Journal of the American Society of Nephrology. 2008;**3**(5):1266–73.

75. Rodrigues F, Papoila AL, Ligeiro D, Gomes MJ, Trindade H. Acute exercise amplifies inflammation in obese patients with COPD. Revista portuguesa de pneumologia. 2016;**22**(6):315–22.

76. Simpson SQ. Oxygen-induced acute hypercapnia in chronic obstructive pulmonary disease: what's the problem? Critical Care Medicine. 2002;**30**(1):258–59.

77. Schulman DS, Matthay RA. The right ventricle in pulmonary disease. Cardiology Clinics. 1992;**10**(1):111–35.

78. Uppot RN, Sahani DV, Hahn PF, Gervais D, Mueller PR. Impact of obesity on medical imaging and image-guided intervention. American Journal of Roentgenology. 2007;**188**(2):433–40.

79. Reynolds A. Obesity and medical imaging challenges. Radiologic Technology. 2011;**82**(3):219–39.

80. von Ungern-Sternberg BS, Regli A, Reber A, Schneider MC. Effect of obesity and thoracic epidural analgesia on perioperative spirometry. British Journal of Anaesthesia. 2005;**94**(1):121–27.

81. Wang J, Olak J, Ferguson MK. Diffusing capacity predicts operative mortality but not long-term survival after resection for lung cancer. Journal of Thoracic and Cardiovascular Surgery. 1999;**117**(3):581–86; discussion 586–87.

82. Fishman A, Martinez F, Naunheim K, et al. A randomized trial comparing lung-volume-reduction surgery with medical therapy for severe emphysema. New England Journal of Medicine. 2003;**348**(21):2059–73.

83. Pierce RJ, Copland JM, Sharpe K, Barter CE. Preoperative risk evaluation for lung cancer resection: predicted postoperative product as a predictor of surgical mortality. American Journal of Respiratory and Critical Care Medicine. 1994;**150**(4):947–55.

84. Fornitano LD, Godoy MF. Exercise testing in individuals with morbid obesity. Obesity Surgery. 2010;**20**(5):583–88.

85. Arena R, Cahalin LP. Evaluation of cardiorespiratory fitness and respiratory muscle function in the obese population. Progress in Cardiovascular Diseases. 2014;**56**(4): 457–64.

86. Kaplan JA, Slinger PD, eds. Thoracic Anesthesia. 3rd ed. Philadelphia, PA: Churchill Livingstone; 2003.

87. Smulders SA, Smeenk FW, Janssen-Heijnen ML, Postmus PE. Actual and predicted postoperative changes in lung function after pneumonectomy: a retrospective analysis. Chest. 2004;**125**(5):1735–41.

88. Ohno Y, Hatabu H, Higashino T, et al. Oxygen-enhanced MR imaging: correlation with postsurgical lung function in patients with lung cancer. Radiology. 2005;**236**(2):704–11.

89. Leo F, Solli P, Spaggiari L, et al. Respiratory function changes after chemotherapy: an additional risk for postoperative respiratory

90. Lapostolle F, Catineau J, Garrigue B, et al. Prospective evaluation of peripheral venous access difficulty in emergency care. Intensive Care Medicine. 2007;**33**(8):1452–57.

91. Nafiu OO, Burke C, Cowan A, Tutuo N, Maclean S, Tremper KK. Comparing peripheral venous access between obese and normal weight children. Paediatric Anaesthesia. 2010;**20**(2):172–76.

92. Costantino TG, Parikh AK, Satz WA, Fojtik JP. Ultrasonography-guided peripheral intravenous access versus traditional approaches in patients with difficult intravenous access. Annals of Emergency Medicine. 2005;**46**(5):456–61.

93. Ottestad E, Schmiessing C, Brock-Utne JG, Kulkarni V, Parris D, Brodsky JB. Central venous access in obese patients: a potential complication. Anesthesia and Analgesia. 2006;**102**(4):1293–94.

94. Thompson EC, Wilkins HE, 3rd, Fox VJ, Fernandez LG. Insufficient length of pulmonary artery introducer in an obese patient. Archives of Surgery (Chicago, IL: 1960). 2004;**139**(7):794–96.

95. Kim SH, Lilot M, Sidhu KS, et al. Accuracy and precision of continuous noninvasive arterial pressure monitoring compared with invasive arterial pressure: a systematic review and meta-analysis. Anesthesiology. 2014;**120**(5):1080–97.

96. Starr JW, Wagner GS, Behar VS, Walston A, 2nd, Greenfield JC, Jr Vectorcardiographic criteria for the diagnosis of inferior myocardial infarction. Circulation. 1974;**49**(5):829–36.

97. Garcia-Labbe D, Ruka E, Bertrand OF, Voisine P, Costerousse O, Poirier P. Obesity and coronary artery disease: evaluation and treatment. Canadian Journal of Cardiology. 2015;**31**(2):184–94.

98. Jense HG, Dubin SA, Silverstein PI, O'Leary-Escolas U. Effect of obesity on safe duration of apnea in anesthetized humans. Anesthesia and Analgesia. 1991;**72**(1):89–93.

99. Bouroche G, Bourgain JL. Preoxygenation and general anesthesia: a review. Minerva Anestesiologica. 2015;**81**(8):910–20.

100. Cullen A, Ferguson A. Perioperative management of the severely obese patient: a selective pathophysiological review. Canadian Journal of Anaesthesia. 2012;**59**(10):974–96.

101. Baraka AS, Taha SK, Siddik-Sayyid SM, et al. Supplementation of pre-oxygenation in morbidly obese patients using nasopharyngeal oxygen insufflation. Anaesthesia. 2007;**62**(8):769–73.

102. Kristensen MS. Airway management and morbid obesity. European Journal of Anaesthesiology. 2010;**27**(11):923–27.

103. Ingrande J, Lemmens HJ. Dose adjustment of anaesthetics in the morbidly obese. British Journal of Anaesthesia. 2010;**105**(Suppl 1):i16–23.

104. Coetzee JF. Total intravenous anaesthesia to obese patients: largely guesswork? European Journal of Anaesthesiology. 2009;**26**(5):359–61.

105. Mahajan V, Hashmi J, Singh R, Samra T, Aneja S. Comparative evaluation of gastric pH and volume in morbidly obese and lean patients undergoing elective surgery and effect of aspiration prophylaxis. Journal of Clinical Anesthesia. 2015;**27**(5):396–400.

106. Busetto L, Enzi G, Inelmen EM, et al. Obstructive sleep apnea syndrome in morbid obesity: effects of intragastric balloon. Chest. 2005;**128**(2):618–23.

107. Malhotra A, Hillman D. Obesity and the lung: 3. Obesity, respiration and intensive care. Thorax. 2008;**63**(10):925–31.

108. Brodsky JB, Lemmens HJ, Brock-Utne JG, Vierra M, Saidman LJ. Morbid obesity and tracheal intubation. Anesthesia and Analgesia. 2002;**94**(3):732–36.

109. Ezri T, Gewurtz G, Sessler DI, et al. Prediction of difficult laryngoscopy in obese patients by ultrasound quantification of anterior neck soft tissue. Anaesthesia. 2003;58(11):1111–14.

110. Collins JS, Lemmens HJ, Brodsky JB, Brock-Utne JG, Levitan RM. Laryngoscopy and morbid obesity: a comparison of the 'sniff' and 'ramped' positions. Obesity Surgery. 2004;14(9):1171–75.

111. Campos JH. Lung isolation techniques for patients with difficult airway. Current Opinion in Anaesthesiology. 2010;23(1):12–17.

112. Campos JH. Lung isolation techniques. Anesthesiology Clinics of North America. 2001;19(3):455–74.

113. Campos JH. Which device should be considered the best for lung isolation: double-lumen endotracheal tube versus bronchial blockers. Current Opinion in Anaesthesiology. 2007;20(1):27–31.

114. de Bellis M, Accardo R, Di Maio M, et al. Is flexible bronchoscopy necessary to confirm the position of double-lumen tubes before thoracic surgery? European Journal of Cardio-Thoracic Surgery. 2011;40(4):912–16.

115. Adams JP, Murphy PG. Obesity in anaesthesia and intensive care. British Journal of Anaesthesia. 2000;85(1):91–108.

116. Petersen VP. Body composition and fluid compartments in normal, obese and underweight human subjects. Acta Medica Scandinavica. 1957;158(2):103–111.

117. Feldschuh J, Enson Y. Prediction of the normal blood volume. Relation of blood volume to body habitus. Circulation. 1977;56(4 Pt 1):605–12.

118. Assaad S, Popescu W, Perrino A. Fluid management in thoracic surgery. Current Opinion in Anaesthesiology. 2013;26(1):31–39.

119. Haas S, Eichhorn V, Hasbach T, et al. Goal-directed fluid therapy using stroke volume variation does not result in pulmonary fluid overload in thoracic surgery requiring one-lung ventilation. Critical Care Research and Practice. 2012;2012:687018.

120. Yuan SY, Breslin JW, Perrin R, et al. Microvascular permeability in diabetes and insulin resistance. Microcirculation (New York, NY: 1994). 2007;14(4–5):363–73.

121. Sharma SK, McCauley J, Cottam D, et al. Acute changes in renal function after laparoscopic gastric surgery for morbid obesity. Surgery for Obesity and Related Diseases. 2006;2(3):389–92.

122. Fan M, Wang DX, Zhu ZH. Alteration in hypoxic pulmonary vasoconstriction during hypothermia in dogs. Journal of Tongji Medical University. 1992;12(3):134–38.

123. Benumof JL, Wahrenbrock EA. Dependency of hypoxic pulmonary vasoconstriction on temperature. Journal of Applied Physiology: Respiratory, Environmental and Exercise Physiology. 1977;42(1):56–58.

124. Fernandes LA, Braz LG, Koga FA, et al. Comparison of peri-operative core temperature in obese and non-obese patients. Anaesthesia. 2012;67(12):1364–69.

125. Purohit A, Bhargava S, Mangal V, Parashar VK. Lung isolation, one-lung ventilation and hypoxaemia during lung isolation. Indian Journal of Anaesthesia. 2015;59(9):606–17.

126. Ranieri VM, Rubenfeld GD, Thompson BT, et al. Acute respiratory distress syndrome: the Berlin Definition. JAMA. 2012;307(23):2526–33.

127. Lohser J. Evidence-based management of one-lung ventilation. Anesthesiology Clinics. 2008;26(2):241–72, v.

128. 130. Lohser J, Slinger P. Lung injury after one-lung ventilation: a review of the pathophysiologic mechanisms affecting the ventilated and the collapsed lung. Anesthesia and Analgesia. 2015;121(2):302–18.

129. Della Rocca G, Coccia C. Acute lung injury in thoracic surgery. Current Opinion in Anaesthesiology. 2013;26(1):40–46.

130. Ishikawa S, Lohser J. One-lung ventilation and arterial oxygenation. Current Opinion in Anaesthesiology. 2011;24(1):24–31.

131. Badner NH, Goure C, Bennett KE, Nicolaou G. Role of continuous positive airway pressure to the non-ventilated lung during one-lung ventilation with low tidal volumes. HSR Proceedings in Intensive Care & Cardiovascular Anesthesia. 2011;3(3):189–94.

132. Michelet P, Roch A, Brousse D, et al. Effects of PEEP on oxygenation and respiratory mechanics during one-lung ventilation. British Journal of Anaesthesia. 2005;95(2):267–73.

133. Lohser J, Kulkarni V, Brodsky JB. Anesthesia for thoracic surgery in morbidly obese patients. Current Opinion in Anaesthesiology. 2007;20(1):10–14.

134. Groth SS, Burt BM, Sugarbaker DJ. Management of complications after pneumonectomy. Thoracic Surgery Clinics. 2015;25(3):335–48.

135. Brodsky JB. Thoracic Anesthesia for Morbidly Obese Patients and Obese Patients with Obstructive Sleep Apnea. **Vol 1**. New York: Springer; 2011.

136. Liu FL, Cherng YG, Chen SY, et al. Postoperative recovery after anesthesia in morbidly obese patients: a systematic review and meta-analysis of randomized controlled trials. Canadian Journal of Anaesthesia. 2015;62(8):907–17.

137. Sudre EC, de Batista PR, Castiglia YM. Longer immediate recovery time after anesthesia increases risk of respiratory complications after laparotomy for bariatric surgery: a randomized clinical trial and a cohort study. Obesity Surgery. 2015;25(11):2205–12.

138. Nazar C, de la Cuadra JC, Munoz H. Neuromuscular blockade monitoring in obese patients: A-131. European Journal of Anaesthesiology. 2005;22(Suppl 34):36.

139. Gaszynski T, Szewczyk T, Gaszynski W. Randomized comparison of sugammadex and neostigmine for reversal of rocuronium-induced muscle relaxation in morbidly obese undergoing general anaesthesia. British Journal of Anaesthesia. 2012;108(2):236–39.

140. Le Corre F, Nejmeddine S, Fatahine C, Tayar C, Marty J, Plaud B. Recurarization after sugammadex reversal in an obese patient. Canadian Journal of Anaesthesia. 2011;58(10):944–47.

141. Van Lancker P, Dillemans B, Bogaert T, Mulier JP, De Kock M, Haspeslagh M. Ideal versus corrected body weight for dosage of sugammadex in morbidly obese patients. Anaesthesia. 2011;66(8):721–25.

142. Pedoto A. Lung physiology and obesity: anesthetic implications for thoracic procedures. Anesthesiology Research and Practice. 2012;2012:154208.

143. Morgan EG Mikhail M, Murray MJ. Anesthesia for Thoracic Surgery. **Vol 1**. 4th ed. New York: McGraw-Hill; 2006.

144. Cullen A, Ferguson A. Perioperative management of the severely obese patient: a selective pathophysiological review. Canadian Journal of Anaesthesia. 2012;59(10):974–96.

145. Ahmad S, Nagle A, McCarthy RJ, Fitzgerald PC, Sullivan JT, Prystowsky J. Postoperative hypoxemia in morbidly obese patients with and without obstructive sleep apnea undergoing laparoscopic bariatric surgery. Anesthesia and Analgesia. 2008;107(1):138–43.

146. Gallagher SF, Haines KL, Osterlund LG, Mullen M, Downs JB. Postoperative hypoxemia: common, undetected, and

unsuspected after bariatric surgery. Journal of Surgical Research. 2010;**159**(2):622–26.

147. Licker MJ, Widikker I, Robert J, et al. Operative mortality and respiratory complications after lung resection for cancer: impact of chronic obstructive pulmonary disease and time trends. Annals of Thoracic Surgery. 2006;**81**(5):1830–37.

148. Whitson BA, Andrade RS, Boettcher A, et al. Video-assisted thoracoscopic surgery is more favorable than thoracotomy for resection of clinical stage I non-small cell lung cancer. Annals of Thoracic Surgery. 2007;**83**(6):1965–70.

149. Gong MN, Bajwa EK, Thompson BT, Christiani DC. Body mass index is associated with the development of acute respiratory distress syndrome. Thorax. 2010;**65**(1):44–50.

150. Lederer DJ, Kawut SM, Wickersham N, et al. Obesity and primary graft dysfunction after lung transplantation: the Lung Transplant Outcomes Group Obesity Study. American Journal of Respiratory and Critical Care Medicine. 2011;**184**(9):1055–61.

151. Muscedere JG, Mullen JB, Gan K, Slutsky AS. Tidal ventilation at low airway pressures can augment lung injury. American Journal of Respiratory and Critical Care Medicine. 1994;**149**(5):1327–34.

152. Ventilation with lower tidal volumes as compared with traditional tidal volumes for acute lung injury and the acute respiratory distress syndrome. The Acute Respiratory Distress Syndrome Network. New England Journal of Medicine. 2000;**342**(18):1301–308.

153. O'Brien JM, Jr, Philips GS, Ali NA, Aberegg SK, Marsh CB, Lemeshow S. The association between body mass index, processes of care, and outcomes from mechanical ventilation: a prospective cohort study. Critical Care Medicine. 2012;**40**(5):1456–63.

154. Wang TJ, Parise H, Levy D, et al. Obesity and the risk of new-onset atrial fibrillation. JAMA. 2004;**292**(20):2471–77.

155. Wong CY, O'Moore-Sullivan T, Leano R, Hukins C, Jenkins C, Marwick TH. Association of subclinical right ventricular dysfunction with obesity. Journal of the American College of Cardiology. 2006;**47**(3):611–16.

156. Vaporciyan AA, Correa AM, Rice DC, et al. Risk factors associated with atrial fibrillation after noncardiac thoracic surgery: analysis of 2588 patients. Journal of Thoracic and Cardiovascular Surgery. 2004;**127**(3):779–86.

157. Chahal H, McClelland RL, Tandri H, et al. Obesity and right ventricular structure and function: the MESA-Right Ventricle Study. Chest. 2012;**141**(2):388–95.

158. Nakatsuka M. Pulmonary vascular resistance and right ventricular function in morbid obesity in relation to gastric bypass surgery. Journal of Clinical Anesthesia. 1996;**8**(3):205–209.

159. Rippey JC, Rao S, Fatovich D. Blunt traumatic rupture of the pericardium with cardiac herniation. CJEM. 2004;**6**(2):126–29.

160. Baisi A, Cioffi U, Nosotti M, De Simone M, Rosso L, Santambrogio L. Intrapericardial left pneumonectomy after induction chemotherapy: the risk of cardiac herniation. Journal of Thoracic and Cardiovascular Surgery. 2002;**123**(6):1206–207.

161. Thomas M, Shen KR. Coagulopathy and anticoagulation during thoracic surgery. Thoracic Surgery Clinics. 2015;**25**(3):309–23.

162. Gerner P. Postthoracotomy pain management problems. Anesthesiology Clinics. 2008;**26**(2):355–67, vii.

163. Gelman S, Laws HL, Potzick J, Strong S, Smith L, Erdemir H. Thoracic epidural vs balanced anesthesia in morbid obesity: an intraoperative and postoperative hemodynamic study. Anesthesia and Analgesia. 1980;**59**(12):902–908.

164. Elmore B, Nguyen V, Blank R, Yount K, Lau C. Pain management following thoracic surgery. Thoracic Surgery Clinics. 2015;**25**(4):393–409.

165. Hodgkinson R, Husain FJ. Obesity, gravity, and spread of epidural anesthesia. Anesthesia and Analgesia. 1981;**60**(6):421–24.

166. Bauer C, Hentz JG, Ducrocq X, et al. Lung function after lobectomy: a randomized, double-blinded trial comparing thoracic epidural ropivacaine/sufentanil and intravenous morphine for patient-controlled analgesia. Anesthesia and Analgesia. 2007;**105**(1):238–44.

167. Oka T, Ozawa Y, Ohkubo Y. Thoracic epidural bupivacaine attenuates supraventricular tachyarrhythmias after pulmonary resection. Anesthesia and Analgesia. 2001;**93**(2):253–59.

168. Ali M, Winter DC, Hanly AM, O'Hagan C, Keaveny J, Broe P. Prospective, randomized, controlled trial of thoracic epidural or patient-controlled opiate analgesia on perioperative quality of life. British Journal of Anaesthesia. 2010;**104**(3):292–97.

169. Joshi GP, Bonnet F, Shah R, et al. A systematic review of randomized trials evaluating regional techniques for postthoracotomy analgesia. Anesthesia and Analgesia. 2008;**107**(3):1026–40.

170. Kotze A, Scally A, Howell S. Efficacy and safety of different techniques of paravertebral block for analgesia after thoracotomy: a systematic review and metaregression. British Journal of Anaesthesia. 2009;**103**(5):626–36.

171. Kramer HJ, Saranathan A, Luke A, et al. Increasing body mass index and obesity in the incident ESRD population. Journal of the American Society of Nephrology. 2006;**17**(5):1453–59.

172. Kim IB, Prowle J, Baldwin I, Bellomo R. Incidence, risk factors and outcome associations of intra-abdominal hypertension in critically ill patients. Anaesthesia and Intensive Care. 2012;**40**(1):79–89.

173. Chagnac A, Weinstein T, Korzets A, Ramadan E, Hirsch J, Gafter U. Glomerular hemodynamics in severe obesity. American Journal of Physiology. Renal Physiology. 2000;**278**(5):F817–22.

174. Amann K, Benz K. Structural renal changes in obesity and diabetes. Seminars in Nephrology. 2013;**33**(1):23–33.

175. Kumar AB, Bridget Zimmerman M, Suneja M. Obesity and post-cardiopulmonary bypass-associated acute kidney injury: a single-center retrospective analysis. Journal of Cardiothoracic and Vascular Anesthesia. 2014;**28**(3):551–56.

176. Soto GJ, Frank AJ, Christiani DC, Gong MN. Body mass index and acute kidney injury in the acute respiratory distress syndrome. Critical Care Medicine. 2012;**40**(9):2601–608.

177. Cirillo M, Anastasio P, De Santo NG. Relationship of gender, age, and body mass index to errors in predicted kidney function. Nephrology, Dialysis, Transplantation. 2005;**20**(9):1791–98.

178. Stevens LA, Schmid CH, Greene T, et al. Comparative performance of the CKD Epidemiology Collaboration (CKD-EPI) and the Modification of Diet in Renal Disease (MDRD) Study equations for estimating GFR levels above 60 mL/min/1.73 m2. American Journal of Kidney Diseases. 2010;**56**(3):486–95.

179. Rocha AT, de Vasconcellos AG, da Luz Neto ER, Araujo DM, Alves ES, Lopes AA. Risk of venous thromboembolism and efficacy of thromboprophylaxis in hospitalized obese medical patients and in obese patients undergoing bariatric surgery. Obesity Surgery. 2006;**16**(12):1645–55.

180. Eichinger S, Hron G, Bialonczyk C, et al. Overweight, obesity, and the risk of recurrent venous thromboembolism. Archives of Internal Medicine. 2008;**168**(15):1678–83.

181. Garcia DA, Baglin TP, Weitz JI, Samama MM. Parenteral anticoagulants: Antithrombotic Therapy and Prevention of Thrombosis, 9th ed: American College of Chest Physicians Evidence-Based Clinical Practice Guidelines. Chest. 2012;**141**(2 Suppl):e24S–43S.

182. World Health Organization. Obesity: Preventing and Managing the Global Epidemic. Report of a WHO consultation (World Health Organization technical report series 894). Geneva: World Health Organization; 2000.

183. Falagas ME, Kompoti M. Obesity and infection. Lancet. Infectious diseases. 2006;**6**(7):438–46.

184. Huttunen R, Syrjanen J. Obesity and the risk and outcome of infection. International Journal of Obesity (2005). 2013;**37**(3):333–40.

185. Compher C, Kinosian BP, Ratcliffe SJ, Baumgarten M. Obesity reduces the risk of pressure ulcers in elderly hospitalized patients. Journals of Gerontology. Series A, Biological Sciences and Medical Sciences. 2007;**62**(11):1310–12.

186. Bochicchio GV, Joshi M, Bochicchio K, Nehman S, Tracy JK, Scalea TM. Impact of obesity in the critically ill trauma patient: a prospective study. Journal of the American College of Surgeons. 2006;**203**(4):533–38.

187. Kaafarani HM, Shikora SA. Nutritional support of the obese and critically ill obese patient. Surgical Clinics of North America. 2011;**91**(4):837–55, viii–ix.

Cardiac surgery in obese patients

Deepu S. Ushakumari and Kelly A. Machovec

Introduction

Obesity is a preventable disease with rising incidence, affecting 13% of the world's adult population. The World Health Organization (WHO) and the National Heart, Lung, and Blood Institute of the National Institutes of Health consider obesity to be a problem of epidemic [1,2] and even pandemic [3] proportion. Several classification schemes are utilized to categorize obesity. The Society of Thoracic Surgeons follows the classification scheme used by American Society for Metabolic and Bariatric Surgery guidelines using body mass index (BMI) [4–6] (Table 13.1). BMI is the most commonly used and validated population-level measure of obesity [7]. A recent National Health and Nutrition Examination Survey evaluation revealed an obesity prevalence of 35% among United States adults older than 20 years [8].

The changing demographic of patients presenting for cardiac surgery reflects obesity in the general population. While we do not know the specific prevalence of obesity among patients presenting for cardiac surgery, obesity is an independent risk factor for cardiovascular diseases [9] and confers a higher risk of cardiac comorbidities, leading to increased likelihood of obesity among those requiring cardiac procedures [9]. The Bypass Angioplasty Revascularization Investigation 2 Diabetes (BARI 2D) trial, in examining a cohort of patients with central obesity, demonstrated that both BMI and waist circumference are independently associated with increased atherothrombotic risk [10]. Frequent comorbid conditions, including diabetes mellitus, hypertension, and hyperlipidaemia, along with obesity-induced systemic inflammation, pose a challenge to care during cardiac surgical procedures, particularly those requiring cardiopulmonary bypass (CPB).

Obesity is associated with significantly reduced quality of life in patients with diabetes and coronary artery disease, independent of comorbidities [11].

The metabolic risk profile of all patients classified as obese (BMI >30 kg/m^2) is not uniform. The vague and misleading term 'metabolically healthy obese', a concept indicating the absence of dyslipidaemia, hypertension, systemic inflammation, and insulin resistance, reflects this variation. Despite the absence of associated ailments, it appears that these patients remain at increased risk for cardiac events [12,13], though this remains controversial [12].

The challenge to the anaesthesiologist caring for an obese cardiac patient includes challenges common to all surgical procedures: potential for difficult ventilation or intubation, increased risk of aspiration, altered pharmacokinetics, and positioning difficulties. Considerations unique to cardiothoracic procedures include difficult vascular access, cannulation site challenges, pump flow alterations, lung isolation difficulties in minimally invasive cardiac procedures, prolonged procedure duration, postoperative arrhythmias, and sternal wound infections [14,15]. Prolonged CPB and cross-clamp times may increase the rate of immediate postoperative complications (Box 13.1). Valve replacement and repair procedures (open, minimally invasive, or percutaneous) may be challenging due to access difficulties, this is compounded by patient–prosthesis mismatch and increased mortality [16,17]. This chapter reviews the perioperative preparation, intraoperative management, postoperative considerations, and pertinent outcomes for the patient with obesity presenting for cardiac surgery.

Table 13.1 Classification of obesity by body mass index

Category	BMI (kg/m^2)
Normal weight	18.9–24.9
Overweight	25–29.9
Obese	≥30
Class I	30–34.9
Class II	35–39.9
Class III	≥40

Box 13.1 Considerations unique to cardiac surgery in obese patients

- Higher number of comorbidities.
- Increased risk of aspiration.
- Difficult airway and shorter safe apnoea time.
- Difficult vascular access.
- Cannulation site challenges.
- Altered CPB pump flow mechanics.
- Prolonged CPB and cross-clamp times.
- Increased postoperative arrhythmias and wound infections.
- Tenuous glycaemic control throughout the perioperative period.

Preoperative preparation

Obese individuals are likely to present for cardiac interventions and procedures due to a higher risk of angina, myocardial infarction, heart failure, and sudden death due to cardiovascular disease [5,18]. Data from the Framingham Heart Study cohort suggests that overweight and obese patients have an increased risk for hypertension, high cholesterol (with elevated triglycerides and low high-density lipoproteins), and diabetes [19]. While obesity must be present for two decades to become an independent risk factor for atherosclerotic disease [20], obesity among young adults accelerates the process, leading to more complex coronary lesions [21]. A clear risk factor for premature non-ST-elevated myocardial infarction is obesity, with obese patients having acute coronary events 4–12 years earlier than normal-weight individuals [22]. The level of visceral adipose tissue plays a key role in cardiovascular risk among obese patients, and therefore a combination of BMI, waist circumference, and waist-to-hip ratio must be employed to assess risk based on excess adiposity [20,23]. Further, obese patients not only exhibit greater platelet reactivity at baseline but are more likely to be resistant to the effects of aspirin and clopidogrel, the two most common drugs that protect against increased thrombosis risk. Purported mechanisms of antiplatelet therapy resistance include insulin resistance, increased intracellular calcium, and oxidative stress [24–26].

Preoperative assessment begins with a complete history and physical examination, evaluating metabolic causes and consequences of obesity and paying specific attention to comorbid conditions of obesity (**Box 13.2**). Subjective historical data such as exertional dyspnoea or orthopnoea, as well as physical findings of peripheral oedema, do not necessarily indicate a cardiac origin in the obese population. Obese patients may have sedentary habits and develop dyspnoea with very little exertion, making the assessment of functional capacity unreliable. In fact, outside of any cardiopulmonary limitations, exercise performance is inversely related to BMI [27]. Comorbid cardiac conditions including hypertension, hyperlipidaemia, diabetes mellitus, and gastro-oesophageal reflux disease should be evaluated. All medications should be reviewed and compliance with the medication regimen should be assessed.

An obese patient presenting for cardiac surgery is likely to have had significant diagnostic evaluation. Review the electrocardiogram (ECG), understanding that increased subcutaneous and epicardial fat may affect findings. Obese patients have high false-positive rates for myocardial infarction [28], repolarization abnormalities, QRS duration, and QT intervals [20]. Certain ECG findings are relatable to body weight: for each increase of 10% in body weight, the heart rate is expected to increase by 0.76 beats per minute, PR interval

increases by 0.5 ms, and axis deviates 1.8 degrees to the left [20]. Following traditional criteria (Sokolow–Lyon index) to diagnose left ventricular hypertrophy (LVH) by ECG leads to underestimation of LVH. The Cornell voltage criteria of R in aVL plus S in V_3 exceeding 28 mm for men or 20 mm for women is more specific to diagnose LVH in obesity [29], though recent data suggest that this too is imperfect [30].

Excess adipose tissue limits echocardiographic evaluation; epicardial fat may appear as pericardial fluid due to similar echogenicity, complicating diagnosis of effusion [31–33]. Interestingly, the presence of epicardial fat reflects the amount of visceral fat [34,35]. LVH is common in obese patients, with a case series suggesting an incidence ranging from 20–85% [36]. Eccentric hypertrophy is more common than concentric hypertrophy, suggesting effects of chronic volume overload [36]. Elevated BMI alone leads to LVH due to effects of increased blood volume on stroke work and cardiac output [37]. Some studies demonstrate an increased incidence of concentric hypertrophy due to pressure overload in the absence of hypertension [38,39]. Moreover, the Framingham Heart Study revealed that obesity correlates with left ventricular mass, as high BMI was associated with increased left ventricular wall thickness and chamber size, even after controlling for hypertension [40]. Echocardiography may show preserved ejection fraction but impaired diastolic function [38]. Cardiac magnetic resonance imaging is an alternative to echocardiography to assess structural heart problems and function [41,42] but this technology is limited by the ability of the patient to fit into the machine, even with the increased limit of 152 kg on modern machines [20].

The challenges of cardiac stress testing are an extension of the limitations of ECG and echocardiography listed previously. Overall poor physical conditioning and a high prevalence of osteoarthritis [43] decrease the ability of obese patients to perform satisfactorily in exercise testing. Patients with obesity have reduced cardiopulmonary reserve due to increased oxygen consumption [44]. Thus, many patients are not even able to achieve the age-predicted maximal heart rate in order to produce a valid result on exercise stress testing [20]. A study of asymptomatic obese individuals revealed a trend towards lower heart rate at peak exercise capacity, reduced heart rate recovery, and decreased chronotropic index compared to normal-weight individuals [45]. Such information may be prognostic: a series of super-obese patients having bariatric surgery found an increased complication rate among those unable to achieve a peak oxygen consumption of at least 15.8 mL/kg/min [46].

However, stress echocardiography (exercise or dobutamine) is sensitive for detection of coronary artery disease in morbidly obese patients [47], though the patients may require more contrast and have poorer acoustic windows [48]. A study in a cohort of patients having bariatric surgery showed that the absence of ischaemia on transoesophageal dobutamine stress echocardiography correlated with a low risk of morbidity in the perioperative period [49].

Nuclear imaging including single-photon emission computed tomography (SPECT) is limited by attenuation artefact in morbidly obese patients. Abnormal chest geometry causes perfusion defects to be missed or to falsely appear, though use of sestamibi and attenuation protocols improve the utility of this technology [50]. SPECT myocardial perfusion imaging successfully predicts long-term outcomes regarding cardiovascular disease in obese patients, as those with normal studies had improved survival compared to

---

Box 13.2 Comorbid conditions associated with obesity

- Diabetes mellitus.
- Coronary artery disease.
- Hypertension.
- Hypercholesterolaemia.
- Asthma.
- Obstructive sleep apnoea.
- Obesity hypoventilation syndrome.
- Osteoarthritis.

those with abnormal studies in a cohort with several-year follow-up after testing [51]. Positron emission tomographic (PET) myocardial perfusion imaging exposes the patient to less radiation compared to SPECT, due to use of radionuclides such as rubidium, with shorter half-lives [52]. PET is better able to attenuate soft tissue and provides coronary circulation information including blood flow per minute per gram of cardiac tissue [52]. A recent evaluation of rubidium PET myocardial perfusion imaging validated this technology as a prognostic tool for predicting cardiac mortality in obese patients. Obese patients with normal PET myocardial perfusion imaging had very low cardiac mortality over a 2-year follow-up period [53].

Angiographic cardiac evaluation in the obese population poses specific challenges. A survey of adult cardiac catheterization laboratories revealed a maximum weight limit of 250 kg for angiography tables [54]. Yet even if the patient meets the weight limit of the table, proper positioning to obtain quality images can be challenging. One recommendation in super-obese patients is to place the individual on a stretcher perpendicular to the imaging device, so that the thorax can be more easily imaged [55]. Access, whether femoral or radial, can be a challenge, though vascular ultrasound devices may facilitate invasive pressure line or sheath placement [56].

Data from the CathPCI Registry indicates increased mortality among obese patients presenting for percutaneous revascularization after ST-elevation myocardial infarction; this study also highlights the enigma of proper heparin dosing guidelines in obesity [57]. A separate registry examining obese patients having percutaneous cardiac revascularization showed an association between severe obesity and increased rates of contrast-induced nephropathy, nephropathy requiring dialysis, and vascular complications [58]. Interestingly, the 'obesity paradox' (see 'Outcomes in cardiac surgery and cardiology') affects percutaneous interventions as well, with patients with a lower BMI having higher morbidity after PCI than patients with a BMI greater than 30 kg/m^2, though patients with a BMI greater than 35 kg/m^2 have the highest rate of complications [59,60]. Regarding cardiac percutaneous interventions, early studies of drug-eluting stents in obese patients suggested that obesity was associated with higher rates of in-stent thrombosis, but this may have been due to inadequate clopidogrel dosing [61]. Subsequent studies of drug-eluting stents in obese patients affirm their safety [62,63].

Challenging vascular access complicates cardiac catheterization procedures in the obese population. Excess subcutaneous fat may occlude visualization and/or palpation of blood vessels. The French Society of Anaesthesia and Intensive Care published guidelines in 2015 regarding use of ultrasound for vascular access in adult patients [64]. While the group found only weak evidence for use of ultrasound in cannulation of peripheral (i.e. radial) arteries, their findings suggest that ultrasound should be utilized if difficulty is anticipated, as it provides a higher chance of success on the first attempt and produces fewer haematomas. However, they found strong evidence based on a meta-analysis that a landmark technique should be abandoned in favour of ultrasound-guided technique for internal jugular vein cannulation [64]. In fact, obese patients exhibit greater overlap of internal jugular and carotid artery compared to normal-weight individuals, both with the neck in the neutral position and particularly when it is rotated 60 degrees, as it is for central venous access placement [65]. Thus, utilizing ultrasound for central venous cannulation may facilitate vein location and lower the risk of carotid puncture and other puncture-related complications

[66]. Interestingly, ultrasound may not improve subclavian vein cannulation; obesity makes the subclavian vein very difficult to locate even with ultrasound guidance, and thus cannulation should not be attempted unless the practitioner is experienced [67]. Ultrasound guidance is of additional benefit in patients with previous vessel cannulation for pacemaker placement or haemodynamic access. Viewing the target vessel prior to puncture with ultrasound allows assessment of vessel size, location, and patency.

Placement of a pulmonary artery catheter (PAC) in obese patients, and indeed in normal-weight patients, remains controversial. Routine PAC use in cardiac surgery has decreased in recent years due to lack of evidence indicating any morbidity or mortality benefit. A Cochrane review of 13 studies examining outcomes in critically ill patients with or without PAC found no difference in intensive care unit (ICU) or hospital length of stay, and no difference in mortality between groups [66]. A criticism of this review is that it did not represent cardiac surgical patients. A recent retrospective database analysis examining this population found that patients with PACs having cardiac surgery experienced increased mortality, more ventilator hours, and increased length of stay, even after adjusting for comorbidities [68]. An economic evaluation of PAC use among intensive care patients in the United Kingdom suggests that elimination of PACs from routine clinical use reduces costs [69].

However, PACs may provide information regarding haemodynamics and shock states as long as the data collected are correctly applied to a given patient [70]. A PAC enables management of complex cardiac and haemodynamic perturbations if the information is utilized appropriately. However, studies examining the use of PACs lack common protocols and management strategies, making the observations difficult to apply across populations [69]. Obese patients in particular may benefit from the information provided by PACs. The chronic inflammation in obesity may increase pulmonary venous resistance even in patients without daytime hypoxia [71], and this information could be utilized for perioperative therapy. Prospective data in the obese population is necessary to evaluate the efficacy of PACs in this cohort.

Intraoperative management

Pre-cardiopulmonary bypass: anaesthetic induction and airway management

Induction of general anaesthesia is preceded by placement of standard American Society of Anesthesiology monitors. Vascular access and invasive monitoring may be obtained with minimal or no sedation before the patient enters the operating room in specially designed preoperative bays. This allows efficient use of operating room time, a decreased chance of haemodynamic instability during line placement, and an opportunity to obtain immediate information regarding cardiac output and arterial blood gas values to establish a baseline prior to induction. Alternatively, access may be obtained after induction of anaesthesia in the operating room, allowing for line placement in a fully anaesthetized, immobile patient, sterile environment, and availability of transoesophageal echocardiography (TOE) to confirm line position. Placement of invasive monitoring lines post induction requires extra personnel to monitor and maintain the haemodynamics while the primary anaesthesiologist places lines. Either approach may be employed in obese patients; there is considerable variability among physicians and practices. The best approach is that which makes the most efficient use of operating room time and causes the least disruption in operating room flow. Additional monitors including core temperature probe, Foley catheter for urinary output, and TOE are typically placed after induction of anaesthesia. Cerebral oximetry and bispectral index monitors are optional. Their use varies widely across institutions and there is no evidence for or against their use in obese patients.

During induction and intubation, obesity-related alterations in cardiac and respiratory physiology make maintenance of stable haemodynamics and avoidance of wide fluctuations in blood pressure more challenging. Avoidance of hypoxia, hypercarbia, and excess sympathetic stimulation is important. Physiological changes in pulmonary function induced by obesity, specifically the decrease in functional residual capacity (FRC), decrease the safe apnoea time to instrument and secure the airway. Effective preoxygenation is of utmost importance prior to induction. Positioning the patient upright (sitting, reverse Trendelenburg, or ramped) improves preoxygenation [65] without haemodynamic perturbations [72,73]. The best strategy is to allow an awake patient to take deep breaths through a mask with limited leaks, augmenting FRC with 5–10 cmH$_2$O continuous positive airway pressure (CPAP), or with the use of a bi-level positive airway pressure device producing a pressure of 7–10 cmH$_2$O above a positive end-expiratory pressure (PEEP) of 7 cmH$_2$O [74–76]. This allows a longer normoxic period in obese patients with potentially challenging airway management. Use of PEEP during induction of anaesthesia is suggested as a mechanism to increase the non-hypoxic apnoea time [77], but this finding has not been replicated in later studies [78]. Prevention of hypoxia is cardinal in the patient with tenuous cardiac oxygen supply–demand ratio, especially in those with right ventricular dysfunction who may not tolerate the increase in pulmonary vascular resistance (PVR) instigated by hypoxia or hypercapnia.

Immediately upon induction of general anaesthesia, efficient airway management is paramount. While elevated BMI with or without comorbid obstructive sleep apnoea (OSA) is not a predictor of difficult laryngoscopy [79,80], obese patients with OSA are at risk for difficult mask ventilation [81]. In addition, obesity is associated with a higher incidence of gastro-oesophageal reflux disease and higher resting gastric volumes despite normal gastric emptying time; this increases the risk of aspiration [82].

Despite this, routine use of succinylcholine and rapid sequence intubation are not specifically recommended. Interestingly, cardiac surgery has a higher incidence of poor laryngoscopic view compared to general surgery, regardless of comorbid obesity [83]. Video laryngoscopy and other advanced airway devices should be immediately available if a difficult airway is expected based on clinical history and examination, as they may be lifesaving in the morbidly obese patient with tenuous cardiac perfusion and short safe apnoea time. Patients with morbid obesity do not require a larger endotracheal tube size; a recent radiographical evaluation of trachea size revealed an inverse relationship between BMI and airway size, likely due to the physical effect of increased adipose tissue on the trachea [84].

Choice of induction agent is based on physician preference, cardiac pathophysiology, planned procedure, planned time of extubation, and does not require special consideration in patients with obesity. However, the altered volumes of distribution and variations in weight-based dosing must be appreciated for each drug considered. The increased body mass in morbidly obese patients is due to both increased fat mass and lean body mass; however, as obesity increases, the ratio of lean body weight (LBW) to total body weight (TBW) decreases [85]. Several equations exist to calculate LBW and ideal body weight (IBW) from TBW [65]. Hypnotic agents including propofol and etomidate should be dosed according to LBW for induction; propofol for maintenance should be dosed according to TBW [86]. Fentanyl, sufentanil, and remifentanil should be dosed by LBW to avoid respiratory and haemodynamic adverse effects; there is no data on dosing of alfentanil in obesity. Non-depolarizing neuromuscular blocking drugs (vecuronium, rocuronium, cisatracurium, atracurium) should be dosed on IBW, as TBW will prolong duration of action [86]. Pancuronium should be dosed per IBW but recognizing that obese patients require much higher doses than non-obese patients to maintain neuromuscular blockade, this drug may not be the preferred agent in obesity [87]. Unlike non-depolarizing neuromuscular blocking drugs, succinylcholine should be dosed on TBW rather than IBW or LBW due to increased levels of pseudocholinesterase and increased extracellular fluid volume in morbid obesity [88] (Table 13.2). Antibiotics for surgical site infection prevention are dosed on TBW. Many institutions have adopted dosing protocols to address increased requirements in morbid obesity. Antibiotics should be documented as per the Surgical Care

Table 13.2 Commonly used anaesthetic drugs: dosage and important considerations

Drug	Loading dose	Maintenance dose	Considerations
Propofol	1–2.5 mg/kg	15–100 mcg/kg/min	Rapid bolus—cardiorespiratory depression
Etomidate	0.3–0.6 mg/kg	Not recommended	Adrenal suppression
Midazolam	0.02–0.05 mg/kg	0.5–3 mg/h	Increased delirium in elderly
Fentanyl	1–5 mcg/kg	50–300 mcg/h	Tachyphylaxis to infusion
Sufentanil	1–2 mcg/kg	0.3–1.5 mcg/kg/h	Prolonged sedation
Morphine	0.05–0.1 mg/kg	PCA 0.02 mg/kg every 10 min	Renal failure metabolites
Hydromorphone	0.005–0.01 mg/kg	PCA 0.002 mg/kg every 10 min	
Dexmedetomidine	0.5–1 mcg/kg over 15–20 min	0.2–0.7 mcg/kg/h	Bradycardia, hypertension on fast infusion

PCA, patient-controlled analgesia.

Box 13.3 SCIP guidelines of importance to obesity

Prophylactic antibiotic received within 1 hour prior to surgical incision (1)—selected based on national guidelines and institutional protocol (2). Antibiotics are to be discontinued within 48 hours for cardiac surgery and 24 hours from surgery end-time for other surgeries (3). Appropriate hair removal as per Association of Peri-Operative Registered Nurses guidelines (4). Maintaining glycaemic control especially on postoperative morning sample (5). Urinary catheters removed at least before postoperative day 2 (6) and good preoperative temperature management (7). Seven out of the ten SCIP measures apply during the peroperative period.

Source: Data from Fry, Donald E., Surgical site infections and the Surgical Care Improvement Project (SCIP): evolution of national quality measures. *Surgical Infections*, 9(6): 578–584, 2008.

Improvement Project (SCIP) guidelines within the appropriate time frame (**Box 13.3**).

Positioning

Positioning of the obese patient for cardiac surgery is challenging. Specialized operating tables with higher weight support capability are required. Most open cardiac procedures are performed with the patient in the supine position, arms tucked at the sides, sometimes with extenders. A roll between the scapular blades may assist in exposure of the anterior chest. Any wedge or ramping material utilized for intubation should be removed once the airway is secured, as extended time in the ramped position increases the risk of peripheral nerve injury. The supine position is associated with 'obesity supine death syndrome', a phenomenon purportedly caused by intrinsic PEEP and extrinsic compression of thorax by the abdominal compartment. These factors lead to collapse of small airways, increased work of breathing, hypoxaemia, increased preload, and decreased cardiac output in an already failing heart [89,90]. Inferior vena cava compression analogous to that which occurs with a gravid uterus has also been described in morbidly obese patients. Long procedure times in the supine position may produce fluid shifts from the legs to other regions of the body including the neck, increasing neck circumference [91], which should be considered if immediate postoperative extubation is planned. Pressure sores and nerve injuries are more likely in diabetic obese patients [92]; pressure injury is exacerbated by hypothermia and decreased perfusion during CPB. Note that obese patients are at greater risk for ulnar neuropathy during surgery than normal body weight patients [93]. Once the patient is in the final position, all pressure points should be checked and padded appropriately, and all intravenous and intra-arterial catheters checked for patency. A dampened arterial waveform may be confirmed by checking a non-invasive blood pressure. Availability of adequately sized cuffs and placement in a conical-shaped upper extremity makes non-invasive blood pressure measurement difficult [94].

The period from intubation through initiation of CPB is marked by wide variations in the level of surgical stimulation. The anaesthesiologist is responsible for maintaining haemodynamic stability during this time. The haemodynamic changes are accentuated in a morbidly obese patient with altered vascular sensitivity and the ventricular morphological changes caused by high systemic and pulmonary vascular pressures. The preoperative TOE is often performed during this period, confirming the findings from earlier evaluations; this is particularly useful in the obese patient with poor transthoracic echocardiographic windows and suboptimal transthoracic images. Specific concerns regarding TOE in morbid obesity were discussed previously in this chapter. The pre-bypass time also includes harvest of vascular conduits, including saphenous veins and the internal mammary artery, which may be time-consuming in an obese patient.

Choice of maintenance agents is based on institutional and personal preference. Halogenated inhalational anaesthetics, narcotics, and intermediate duration muscle relaxants are used most commonly. Any inhalational agent may be used. Desflurane has the theoretical benefit of decreased lipophilicity and solubility, but studies do not conclusively indicate that morbidly obese patients have faster awakening or emergence if desflurane is used instead of sevoflurane or isoflurane [86]. Nitrous oxide is not specifically contraindicated in cardiac surgery, though patients with baseline elevated PVR and mitral stenosis experience a clinically significant increase in PVR with use of nitrous oxide [95]. Exercise caution when utilizing nitrous oxide in the obese cardiac surgical patient with diagnosed or undiagnosed increased PVR and elevated right ventricular pressures. In terms of ventilation strategy, it has been demonstrated in bariatric procedures that intraoperative ventilation using a high PEEP with the addition of periodic recruitment manoeuvres or vital capacity improves oxygenation better than the application of PEEP alone [96,97]. However, the haemodynamic changes (specifically, reduction in right ventricular preload and increase in PVR, leading to hypotension) produced by such manoeuvres, in addition to interference of an inflated lung into the surgical field, make these strategies less useful in cardiac anaesthesia. Interestingly, the recruitment manoeuvres and high PEEP may not significantly alter haemodynamics in an adequately volume-loaded morbidly obese patient [98].

Cardiopulmonary bypass

See **Box 13.4** for CPB considerations.

Box 13.4 Cardiopulmonary bypass considerations

Pre-cardiopulmonary bypass checklist
- Anticoagulation.
- Anaesthetic agents.
- Pump flow mechanics—good flows, no air.
- Infusions—vasoactive and others.

During cardiopulmonary bypass
- Anaesthetic ventilator on standby when ejection stops/full flow.
- Muscle relaxant/opioid/amnestic additional doses, if required.
- Monitor mean arterial pressure while on pump.
- Processed electroencephalography monitors and cerebral oximetry monitors.
- Anaesthetic agent via CPB machine.
- Glucose/arterial blood gas/haemoglobin monitor while on pump.

Weaning considerations in obese
- Slow rewarming because of increased circulatory volume.
- Complications of prolonged pump run—bleeding, myocardial dysfunction.
- Glycaemic control.
- Vasoplegic syndrome.
- Increased atrial fibrillation.

Anticoagulation management

Adequate anticoagulation is necessary prior to initiation of CPB. Heparin is the most commonly used anticoagulant, at an initial dose of 300–400 U/kg. This dosing strategy is based on the assumption that heparin metabolism is the same for lean and fat tissue [99]. However, in the obese patient fat tissue is poorly perfused compared to lean body tissue; using this standard dosing strategy with TBW leads to an approximately 25% overdose of heparin in the obese patient [100,101]. Use of LBW instead of TBW for the heparin loading dose reduces transfusion rates and adverse events associated with heparin and protamine [20,102]. Specialized devices to calculate heparin dosing based on projected blood heparin concentrations are shown to suppress the activation of the coagulation system and inflammatory responses induced by CPB more effectively than activated clotting time monitoring alone [103]. However, a retrospective database review of nearly 4000 patients having cardiac surgery suggests that use of devices that measure blood heparin concentration do not reliably predict heparin bolus dose requirements prior to bypass [104]. The authors of this study identify errors in estimation of blood volume as a potential source of error in utilizing these devices to manage anticoagulation. Further prospective analyses, particularly in obese subjects, is warranted. Regardless of institutional differences in anticoagulation management, the traditional strategy of administering heparin to achieve an activated clotting time greater than 480 seconds before initiation of bypass remains the standard practice in many institutions.

Cannulation and maintenance of cardiopulmonary bypass

Arterial and venous cannulation may commence after adequate anticoagulation. Careful consideration should be given to the size of the cannula due to the increased flow requirements in obese patients on CPB. The minimal safe pump flow required for optimal tissue perfusion depends on body surface area (BSA), degree of hypothermia, pH status, balance of oxygen delivery and consumption, depth of anaesthesia, and degree of neuromuscular blockade. However, the 'safe' pump flow is highly variable between patients due each individual's ischaemic tolerance. At CPB initiation, the perfusionist determines an initial flow rate based on BSA and projected temperature [105]. The potential for organ hypoperfusion with low flow must be balanced with the risks of air embolism and systemic inflammatory response with higher flows [106]. A flow rate of 2.2–2.5 L/min/m² of BSA approximates the cardiac index of an anaesthetized patient with normal temperature and haematocrit [107]. The use of BSA to calculate flow rates is based on the assumption that each square metre of body mass has the same metabolic rate, irrespective of the tissue composition [99]. However, the relationship between BSA and metabolic rate is not linear; lean tissue (e.g. muscle) is the main determinant of metabolic rate. In obese patients, in whom fat contributes to a greater proportion of body mass than lean tissue or muscle, a BSA-based calculation may overestimate metabolic rate. In addition, adipocyte perfusion may not be uniform, as increased vascularization does not parallel adipocyte hyperplasia [108]. Results of a small cohort of 50 patients with BMIs greater than 30 kg/m² indicate that calculating CPB flow rate based on ideal BSA produced fewer complications and perioperative blood transfusions compared to calculating CPB flow rate based on

TBW [109]. However, larger studies have not validated this claim. Management of CPB during deep hypothermic circulatory arrest in morbid obesity can be especially challenging. The exsanguination phase requires a large capacity venous reservoir to collect the large circulating blood volume. In addition, standard CPBs are not designed for very high CPB flow rates (when calculated using TBW) required to maintain perfusion in the morbidly obese patient [110]. Finally, volume of distribution is increased in the rewarming phase and additional doses of muscle relaxants or sedative-hypnotic agents may be required. Maintenance of anaesthesia on CPB is commonly achieved by volatile agents administered through the CPB circuit.

Morbidly obese patients are more susceptible to inadequate myocardial protection during coronary artery bypass graft (CABG) procedures, leading to acute ischaemia and reperfusion injury. Inadequate protection is a proposed mechanism for increased perioperative myocardial infarction [111]. Interestingly, despite the surgical challenges posed by the morbidly obese patient and potential for over-heparinization, obese patients have a lower chance of intraoperative transfusion than normal-weight individual [101,112].

Maintenance of glycaemic control during cardiac bypass procedures deserves special attention. Diabetes mellitus is a frequent comorbid condition in obesity. Combined effects of the systemic inflammatory response induced by CPB and the inflammatory substrate provided by obesity makes maintenance of normoglycaemia challenging in obese patients [113]. Hyperglycaemia was an independent risk factor for death after CABG in the Portland Diabetic Project, a prospective, non-randomized trial of nearly 5000 patients examining effects of intravenous insulin to maintain normoglycaemia in cardiac surgical patients [114]. Strict glucose control is shown to decrease the incidence of sternal wound infection in diabetics after open heart surgery [115]. Insulin therapy has also been found to be effective in reducing the incidence of postoperative atrial arrhythmia [116].

Post-cardiopulmonary bypass

Separation from CPB necessitates a team approach with clear communication among anaesthesiologist, surgeon, and perfusionist. Requirements in preparation for separation include normothermia, presence of a perfusing cardiac rhythm, adequate ventilation, optimized cardiac function, correction of acid–base disturbances, and correction of coagulopathy (where applicable) [117]. Mnemonics such as 'CVP' [118] have been in use for decades. More recently, simulation-based training has been shown to improve physician performance in weaning CPB [119].

TOE is an invaluable monitor during separation from bypass. TOE is utilized to assess valvular integrity, myocardial perfusion, presence of air, and real-time imaging of cardiac function. Skilled interpretation of TOE can quickly identify existing pathology and lead to goal-directed therapeutic decision-making [117]. Detailed explanation of issues related to separation from bypass is beyond the scope of this discussion and readers are referred to algorithms available in the literature [120]. While the steps in separation from bypass in the morbidly obese patient do not differ from the normal-weight patient, there are problems unique to the obese cardiac surgical patient. Consider excess circulatory volume may slow the rewarming process, challenging surgical exposure due to large body mass may prolong the on-pump and cross-clamp times, and glycaemic control may be more difficult, as discussed earlier.

In addition, obese patients are at increased risk for vasoplegic syndrome, making difficulty in weaning from CPB more likely. Risk factors for norepinephrine-resistant vasoplegia include long-term use of angiotensin receptor blockers or calcium channel blockers, pre-existing heart failure, diabetes mellitus, prolonged CPB times, and residual hypothermia; obese patients are likely to have more than one of these factors. The proposed mechanism for vasoplegia is overexpression of inflammatory mediators and endothelial dysfunction [120]. Morbidly obese patients exist in a proinflammatory state as a result of their physiology, creating a predisposition for vasoplegia. Correlating the blood pressure measurement from the radial arterial line with the aortic root pressure may be helpful in cases with prolonged CPB and suspicion of vasoplegia.

Finally, obesity-induced alterations in the myocardium, including LVH and increased PVR with accompanying right ventricular dysfunction, must be recognized when separating from CPB. Obese patients have a higher incidence of pulmonary hypertension than normal-weight patients; pulmonary hypertension is an independent risk factor for increased mortality after cardiac surgery [121]. CPB may acutely worsen pulmonary hypertension and precipitate right ventricular failure. Given these challenges, a vigilant anaesthesiologist skilled in TOE is invaluable during separation from CPB.

After successful termination of CPB, the anaesthesiologist must remain vigilant, as dysrhythmias, pulmonary complications, and cardiovascular decompensation may occur at any time. Metabolic perturbations and coagulopathy are common and must be aggressively treated. There is no evidence that post-CPB complications are any different in obese patients, with the exceptions noted previously.

Placement of chest tubes and sternal closure may be more time-consuming in a morbidly obese patient due to increased subcutaneous tissue. Following chest closure, the patient is transported to the ICU per institution protocol. Most patients remain intubated and sedated for ICU transport and convalescence, though extubation in the operating room leads to improved patient outcomes [122] including long-term and short-term morbidity benefit and decreased length of hospital stay. In fact, fast-track management of cardiac surgery patients with early extubation decreases hospital length of hospital stay and reduces costs. Obesity is not a predictor for failure of fast-track management [123].

Postoperative management

Transport to the ICU is a critical time, with potential for haemodynamic change and inadvertent disconnection of airway support, invasive lines, or vasoactive infusions. The anaesthesiologist should travel with emergency medications and airway equipment, continuing intravenous vasopressors or inotropes as needed. Sedation should be provided during transport in the intubated patient. On arrival to the ICU, serial disconnection of monitors is recommended if there is no brick system allowing continuous monitoring and smooth transition from transport monitor to ICU monitor. A check list or protocol for transfer of care tailored to the institution will ensure accurate comprehensive communication and continuity of care. The immediate postoperative period is marked by attention to several possible complications, including low cardiac output syndrome

(LCOS), arrhythmia, renal insufficiency, cognitive dysfunction, respiratory failure, and postoperative haemorrhage.

Low cardiac output syndrome

The phenomenon of LCOS is created in part by ischaemia–perfusion injury to the myocardium, which creates a myocardial energy deficit, compounded by the inability of the myocardium to utilize exogenous energy substrates [124,125]. Diagnostic criteria for LCOS include cardiac index less than 2.4 L/min/m², elevated lactate level, urine output less than 0.5 m/kg/h for more than 1 hour, and low mixed venous oxygen saturation. Supportive measures, including administration of inotropes, vasopressors, or afterload-reducing agents and optimization of the myocardial oxygen supply–demand ratio, serve as initial treatment strategies. Pre-existing diastolic dysfunction is associated with difficult weaning from CPB and increased vasopressor requirement in the ICU [126]. While obesity per se is not an independent risk factor for LCOS, obese patients are more likely to have one of these risk factors than patients with a normal BMI. The preoperative independent predictors for LCOS after aortic valve surgery are the same as for CABG with the addition of renal failure [127]. Surprisingly, the independent predictors for LCOS after mitral valve surgery are the same, with the addition of BSA less than 1.7 m², ischaemic mitral valve pathology, and CPB time [128]. The preoperative independent predictors for LCOS after CABG include poor left ventricular function (left ventricular ejection fraction <20%), cardiogenic shock, emergent procedure, reoperative CABG, earlier year of operation, and female sex [129,130]. Obese patients with preoperative renal insufficiency have an increased risk for LCOS and postoperative myocardial infarction [131].

Arrhythmia

The most common arrhythmia after cardiac surgery is atrial fibrillation (postoperative atrial fibrillation (POAF)). Despite advances in treatment, 20–40% of patients undergoing cardiac surgery develop POAF. POAF is associated with increased morbidity and mortality, including stroke, ventricular arrhythmias, postoperative myocardial infarction, congestive heart failure, renal failure, inotropic requirement, mechanical circulatory support device requirement, increased hospital length of stay, and increased cost [132].

Wang and colleagues initially reported elevated BMI as an independent risk factor for atrial fibrillation [133]. The results of this prospective observational cohort study suggested that atrial fibrillation in obesity is due to increase in left atrial size. Subsequent studies have investigated this association after cardiac surgery; two meta-analyses report conflicting results. In 2008, Wanahita et al. reported that obesity is not associated with an increased risk of POAF. Of note, this meta-analysis involved patients with pre-existing atrial fibrillation [134]. In 2013, Hernandez et al. published a meta-analysis excluding trials of patients with preoperative atrial fibrillation; results showed a higher incidence of POAF in obese versus non-obese patients [14]. In patients younger than 50 years, metabolic syndrome, increased waist circumference, and increased levels of C-reactive protein are all risk factors for atrial fibrillation [135,136]. Further, obese patients with OSA may have an additional, non-cardiac mechanism of POAF. Negative tracheal pressure against an obstructed airway is a mechanism for vagally mediated increased susceptibility to atrial fibrillation in a pig model of OSA [137]. Other arrhythmias, including bradyarrhythmias and ventricular arrhythmias, have not been shown to be increased in the obese population.

Renal insufficiency

The increased prevalence of comorbidities (e.g. hypertension and diabetes mellitus) combined with renal structural changes in obese patients confer an increased risk of perioperative acute kidney injury (AKI) [138–140]. There also exists a positive correlation between high BMI and chronic kidney disease [141]. Comorbid obesity and preoperative renal insufficiency confers an increased risk of poor postoperative outcomes, including postoperative myocardial infarction, LCOS, stroke, postoperative chronic renal failure, ventilator dependence, sternal wound infection, and increased hospital length of stay after primary CABG surgery [131]. A swine study suggested that an obesogenic, high-fat diet protected the animals against post-bypass AKI, but this has not been replicated nor demonstrated in humans [142]. Further, obese patients are more likely to be on drugs that affect the renin–angiotensin–aldosterone system, which in itself is associated with increased incidence of postoperative AKI; changes in glomerular pressure induced by these drugs are a proposed a causative factor [143]. Unfortunately, as the studies examining obesity and postoperative AKI are varied in designs and end points, no evidence of causality exists, despite evidence of association between obesity and postoperative AKI.

Central nervous system dysfunction

A prospective multicentre study examining cerebral injury after cardiac surgery found that one out of six patients undergoing intracardiac surgery with coronary revascularization is at increased risk for central nervous system dysfunction [144]. Although obesity was not an independent risk factor for central nervous system dysfunction in this study, perioperative dysrhythmia, uncontrolled hypertension, and LCOS after CPB were all risk factors for new-onset cognitive dysfunction or seizures persisting at hospital discharge [144]. Obese patients are more likely to have one or more of these risk factors. This problem has both immediate and long-term clinical and financial implications. A Neurological Outcome Research Group study demonstrated a 53% incidence of cognitive decline after CABG, with an incidence of 42% at 5 years. The authors concluded that early postoperative central nervous system dysfunction predicts long term cognitive outcome [145]. Interventions for neuroprotection, including epiaortic imaging to identify and avoid manipulation of aortic atheroma, maintenance of higher mean arterial pressures during CPB, alpha-stat blood gas management, and employing a pulsatile perfusion strategy may be beneficial, particularly in the geriatric obese patient presenting for cardiac surgery [146].

Respiratory failure

Traditionally, cardiac surgical patients were maintained on overnight mechanical ventilation after their procedure. However, fast-track cardiac surgery protocols, aiming to extubate patients within 2–6 hours postoperatively, have become commonplace. Studies inconsistently predict the outcome of fast-tracking after cardiac surgery in obese patients. Although an early study predicted higher chance of failure of early extubation in obese versus non-obese, more recent literature does not include obesity as a predictor of failure in fast-track cardiac surgery [123,147]. Off-pump CABG has been shown to be more efficient than on-pump CABG [148]; this

should enhance fast-tracking protocols. However, caution is recommended in following ultra-fast-track (immediate extubation) protocols in obese patients with haemodynamic instability after off-pump CABG [149]. A patient should only be extubated after meeting all extubation criteria with measures to immediately re-secure the airway readily available, especially in patients with a difficult airway, as the time to desaturation will be extremely low in obese, post-sternotomy patients.

After extubation, immediate application of CPAP with minimal or no supplemental oxygen is recommended for the morbidly obese. Oxygen supplementation alone may worsen the apnoea or hypopnea in patients with OSA [94]. Median sternotomy causes significant reduction in total lung capacity, vital capacity, forced expiratory volume in 1 minute, and FRC, leading to postoperative atelectasis and hypoxaemia [150]. The relationship between FRC and closing capacity in obese patients renders them particularly susceptible to hypoxaemia, which may have significant haemodynamic consequences in the tenuous postoperative period.

Bleeding/coagulopathy

Morbidly obese patients show lower postoperative blood loss, lower risk of reoperation for bleeding, and fewer blood transfusions after both CABG and valvular cardiac procedures [6,151]. The reduced blood loss among obese compared to normal-weight patients has been attributed to a higher baseline fibrinogen concentration and prothrombotic status conferred by obesity. This prothrombotic state is due to proinflammatory leptin and cytokines, upregulation of tissue factor production, increased factor VII and VIII production, and increased plasminogen activator inhibitors. An exaggerated inflammatory response to CPB and higher postoperative platelet counts also contribute. Interestingly, this prothrombotic state is not associated with increased risk of thromboembolic events [152,153]. However, even though these trends are observed, caution is warranted in interpreting these studies, as the end points and procedures evaluated are heterogeneous, making it difficult to draw a clear conclusion [152].

Critical care management

Postoperative pain medication requirements are not expected to be higher for obese patients, but caution should be exercised when determining dosage. Administration of opioid or sedative medication based on TBW may result in inadvertent overdose with exaggerated side effects. Patient-controlled analgesia is recommended [154], without a continuous background infusion to minimize respiratory effects. Morbidly obese patients are more likely to have a prolonged intensive care length of stay and resultant increased resource utilization, in part due to ventilator dependence, wound infection, or arrhythmias [155]. Obese patients are more susceptible to infections, including mediastinitis and sternal wound infections, due to obesity-induced immune dysfunction and inadequate tissue perfusion [156]. Alteration in number and function of dendritic epidermal T cells caused by obesity impeding skin barrier function and hindering wound re-epithelialization slows wound healing [156,157]. The perioperative antibiotic regimen should be thoughtfully administered, with careful attention to timing and dosage.

Finally, glycaemic control must extend into the postoperative period. Achieving normoglycaemia may be arduous in obese patients with coexisting diabetes mellitus, with or without insulin resistance.

Hyperglycaemia, particularly in the first few postoperative days, has been correlated with increased morbidity [113]. Protocols targeting euglycaemia will improve outcomes in the obese patients. Early mobility after cardiac surgery, as a part of fast-track programme, should be encouraged in obese patients [65].

Outcomes in cardiac surgery and cardiology

The 'obesity paradox' was initially used to describe the superior outcomes in overweight and obese haemodialysis patients compared to their normal-weight counterparts [158]. This phenomenon has been witnessed in other disease states, including cardiac disease—heart failure, myocardial infarction, acute coronary syndrome, cardiac surgery, and cardiac interventional procedures. The obesity paradox and the more inclusive term 'reverse epidemiology' [159] refers to the concept that obese patients have better outcomes than normal-weight patients in a variety of clinical contexts, including cardiac surgery and other cardiac interventions. Supporting this theory is epidemiological evidence of a surprisingly longer life expectancy in societies with high prevalence of overweight and obesity, compared to societies with low prevalence [160,161].

While a review of the obesity paradox in cardiac surgery is beyond the scope of this chapter, some discussion is warranted. Interestingly, in cardiac surgery this phenomenon was noted by Birkmeyer et al. prior to introduction of the term 'obesity paradox' [151]. Results of several studies seem to indicate a protective effect of high BMI. In a cohort study of more than 2400 patients having CABG surgery, overweight patients (those with BMIs of 25–29.9 kg/m^2) had better 5-year survival than normal-weight patients, though this did not extend to obese patients (BMIs of at least 30 kg/m^2) [6]. However, another retrospective database study showed that both 30-day and long-term mortality after CABG were similar in overweight (BMI 25–29.9 kg/m^2) compared to normal-weight patients; obese and morbidly obese patients had higher long-term mortality than normal-weight patients [162]. Among studies comparing obese to normal-weight patients, a retrospective analysis of nearly 2000 patients found no difference in complication rate or hospital mortality after CABG surgery in obese compared to normal-weight patients [163].

Similar outcomes are noted in the cardiac catheterization laboratory and minimally invasive cardiac surgery. The BARI (Bypass Angioplasty Revascularization Investigation) Trial examined the impact of BMI on short- and long-term outcomes after coronary revascularization procedures, both percutaneous transluminal coronary angioplasty and CABG. Results demonstrated that in the percutaneous transluminal coronary angioplasty group, the risk of having a major post-procedure event was inversely proportional to BMI; in the CABG group, outcomes were not correlated with BMI [164]. In addition, a study of patients with coronary artery disease having percutaneous coronary intervention noted that underweight (BMI <18.5 kg/m^2) and normal weight (BMI 18.5–24.5 kg/m^2) individuals had the highest risk for in-hospital complications, and 1-year mortality when compared to overweight and obese patients [165]. Overweight and obese patients were also observed to have a lower risk for major morbidity, and 30-day and 1-year mortality following transcatheter aortic valve implantation [166,167].

Several reasons exist for the apparent survival benefit of high BMI. First, as demonstrated by some of the aforementioned studies, overweight patients may have a survival benefit, but this may not extend to obese. Second, a criticism of such retrospective analyses is that the age of the patients in each weight category may not be well matched, as the normal-weight cohort often consists of older patients than the overweight or obese cohort. This produces a lead-time bias in the data [167]. The CRUSADE registry (Can Rapid Risk Stratification of Unstable Angina Patients Suppress Adverse Outcomes With Early Implementation of the American College of Cardiology/American Heart Association Guidelines), a project examining outcomes of over 80,000 patients, illustrated that obese patients (BMI >30 kg/m^2) were on average younger than normal-weight patients at the time of presentation with an acute coronary event [168]. Obese patients are also more likely to present earlier and require more intensive intervention [169]. Finally, studies providing evidence in favour of the obesity paradox may be of insufficient power and length of follow-up to provide meaningful results [170]. Collaborative data examining 57 studies of outcomes between obesity and BMI demonstrated that mortality is lowest with a BMI of 22.5–25 kg/m^2 supporting the need for large, prospective studies with sufficient long-term follow-up to determine if the obesity paradox is a true entity [171].

The parabolic relationship between BMI and survival after CABG surgery is clearly defined with underweight and morbidly obese patients having poor survival [169]. A retrospective analysis of more than 500,000 patients in the Society of Thoracic Surgeons Database noted a markedly increased risk for extremely obese patients (BMI >40 kg/m^2) to have major perioperative complications, including renal failure, prolonged ventilation, sternal infection, reoperation, and prolonged length of stay [172]. This series suggested a 50% risk-adjusted increase in mortality among extremely obese patients; even moderately obese patients (BMI 35–39.9 kg/m^2) had a slight increase in risk-adjusted mortality [172]. In both cardiac surgery and other surgical and medical specialties, obesity has been linked to greater resource utilization [173]. Vigorous participation in weight loss programmes is strongly recommended after CABG surgery to decrease long-term morbidity and mortality [162].

Conclusion

The growing epidemic of obesity, combined with the comorbid cardiac pathology associated with obesity, guarantees that anaesthesiologists will continue to encounter more of this population subset in the cardiac operating room and interventional cardiology suite. A solid knowledge base of metabolic syndrome, physiological consequences of obesity, and potential challenges when caring for this population is necessary to provide optimal care to them. Future directions in this field include examination of outcomes in obesity and cardiac interventions, including outcomes potentially altered by anaesthetic management.

CASE REPORT

A 69-year-old, 160 cm, 139.5 kg female started experiencing severe chest pain this afternoon and took aspirin and sublingual nitroglycerine, to no avail. She was seen in the emergency department, noted to have a widened mediastinum on her chest X-ray, and a computed tomography angiogram of her chest was performed which showed a Stanford type A aortic dissection. She is scheduled for an emergency thoracic aortic dissection repair with deep hypothermic circulatory arrest.

How would you evaluate and prepare this patient for surgery?

Initial management of thoracic aortic dissection is directed at decreasing the aortic wall stress and preventing the propagation of dissection while ensuring vital organ perfusion. This is done by using vasodilators (nitroprusside, nitroglycerine, or fenoldopam) and decreasing left ventricular ejection force (dP/dt) using intravenous beta blockers or calcium channel blockers. Once the target heart rate of less than 60 beats/min is attained, vasodilators are used to titrate systolic blood pressure to less than 100–120 mmHg.

History of anaesthetic problems, quick airway assessment and plan to secure the airway without major haemodynamic perturbations, medication allergies, availability of at least 8–10 units of typed and cross-matched blood products and cell-saver techniques, and fasting history should all be established prior to surgery. A focused review of the computed tomography angiogram to identify coronary, cerebral, or renal vascular impairment should be done. Morbidly obese patients in a high-stress situation like this should be considered at high risk for aspiration. Anxiolytics and pain medications should be titrated to target blood pressure levels.

Standard ASA monitors precede establishment of two arterial lines—a left radial artery (right subclavian may be involved in the disease process or used by the surgeon for axillary artery cannulation) and femoral artery lines (if time permits). Large bore central venous access with or without PACs can also be done prior to induction and intubation. TOE and neurological monitoring is usually established after induction of anaesthesia.

What is your plan for anaesthetic induction and intubation?

Use of modified rapid sequence induction balances airway protection and haemodynamic fluctuation. A 25-degree head-elevated position, preoxygenation with CPAP, and use of video laryngoscopy may help decrease the chance of desaturation and enable expeditious securing of the airway. Use of non-particulate antacids and H2-blockers will help decrease the risk of aspiration. Intravenous vasopressors and vasodilators are titrated to avoid changes in blood pressure.

Does this patient's morbid obesity affect your anaesthetic plan and decision-making?

Yes. Morbid obesity makes this patient highly likely to have other comorbidities such as diabetes mellitus, hypertension, hyperlipidaemia, gastro-oesophageal reflux disease, OSA syndrome, obesity hypoventilation syndrome, deep venous thrombosis, and pulmonary artery hypertension. All these conditions can have a significant effect on the perioperative management and morbidity and mortality of this patient after an emergent cardiac surgical procedure. Diagnostic interpretations of ECGs and TOEs can be altered by obesity. The respiratory changes of obesity will affect ventilator management both intra- and postoperatively. Altered volumes of distribution of drugs and variations in weight-based dosing must be appreciated for each drug administered. Timely administration of adequate weight-based antibiotics should be done prior to the start of surgery and re-dosing should be considered for the alterations in blood volumes caused by blood loss and transfusions.

Do you foresee any challenges in cardiopulmonary bypass management or circulatory arrest?

An optimal pump flow rate balances the risks of hypoperfusion and overperfusion. The traditional 2.4 L/min/m² of BSA does not take into account the lean body mass of the patient and can be replaced by controlling the flow rate to indices of tissue perfusion (mixed venous oxygen saturation, urine output, and cerebral oximetry). Arterial and venous cannulas should be capable of high flow rates. Reservoir capacity should tolerate the huge circulation volume during the exsanguination phase of circulatory arrest. Temperature management using alpha-stat should allow for a longer time to achieve hypothermia and for rewarming. Heparin management systems will help with adequate dosing of heparin and protamine. Deep hypothermic circulatory arrest with antegrade or retrograde cerebral perfusion and slow rewarming will decrease the risk of cerebrovascular accidents.

Is this patient at higher risk for postoperative complications?

She is more likely to have a prolonged CPB and its inherent higher risk for postoperative complications. These complications include coagulopathy, stroke, renal dysfunction, arrhythmias, pulmonary dysfunction, multiple blood transfusions, and cognitive dysfunction. In addition, obesity itself predisposes this patient to a higher risk of sternal wound infections, challenging glycaemic control, deep vein thrombosis, postoperative ventilator dependence, and prolonged ICU stay.

REFERENCES

1. National Institutes of Health. Clinical guidelines on the identification, evaluation, and treatment of overweight and obesity in adults—the evidence report. National Institutes of Health. Obesity Research. 1998;6 Suppl 2:51–209S.
2. World Health Organization. Obesity: Preventing and Managing the Global Epidemic. Report of a WHO Consultation. World Health Organization Technical Report Series 894. Geneva: World Health Organization; 2000.
3. Swinburn BA, Sacks G, Hall KD, et al. The global obesity pandemic: shaped by global drivers and local environments. Lancet. 2011;**378**(9793):804–14.
4. Standards Committee, American Society for Bariatric Surgery. Guidelines for reporting results in bariatric surgery. Obesity Surgery. 1997;**7**(6):521–22.
5. Hubert HB, Feinleib M, McNamara PM, Castelli WP. Obesity as an independent risk factor for cardiovascular disease: a 26-year follow-up of participants in the Framingham Heart Study. Circulation. 1983;**67**(5):968–77.
6. Stamou SC, Nussbaum M, Stiegel RM, et al. Effect of body mass index on outcomes after cardiac surgery: is there an obesity paradox? Ann Thorac Surg. 2011;**91**(1):42–47.
7. World Health Organization. Obesity and overweight. Fact sheet no. 311. Updated 2016. https://www.who.int/news-room/fact-sheets/detail/obesity-and-overweight
8. National Center for Health Statistics. Obesity. 2014. http://www.cdc.gov/nchs/data/factsheets/factsheet_obesity.htm
9. Fontaine KR, Redden DT, Wang C, Westfall AO, Allison DB. Years of life lost due to obesity. JAMA. 2003;**289**(2):187–93.

10. Albu JB, Lu J, Mooradian AD, et al. Relationships of obesity and fat distribution with atherothrombotic risk factors: baseline results from the Bypass Angioplasty Revascularization Investigation 2 Diabetes (BARI 2D) trial. Obesity. 2010;**18**(5):1046–54.

11. Hlatky MA, Chung SC, Escobedo J, et al. The effect of obesity on quality of life in patients with diabetes and coronary artery disease. American Heart Journal. 2010;**159**(2):292–300.

12. Roberson LL, Aneni EC, Maziak W, et al. Beyond BMI: the 'metabolically healthy obese' phenotype & its association with clinical/subclinical cardiovascular disease and all-cause mortality—a systematic review. BMC Public Health. 2014;**14**:14.

13. Kramer CK, Zinman B, Retnakaran R. Are metabolically healthy overweight and obesity benign conditions?: A systematic review and meta-analysis. Annals of Internal Medicine. 2013;**159**(11):758–69.

14. Hernandez AV, Kaw R, Pasupuleti V, et al. Association between obesity and postoperative atrial fibrillation in patients undergoing cardiac operations: a systematic review and meta-analysis. Annals of Thoracic Surgery. 2013;**96**(3):1104–16.

15. Akinnusi ME, Pineda LA, El Solh AA. Effect of obesity on intensive care morbidity and mortality: a meta-analysis. Critical Care Medicine. 2008;**36**(1):151–58.

16. Wang B, Yang H, Zhu W, Zhang X, Cao G, Wu S. Obesity is associated with higher long-term mortality after aortic valve replacement with small prosthesis. Heart, Lung & Circulation. 2013;**22**(9):731–37.

17. Bakir I, Casselman FP, Onan B, Van Praet F, Vermeulen Y, Degrieck I. Does a minimally invasive approach increase the incidence of patient-prosthesis mismatch in aortic valve replacement? Journal of Heart Valve Disease. 2014;**23**(2):161–67.

18. Plourde B, Sarrazin JF, Nault I, Poirier P. Sudden cardiac death and obesity. Expert Review of Cardiovascular Therapy. 2014;**12**(9):1099–10.

19. Wilson PW, D'Agostino RB, Sullivan L, Parise H, Kannel WB. Overweight and obesity as determinants of cardiovascular risk: the Framingham experience. Archives of Internal Medicine. 2002;**162**(16):1867–72.

20. Garcia-Labbe D, Ruka E, Bertrand OF, Voisine P, Costerousse O, Poirier P. Obesity and coronary artery disease: evaluation and treatment. Canadian Journal of Cardiology. 2015;**31**(2):184–94.

21. McGill HC, Jr, McMahan CA, Herderick EE, et al. Obesity accelerates the progression of coronary atherosclerosis in young men. Circulation. 2002;**105**(23):2712–18.

22. Madala MC, Franklin BA, Chen AY, et al. Obesity and age of first non-ST-segment elevation myocardial infarction. Journal of the American College of Cardiology. 2008;**52**(12):979–85.

23. Emerging Risk Factors Collaboration, Wormser D, Kaptoge S, et al. Separate and combined associations of body-mass index and abdominal adiposity with cardiovascular disease: collaborative analysis of 58 prospective studies. Lancet. 2011;**377**(9771):1085–95.

24. Anfossi G, Russo I, Trovati M. Platelet dysfunction in central obesity. Nutrition, metabolism, and cardiovascular diseases: NMCD. 2009;**19**(6):440–49.

25. Salama MM, Morad AR, Saleh MA, Sabri NA, Zaki MM, ElSafady LA. Resistance to low-dose aspirin therapy among patients with acute coronary syndrome in relation to associated risk factors. Journal of Clinical Pharmacy and Therapeutics. 2012;**37**(6):630–36.

26. Feher G, Koltai K, Alkonyi B, et al. Clopidogrel resistance: role of body mass and concomitant medications. International Journal of Cardiology. 2007;**120**(2):188–92.

27. Gallagher MJ, Franklin BA, Ehrman JK, et al. Comparative impact of morbid obesity vs heart failure on cardiorespiratory fitness. Chest. 2005;**127**(6):2197–2203.

28. Starr JW, Wagner GS, Behar VS, Walston A, 2nd, Greenfield JC, Jr Vectorcardiographic criteria for the diagnosis of inferior myocardial infarction. Circulation. 1974;**49**(5):829–36.

29. Abergel E, Tase M, Menard J, Chatellier G. Influence of obesity on the diagnostic value of electrocardiographic criteria for detecting left ventricular hypertrophy. American Journal of Cardiology. 1996;**77**(9):739–44.

30. Rodrigues JC, McIntyre B, Dastidar AG, et al. The effect of obesity on electrocardiographic detection of hypertensive left ventricular hypertrophy: recalibration against cardiac magnetic resonance. Journal of Human Hypertension. 2016; **30**(3):197–203.

31. Ansari A, Rholl AO. Pseudopericardial effusion: echocardiographic and computed tomographic correlations. Clinical Cardiology. 1986;**9**(11):551–55.

32. Savage DD, Garrison RJ, Brand F, et al. Prevalence and correlates of posterior extra echocardiographic spaces in a free-living population based sample (the Framingham study). American Journal of Cardiology. 1983;**51**(7):1207–12.

33. House AA, Walley VM. Right heart failure due to ventricular adiposity: 'adipositas cordis'—an old diagnosis revisited. Canadian Journal of Cardiology. 1996;**12**(5):485–89.

34. Iacobellis G, Willens HJ. Echocardiographic epicardial fat: a review of research and clinical applications. Journal of the American Society of Echocardiography. 2009;**22**(12):1311–19.

35. Iacobellis G, Willens HJ, Barbaro G, Sharma AM. Threshold values of high-risk echocardiographic epicardial fat thickness. Obesity. 2008;**16**(4):887–92.

36. Cuspidi C, Rescaldani M, Sala C, Grassi G. Left-ventricular hypertrophy and obesity: a systematic review and meta-analysis of echocardiographic studies. Journal of Hypertension. 2014;**32**(1):16–25.

37. Lavie CJ, Milani RV, Ventura HO. Obesity and cardiovascular disease: risk factor, paradox, and impact of weight loss. Journal of the American College of Cardiology. 2009;**53**(21):1925–32.

38. Wong CY, O'Moore-Sullivan T, Leano R, Byrne N, Beller E, Marwick TH. Alterations of left ventricular myocardial characteristics associated with obesity. Circulation. 2004;**110**(19):3081–87.

39. Lavie CJ, Milani RV, Ventura HO, Cardenas GA, Mehra MR, Messerli FH. Disparate effects of left ventricular geometry and obesity on mortality in patients with preserved left ventricular ejection fraction. American Journal of Cardiology. 2007;**100**(9):1460–64.

40. Lauer MS, Anderson KM, Kannel WB, Levy D. The impact of obesity on left ventricular mass and geometry. The Framingham Heart Study. JAMA. 1991;**266**(2):231–36.

41. Rider OJ, Francis JM, Ali MK, et al. Beneficial cardiovascular effects of bariatric surgical and dietary weight loss in obesity. Journal of the American College of Cardiology. 2009;**54**(8):718–26.

42. Avelar E, Cloward TV, Walker JM, et al. Left ventricular hypertrophy in severe obesity: interactions among blood pressure, nocturnal hypoxemia, and body mass. Hypertension. 2007;**49**(1):34–39.

43. Palazzo C, Nguyen C, Lefevre-Colau MM, Rannou F, Poiraudeau S. Risk factors and burden of osteoarthritis. Annals of Physical and Rehabilitation Medicine. 2016; **59**(3):134–38.

44. Gondoni LA, Liuzzi A, Titon AM, et al. A simple tool to predict exercise capacity of obese patients with ischaemic heart disease. Heart. 2006;**92**(7):899–904.

45. Aneni EC, Oni ET, Osondu CU, et al. Obesity modifies the effect of fitness on heart rate indices during exercise stress testing in asymptomatic individuals. Cardiology. 2015;**132**(4):242–48.

46. McCullough PA, Gallagher MJ, Dejong AT, et al. Cardiorespiratory fitness and short-term complications after bariatric surgery. Chest. 2006;**130**(2):517–25.

47. Madu EC. Transesophageal dobutamine stress echocardiography in the evaluation of myocardial ischemia in morbidly obese subjects. Chest. 2000;**117**(3):657–61.

48. Supariwala A, Makani H, Kahan J, et al. Feasibility and prognostic value of stress echocardiography in obese, morbidly obese, and super obese patients referred for bariatric surgery. Echocardiography. 2014;**31**(7):879–85.

49. Legault S, Senechal M, Bergeron S, et al. Usefulness of an accelerated transoesophageal stress echocardiography in the preoperative evaluation of high risk severely obese subjects awaiting bariatric surgery. Cardiovascular Ultrasound. 2010;**8**:30.

50. Barnden LR, Ong PL, Rowe CC. Simultaneous emission transmission tomography using technetium-99m for both emission and transmission. European Journal of Nuclear Medicine. 1997;**24**(11):1390–97.

51. Korbee RS, Boiten HJ, Ottenhof M, Valkema R, van Domburg RT, Schinkel AF. What is the value of stress (99m)Tc-tetrofosmin myocardial perfusion imaging for the assessment of very long-term outcome in obese patients? Journal of Nuclear Cardiology. 2013;**20**(2):227–33.

52. Flachskampf FA, Dilsizian V. Leaning heavily on PET myocardial perfusion for prognosis. JACC. Cardiovascular Imaging. 2014;**7**(3):288–91.

53. Chow BJ, Dorbala S, Di Carli MF, et al. Prognostic value of PET myocardial perfusion imaging in obese patients. JACC. Cardiovascular Imaging. 2014;**7**(3):278–87.

54. Vanhecke TE, Berman AD, McCullough PA. Body weight limitations of United States cardiac catheterization laboratories including restricted access for the morbidly obese. American Journal of Cardiology. 2008;**102**(3):285–86.

55. Kussmaul WG, 3rd, Bowers B, Dairywala I. Method for coronary angiography in morbidly obese patients. Catheterization and Cardiovascular Interventions. 2005;**65**(2):268–70.

56. Zaremski L, Quesada R, Kovacs M, Schernthaner M, Uthoff H. Prospective comparison of palpation versus ultrasound-guided radial access for cardiac catheterization. Journal of Invasive Cardiology. 2013;**25**(10):538–42.

57. Payvar S, Kim S, Rao SV, et al. In-hospital outcomes of percutaneous coronary interventions in extremely obese and normal-weight patients: findings from the NCDR (National Cardiovascular Data Registry). Journal of the American College of Cardiology. 2013;**62**(8):692–96.

58. Buschur ME, Smith D, Share D, et al. The burgeoning epidemic of morbid obesity in patients undergoing percutaneous coronary intervention: insight from the Blue Cross Blue Shield of Michigan Cardiovascular Consortium. Journal of the American College of Cardiology. 2013;**62**(8):685–91.

59. Lancefield T, Clark DJ, Andrianopoulos N, et al. Is there an obesity paradox after percutaneous coronary intervention in the contemporary era? An analysis from a multicenter Australian registry. JACC. Cardiovascular Interventions. 2010;**3**(6):660–68.

60. Mehta L, Devlin W, McCullough PA, et al. Impact of body mass index on outcomes after percutaneous coronary intervention in patients with acute myocardial infarction. American Journal of Cardiology. 2007;**99**(7):906–10.

61. Sarno G, Garg S, Onuma Y, et al. The impact of body mass index on the one year outcomes of patients treated by percutaneous coronary intervention with Biolimus- and Sirolimus-eluting stents (from the LEADERS Trial). American Journal of Cardiology. 2010;**105**(4):475–79.

62. Wang ZJ, Zhou YJ, Zhao YX, et al. Effect of obesity on repeat revascularization in patients undergoing percutaneous coronary intervention with drug-eluting stents. Obesity. 2012;**20**(1):141–46.

63. Akin I, Tolg R, Hochadel M, et al. No evidence of 'obesity paradox' after treatment with drug-eluting stents in a routine clinical practice: results from the prospective multicenter German DES.DE (German Drug-Eluting Stent) Registry. JACC. Cardiovascular Interventions. 2012;**5**(2):162–69.

64. Bouaziz H, Zetlaoui PJ, Pierre S, et al. Guidelines on the use of ultrasound guidance for vascular access. Anaesthesia, Critical Care & Pain Medicine. 2015;**34**(1):65–69.

65. Cullen A, Ferguson A. Perioperative management of the severely obese patient: a selective pathophysiological review. Canadian Journal of Anaesthesia. 2012;**59**(10):974–96.

66. Rajaram SS, Desai NK, Kalra A, et al. Pulmonary artery catheters for adult patients in intensive care. Cochrane Database of Systematic Reviews. 2013;**2**:CD003408.

67. McGrath TM, Farabaugh EA, Pickett MJ, Wagner DK, Griswold-Theodorson S. Obesity hinders ultrasound visualization of the subclavian vein: implications for central venous access. Journal of Vascular Access. 2012;**13**(2):246–50.

68. Chiang Y, Hosseinian L, Rhee A, Itagaki S, Cavallaro P, Chikwe J. Questionable benefit of the pulmonary artery catheter after cardiac surgery in high-risk patients. Journal of Cardiothoracic and Vascular Anesthesia. 2015;**29**(1):76–81.

69. Harvey S, Harrison DA, Singer M, et al. Assessment of the clinical effectiveness of pulmonary artery catheters in management of patients in intensive care (PAC-Man): a randomised controlled trial. Lancet. 2005;**366**(9484):472–77.

70. Evans DC, Doraiswamy VA, Prosciak MP, et al. Complications associated with pulmonary artery catheters: a comprehensive clinical review. Scandinavian Journal of Surgery. 2009;**98**(4):199–208.

71. Her C, Cerabona T, Baek SH, Shin SW. Increased pulmonary venous resistance in morbidly obese patients without daytime hypoxia: clinical utility of the pulmonary artery catheter. Anesthesiology. 2010;**113**(3):552–59.

72. Perilli V, Sollazzi L, Bozza P, et al. The effects of the reverse Trendelenburg position on respiratory mechanics and blood gases in morbidly obese patients during bariatric surgery. Anesthesia and Analgesia. 2000;**91**(6):1520–25.

73. Lane S, Saunders D, Schofield A, Padmanabhan R, Hildreth A, Laws D. A prospective, randomised controlled trial comparing the efficacy of pre-oxygenation in the 20 degrees head-up vs supine position. Anaesthesia. 2005;**60**(11):1064–67.

74. Herriger A, Frascarolo P, Spahn DR, Magnusson L. The effect of positive airway pressure during pre-oxygenation and induction of anaesthesia upon duration of non-hypoxic apnoea. Anaesthesia. 2004;**59**(3):243–47.

75. Futier E, Constantin JM, Pelosi P, et al. Noninvasive ventilation and alveolar recruitment maneuver improve respiratory function during and after intubation of morbidly obese patients: a randomized controlled study. Anesthesiology. 2011;**114**(6):1354–63.

76. Harbut P, Gozdzik W, Stjernfalt E, Marsk R, Hesselvik JF. Continuous positive airway pressure/pressure support pre-oxygenation of morbidly obese patients. Acta Anaesthesiologica Scandinavica. 2014;**58**(6):675–80.

77. Gander S, Frascarolo P, Suter M, Spahn DR, Magnusson L. Positive end-expiratory pressure during induction of general anesthesia increases duration of nonhypoxic apnea in morbidly obese patients. Anesthesia and Analgesia. 2005;**100**(2):580–84.

78. Coussa M, Proietti S, Schnyder P, et al. Prevention of atelectasis formation during the induction of general anesthesia in morbidly obese patients. Anesthesia and Analgesia. 2004;**98**(5):1491–95.

79. Ezri T, Medalion B, Weisenberg M, Szmuk P, Warters RD, Charuzi I. Increased body mass index per se is not a predictor of difficult laryngoscopy. Canadian Journal of Anaesthesia. 2003;**50**(2):179–83.

80. Neligan PJ, Porter S, Max B, Malhotra G, Greenblatt EP, Ochroch EA. Obstructive sleep apnea is not a risk factor for difficult intubation in morbidly obese patients. Anesthesia and Analgesia. 2009;**109**(4):1182–86.

81. Leoni A, Arlati S, Ghisi D, et al. Difficult mask ventilation in obese patients: analysis of predictive factors. Minerva Anestesiologica. 2014;**80**(2):149–57.

82. Mahajan V, Hashmi J, Singh R, Samra T, Aneja S. Comparative evaluation of gastric pH and volume in morbidly obese and lean patients undergoing elective surgery and effect of aspiration prophylaxis. Journal of Clinical Anesthesia. 2015;**27**(5):396–400.

83. Heinrich S, Ackermann A, Prottengeier J, Castellanos I, Schmidt J, Schuttler J. Increased rate of poor laryngoscopic views in patients scheduled for cardiac surgery versus patients scheduled for general surgery: a propensity score-based analysis of 21,561 cases. Journal of Cardiothoracic and Vascular Anesthesia. 2015; **29**(6):1537–43.

84. D'Anza B, Knight J, Greene JS. Does body mass index predict tracheal airway size? Laryngoscope. 2015;**125**(5):1093–97.

85. Janmahasatian S, Duffull SB, Ash S, Ward LC, Byrne NM, Green B. Quantification of lean bodyweight. Clinical Pharmacokinetics. 2005;**44**(10):1051–65.

86. Ingrande J, Lemmens HJ. Dose adjustment of anaesthetics in the morbidly obese. British Journal of Anaesthesia. 2010;105 Suppl 1:i16–23.

87. Tsueda K, Warren JE, McCafferty LA, Nagle JP. Pancuronium bromide requirement during anesthesia for the morbidly obese. Anesthesiology. 1978;**48**(6):438–39.

88. Bentley JB, Borel JD, Vaughan RW, Gandolfi AJ. Weight, pseudocholinesterase activity, and succinylcholine requirement. Anesthesiology. 1982;**57**(1):48–49.

89. Lemyze M, Guerry MJ, Mallat J, Thevenin D. Obesity supine death syndrome revisited. European Respiratory Journal. 2012;**40**(6):1568–69.

90. Tsueda K, Debrand M, Zeok SS, Wright BD, Griffin WO. Obesity supine death syndrome: reports of two morbidly obese patients. Anesthesia and Analgesia. 1979;**58**(4):345–47.

91. Jafari B, Mohsenin V. Overnight rostral fluid shift in obstructive sleep apnea: does it affect the severity of sleep-disordered breathing? Chest. 2011;**140**(4):991–97.

92. Adams JP, Murphy PG. Obesity in anaesthesia and intensive care. British Journal of Anaesthesia. 2000;**85**(1):91–108.

93. Warner MA, Warner ME, Martin JT. Ulnar neuropathy. Incidence, outcome, and risk factors in sedated or anesthetized patients. Anesthesiology. 1994;**81**(6):1332–40.

94. Sinha AC, Singh PM. Controversies in perioperative anesthetic management of the morbidly obese: I am a surgeon, why should I care? Obesity Surgery. 2015;**25**(5):879–87.

95. Schulte-Sasse U, Hess W, Tarnow J. Pulmonary vascular responses to nitrous oxide in patients with normal and high pulmonary vascular resistance. Anesthesiology. 1982;**57**(1):9–13.

96. Futier E, Constantin JM, Pelosi P, et al. Intraoperative recruitment maneuver reverses detrimental pneumoperitoneum-induced respiratory effects in healthy weight and obese patients undergoing laparoscopy. Anesthesiology. 2010;**113**(6):1310–19.

97. Chalhoub V, Yazigi A, Sleilaty G, et al. Effect of vital capacity manoeuvres on arterial oxygenation in morbidly obese patients undergoing open bariatric surgery. European Journal of Anaesthesiology. 2007;**24**(3):283–88.

98. Bohm SH, Thamm OC, von Sandersleben A, et al. Alveolar recruitment strategy and high positive end-expiratory pressure levels do not affect hemodynamics in morbidly obese intravascular volume-loaded patients. Anesthesia and Analgesia. 2009;**109**(1):160–63.

99. Du Bois D, Du Bois EF. A formula to estimate the approximate surface area if height and weight be known. 1916. Nutrition. 1989;**5**(5):303–11; discussion 312–303.

100. Cheymol G. Clinical pharmacokinetics of drugs in obesity. An update. Clinical Pharmacokinetics. 1993;**25**(2):103–14.

101. Baker MS, Skoyles JR, Shajar FM, Skinner H, Richens D, Mitchell IM. Can lean body mass be used to reduce the dose of heparin and protamine for obese patients undergoing cardiopulmonary bypass? Journal of Extra-Corporeal Technology. 2005;**37**(2):153–56.

102. Lindblad B. Protamine sulphate: a review of its effects: hypersensitivity and toxicity. European Journal of Vascular Surgery. 1989;**3**(3):195–201.

103. Koster A, Fischer T, Praus M, et al. Hemostatic activation and inflammatory response during cardiopulmonary bypass: impact of heparin management. Anesthesiology. 2002;**97**(4):837–41.

104. Garvin S, FitzGerald DC, Despotis G, Shekar P, Body SC. Heparin concentration-based anticoagulation for cardiac surgery fails to reliably predict heparin bolus dose requirements. Anesthesia and Analgesia. 2010;**111**(4):849–55.

105. Murphy GS, Hessel EA, 2nd, Groom RC. Optimal perfusion during cardiopulmonary bypass: an evidence-based approach. Anesthesia and Analgesia. 2009;**108**(5):1394–1417.

106. Paparella D, Yau TM, Young E. Cardiopulmonary bypass induced inflammation: pathophysiology and treatment. An update. European Journal of Cardio-Thoracic Surgery. 2002;**21**(2):232–44.

107. Cook DJ, Proper JA, Orszulak TA, Daly RC, Oliver WC, Jr Effect of pump flow rate on cerebral blood flow during hypothermic cardiopulmonary bypass in adults. Journal of Cardiothoracic and Vascular Anesthesia. 1997;**11**(4):415–19.

108. Sotornik R, Brassard P, Martin E, Yale P, Carpentier AC, Ardilouze JL. Update on adipose tissue blood flow regulation. American Journal of Physiology. Endocrinology and Metabolism. 2012;**302**(10):E1157–70.

109. Santambrogio L, Leva C, Musazzi G, et al. Determination of pump flow rate during cardiopulmonary bypass in obese patients avoiding hemodilution. Journal of Cardiac Surgery. 2009;**24**(3):245–49.

110. Molnar J, Colah S, Larobina M, Large SR, Arrowsmith JE, Klein AA. Cardiopulmonary bypass and deep hypothermic circulatory arrest in a massively obese patient. Perfusion. 2008;**23**(4):243–45.

111. Hausenloy DJ, Boston-Griffiths E, Yellon DM. Cardioprotection during cardiac surgery. Cardiovascular Research. 2012;**94**(2):253–65.

112. Nolan HR, Davenport DL, Ramaiah C. BMI is an independent preoperative predictor of intraoperative transfusion and postoperative chest-tube output. International Journal of Angiology. 2013;**22**(1):31–36.

113. Cunningham GR, Daoud D, Baimbridge S, Baimbridge C, Abdelnour S. Effects of glycemia on immediate complications following CABG. Endocrine Practice. 2013;**19**(6):928–36.

114. Furnary AP, Wu Y, Bookin SO. Effect of hyperglycemia and continuous intravenous insulin infusions on outcomes of cardiac surgical procedures: the Portland Diabetic Project. Endocrine Practice. 2004;10 Suppl 2:21–33.

115. Zerr KJ, Furnary AP, Grunkemeier GL, Bookin S, Kanhere V, Starr A. Glucose control lowers the risk of wound infection in diabetics after open heart operations. Annals of Thoracic Surgery. 1997;**63**(2):356–61.

116. Kirdemir P, Yildirim V, Kiris I, et al. Does continuous insulin therapy reduce postoperative supraventricular tachycardia incidence after coronary artery bypass operations in diabetic patients? Journal of Cardiothoracic and Vascular Anesthesia. 2008;**22**(3):383–87.

117. Cui WW, Ramsay JG. Pharmacologic approaches to weaning from cardiopulmonary bypass and extracorporeal membrane oxygenation. Best practice & research. Clinical Anaesthesiology. 2015;**29**(2):257–70.

118. Romanoff ME aLD. Weaning from cardiopulmonary bypass. In: Hensley FA Jr, Martin DE, Gravlee GP, ed. A Practical Approach to Cardiac Anesthesia. 3rd ed. Philadelphia, PA: Lippincott Williams and Wilkins; 2003.

119. Bruppacher HR, Alam SK, LeBlanc VR, et al. Simulation-based training improves physicians' performance in patient care in high-stakes clinical setting of cardiac surgery. Anesthesiology. 2010;**112**(4):985–92.

120. Licker M, Diaper J, Cartier V, et al. Clinical review: management of weaning from cardiopulmonary bypass after cardiac surgery. Annals of Cardiac Anaesthesia. 2012;**15**(3):206–23.

121. Roques F, Nashef SA, Michel P, et al. Risk factors and outcome in European cardiac surgery: analysis of the EuroSCORE multinational database of 19,030 patients. European Journal of Cardio-Thoracic Surgery. 1999;**15**(6):816–22; discussion 822–813.

122. Badhwar V, Esper S, Brooks M, et al. Extubating in the operating room after adult cardiac surgery safely improves outcomes and lowers costs. Journal of Thoracic and Cardiovascular Surgery. 2014;**148**(6):3101–109.

123. Youssefi P, Timbrell D, Valencia O, et al. Predictors of failure in fast-track cardiac surgery. Journal of Cardiothoracic and Vascular Anesthesia. 2015; **29**(6):1466–71.

124. Hakanson E, Svedjeholm R, Vanhanen I. Physiologic aspects in postoperative cardiac patients. Annals of Thoracic Surgery. 1995;**59**(2 Suppl):S12–14.

125. Gillies M, Bellomo R, Doolan L, Buxton B. Bench-to-bedside review: Inotropic drug therapy after adult cardiac surgery—a systematic literature review. Critical Care. 2005;**9**(3):266–79.

126. Bernard F, Denault A, Babin D, et al. Diastolic dysfunction is predictive of difficult weaning from cardiopulmonary bypass. Anesthesia and Analgesia. 2001;**92**(2):291–98.

127. Maganti MD, Rao V, Borger MA, Ivanov J, David TE. Predictors of low cardiac output syndrome after isolated aortic valve surgery. Circulation. 2005;**112**(9 Suppl):I448–52.

128. Maganti M, Badiwala M, Sheikh A, et al. Predictors of low cardiac output syndrome after isolated mitral valve surgery. Journal of Thoracic and Cardiovascular Surgery. 2010;**140**(4):790–96.

129. Algarni KD, Maganti M, Yau TM. Predictors of low cardiac output syndrome after isolated coronary artery bypass surgery: trends over 20 years. Annals of Thoracic Surgery. 2011;**92**(5):1678–84.

130. Ding W, Ji Q, Shi Y, Ma R. Predictors of low cardiac output syndrome after isolated coronary artery bypass grafting. International Heart Journal. 2015;**56**(2):144–49.

131. Tolpin DA, Collard CD, Lee VV, Elayda MA, Pan W. Obesity is associated with increased morbidity after coronary artery bypass graft surgery in patients with renal insufficiency. Journal of Thoracic and Cardiovascular Surgery. 2009;**138**(4):873–79.

132. Shantsila E, Watson T, Lip GY. Atrial fibrillation post-cardiac surgery: changing perspectives. Current Medical Research and Opinion. 2006;**22**(8):1437–41.

133. Wang TJ, Parise H, Levy D, et al. Obesity and the risk of new-onset atrial fibrillation. JAMA. 2004;**292**(20):2471–77.

134. Wanahita N, Messerli FH, Bangalore S, Gami AS, Somers VK, Steinberg JS. Atrial fibrillation and obesity—results of a meta-analysis. American Heart Journal. 2008;**155**(2):310–15.

135. Echahidi N, Mohty D, Pibarot P, et al. Obesity and metabolic syndrome are independent risk factors for atrial fibrillation after coronary artery bypass graft surgery. Circulation. 2007;**116**(11 Suppl):I213–19.

136. Girerd N, Pibarot P, Fournier D, et al. Middle-aged men with increased waist circumference and elevated C-reactive protein level are at higher risk for postoperative atrial fibrillation following coronary artery bypass grafting surgery. European Heart Journal. 2009;**30**(10):1270–78.

137. Linz D, Schotten U, Neuberger HR, Bohm M, Wirth K. Negative tracheal pressure during obstructive respiratory events promotes atrial fibrillation by vagal activation. Heart Rhythm. 2011;**8**(9):1436–43.

138. Chagnac A, Weinstein T, Korzets A, Ramadan E, Hirsch J, Gafter U. Glomerular hemodynamics in severe obesity. American Journal of Physiology. Renal Physiology. 2000;**278**(5):F817–22.

139. Amann K, Benz K. Structural renal changes in obesity and diabetes. Seminars in Nephrology. 2013;**33**(1):23–33.

140. Kumar AB, Bridget Zimmerman M, Suneja M. Obesity and post-cardiopulmonary bypass-associated acute kidney injury: a single-center retrospective analysis. Journal of Cardiothoracic and Vascular Anesthesia. 2014;**28**(3):551–56.

141. Kramer HJ, Saranathan A, Luke A, et al. Increasing body mass index and obesity in the incident ESRD population. Journal of the American Society of Nephrology. 2006;**17**(5):1453–59.

142. Sleeman P, Patel NN, Lin H, et al. High fat feeding promotes obesity and renal inflammation and protects against post cardiopulmonary bypass acute kidney injury in swine. Critical Care. 2013;**17**(5):R262.

143. Arora P, Rajagopalam S, Ranjan R, et al. Preoperative use of angiotensin-converting enzyme inhibitors/angiotensin receptor blockers is associated with increased risk for acute kidney injury after cardiovascular surgery. Clinical Journal of the American Society of Nephrology. 2008;**3**(5):1266–73.

144. Wolman RL, Nussmeier NA, Aggarwal A, et al. Cerebral injury after cardiac surgery: identification of a group at extraordinary risk. Multicenter Study of Perioperative Ischemia Research Group (McSPI) and the Ischemia Research Education Foundation (IREF) Investigators. Stroke. 1999;**30**(3):514–22.

145. Newman MF, Kirchner JL, Phillips-Bute B, et al. Longitudinal assessment of neurocognitive function after coronary-artery bypass surgery. New England Journal of Medicine. 2001;**344**(6):395–402.

146. Hogue CW, Jr, Palin CA, Arrowsmith JE. Cardiopulmonary bypass management and neurologic outcomes: an evidence-based appraisal of current practices. Anesthesia and Analgesia. 2006;**103**(1):21–37.

147. Parlow JL, Ahn R, Milne B. Obesity is a risk factor for failure of 'fast track' extubation following coronary artery bypass surgery. Canadian Journal of Anaesthesia. 2006;**53**(3):288–94.

148. Scott BH, Seifert FC, Grimson R, Glass PS. Resource utilization in on- and off-pump coronary artery surgery: factors influencing postoperative length of stay—an experience of 1,746 consecutive patients undergoing fast-track cardiac anesthesia. Journal of Cardiothoracic and Vascular Anesthesia. 2005;**19**(1):26–31.

149. Borracci RA, Dayan R, Rubio M, Axelrud G, Ochoa G, Rodriguez LD. [Operating room extubation (ultra fast-track anesthesia) in patients undergoing on-pump and off-pump cardiac surgery]. Archivos de Cardiologia de Mexico. 2006;**76**(4):383–89.

150. van Belle AF, Wesseling GJ, Penn OC, Wouters EF. Postoperative pulmonary function abnormalities after coronary artery bypass surgery. Respiratory Medicine. 1992;**86**(3):195–99.

151. Birkmeyer NJ, Charlesworth DC, Hernandez F, et al. Obesity and risk of adverse outcomes associated with coronary artery bypass surgery. Northern New England Cardiovascular Disease Study Group. Circulation. 1998;**97**(17):1689–94.

152. Kindo M, Minh TH, Gerelli S, et al. The prothrombotic paradox of severe obesity after cardiac surgery under cardiopulmonary bypass. Thrombosis Research. 2014;**134**(2):346–53.

153. Faber DR, de Groot PG, Visseren FL. Role of adipose tissue in haemostasis, coagulation and fibrinolysis. Obesity Reviews. 2009;**10**(5):554–63.

154. Grodofsky SR, Sinha AC. The association of gender and body mass index with postoperative pain scores when undergoing ankle fracture surgery. Journal of Anaesthesiology, Clinical Pharmacology. 2014;**30**(2):248–52.

155. Kuduvalli M, Grayson AD, Oo AY, Fabri BM, Rashid A. Risk of morbidity and in-hospital mortality in obese patients undergoing coronary artery bypass surgery. European Journal of Cardio-Thoracic Surgery. 2002;**22**(5):787–93.

156. Falagas ME, Kompoti M. Obesity and infection. Lancet Infectious Diseases. 2006;**6**(7):438–46.

157. Cheung KP, Taylor KR, Jameson JM. Immunomodulation at epithelial sites by obesity and metabolic disease. Immunologic Research. 2012;**52**(3):182–99.

158. Schmidt DS, Salahudeen AK. Obesity-survival paradox—still a controversy? Seminars in Dialysis. 2007;**20**(6):486–92.

159. Kalantar-Zadeh K, Block G, Humphreys MH, Kopple JD. Reverse epidemiology of cardiovascular risk factors in maintenance dialysis patients. Kidney International. 2003;**63**(3):793–808.

160. Murray CJ, Lopez AD. Alternative projections of mortality and disability by cause 1990–2020: Global Burden of Disease Study. Lancet. 1997;**349**(9064):1498–504.

161. Menotti A, Blackburn H, Kromhout D, Nissinen A, Adachi H, Lanti M. Cardiovascular risk factors as determinants of 25-year all-cause mortality in the seven countries study. European Journal of Epidemiology. 2001;**17**(4):337–46.

162. Benedetto U, Danese C, Codispoti M. Obesity paradox in coronary artery bypass grafting: myth or reality? Journal of Thoracic and Cardiovascular Surgery. 2014;**147**(5):1517–23.

163. Le-Bert G, Santana O, Pineda AM, Zamora C, Lamas GA, Lamelas J. The obesity paradox in elderly obese patients undergoing coronary artery bypass surgery. Interactive Cardiovascular and Thoracic Surgery. 2011;**13**(2):124–27.

164. Gurm HS, Whitlow PL, Kip KE. The impact of body mass index on short- and long-term outcomes in patients undergoing coronary revascularization. Insights from the bypass angioplasty revascularization investigation (BARI). Journal of the American College of Cardiology. 2002;**39**(5):834–40.

165. Gruberg L, Weissman NJ, Waksman R, et al. The impact of obesity on the short-term and long-term outcomes after percutaneous coronary intervention: the obesity paradox? Journal of the American College of Cardiology. 2002;**39**(4):578–84.

166. Yamamoto M, Mouillet G, Oguri A, et al. Effect of body mass index on 30- and 365-day complication and survival rates of transcatheter aortic valve implantation (from the FRench Aortic National CoreValve and Edwards 2 [FRANCE 2] registry). American Journal of Cardiology. 2013;**112**(12):1932–37.

167. van der Boon RM, Chieffo A, Dumonteil N, et al. Effect of body mass index on short- and long-term outcomes after transcatheter aortic valve implantation. American Journal of Cardiology. 2013;**111**(2):231–36.

168. Diercks DB, Roe MT, Mulgund J, et al. The obesity paradox in non-ST-segment elevation acute coronary syndromes: results from the Can Rapid risk stratification of Unstable angina patients Suppress ADverse outcomes with Early implementation of the American College of Cardiology/American Heart Association Guidelines Quality Improvement Initiative. American Heart Journal. 2006;**152**(1):140–48.

169. Hastie CE, Padmanabhan S, Slack R, et al. Obesity paradox in a cohort of 4880 consecutive patients undergoing percutaneous coronary intervention. European Heart Journal. 2010;**31**(2):222–26.

170. Amundson DE, Djurkovic S, Matwiyoff GN. The obesity paradox. Critical Care Clinics. 2010;**26**(4):583–96.

171. Whitlock G, Lewington S, Sherliker P, et al. Body-mass index and cause-specific mortality in 9,00,000 adults: collaborative analyses of 57 prospective studies. Lancet. 2009;**373**(9669):1083–96.

172. Prabhakar G, Haan CK, Peterson ED, Coombs LP, Cruzzavala JL, Murray GF. The risks of moderate and extreme obesity for coronary artery bypass grafting outcomes: a study from the Society of Thoracic Surgeons' database. Annals of Thoracic Surgery. 2002;**74**(4):1125–30.

173. Totaro P. Obesity and coronary surgery: new concepts for an old problem. Expert Review of Cardiovascular Therapy. 2008;**6**(6):897–903.

Obesity and anaesthesia for spine and neurosurgery

Anurag Tewari, Mahmood Ghazanwy, and Eugenia Ayrian

Definitions

Obesity has several definitions, including body weight greater than 120% of the ideal body weight (IBW). The National Center for Health Statistics defined obesity as a body mass index (BMI) of more than the 85th percentile. This value corresponds to a BMI of more than 27.8 kg/m² for men and more than 27.3 kg/m² for women aged 20–29 years. A BMI of more than 27 kg/m² is commonly used to define obesity for all ages. The World Health Organization defined overweight as a BMI of 25–30 kg/m² and obesity as a BMI of more than 30 kg/m² (Table 14.1) [1].

BMI is the most commonly used method of measurement of obesity besides methods such as skinfold thickness, dual-energy X-ray absorptiometry, deuterium dilution, total body potassium, underwater weighing, computed tomography, and magnetic resonance imaging [2], but most of these are not very practical for routine use.

Epidemiology

Obesity is the most common chronic health condition in the United States [3]. Medicare classifies it as a disease, which assists people in obtaining medical coverage for illness related to obesity. However, it is controversial to classify obesity as a disease [4,5]. Half the population of the United States over the age of 20 years is overweight and approximately one-third are obese [6,7]. Poor diet and lack of physical activity contribute to overweight and obesity. Obesity is also related to the leading causes of death in the United States (ischaemic heart disease, stroke, and cancer). In 1998, Finkelstein et al. noted that the medical expenses of obesity were projected to around US$78.5 billion. The augmented occurrence of obesity is accountable for almost US$40 billion of increased medical expenditure through 2006. They projected that the medical costs of obesity would increase to US$147 billion per year by 2008 [8].

Aetiology

The causes of obesity are complex and multiple (mechanisms of fat storage, genetic, and psychological) (Table 14.2) [9].

Control of eating is regulated by endocrine and neural impulses from fat and the endocrine, neurological, and gastrointestinal systems [10]. The arcuate and paraventricular nuclei of the ventromedial hypothalamus are particularly important in regulation of body weight. They receive input from the vagus nerve, catecholaminergic nerves, and hormones (insulin, cholecystokinin, leptin, and glucocorticoids). In response, they modulate the release of peptides that affect food intake, signal to the pituitary to modify how calories are used and affect the autonomic nervous system that influences energy expenditure and insulin release.

Hypothalamic damage after surgery for lesions in the region of the third ventricle, particularly craniopharyngioma, may be associated with obesity. Bilateral destruction of the ventromedial hypothalamus leads to hyperphagia, obesity, and rage behaviour [11]. Hoffman et al. noted that radical resection of craniopharyngiomas causes obesity in 52% of children at the time of follow-up [12]. The extent of hypothalamic injury based

Table 14.1 Body mass index-based classification of weight

Classification	BMI (kg/m²)	Risk of comorbidities
Underweight	<18.5	Low (relevant risk of other clinical problem)
Normal weight	18.5–24.9	Standard
Overweight	25.0–29.9	Increased
Obese		
Class 1	30.0–34.9	Moderate
Class 2	35.0–39.9	Severe
Class 3	40.0–49.9	Highest

Body mass index (BMI) is the patient's weight in kilograms divided by the square of the height of the patient in metres (kg/m²).

Table 14.2 Aetiology of obesity

Causes	
Genetic	Prader–Willi syndrome, Lawrence–Moon–Biedl syndrome, Alström syndrome, hyperostosis frontalis interna, pseudohypoparathyroidism
Menstrual/ reproductive	Pregnancy, post-menopausal, polycystic ovary syndrome, Turner syndrome
Endocrine	Diabetes mellitus, insulinoma, pituitary dysfunction, hypogonadotropic hypogonadism (Kallman's syndrome), Cushing's disease, hypopituitarism, growth hormone deficiency, primary hypothyroidism, Cushing's syndrome, Klinefelter's syndrome, Noonan's syndrome
Hypothalamic	Hypothalamic tumours, hypothalamic hypogonadism, iatrogenic or spontaneous trauma
Drugs	Corticosteroids, insulin, sulfonylureas, alcohol, phenothiazines, sodium valproate, carbamazepine, gabapentin, benzodiazepines, pizotifen
Other	Down's syndrome, familial obesity

Reproduced with permission from Knecht, S., Ellger, T., Levine, J. A. Obesity in Neurobiology, *Progress in Neurobiology*, 84(1): 85–103. Copyright © 2008 Elsevier. https://doi.org/10.1016/j.pneurobio.2007.09.003

on magnetic resonance imaging was correlated with postoperative weight gain [13].

Various pharmacological options (phentermine, sibutramine, and orlistat) and surgical management of obesity include obstructive and restrictive procedures to reduce the size of the stomach and to create an intestinal bypass to reduce food absorption.

Physiological effects

Obesity and the associated physiological and anatomical disturbances prompt for careful anaesthetic considerations as changes in body structure challenge the access for both anaesthesiologist and surgeon, increase the complexity of intraoperative management, and increase the incidence of postoperative complications. Obesity is associated with various effects on many organ systems (Table 14.3) [9,14–16]. There is a direct correlation between increasing BMI and increasing morbidity and mortality. Conversely, the lower the BMI, the lower the rate of mortality [17].

The sum of metabolic and physical abnormalities known as metabolic syndrome has abdominal obesity, reduced levels of high-density lipoprotein, hyperinsulinaemia, glucose intolerance, hypertension, and other characteristic features [18]. The diagnosis of metabolic syndrome requires at least three clinical criteria from the following: abdominal obesity, elevated fasting glucose, hypertension, low high-density lipoprotein levels, and hypertriglyceridemia (Table 14.4) [19].

Airway control is potentially limited by reduced neck mobility and narrowed oropharyngeal anatomy due to increased soft tissue [20,21]. Impaired pulmonary mechanics and decreased chest wall compliance interfere with oxygenation and ventilations [22]. Morbid obesity causes a larger reduction in functional residual capacity and expiratory reserve volume in the supine position. The work of breathing is increased because of decreased chest wall compliance [23]. In obese patients, intraoperative and postoperative

Table 14.3 Physiological disturbances due to obesity

System	Effects
Respiratory	Obstructive sleep apnoea, obesity hypoventilation syndrome, restrictive lung disease
Cardiovascular	Systemic hypertension, cardiomegaly, congestive heart failure, ischaemic heart disease, myocardial infarction, ischaemic and haemorrhagic stroke, peripheral vascular disease, pulmonary hypertension, deep vein thrombosis, pulmonary embolism, sudden death
Endocrine	Polycystic ovary syndrome, Cushing syndrome, hypothyroidism, male hypogonadism
Metabolic	Impaired glucose tolerance, type 2 diabetes, hypercholesterolaemia, hypertriglyceridemia
Gastrointestinal	Non-alcoholic fatty liver, gastro-oesophageal reflux, cholelithiasis, inguinal hernia, hiatal hernia
Musculoskeletal	Lumbar disc disease, back pain, osteoarthritis of weight-bearing joints
Neurological	Carpal tunnel syndrome, pseudotumor cerebri, dementia
Tumour	Hepatic carcinoma, colorectal carcinoma, cancer of cervix, endometrium, breast, ovary, pancreas and prostate
Psychological	Body image disturbance, eating disorders, depression
Skin	Intertriginous dermatitis
Reproductive	Primary infertility

Source: Data from Knecht, S., Ellger, T., Levine, J. A., Obesity in neurobiology. *Prog Neurobiol* 2008, 84(1):85–103; data from Beydoun, M. A., Beydoun, H. A., Wang, Y., Obesity and central obesity as risk factors for incident dementia and its subtypes: A systematic review and meta- analysis. *Obes Rev* 2008;9:204–218; data from Nigam, A., Wright, R. S., Allison, T. G. et al., Excess weight at time of presentation of myocardial infarction is associated with lower initial mortality risks but higher longterm risks including recurrent re-infarction and cardiac death. *Int J Cardiol* 2006;110:153–159; data from World Health Organization: Obesity: Preventing and Managing the Global Epidemic. Report on a WHO Consultation Technical Report Series. Geneva, World Health Organization, 1997.

oxygen tension may be significantly reduced as compared with baseline even with increased oxygenation [24]. Closing capacity in obese individuals is close to or may decrease below functional residual capacity, particularly in the supine or recumbent position. As a result of this underlying physiology, an obese patient is more prone for rapid oxygen desaturation, especially during periods of apnoea such as that which occurs during the induction of general anaesthesia.

Table 14.4 Clinical criteria for diagnosing metabolic syndrome

Criteria	Defining values
Abdominal obesity	Waist circumference >102 cm in men and >88 cm in women
Triglycerides	≥ 150 mg/dL
High-density lipoprotein cholesterol	<40 mg/dL in men and <50 mg/dL in women
Blood pressure	≥130/85 mmHg
Fasting glucose	≥110 mg/dL

Note: three of the five criteria must be met.
Reproduced with permission from National Heart, Lung, and Blood Institute; National Institutes of Health; U.S. Department of Health and Human Services.

Anaesthetic considerations

Preoperative evaluation

Preoperative assessment of obesity for spine and neurosurgery includes consideration of coronary artery disease, hypertension, diabetes mellitus, osteoarthritis, and obstructive sleep apnoea. Patients should be optimally managed perioperatively for better outcomes. Sleep study is important in diagnosing obstructive sleep apnoea. An apnoea–hypopnea index more than 30 indicates severe sleep apnoea [25]. This is an important and dangerous sign and predicts rapid and severe desaturation during induction. The use of continuous positive airway pressure greater than $10\,cmH_2O$ for breathing in patients may lead to potential difficult mask ventilation. Non-alcoholic fatty liver disease is common in obesity with the extent of disease being a predictive factor for perioperative risk and postoperative outcomes.

Examining the history of previous surgeries, their anaesthetic challenges (ease or difficulty in securing the airway, intravenous access), need for intensive care unit (ICU) admission, surgical outcomes, and the weight of the patient at that time may help anaesthesiologists for better preparation of the patient for upcoming surgery. Laboratory evaluations required preoperatively are fasting blood glucose, lipid profile, serum chemistries, complete blood count, ferritin, vitamin B_{12}, thyrotropin, and 25-hydroxyvitamin D.

Intraoperative management

Obesity poses specific challenges during intraoperative period such as airway management, patient positioning, monitoring, choice of anaesthetic drugs and dosing, fluid management, pain control, and various complications. The most critical step is airway management which includes endotracheal intubation, pulmonary physiology, and techniques of maintaining adequate blood oxygenation and lung volume.

Airway management

Obesity has a higher potential for difficult mask ventilation, laryngoscopy, and intubation. This is due to a short, thick neck, atlantoaxial joint limitation, pre-sternal fat deposits, a large tongue, and significant oropharyngeal soft tissue. Weight or BMI is just one of several factors to consider for airway assessment [26]. A neck circumference at the level of the thyroid cartilage of more than 43 cm is associated with an increased threat of difficult intubation [21]. The decision to secure the airway by means of awake intubation, rapid sequence intubation, or conventional intubation depends on evaluation of the patient [27] not just the presence of obesity. As predictors of difficult intubation such as the Mallampati classification, thyromental distance, and range of movement in the neck are normal despite high BMI, the risk of difficult intubation remains low [26].

Obese patients have a reduced oxygen supply during periods of apnoea at the time of induction. Hypoxaemia and further hypercarbia during periods of apnoea are strong stimuli of cerebral blood flow and intracranial pressure increases. Stosic et al. have found that a 30-degree reverse Trendelenburg's position provides a longer safe period of apnoea as compared to horizontal-supine positions [28]. This extra time may preclude adverse sequelae resulting from hypoxaemia during induction of obese neurosurgical patients.

Positioning of an obese individual for laryngoscopy and endotracheal intubation is an important and critical step. Ramped positioning or elevating the upper body and head of morbidly obese patients to align the ear with the sternum horizontally has been shown to improve the laryngoscopic view [29]. Collins and colleagues studied morbidly obese patients who were assigned to be placed in a sniffing position or in a ramped position for airway management and demonstrated a statistically significant difference in laryngeal view, with the ramped position providing the better view.

Another area where these patients require specific care during the perioperative period is their disturbed respiratory physiology, as they are more prone for more rapid and larger oxygen desaturation during induction and extubation. To overcome these issues, patients should be denitrogenated with 100% oxygen prior to induction, receive continuous positive airway pressure during preoxygenation and immediately after extubation, and receive positive end-expiratory pressure with mechanical ventilation maintain oxygenation and lung volume perioperatively [30–32].

Patient positioning

Morbidly obese patients need extra care in positioning during craniotomy and spine surgery. In the supine position, rhabdomyolysis from pressure on the gluteal muscles leading to renal failure and even death has occurred [33,34]. Even if pressure points are carefully padded, skin breakdown can still occur. This leads to tissue necrosis and infections especially in prolonged surgery [35]. Obese patients have excess axillary tissue, which imposes difficulty in placing an axillary roll in the lateral decubitus position.

The prone position is required for surgical exposure in spine surgery. Changing position from supine to prone may have adverse effects on epidural venous pressure and airway pressure more in obese patients because pressure on the abdominal wall may exacerbate the restrictive nature of pulmonary disease [36,37]. Major issues noted in obese patients are difficulties with cardiac dysfunction and ventilation due to restriction of chest and abdominal movement. Obesity exacerbates the decrease in pulmonary compliance in the prone position. A very high airway pressure may be required for adequate ventilation in such patients. In turn, high airway pressures may impair venous return to the heart, decrease cardiac output, and increase systemic venous pressure which may exacerbate surgical bleeding and decrease spinal cord perfusion pressure, increasing the risk of neurological complications. Various surgical frames have been designed to minimize the adverse cardiopulmonary response to the prone position.

Severely obese patients have brachial plexus injuries when in the prone position during spine surgery [38]. These positional palsies may develop because of the increased weight of each upper extremity causing tractional stress on the affected neurovascular bundle. Minimizing these potential complications requires specific attention to perioperative positioning, with support and immobilization to the upper extremities and excess padding around all pressure points in the upper and lower extremities.

Anaesthetic drugs and dosing

Increased incidence of comorbidities such as diabetes, hypertension, obstructive sleep apnoea, and cardiopulmonary disease in the obese population decreases the margin of safety of anaesthetic drugs.

The change in pharmacokinetics and pharmacodynamics of anaesthetic agents in obese patients are due to increased cardiac output, increased lean body weight, increased fat mass, and increased extracellular fluid volume. With the increased practice of awake craniotomy in neurosurgery, it becomes attractive to use short-acting drugs and non-depressors of ventilation such as the alpha-2-agonist dexmedetomidine. It acts as an adjunct to anaesthesia as it reduces intraoperative as well as postoperative opioid requirements [39].

Lean body mass (120% of IBW) is a good weight approximation to use when dosing hydrophilic medications. Anaesthetic drugs which are commonly used can be dosed as per total body weight (TBW) or IBW based on lipid solubility. Drug dosing of propofol, vecuronium, rocuronium, and remifentanil is based on IBW. In contrast, thiopental, midazolam, succinylcholine, atracurium, cisatracurium, fentanyl, and sufentanil should be dosed based on TBW. The maintenance doses of propofol should be based on TBW and on IBW for sufentanil [40]. Vecuronium and rocuronium are re-dosed as per the state of neuromuscular blockade. Volume of distribution is changed in obese patients with reference to lipophilic drugs. Three exceptions are digoxin, procainamide, and remifentanil, which have no relationship between properties of the drug and their volume of distribution [40–43].

Nitrous oxide provides some analgesic effect and is eliminated rapidly, but because of high oxygen demand in obesity it is probably best avoided. Volatile agent choice is based on blood–gas partition coefficients and fat–blood partition coefficients.

Overweight and obese patients pose a high risk for delayed awakening after general surgery [44–46]. In obesity, the early post-anaesthesia period is commonly complicated by an increase in the arterial pressure of carbon dioxide ($PaCO_2$) that leads to hypercapnia and cerebral hyperaemia [47]. In neurosurgical procedures, cerebral hyperaemia may contribute to adverse cerebral outcomes by increasing cerebral oedema, intracranial pressure, and the risk of cerebral haemorrhage [48–50]. Bilotta et al. [51] concluded that in overweight and obese patients undergoing craniotomy for supratentorial expanding brain lesions, both sevoflurane and desflurane inhalational anaesthetics provide optimum intraoperative haemodynamic conditions and are suitable for fast-track neuroanaesthesia.

Fluid management

Euvolemia is poorly defined in obese patients. Measures of volume status and tissue perfusion are the most important determining factors. Intraoperative and perioperative fluid strategies in severely obese patients aim to maintain euvolemia [52].

Monitoring

The patient's comorbidities and type of surgery guides the extent of intraoperative monitoring [52]. For most patients, standard intraoperative monitoring includes oxygenation, ventilation, blood pressure, heart rate, and body temperature. The threshold for invasive blood pressure monitoring should be kept low in case of cardiovascular comorbidities and neuromuscular procedures. Processed electrocorticography to assess depth of anaesthesia can provide useful information during anaesthesia delivery and recovery in morbidly obese patients [53,54]. These devices can help in titrating anaesthetic drugs to achieve and maintain an optimal level of anaesthesia.

Pain control

A multimodal approach to pain control reduces the adverse events of respiratory complications and opioid-related side effects. Multimodal analgesia includes potent non-steroidal anti-inflammatory analgesics, such as ketorolac, local anaesthetic infiltration, and scalp block. To further augment multimodal analgesia, ketamine, alpha-2 agonists, and ultra-short acting opioid (remifentanil) are used. The success of scalp block has been elucidated by Hansen et al. [54] in awake craniotomies based on cranial nerve blocks, permanent presence of an intraoperative contact person and constant reassuring, and therapeutic communication. No sedation was necessary for any of the patients and only two-thirds of the patients requested remifentanil.

Dexmedetomidine is given by continuous infusion and has been used as an adjunct to general anaesthesia for morbidly obese patients. It decreases perioperative opioid requirements and length of recovery room stay [54]. A perspective study done by Ard et al. [56] for patients undergoing awake craniotomy confirmed dexmedetomidine's ability in reducing the incidence of adverse events. They also found that dexmedetomidine administration reduced the necessary amounts of other drugs and improved surgical work, probably related to induced cerebral flux decrease [57]. Hassan et al. have used a combination of dexmedetomidine and remifentanil with scalp block for a case series of awake craniotomy for brain tumours [58]. They found that patients were comfortable throughout the surgery without any adverse neurological deficits. All tumours were successfully excised while all patients were in an arousable and cooperative state. Rajan et al. [59] in a retrospective review comparing patients undergoing an awake craniotomy to patients undergoing craniotomy under general anaesthesia. They observed that craniotomies with propofol–dexmedetomidine infusion had stable haemodynamic responses to pinning and emergence and less overall narcotic use compared to general anaesthesia, but higher incidences of temporary episodes of desaturation and hypoventilation were observed.

Lettieri et al. [60] have used a ketamine-based anaesthetic protocol for general anaesthesia and have shown that it provides good clinical conditions for deep brain stimulation surgery for Parkinson disease without interfering with microelectrode recordings.

Effects of obesity on extraneural surgery

Obesity increases the risk of perioperative mortality and complications and risk of infections such as pneumonia, catheter infection, urinary tract infection, and multiorgan failure in patients in ICUs [4,61–63]. Strandberg et al. noted an association between obesity and the area of lung opacities seen immediately after induction of anaesthesia [64]. A study found that during general anaesthesia, morbidly obese patients suffer more atelectasis than non-obese patients that persists for 24 hours [65]. Atelectasis may result in arterial hypoxaemia and marked alterations in respiratory mechanics which can lead to more postoperative complications. A retrospective analysis of 7271 complications within 30 days of surgery among 94,853 patients who underwent non-cardiac surgery showed an increased risk of myocardial infarction, peripheral nerve injury, wound infection, and urinary tract infection among obese patients [66]. Mortality, tracheal reintubation, and cardiac arrest were also higher in the morbidly obese. The overall complication rate in obese (2.1%)

and non-obese (2%) neurosurgery patients were not high, but obese patients have an increased risk of infection [67]. Extremely obese patients undergoing cardiac procedures have a longer recovery time and higher incidence of postoperative complications than normal-weight patients [68]. Wound complications postoperatively are the main adverse complications in obese patients. The 30-day mortality rate after bariatric surgery is as low as 0.3% despite associated comorbidities [69]. Few studies found that elective surgery in obese patients tends to be associated with a small increase in perioperative complications, mainly wound complications [4]. The risk of occurrence of postoperative thromboembolism, atelectasis, and pneumonia are higher in morbidly obese patients [70].

A retrospective study of 1471 patients noted that morbid obesity was associated with increased mortality in patients with an ICU stay longer than 4 days [71]. Mortality in 1167 trauma patients admitted to an ICU was seven times higher for patients with a BMI of greater than 30 kg/m^2 [61]. The nature of injury differs in trauma patients who are obese, with a lower risk of head injury and a higher risk of thoracic injury [72,73]. Brown et al. noted that obese patients with neurological disease (e.g. head injury) had the same outcome and mortality as patients who were not obese [73].

Anaesthetic considerations in the obese paediatric population are also of paramount importance and per Chidambaran et al. there is an increased demand for upgraded strategies for perioperative management in this patient population [74].

Effects of obesity on neural surgery

Aghi et al. retrospectively reviewed male patients who underwent craniotomy for benign meningiomas [75]. They found that men with meningiomas were more often obese, suggesting a hormonal influence on meningiomas in men as well as women. They also concluded that these patients had a high risk of postoperative complications.

Obesity increases the risk of infection after spine surgery [76,77]. Gepstein et al. [78] and Telfeian et al. [79] reported a higher complication incidence in lumbar decompressive surgery with increasing BMI but no difference in overall clinical outcomes. Wound infection rates and pulmonary embolism occurrence may be higher in obese patients [78–82]. In a retrospective review of elective thoracolumbar fusion procedures, Patel et al. [38] reported an association between increasing BMI and the increased incidence of significant perioperative complications. They performed a review of 332 patients for elective thoracic and lumbar spine surgery for degenerative disease and reported an association between increased BMI and major complications. Takrouri et al. [83] also reported an incidence of femoral vein thrombosis and restricted ventilation after prone positioning in a morbidly obese patient with cervical spine fixation.

Shamji et al. [84] performed a population-based assessment of complications in thoracolumbar spine fusion procedures and concluded that obese patients are at a higher risk of associated comorbidities and are more likely to suffer wound complications and postoperative infections. Interestingly, they also mentioned that overall complication rates were similar, with a limited influence of BMI. Rosen et al. [85] reported on a series of 110 patients undergoing minimally invasive lumbar arthrodesis procedures and found that BMI had no impact on complications and patient outcomes. Another review of 404 patients undergoing spinal neurosurgical procedures did not find a correlation of BMI with postoperative morbidity, including wound infection [84].

Schultheiss et al. [86] found in a retrospective and perspective study that obesity was not associated with poor outcome after subarachnoid haemorrhage (SAH). Rather, they found that the outcomes were worse among patients with a lower BMI (31%) as compared to obese patients (27%)—the obesity paradox. Juvela et al. [87,88] found no effect of increased BMI on outcome after SAH, but increased BMI was associated with cerebral infarction on follow-up computed tomography scans. Obesity may influence the risk of aneurysm formation and rupture and/or the outcome of patients who have aneurysmal SAH. The most consistently identified risk factors for SAH include cigarette smoking and hypertension. A review of 26 prospective cohort studies from the Asia-Pacific region involving 306,620 patients reported 236 cases of SAH during a median follow-up period of 8.2 years [89]. For these patients, smoking and hypertension were risk factors for SAH, but not BMI, alcohol intake, or serum cholesterol. There were similar outcomes in a study of Korean patients [90]. Low BMI tends to be associated with SAH [91]. In a large study of Japanese patients dying of SAH, low BMI was found to be a risk factor only in men [92].

Conclusion

Optimum anaesthetic management of the obese patient population who present for neurosurgery requires considerate pre-procedure evaluation and scrupulous perioperative management. The anaesthetic regimen should be personalized to related comorbidities, with increased cognizance of possible perioperative risks and complications.

CASE REPORT

A 52-year-old female with a past medical history of hypertension, diabetes, frequent headaches, and morbid obesity with BMI of 48 kg/m^2 presented to the emergency department with a primary complaint of 'the worst headache of her life' accompanied by episodes of right-sided facial pain and sensitivity. The patient's initial vital signs were a blood pressure of 174/89 mmHg, pulse 92 beats/min, respirations 21 breaths/min, temperature 37.6°C, and SpO$_2$ 100% (on room air).

Immediate computed tomography angiography of the head and neck revealed a ruptured right posterior communicating artery (PCOM) aneurysm and a SAH. The patient was admitted to the ICU where an external ventricular drain was placed by the surgeon. The patient's condition continued to deteriorate.

The patient was brought to the operating room emergently for right-sided craniotomy for clipping of the ruptured PCOM aneurysm. By the time the patient arrived in the operating room she was not arousable. She was placed on the operating table with the head secured in the sniffing position and underwent modified rapid sequence induction with propofol and rocuronium. After rapid sequence induction the trachea was successfully intubated with the assistance of the video laryngoscope. The airway was secured with a 7.5 mm endotracheal tube at a depth of 22 cm. An arterial line and an additional peripheral intravenous catheter were placed, and the patient was positioned with the head turned to the right and placed in the Mayfield head holder. After careful retraction and delicate dissection, the PCOM aneurysm was located.

Brain protection was achieved by the administration of mannitol after the dura was opened, along with maintaining the $PaCO_2$ at 37 mmHg, and keeping the patient in burst suppression with propofol. Blood pressure was maintained at 10% above her normal level. After application of the temporary clip for 8 minutes, the aneurysm was successfully clipped. The patient was taken out from the burst suppression, and the dura and skin were closed. The patient was taken out of the Mayfield head holder and placed in the supine position.

At this time the oxygen saturation started declining rapidly. The patient was immediately placed on 100% oxygen, taken off the mechanical ventilation, and ventilated manually. Despite the manual ventilation, oxygen saturation did not increase above 84%. The lungs ware auscultated, and decreased breath sounds were heard on the left side of the chest. The diagnosis of tube migration to the right main bronchus was made. The patient was disconnected from the ventilator, the cuff was deflated, and the tube was withdrawn 2 cm. After the reinflation of the endotracheal tube cuff and connecting the patient to the ventilator, the oxygen saturation came back up to 100%. The decision was made to leave the patient on the ventilator and transfer to the ICU. The patient was successfully extubated in the ICU 24 hours later. She appeared mentally intact but complained of remnant headache, which resolved over the next day. She recovered successfully without symptoms of postoperative vasospasm and was discharged from the hospital a few days later.

REFERENCES

1. WHO Expert Consultation. Appropriate body mass index for Asian populations and its complications for policy and intervention strategies. Lancet. 2004;**363**:157–63.
2. Kopelman PG. Investigation of obesity. Clin Endocrinol (Oxf). 2004;**41**:703–708.
3. Choban PS, Flancbaum L. The impact of obesity on surgical outcomes: a review. J Am Coll Surg. 1997;**185**:593–603.
4. Heshka S, Allison DB. Is obesity a disease? Int J Obes Relat Metab Disord. 2001;**25**:1401–1404.
5. Kopelman PG, Finer N. Reply: Is obesity a disease? Int J Obes Relat Metab Disord. 2001;**25**:1405–406.
6. World Health Organization. Obesity and overweight. Fact sheet no. 311. Updated March 2013. https://www.who.int/news-room/fact-sheets/detail/obesity-and-overweight
7. Ogden CL, Carroll MD, Curtin LR, McDowell MA, Tabak CJ, Flegal KM. Prevalence of overweight and obesity in the United States, 1999–2004. JAMA. 2006;**295**:1549–55.
8. Finkelstein EA, Trogdon JG, Cohen JW, et al. Annual medical spending attributable to obesity: payer-and service-specific estimates. Health Affairs. 2009;**5**:822–31.
9. Knecht S, Ellger T, Levine JA. Obesity in neurobiology. Prog Neurobiol. 2008;**84**:85–103.
10. Rosenbaum M, Leibel RL, Hirsch J. Obesity. N Engl J Med. 1997;**337**:396–407.
11. Reeves AG, Plum F. Hyperphagia, rage, and dementia accompanying a ventromedial hypothalamic neoplasm. Arch Neurol. 1969;**20**:616–24.
12. Hoffman HJ, De Silva M, Humphreys RP, Drake JM, Smith ML, Blaser SI. Aggressive surgical management of craniopharyngiomas in children. J Neurosurg. 1992;**76**:47–52.
13. de Vile CJ, Grant DB, Hayward RD, Kendall BE, Neville BG, Stanhope R. Obesity in childhood craniopharyngioma: relation to post-operative hypothalamic damage shown by magnetic resonance imaging. J Clin Endocrinol Metab. 1996;**81**:2734–37.
14. Beydoun MA, Beydoun HA, Wang Y. Obesity and central obesity as risk factors for incident dementia and its subtypes: a systematic review and meta- analysis. Obes Rev. 2008;**9**:204–18.
15. Nigam A, Wright RS, Allison TG, et al. Excess weight at time of presentation of myocardial infarction is associated with lower initial mortality risks but higher longterm risks including recurrent re-infarction and cardiac death. Int J Cardiol. 2006;**110**:153–59.
16. World Health Organization. Obesity: Preventing and Managing the Global Epidemic. Report on a WHO Consultation Technical Report Series 894. Geneva: World Health Organization; 1997.
17. Stevens J, Cai J, Pamuk ER, Williamson DF, Thun MJ, Wood JL. The effect of age on the association between body-mass index and mortality. N Engl J Med. 1998;**338**:1–7.
18. Liberopoulos EN, Mikhailidis DP, Elisaf MS. Diagnosis and management of the metabolic syndrome in obesity. Obes Rev. 2005;**6**:283–96.
19. National Heart, Lung, and Blood Institute. Third Report of the National Cholesterol Education Program (NCEP) Expert Panel on Detection, Evaluation, and Treatment of High Blood Cholesterol in Adults (Adult Treatment Panel III). Final Report. NIH Publication No. 02-5215. Bethesda, MD: National Heart, Lung, and Blood Institute; 2002.
20. Gonzalez H, Miniville V, Delanoue K, et al. The importance of increased neck circumference to intubation difficulties in obese patients. Anesth Analg. 2008;**106**:1132–36.
21. Isono S. Obstructive sleep apnea of obese adults: pathophysiology and perioperative airway management. Anesthesiology. 2009;**110**:908–21.
22. Pelosi P, Gregoretti C. Perioperative management of obese patients. Best Pract Res Clin Anaesthesiol. 2010;**24**:211–25.
23. Ladosky W, Botelho MA, Albuquerque JP Jr. Chest mechanics in morbidly obese non-hypoventilated patients. Respir Med. 2001;**95**:281–86.
24. Kabon B, Nagele A, Reddy D, et al. Obesity decreases perioperative tissue oxygenation. Anesthesiology. 2004;**100**:274–80.
25. Patil SP, Schneider H, Schwartz AR, Smith PL. Adult obstructive sleep apnea. Chest. 2007;**132**:325–37.
26. El-Ganzouri AR, McCarthy RJ, Tuman KJ, et al. Preoperative airway assessment: predictive value of a multivariate risk index. Anesth Analg. 1996;**82**:1119–204.
27. American Society of Anesthesiologists Task Force on Management of the Difficult Airway. Practice guidelines for management of the difficult airway: an updated report by the American Society of Anesthesiologists Task Force on Management of the Difficult Airway. Anesthesiology. 2003;**98**:1269–77.
28. Stosic M, Milakovic B, Dostanic M, Baljozovic B. Reverse Trendelenburg's position vs. supine-horizontal position for induction of general anesthesia in obese neurosurgical patients. Srp Arh Celok Lek. 2006;**134**:208–12.
29. Collins JS, Lemmens HJ, Brodsky JB, et al. Laryngoscopy and morbid obesity: a comparison of the 'sniff' and 'ramped' positions. Obes Surg. 2004;**14**:1171–75.
30. Coussa M, Proietti S, Schnyder P, et al. Prevention of atelectasis formation during the induction of general anesthesia in morbidly obese patients. Anesth Analg. 2004;**98**:1491–95.
31. Cressey DM, Berthoud MC, Reilly CS. Effectiveness of continuous positive airway pressure to enhance pre-oxygenation in morbidly obese women. Anaesthesia. 2001;**56**:680–84.

32. Gander S, Frascarolo P, Suter M, et al. Positive end-expiratory pressure during induction of general anesthesia increases duration of nonhypoxic apnea in morbidly obese patients. Anesth Analg. 2005;**100**:580–84.

33. Bostanjian D, Anthone GJ, Hamouti N, et al. Rhabdomyolysis of gluteal muscles leading to renal failure: a potentially fatal complication of surgery in the morbidly obese. Obes Surg. 2003;**13**:302–305.

34. Collier B, Goreja MA, Duke III BE. Postoperative rhabdomyolysis with bariatric surgery. Obes Surg. 2003;**13**:941–43.

35. Passannante AN, Rock P. Anesthetic management of patients with obesity and sleep apnea. Anesthesiol Clin North Am. 2005;**23**:479–91.

36. Pearce DJ. The role of posture in laminectomy. Proc R Soc Med. 1957;**50**:109–12.

37. Smith RH, Gramling ZW, Volpitto PP. Problems related to the prone position for surgical operations. Anesthesiology. 1961;**22**:189–93.

38. Patel N, Bagan B, Vadera S, et al. Obesity and spine surgery: relation to perioperative complications. J Neurosurg Spine. 2007;**6**:291–97.

39. Pawlik MT, Hansen E, Waldhauser D, et al. Clonidine premedication in patients with sleep apnea syndrome: a randomized, double blind, placebo-controlled study. Anesth Analg. 2005;**101**:1374–80.

40. Ogunnaike BO, Jones SB, Jones DB, et al. Anesthetic considerations for bariatric surgery. Anesth Analg. 2002;**95**:1793–805.

41. Abernethy DR, Greenblatt DJ, Smith TW. Digoxin disposition in obesity: clinical pharmacokinetic investigation. Am Heart J. 1981;**102**:740–44.

42. Christoff PB, Conti DR, Naylor C, Jusko WJ. Procainamide disposition in obesity. Drug Intell Clin Pharm. 1983;**17**:516–22.

43. Egan TD, Huizinga B, Gupta SK, et al. Remifentanil pharmacokinetics in obese versus lean patients. Anesthesiology. 1998;**89**:562–73.

44. Suzuki T, Masaki G, Ogawa S. Neostigmine-induced reversal of vecuronium in normal weight, overweight and obese female patients. Br J Anaesth. 2006;**97**:160–63.

45. Deepak R, Biswas G. Morbid obesity and anaesthesia. Anaesthesia. 2007;**62**:1299–1300.

46. La Colla L, Albertin A, La Colla G, et al. Faster wash-out and recovery for desflurane versus sevoflurane in morbidly obese patients when no premedication is used. Br J Anaesth. 2007;**99**:353–58.

47. Ito H, Kanno I, Ibaraki M, et al. Changes in human cerebral blood flow and cerebral blood volume during hypercapnia and hypocapnia measured by positron emission tomography. J Cereb Blood Flow Metab. 2003;**23**:665–70.

48. Bruder N, Pellissier D, Grillot P, et al. Cerebral hyperemia during recovery from general anesthesia in neurosurgical patients. Anesth Analg. 2002;**94**:650–54.

49. Constantini S, Cotev S, Rappaport ZH, et al. Intracranial pressure monitoring after elective intracranial surgery. A retrospective study of 514 consecutive patients. J Neurosurg. 1988;**69**:540–44.

50. Young WL, Kader A, Ornstein E, et al. Cerebral hyperemia after arteriovenous malformation resection is related to "breakthrough" complications but not to feeding artery pressure. The Columbia University Arteriovenous Malformation Study Project. Neurosurgery. 1996;**38**:1085–93.

51. Bilotta F, Doronzio A, Cuzzone V et al. Early postoperative cognitive recovery and gas exchange patterns after balanced anesthesia with sevoflurane or desflurane in overweight and obese patients undergoing craniotomy: a prospective randomized trial. J Neurosurg Anesthesiol. 2009;**21**:207–13.

52. Schumann R, Jones SB, Cooper B, et al. Update on best practice recommendations for anesthetic perioperative care and pain management in weight loss surgery, 2004–2007. Obesity. 2009;**17**:889–994.

53. Feld JM, Hoffman WE, Stechert MM, et al. Fentanyl or dexmedetomidine combined with desflurane for bariatric surgery. J Clin Anesth. 2006;**18**:24–28.

54. Tufanogullari B, White PF, Peixoto MP, et al. Dexmedetomidine infusion during laparoscopic bariatric surgery: the effect on recovery outcome variables. Anesth Analg. 2008;**106**:1741–48.

55. Hansen E, Seemann M, Zech N, Doenitz C, Luerding R, Brawanski A. Awake craniotomies without any sedation: the awake-awake-awake technique. Acta Neurochir. 2013;**155**:1417–24.

56. Ard JL, Bekker AY, Doyle WK. Dexmedetomidine in awake craniotomy: a technical note. Surg Neurol. 2005;**63**:114–17.

57. Zornow MH, Maze M, Dyck JB, Shaker SL. Dexmedetomidine decreases cerebral blood flow velocity in humans. J Cereb Blood Flow Metab. 1993;**13**:350–53.

58. Hassan WMZW, Lukman MH, Mukmin LA, Idris Z, Ghani ARI, Zaini RHM. Awake craniotomy: a case series of anaesthetic management using a combination of scalp block, dexmedetomidine and remifentanil in hospital University Sains Malaysia. Med J Malaysia. 2013;**68**:64–66.

59. Rajan S, Cata JP, Nada E, Weil R, Pal R, Avitsian R. Asleep-awake-asleep craniotomy: a comparison with general anesthesia for resection of supratentorial tumors. J Clin Neurosci. 2013;**20**:1068–73.

60. Lettieri C, Rinaldo S, Devigili G, et al. Deep brain stimulation: subthalamic nucleus electrophysiological activity in awake and anesthetized patients. Clin Neurophysiol. 2012;**123**:2406–13.

61. Bochicchio GV, Joshi M, Bochicchio K, et al. Impact of obesity in the critically ill trauma patient: a prospective study. J Am Coll Surg. 2006;**203**:533–38.

62. Choban PS, Heckler R, Burge JC, Flancbaum L. Increased incidence of nosocomial infections in obese surgical patients. Am Surg. 1995;**61**:1001–1005.

63. Ciesla DJ, Moore EE, Johnson JL, Burch JM, Cothren CC, Sauaia A. Obesity increases risk of organ failure after severe trauma. J Am Coll Surg. 2006;**203**:539–45.

64. Strandberg A, Tokics L, Brismar B, et al. Constitutional factors promoting developmental of atelectasis during anesthesia. Acta Anesthesiol Scand. 1987;**31**:21–24

65. Eichenberger A, Proietti S, Wicky S, et al. Morbid obesity and postoperative pulmonary atelectasis: an underestimated problem. Anesth Analg. 2002;**95**:1788–92.

66. Bamgbade OA, Rutter TW, Nafiu OO, Dorje P. Postoperative complications in obese and nonobese patients. World J Surg. 2007;**31**:556–61.

67. Namba RS, Paxton L, Fithian DC, Stone ML. Obesity and perioperative morbidity in total hip and total knee arthroplasty patients. J Arthroplasty. 2005;**20**:46–50.

68. Wigfield CH, Lindsey JD, Munoz A, et al. Is extreme obesity a risk factor for cardiac surgery? An analysis of patients with a BMI >40. Eur J Cardiothorac Surg. 2006;**9**:34–40.

69. Flum DR, Belle SH, King WC, et al. Perioperative safety in the longitudinal assessment of bariatric surgery. N Engl J Med. 2009;**361**:445–54.

70. Flier S, Knape JT. How to inform a morbidly obese patient on the specific risk to develop postoperative pulmonary complications

using evidence-based methodology. Eur J Anaesthesiol. 2006;**23**:154–59.

71. Nasraway SA Jr, Albert M, Donnelly AM, et al. Morbid obesity is an independent determinant of death among surgical critically ill patients. Crit Care Med. 2006;**34**:964–70.

72. Boulanger BR, Milzman D, Mitchell K, Rodriguez A. Body habitus as a predictor of injury pattern after blunt trauma. J Trauma. 1992;**33**:228–32.

73. Brown CV, Rhee P, Neville AL, Sangthong B, Salim A, Demetriades D. Obesity and traumatic brain injury. J Trauma. 2006;**61**:572–76.

74. Chidambaran V, Tewari A, Mahmoud M. Anesthetic and pharmacologic considerations in perioperative care of obese children. J Clin Anesth. 2018;**45**:39–50.

75. Aghi MK, Eskandar EN, Carter BS, Curry WT Jr, Barker FG 2nd. Increased prevalence of obesity and obesity-related postoperative complications in male patients with meningiomas. Neurosurgery. 2007;**61**:754–60.

76. Capen DA, Calderone RR, Green A. Perioperative risk factors for wound infections after lower back fusions. Orthop Clin North Am. 1996;**27**:83–86.

77. Friedman ND, Sexton DJ, Connelly SM, Kaye KS. Risk factors for surgical site infection complicating laminectomy. Infect Control Hosp Epidemiol. 2007;**28**:1060–65.

78. Gepstein R, Shabat S, Arinzon ZH, et al. Does obesity affect the results of lumbar decompressive spinal surgery in the elderly? Clin Orthop Relat Res. 2004;**426**:138–44.

79. Telfeian A, Reiter T, Durham SR, Marcotte P. Spine surgery in morbidly obese patients. J Neurosurg. 2002;**97**:20–24.

80. Olsen MA, Nepple JJ, Riew KD, et al. Risk factors for surgical site infection following orthopaedic spinal operations. J Bone Joint Surg Am. 2008;**90**:62–69.

81. Wimmer C, Gluch H, Franzreb M, Ogon M. Predisposing factors for infection in spine surgery: a survey of 850 spinal procedures. J Spinal Disord. 1998;**11**:124–28.

82. Olsen MA, Mayfield J, Lauryssen C, et al. Risk factors for surgical site infection in spinal surgery. J Neurosurg. 2003;**98**:149–55.

83. Takrouri MSM, Shubbak F, Al-Musrea K, Ghanem N. Problems faced during anesthesia in morbidly obese patient with cervical injury presented for fixation in prone position. Internet J Anesthesiol. 2008;**19**:1–4.

84. Shamji M, Parker S, Cook C, et al. Impact of body habitus on perioperative morbidity associated with fusion of the thoracolumbar and lumbar spine. Neurosurgery. 2009;**65**:490–98.

85. Rosen D, Ferguson S, Ogden A, et al. Obesity and self-reported outcome after minimally invasive lumbar spinal fusion surgery. Neurosurgery. 2008;**63**:956–60.

86. Schultheiss KE, Jang YG, Yanowitch RN, et al. Fat and neurosurgery: does obesity affect outcome after intracranial surgery? Neurosurgery. 2009;**64**:316–27.

87. Juvela S, Siironen J, Kuhmonen J. Hyperglycemia, excess weight, and history of hypertension as risk factors for poor outcome and cerebral infarction after aneurysmal subarachnoid hemorrhage. J Neurosurg. 2005;**102**:998–1003.

88. Juvela S, Siironen J, Varis J, Poussa K, Porras M. Risk factors for ischemic lesions following aneurysmal subarachnoid hemorrhage. J Neurosurg. 2005;**102**:194–201.

89. Feigin V, Parag V, Lawes CM, et al. Smoking and elevated blood pressure are the most important risk factors for subarachnoid hemorrhage in the Asia-Pacific region: an overview of 26 cohorts involving 306,620 participants. Stroke. 2005;**36**:1360–65.

90. Suh I, Jee SH, Kim HC, et al. Low serum cholesterol and haemorrhagic stroke in men: Korea Medical Insurance Corporation Study. Lancet. 2001;**357**:922–25.

91. Broderick JP, Viscoli CM, Brott T, et al. Major risk factors for aneurysmal subarachnoid hemorrhage in the young are modifiable. Stroke. 2003;**34**:1375–81.

92. Yamada S, Koizumi A, Iso H, et al. Japan Collaborative Cohort Study Group: Risk factors for fatal subarachnoid hemorrhage: the Japan Collaborative Cohort Study. Stroke. 2003;**34**:2781–88.

SECTION 4
Bariatric surgery

Patient selection and overview of selected procedures

Matthew E. Pontell, Alvaro Galvez, Elizabeth Renza-Stigone, and Andres Castellanos[†]

Patient selection

The surgical management of morbid obesity is a rapidly evolving practice, the indications for which continue to be the subject of discussion as long-term outcomes from these procedures become available. In the United States, the National Institutes of Health published an initial consensus statement in 1991 regarding the indications for bariatric surgery [1]. In 2013, the American Association of Clinical Endocrinologists, The Obesity Society and the American Society for Metabolic and Bariatric Surgery published a consensus update [2]. Current indications for bariatric surgery include the following: patients with a body mass index (BMI) of at least 40 kg/m² who are reasonable candidates for surgery (grade A), patients with a BMI of at least 35 kg/m² with at least one severe comorbid condition associated with morbid obesity (Table 15.1) [3–8], and patients with a BMI between 30 and 34.9 kg/m² with type 2 diabetes mellitus or metabolic syndrome [2–6]. It should be noted that there is a lack of long-term data demonstrating a net benefit for those patients who fall within the last indication, and there is insufficient evidence to recommend weight loss surgery for the management of cardiovascular disease risk, glycaemic control, and/or lipid control [3–6].

Table 15.1 Table depicting the comorbid conditions qualifying a patient for bariatric surgery when their BMI falls between 35 and 39.9 kg/m²

Comorbid conditions associated with morbid obesity	
Diabetes mellitus type 2	Non-alcoholic fatty liver disease
Hypertension	Non-alcoholic steatohepatitis
Obstructive sleep apnoea	Debilitating arthritis
Obesity hypoventilation syndrome	Severe urinary incontinence
Pickwickian syndrome (obstructive sleep apnoea and obesity hypoventilation syndrome)	Pseudotumor cerebri
	Gastro-oesophageal reflux disease
	Hyperlipidaemia
Severe asthma	
Polycystic ovary syndrome	

This consensus statement also recommends weight reduction surgery for patients with a BMI greater than 35 kg/m² with therapeutic goals that consist of weight control and reduction of cardiovascular risk factors (grade A) [2]. Grade B evidence supports offering bariatric surgery with the same therapeutic intention for patients with a BMI between 30 and 34.9 kg/m², while grade C evidence supports bariatric surgery for patients within this BMI range with the intention to improve glycaemic control [2]. As of 2014, new recommendations from the National Institute for Health and Care Excellence (United Kingdom) have expanded the criteria for patient selection to include any patient with a BMI of at least 35 kg/m² with type 2 diabetes diagnosed within the last 10 years [7]. Other authors also advocate for weight loss surgery in patients with a BMI between 30 and 34.9 kg/m² [7].

The aforementioned criteria for selection do not ensure the best outcomes and these recommendations require a thorough, multidisciplinary preoperative assessment. The multidisciplinary team should, at a minimum include nutritionists, mental health professionals (psychologists and/or psychiatrists), and medical subspecialists with specialized training in bariatric medicine and surgery. All known comorbidities should be assessed and treatment plans should be optimized prior to surgery. Workup should also be undertaken in attempts to unmask occult cardiopulmonary, gastrointestinal, psychological, and psychiatric disease processes [1,8].

At our institution, preoperative planning takes anywhere from 3 to 6 months, depending on the patient's insurance requirements and the length of mandatory nutritional counselling suggested. All patients must attend a weight loss surgery seminar prior to initial consultation. We find this helps to select out patients who are simply looking for a quick solution to their problem. All patients undergo a comprehensive medical evaluation during this time period and are evaluated by cardiology, pulmonology, psychiatry, and gastroenterology specialists who then dictate the appropriate workup required before proceeding with surgery.

---

† It is with great regret that we report the death of Andres Castellanos during the production of this textbook.

In the immediate preoperative period, we recommend 'liver-shrinking', high-protein, liquid diets for 2 weeks prior to surgery for patients with BMIs of 40–55 kg/m², based on surgeon preference. We routinely administer weight-based enoxaparin 30 minutes prior to incision, apply sequential compression devices perioperatively, and encourage early postoperative ambulation in all patients to decrease the risk of pulmonary embolism. Postoperatively, follow-up appointments are conducted at 1–2 weeks, 4 weeks, 3 months, 6 months, 9 months, 1 year, and anywhere in between should the patients be experiencing difficulty. Support groups are run monthly by our bariatric nurse coordinator and they are routinely attended by patients in the post- and preoperative periods.

Contraindications to bariatric surgery are only relative and are similar to most other elective procedures. They include severe heart failure, unstable coronary artery disease, uncontrolled drug and/or alcohol dependency, active psychiatric disease, severe intellectual dysfunction, cirrhosis with concomitant portal hypertension, end-stage lung disease, and an active diagnosis of cancer. With regard to bariatric surgery specifically, preoperative factors indicating a high-risk for postoperative complications include male sex, BMI greater than 45 kg/m², hypertension, right heart failure, obesity hypoventilation syndrome, or a history of inferior vena cava filter placement [9]. Additionally, the morbidly obese have increased risk for pulmonary embolism; prior diagnoses of vascular thrombosis and/or pulmonary embolus confer elevated risks to individual patients.

Overview of selected procedures

Introduction

The field of weight loss surgery has evolved appreciably over the past years, and it continues to do so. The surgical procedures that served as the forefront of this field have been continuously modified to create those that are employed in current practice. Despite the numerous options available to the surgeon, there is still no evidence-based algorithm recommending one procedure over another, nor is there a proven, single best surgical option [8]. Procedure selection ultimately depends on many factors, including goals of therapy, weight loss desired, metabolic and/or glycaemic control, personalized risk stratification, presence or absence of certain comorbidities, and the expertise of the attending surgeon [10–12]. In general, the laparoscopic approach is favoured over the open approach due to the lower morbidity in the postoperative period and the lower risk of mortality [9]. In addition, the laparoscopic approach also offers the benefit of a decreased incidence of wound infection and postoperative incisional hernias, which are exceptionally common in the morbidly obese population [8]. It is generally accepted that those patients starting with a BMI greater than 50 kg/m² have high rates of weight loss failure with restrictive procedures and, as such, are often recommended procedures with at least some component of malabsorption [8]. Ultimately, the final decision rests in the hands of the patient and the surgeon should recommend deciding only after proper information has been obtained from official seminars, preoperative consultations, and independent research [13]. Family support also plays a critical role in the preoperative and postoperative periods. The three most commonly practised procedures are the laparoscopic adjustable gastric band (LAGB), the laparoscopic

sleeve gastrectomy (LSG), and the laparoscopic Roux-en-Y gastric bypass (RYGB) [14,15].

Common practice

Laparoscopic adjustable gastric band

The LAGB was introduced in the 1920s, and it was one of the three most commonly practised procedures in the field of surgical weight loss. Nationally, the rates of LAGB have fallen in the past 10 years as the sleeve gastrectomy has become more common. The operation begins with the creation of a retrogastric tunnel. An orogastric calibration balloon is then inserted through the oral cavity and inflated with 15 mL of normal saline once the balloon has passed into the stomach. The calibration balloon is withdrawn until it catches at the gastro-oesophageal junction. The gastric band is then placed through the retrogastric window around the proximal stomach just below the intragastric calibration balloon. The calibrator is deflated and extracted and the laparoscopic band is secured in place. Using interrupted sutures, the stomach is imbricated over the band to further secure it in place. The tubing connected to the band is then brought out through one of the port incisions and connected to a subcutaneous calibration port (**Fig. 15.1**) [16].

The LAGB is attractive to patients as it is completely reversible. This allows the patient to opt for a conversion to an alternate procedure, should it be recommended or required later [17,18]. The band functions in a restrictive manner by inducing the sensation of early satiety secondary to a decreased functional stomach capacity.

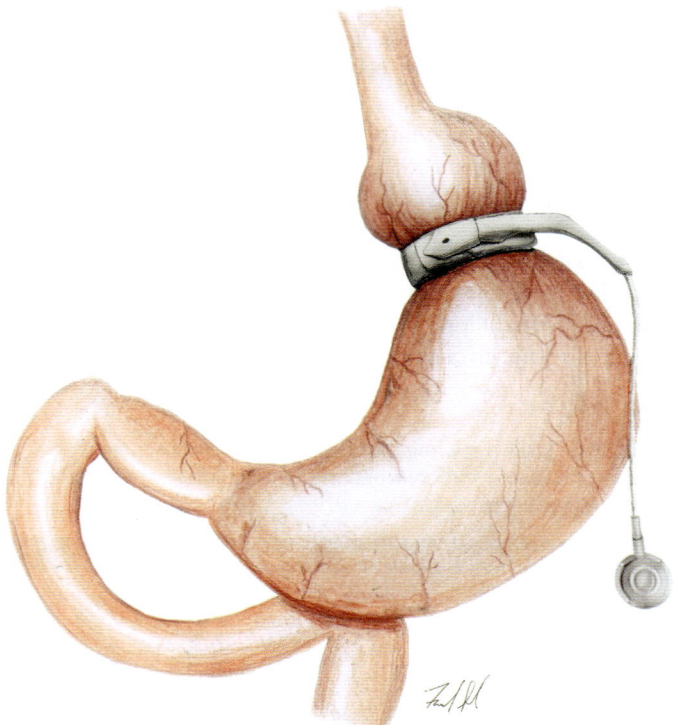

Fig. 15.1 Artist's representation of the LAGB. A resizable band (a) is secured around the stomach below the gastro-oesophageal junction creating a restricted gastric pouch (b). The band is connected to the subcutaneous port via saline-filled tubing.

Reproduced courtesy of Frank Scali, Matthew E. Pontell, and Alvaro Galvez.

The port is accessed by the clinician on subsequent follow-up visits, and saline is added to adjust the size of the patient's band based on satiety and/or weight loss progression. These adjustments amplify weight loss throughout the postoperative period as the body adapts to the change in stomach size [9]. As expected, this procedure mandates close and lifelong follow-up, an often-difficult request [9]. The LAGB is an effective option for patients of any BMI [9]; however, we do not routinely offer the procedure at our institution due to the high rate of complications, loss to follow-up, and lack of successful weight loss. Additionally, it is highly dependent on patient eating habits and the restrictive component can be overcome by maintaining a diet rich in high-calorie liquids and soft foods that undergo substantial liquefaction prior to reaching the gastro-oesophageal junction. These foods are digested early on and are not restricted by the newly constructed gastric outlet.

Laparoscopic sleeve gastrectomy

The LSG was first performed in the late 1980s as a first-step procedure prior to the completion of the biliopancreatic diversion. In the late 1990s it became a primary procedure and is now routinely offered to those patients considering weight loss surgery [8]. The LSG is performed by entering the abdomen laparoscopically and identifying the pylorus. In an area roughly 5–6 cm proximal to the pylorus, the short gastric vessels are ligated, often with electrocautery or ultrasound technology. Once haemostasis has been achieved, the temperature probe and nasogastric tube are removed and a bougie catheter is inserted through the oral cavity to the pylorus. The exact size of the bougie catheter is a matter of debate; however, anywhere from a 32- to a 40-French catheter is considered acceptable in current practice. A cutting stapler is than used to excise the lateral stomach, using the bougie catheter to calibrate the size of the remaining 'gastric sleeve'. Special care is taken to ensure that the bougie catheter is not included in the staple line, and some surgeons will also perform a leak test using insufflation (**Fig. 15.2**) [19].

This procedure induces weight loss in a restrictive fashion by decreasing stomach capacity. It also removes the majority of the stomach fundus which houses the glands responsible for ghrelin-mediated appetite stimulation [8]. LSG also may be performed as a primary weight loss procedure or as a first step in high-risk patients eventually being considered for RYGB or biliopancreatic diversion with duodenal switch (BPD-DS) [20]. It also plays a special role in patients considered relatively poor surgical candidates or those who do not wish to undergo intestinal rearrangement. Certain centres will also offer LSG to patients requiring organ transplantation or joint replacement, as transplant surgeons and orthopaedists will often not operate on patients with a BMI of 40 kg/m² or greater. LSG has been safely performed in patients with cirrhosis without severe portal hypertension, patients with dense adhesions from multiple past abdominal surgeries, and it is also an excellent option for patients anticipating future intestinal surgery secondary to a history of diverticulosis or inflammatory bowel disease. Complications such as marginal ulceration and internal herniation are non-existent; whereas with RYGB, micronutrient and pharmacological malabsorption are frequently a concern [21]. The LSG offers less alteration to the normal digestive process.

Relative contraindications to the LSG include severe gastro-oesophageal reflux disease with or without concomitant Barrett's

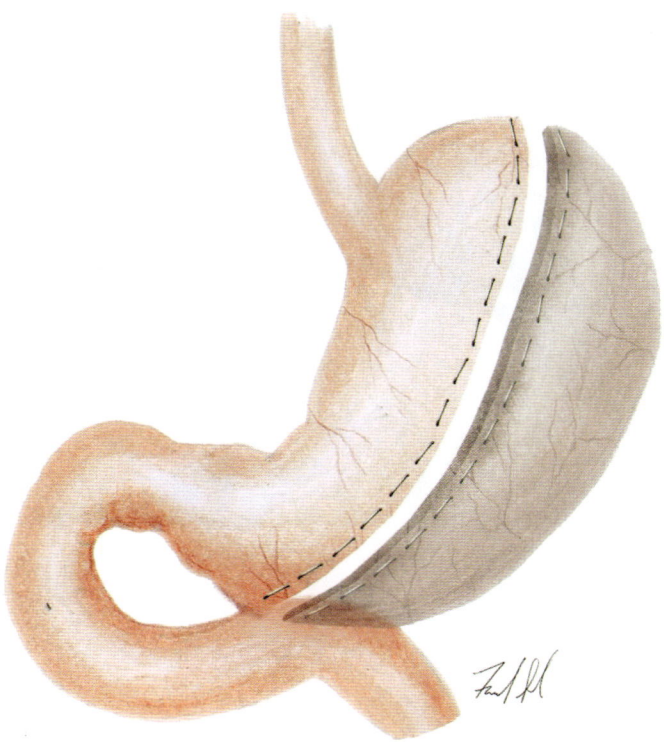

Fig. 15.2 Artist's representation of the LSG. The stomach is devascularized from the short gastric blood supply (a) and a cutting stapler is passed from a point 5–6 cm proximal to the pylorus (b) towards the angle of His (c) alongside a calibrating bougie catheter.
Reproduced courtesy of Frank Scali, Matthew E. Pontell, and Alvaro Galvez.

oesophagus. The sleeve is thought to create a high-pressure system thereby exaggerating pre-existing gastro-oesophageal reflux disease. Any condition which may eventually necessitate an esophagectomy, that is, Barrett's oesophagus with high-grade dysplasia or an oesophageal neoplasm, is also a contraindication for LSG. Aside from the general increase in mortality, patients with Child's B or C cirrhosis with coexisting severe portal hypertension are not good candidates for LSG due to the potential increase in portal pressures once the venous capacitance is decreased with ligation of the short gastric vessels [8].

Roux-en-Y gastric bypass

The first version of the gastric bypass was performed in the late 1960s. The procedure began with a partial gastrectomy, creating a 150 mL gastric pouch, and was completed with the creation of a loop gastrojejunostomy [8]. This version of the procedure was frequently complicated by bile reflux gastritis and was subsequently converted to its current form. The RYGB is most commonly performed by entering the abdomen laparoscopically and may be performed as a primary procedure or secondarily due to a failed primary procedure (i.e. vertical banded gastroplasty (VBG) or LAGB).

The RYGB begins with the identification of the ligament of Treitz. The jejunum is then divided 30–50 cm distal to the ligament and the biliopancreatic limb is anastomosed in an end-to-side fashion 75–150 cm distal to the initial jejunal transection. This allows for a common channel of several metres. The Roux limb is then brought into the epigastrium via an ante- or retrocolic route.

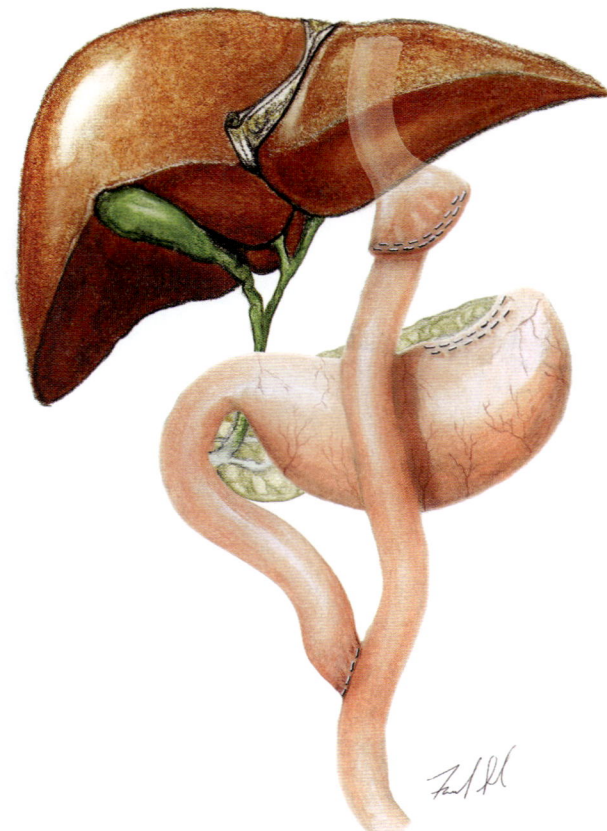

Fig. 15.3 Artist's representation of the Roux-en-Y gastric bypass as it is performed today. The jejunum is transected 30–50 cm distal to the ligament of Treitz and the jejuno-jejunostomy is created 75–150 cm distal to the original jejunal transection (a). A 15–20 mL gastric pouch is created (b) and the gastric remnant is left in its anatomical position (c). The Roux limb is then anastomosed to the gastric pouch (d).
Reproduced courtesy of Frank Scali, Matthew E. Pontell, and Alvaro Galvez.

The Roux limb can be adjusted based on patient BMI (i.e. longer Roux limbs are created for more obese patients). At this point, the gastro-oesophageal junction is exposed, a retrogastric window is created, all temperature probes and nasogastric tubes are extracted, and using a cutting stapler a 15–20 mL gastric pouch is created. The gastric remnant is left in its anatomical position. The Roux limb is anastomosed to the gastric pouch and a leak test is frequently performed by submerging the gastrojejunostomy in sterile saline and insufflating the anastomosis with an endoscope or an orogastric tube (**Fig. 15.3**) [8].

This intestinal configuration combines the restrictive effects of a small gastric pouch with the malabsorptive effects of the Roux-en-Y anastomosis. Aside from bypassing 75–150 cm of intestinal absorption, delivery of nutrients to the distal small bowel has been shown to trigger an amplified incretin response, thereby stimulating pancreatic beta cells as well as mediators of satiety [8]. There currently exists level II evidence suggesting that the creation of long Roux limbs (>150 cm) may improve weight loss in the immediate postoperative period. However, long Roux limbs may also be associated with more severe nutritional complications [9]. The National Institutes of Health currently recommends the RYGB as the 'gold standard' for patients with BMI's greater than 40 kg/m² with or without comorbid conditions

[1,8]. Given the theoretical 'low-pressure' gastrojejunostomy, it is frequently recommended for candidates with severe preoperative gastro-oesophageal reflux disease [8]. At our institution we routinely offer this procedure to those who are reasonable surgical candidates and have severe preoperative gastro-oesophageal reflux disease and/ or a propensity towards snacking on foods with high caloric and sugar contents. We find that postoperative dumping syndrome serves as a strong deterrent of dietary relapses.

Biliopancreatic diversion with duodenal switch

The biliopancreatic diversion was further modified from its initial form to include a duodenal switch (BPD-DS). The addition of the duodenal switch component assists in reducing postoperative marginal ulceration and dumping syndrome, side effects frequently seen with BPD [9]. The BPD-DS was first performed in the late 1990s and can be performed as either a single-stage procedure or a two-stage procedure, the first stage consisting of a vertical sleeve gastrectomy alone [8,9]. The remainder of the procedure involves first transecting the duodenum just distal to the first portion and then transecting the ileum at a site roughly 150–200 cm distal to the ligament of Treitz. The first portion of the duodenum remains in continuity with the stomach 'sleeve' and it is then anastomosed to the distal aspect of the transected ileum. The biliopancreatic limb is then anastomosed in an end-to-side fashion with the distal ileum leaving a common channel of roughly 50–100 cm [9,22] (**Fig. 15.4**).

The BPD-DS has both a restrictive and large malabsorptive component and while beneficial, these patients are at a greater risk of nutrient deficiency due to the large amount of small intestinal absorptive surface area that is bypassed [9,22]. As such, these patients are required to demonstrate understanding of these risks preoperatively and undergo close postoperative surveillance with rigorous nutrient supplementation and dietary modification [8,9]. The BPD-DS is a very effective weight loss procedure, especially in the super-obese and those who have failed previous attempts at weight loss surgery [23,24]. Despite the potential for a greater degree of weight loss, the BPD-DS is associated with significant perioperative morbidity and it claims the highest mortality rate of any bariatric procedure [9]. For the aforementioned reasons, this procedure is not routinely performed at our institution, but is performed with success at other institutions in the region.

Historical perspectives

Jejunoileal bypass

It is worthwhile to mention the procedures that have fallen out of favour, as they serve as the foundations of the more commonplace operations performed today. One of the first procedures in the field of weight loss surgery was the jejunoileal bypass. This procedure was performed by identifying the ligament of Treitz and dividing the jejunum at a point roughly 35 cm distal to this site. The jejunal segment in continuity with the duodenum was then anastomosed to a segment of ileum at about 10 cm proximal to the ileocecal valve (**Fig. 15.5**). This procedure's efficacy was based on the significant malabsorptive component; however, it was fraught with severe side effects such as bacterial overgrowth of the bypassed intestinal segment, vitamin deficiency, and hepatic and/or renal failure. As a result of the morbidity associated with this operation, it was largely abandoned in the 1960s [8].

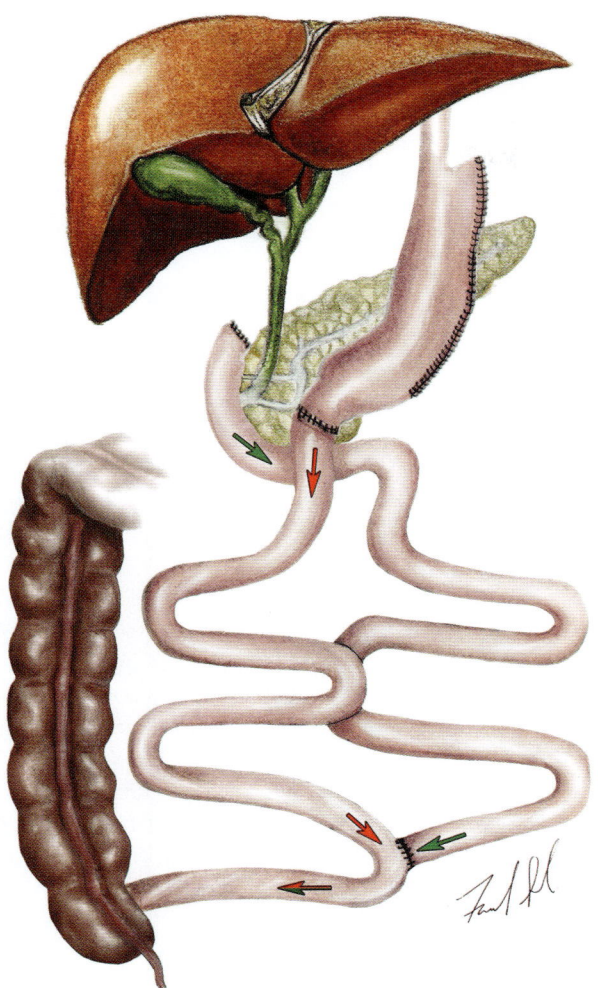

Fig. 15.4 Artist's representation of the biliopancreatic diversion with duodenal switch. A sleeve gastrectomy is performed (a) followed by a duodenal transection between the first and second portions. The ileum is also transected at a location roughly 150–200 cm distal from the ligament of Treitz. A duodeno-ileostomy (b) and a jejuno-ileostomy (c) are then created leaving a common channel of 50–100 cm (d).
Reproduced courtesy of Frank Scali, Matthew E. Pontell, and Alvaro Galvez.

Biliopancreatic diversion

The BPD was a procedure developed to ameliorate the postoperative complications of the jejunoileal bypass, while maximizing the efficacious components. It involves performing a distal gastrectomy with division of the pyloroduodenal junction. The jejunum is than divided at a site roughly 30–40 cm from the ligament of Treitz and a Roux limb is then brought up and anastomosed to the remaining stomach. The biliopancreatic limb is than anastomosed to the Roux limb 250 cm distal to the gastrojejunal anastomosis, leaving roughly 50 cm of a common channel proximal to the ileocecal valve. This procedure maintained the malabsorptive component of the jejunoileal bypass while also adding a restrictive component by including a partial gastrectomy. In addition, the blind loop was eliminated therefore decreasing the risk of bacterial overgrowth and the antral resection also afforded the benefit of decreased gastric acid secretion and subsequently a lesser risk of marginal ulceration. This procedure was further revised prior to its currently adopted form [8].

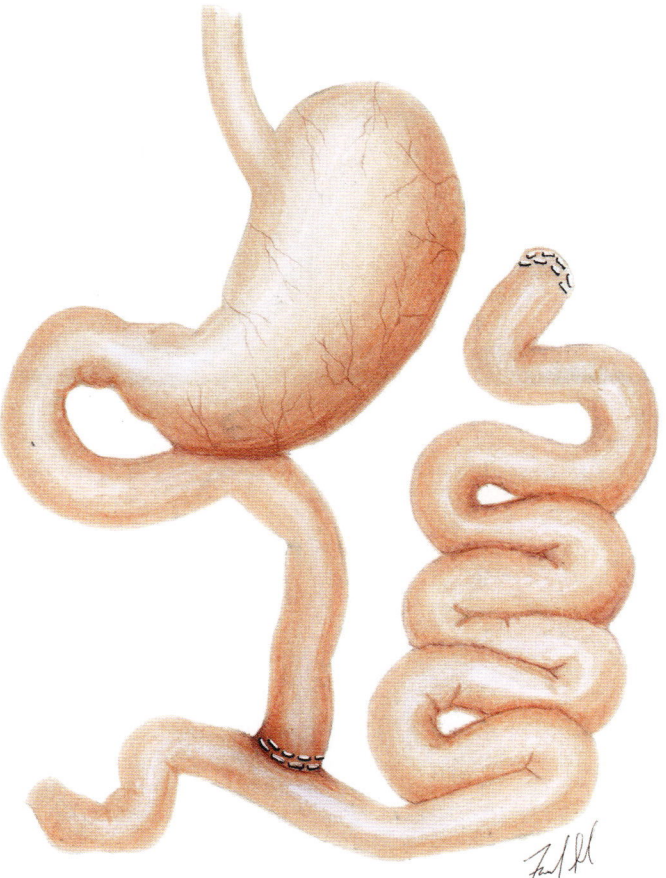

Fig. 15.5 Artist's representation of the jejunoileal bypass. The jejunum is divided at roughly 35 cm from the ligament of Treitz and anastomosed to a segment of ileum approximately ten cm proximal to the ileocecal valve (a).
Reproduced courtesy of Frank Scali, Matthew E. Pontell, and Alvaro Galvez.

Vertical banded gastroplasty

The final procedure worth mentioning in this section is the VBG. Created in 1982, the technique involved first making a small passage through the stomach several centimetres inferior and lateral to the gastro-oesophageal junction using a circular stapler. A non-cutting stapler is then fired superior to the circular window towards the angle of His. A piece of mesh, often polypropylene, is then passed through the circular passage and wrapped round the medial portion of the stomach below the gastro-oesophageal junction creating a gastric 'pouch' which is roughly 10% of the size of the normal stomach (**Fig. 15.6**). This restrictive procedure induces early satiety without affecting the normal physiology of digestion. However, patients can overcome the restrictive component by adopting poor eating habits, similar to those mentioned in the section on LAGB. VBG was abandoned due to high failure rates resulting from maladaptive eating patterns and complications such as staple line dehiscence, pouch enlargement, and mesh erosion. Patients with a history of VBG are frequently seen in clinic with a chief complaint of persistent weight gain or chronic abdominal pain and revision to either a RYGB or a duodenal switch is recommended at that time [25,26].

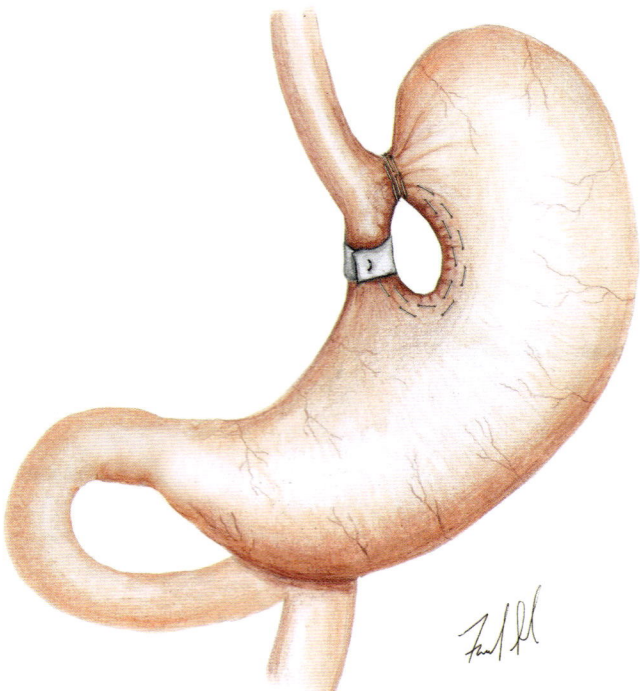

Fig. 15.6 A diagrammatic representation of the vertical banded gastroplasty. A window is created through the stomach using a circular stapler (a). A non-cutting stapler is then passed from the window towards the angle of His (b) creating two lumens. A polypropylene mesh is than inserted through the window (c) and passed medially creating a functional stomach roughly 10% of the size of the normal stomach (d). Reproduced courtesy of Frank Scali, Matthew E. Pontell, and Alvaro Galvez.

CASE REPORT Oesophageal dilatation and Barrett's oesophagus after laparoscopic adjustable gastric banding

Introduction
LAGB is a procedure practised for the treatment of obesity, gaining approval from the Food and Drug Administration in the United States in 2001. Although it enjoyed huge success during its introduction due to minimal invasiveness, reversibility, and adjustability, it has now fallen out of favour due to growing reports of complications and unsatisfactory long-term weight loss [27].

Case presentation
We present a 49-year-old female who underwent gastric banding in 2008. She lost approximately 45 kg in 5 years, but comes to bariatric clinic complaining of pyrosis, dyspepsia, epigastric pain, and intermittent nausea and vomiting despite proton pump inhibitor therapy. She weighed 76.5 kg lbs, her BMI was 27.4 kg/m². Band intolerance was diagnosed and 4 mL of saline were removed, completely deflating her band. All symptoms resolved.

She would return to clinic several times for 2 years requesting band reinflation due to weight gain and deflation due to intolerance. Finally, the band was completely deflated and removal was discussed.

Three years from her initial visit she is admitted with an unrelated problem but the bariatric surgical team was consulted given continued band intolerance despite complete deflation. An oesophagogastroduodenoscopy 3 months prior found Barrett's

oesophagus without dysplasia, distal oesophageal dilatation, and pooling of alimentary content on the gastric pouch proximal to the gastric band.

A repeat oesophagogastroduodenoscopy reported the same findings and removal was offered to resolve her symptoms and halt Barrett's oesophagus progression. The patient refused conversion to another bariatric procedure. She underwent uneventful laparoscopic removal and was discharged the next day.

An outpatient visit 2 weeks later showed healing of incision sites and complete resolution of pain, regurgitation, and nausea.

Discussion
Gastric banding is a restrictive bariatric procedure that limits food intake for weight loss. An adjustable silicone belt is laparoscopically implanted around the gastric cardia to create a gastric 'pouch'. The band is connected to a silicone port, implanted in the subcutaneous tissue of the abdomen. The amount of restriction can be adjusted by injecting saline into the port.

Gastric banding currently accounts for 17.8% of all bariatric procedures performed in the United States, third after the RYGB (46.6%) and the LSG (27.8%). It has steeply fallen out of favour (42.3% of all procedures performed up to 2008 to 17.8% reported in 2011), mainly due to concerns with weight regain and a high rate of early and late complications [28].

Early complications include acute stomal obstruction, band infection, gastric perforation, haemorrhage, intractable nausea and vomiting, and delayed gastric emptying due to dyskinesia. Late complications described include band erosion, slippage, infection, port and band malfunction, and oesophageal dilatation with esophagitis [29]. Reoperation rates range from 16% to 60% and have been shown to increase proportionally with time [30–32]. Weight loss has also overall proven unsatisfactory, especially with patients suffering super-obesity (BMI >50 kg/m²). A study published in 2011 mentions only 8% of 144 patients achieving 50% of the estimated weight loss in 1 year [32]. If the patient needs a reoperation to remove the band, a conversion to another bariatric procedure can be safely performed and is typically offered.

We present a patient who suffered two well-described late mechanical complications of LAGB, for which we performed laparoscopic removal. Given recent literature we encourage surgeons to inform patients of recent data and suggest either LSG or RYGB to patients, especially those with higher BMIs, in hopes of better long-term outcomes and fewer complications.

REFERENCES

1. National Institutes of Health. Gastrointestinal surgery for severe obesity: consensus statement. NIH Consens Dev Conf Consens Statement. 1991;**9**(1):1–10.

2. Mechanick JI, Youdim A, Jones DB, et al. Clinical practice guidelines for the perioperative nutritional, metabolic and nonsurgical support of the bariatric surgery patient—2013 Update: cosponsored by American Association of Clinical Endocrinologists, The Obesity Society, and American Society for Metabolic and Bariatric Surgery. Surg Obes Relat Dis. 2013;**9**(2):159–91.

3. Ogden CL, Carroll MD, Kit BK, et al. Prevalence of obesity in the United States, 2009–2020. NCHS Data Brief. 2012;**82**:1–8.

4. Berrington de Gonzalez A, Hartge P, Cerhan JR, et al. Body-mass index and mortality among 1.46 million white adults. N Engl J Med. 2010;**363**(23):2211–19. Erratum in: N Engl J Med. 2011;365(9):869.

5. Mechanick JI, Garber AJ, Handelsman Y, et al. American Association of Clinical Endocrinologists (AACE) position paper on obesity and obesity medicine. Endocr Pract. 2012;**18**(5):642–48.

6. Ryan DH, Johnson WD, Myers VH, et al. Nonsurgical weight loss for extreme obesity in primary care settings: results of the Louisiana Obese Subjects Study. Arch Intern Med. 2010;**170**(2):146–54.

7. National Institute for Health and Care Excellence. Obesity: Identification, Assessment and Management of Overweight and Obesity in Children, Young People and Adults. Clinical Guideline 43. London: National Institute for Health and Care Excellence; 2014.

8. Fischer JE. Morbid obesity. In: Fischer JE, ed. Fischer's Mastery of Surgery. 6th ed. Philadelphia, PA: Wolters Kluwer Health/ Lippincott Williams & Wilkins; 2012:1097–50.

9. SAGES. Guidelines for clinical application of laparoscopic bariatric surgery. 2008. http://www.sages.org/publications/guidelines/guidelines-for-clinical-application-of-laparoscopic-bariatric-surgery/

10. Livingston EH. The incidence of bariatric surgery has plateaued in the U.S. Am J Surg. 2010;**200**(3):378–85.

11. American Society for Metabolic and Bariatric Surgery. Metabolic and bariatric surgery. 2013. https://asmbs.org/resources/metabolic-and-bariatric-surgery

12. Mechanick JI, Kushner RF, Sugerman HJ, et al. American Association of Clinical Endocrinologists, The Obesity Society, and the American Society for Metabolic & Bariatric Surgery medical guidelines for clinical practice for the perioperative nutritional, metabolic, and nonsurgical support of the bariatric surgery patient. Endocr Pract. 2008;14 Suppl 1:1–83.

13. Weinstein AL, Marascalchi BJ, Spiegel MA, et al. Patient preferences and bariatric surgery procedure selection; the need for shared decision-making. Obes Surg. 2014;**24**(11):1933–39.

14. Hutter MM, Schirmer BD, Jones D, et al. First report from the American College of Surgeons Bariatric Surgery Center network: laparoscopic sleeve gastrectomy has morbidity and effectiveness positioned between the band and the bypass. Ann Surg. 2011;**254**(3):410–20.

15. Tice J, Karliner L, Walsh J, et al. Gastric banding or bypass? A systematic review comparing the two most popular bariatric procedures. Am J Med. 2008;**121**(10):885–93.

16. Ren CJ, Fielding GA. Laparoscopic adjustable gastric banding: surgical technique. J Laparoendosc Adv Surg Tech A. 2003;**13**(4):257–63.

17. Allen JW, Coleman MG, Fielding GA. Lessons learned from laparoscopic gastric banding for morbid obesity. Am J Surg. 2001;**182**(1):10–14.

18. Dixon JB, O'Brien PE. Selecting the optimal patient for lap-band placement. Am J Surg. 2002;184 Suppl 6B:S17–20.

19. Roa PE, Kaldar-Person O, Pinto D, et al. Laparoscopic sleeve gastrectomy as treatment for morbid obesity: technique and short-term outcome. Obes Surg. 2006;**16**(10):1323–26.

20. Regan JP, Inabnet WB, Gagner M, et al. Early experience with two-stage laparoscopic Roux-en-Y gastric bypass as an alternative in the super-super obese patient. Obes Surg. 2003;**13**(6):861–64.

21. Tucker O, Szomstein S, Rosenthal RJ. Indications for sleeve gastrectomy as a primary procedure for weight loss in the morbidly obese. J Gastrointest Surg. 2008;**12**(4):662–67.

22. Anthone GJ, Lord R, DeMeester TR, et al. The duodenal switch operation for the treatment of morbid obesity. Ann Surg. 2003;**238**(4):618–27.

23. Prachand VN, DaVee RT, Alverdy JC. Duodenal switch provides superior weight loss in the super-obese (BMI > or = 50 kg/m²) compared with gastric bypass. Ann Surg. 2006;**244**(4):611–19.

24. Suvik TT, Taha O, Aasheim ET, et al. Randomized clinical trial of laparoscopic gastric bypass versus laparoscopic duodenal switch for super obesity. Br J Surg. 2010;**97**(2):160–66.

25. Behrns KE, Smith CD, Kelly KA, et al. Reoperative bariatric surgery. Lessons learned to improve patient selection and results. Ann Surg. 1993:**218**(5):646–53.

26. Sugerman HJ, Kellum JM, DeMaria EJ, et al. Conversion of failed or complicated vertical banded gastroplasty to gastric bypass in morbid obesity. Am J Surg. 1996;**171**(2):263–69.

27. Chiapaikeo D, Schultheis M, Protyniak B, Pearce P, Borao FJ, Binenbaum SJ. Analysis of reoperations after laparoscopic adjustable gastric banding. JSLS. 2014;**18**(4):e2014.

28. Buchwald H, Oien DM. Metabolic/bariatric surgery worldwide 2011. Obes Surg. 2013;**23**(4):427–36.

29. DeMaria EJ, Sugerman HJ, Meador JG, et al. High failure rate after laparoscopic adjustable silicone gastric banding for treatment of morbid obesity. Ann Surg. 2001;**233**(6):809–18.

30. Singhal R, Super P. Role of laparoscopic adjustable gastric banding in the treatment of obesity and related disorders. Br J Diabetes Vasc Dis. 2009;**9**(3):131–33.

31. Lanthaler M, Aigner F, Kinzl J, Sieb M, Cakar-Beck F, Nehoda H. Long-term results and complications following adjustable gastric banding. Obes Surg. 2010;**20**(8):1078–85.

32. Kasza J, Brody F, Vaziri K, et al. Analysis of poor outcomes after laparoscopic adjustable gastric banding. Surg Endosc. 2011;**25**(1):41–7.

Outcomes in bariatric surgery

Gabriel Mekel, Elizabeth Renza-Stingone, and Andres Castellanos†

Introduction

Laparoscopic Roux-en-Y gastric bypass (RYGB) is the second-most commonly performed bariatric procedure in the United States, and even though it is not considered by all weight-loss surgeons as the 'gold standard', it is the benchmark by which all other bariatric procedures are currently compared [1]. RYGB has been surpassed in recent years by laparoscopic (vertical) sleeve gastrectomy (LSG) and its success and complication rates have placed it between the laparoscopic RYGB and the laparoscopic adjustable gastric band (LAGB) [2]. A report in 2015 by Altieri and colleagues demonstrated 20% of patients required band removal or revision, with a conversion to LSG and laparoscopic RYGB in 5% and 12% of cases, respectively [3]. Initially, the band was favoured by patients and surgeons alike due to its high safety profile and reversible nature [3]; however, of late, the LAGB has been losing favour and is being implanted with less and less frequency (17% compared to 28% and 46% for LSG and laparoscopic RYGB, respectively in 2011) [4]. This is likely related to its lower percentage of excess weight loss (%EWL) as well as complications associated with a long-term implanted device that include but are not limited to gastric prolapse ('slipped band'), gastro-oesophageal dilation, band loosening, and erosion of band [5]. In a similar fashion, the number of RYGBs has decreased whereas the number of LSGs has increased over the past decade [4].

Outcome measures

The %EWL is one of the most common outcome measures used in bariatric surgery. Improvement and resolution of comorbidities has been directly associated with %EWL [6]. Weight loss after LAGB is gradual and steady for up to 3 years after which a steady state of approximately 50% EWL is reached at 5 years [6–8]. When compared to laparoscopic RYGB, estimated weight loss ranges from 50% to 80% 5 years after surgery in most major series [1,9]. Christou et al. reported the greatest weight loss to occur 2 years after RYGB and a slow and steady increase in the subsequent years in their 12-year follow-up study [10]. A literature review by Shi and colleagues demonstrated

an estimated 59% EWL at 1 year after LSG that increased to 66% at 3 years [11]. These findings are consistent with a report from the American College of Surgeons that situated the LSG weight loss reduction between the LAGB and the gastric bypass [2] and is also consistent with the results obtained by Bohdjalian and colleagues who reported 60% EWL 5 years after surgery with the greatest impact seen in the first year [12].

The number of patients undergoing revision or removal of gastric bands has increased over the past few years and despite of the lack of long-term follow-up studies, there is some controversy as to the complication rates after conversion surgery from LAGB to either LGS or RYGB [13]. In one study, revision surgery was associated with more complications; however, patients undergoing primary surgery were younger, weighted more, and had more comorbidity [14]. Conversely, Courcoulas et al. found that conversion from LAGB to RYGB occurred more frequently in younger females with less comorbidity and, hence, was associated with fewer complications [15]. Therefore, longer-term studies with comparable groups are needed before making conclusions regarding the outcomes of primary versus revisional bariatric surgery [13].

Insulin resistance and diabetes mellitus are directly related to obesity. However, beneficial effects of RYGB on diabetes cannot be accounted for by weight loss alone, but are also due to the reduced oral intake, lack of passage of food through the duodenum, and hormonal influences [16,17]. A systematic meta-analysis of 136 studies, involving over 22,000 patients, reported that RYGB completely resolved diabetes in 84% of cases [18]. LAGB causes resolution of diabetes in two-thirds of patients and improved glucose control for the remainder [6]. This is consistent with the results of Tice and colleagues, who compared LAGB with RYGB and reported blood glucose normalization in 40% with LAGB as opposed to 100% resolution in those undergoing RYGB [19]. Despite the scarce data on long-term follow-up for LSG, complete remission of diabetes has been reported to be 50.7% 1 year after surgery with a significant weight regain and decrease in remission rate over time [20]. However, remission rates up to 78% have been described [21]. The durability of remission of diabetes for LSG is still to be determined by studies with longer follow-up.

---

† It is with great regret that we report the death of Andres Castellanos during the production of this textbook.

Table 16.1. Estimated percentage of resolution of comorbidities after bariatric surgery

	LAGB (%)	LSG (%)	RYGB (%)
Hypertension	18	40	45
Diabetes mellitus	40	50	84
Hyperlipidaemia	33	35	66
Obstructive sleep apnoea	38	62	66

Despite the high rate of diabetes resolution after bariatric surgery, gastric dilation and changes in gastric emptying may lead in the long term to increased fat mass, insulin resistance, and ultimately diabetes recurrence [22]. At the present time, there are not many options to treat recurrent weight gain and diabetes after RYGB. They include the duodenal switch, which also entails a high morbidity and the fact that it can only be performed in a highly selected group of patients; and more recently, laparoscopic jejunal sleeve, which has shown up to a 5–10-point reduction in body mass index in the short term [23]. Since diabetes is a chronic disease, and the fact that RYGB has a higher resolution rate of diabetes only in the 5–10-year period compared to LSG, probably the latter procedure may become the best first approach to resolve and prevent recurrences of diabetes in obese patients as studies with longer follow-up take place [22]. In a study that compared remission rates of diabetes in patients with super obesity (body mass index >50 kg/m²) who underwent LSG followed by duodenal switch versus single-staged duodenal switch, there was no statistical difference between comorbidities resolution after LSG in the two-staged arm when compared to the single-stage group [24]. This may suggest that LSG alone may account for resolution of comorbidities without the complications entailed by the duodenal switch.

Hypertension is also improved significantly after bariatric surgery and its impact is directly related to the percentage of weight lost [6]. Rates of hypertension resolution hover around 21% 5 years after LAGB but rates up to 70% rates have been reported in small series [7,8]. The Swedish Obesity Study demonstrated a marked improvement in diabetes and hypertension after bypass; however, after 10 years, the impact on hypertension tends to be significantly decreased [1]. Similar results have been reported by Golomb and colleagues for the LSG. While 80% of patients achieved partial remission of hypertension at 3 years, only 54% maintained partial remission at 5 years. Forty-five per cent of patients had a complete remission at 5 years [20].

In terms of hyperlipidaemia, it had resolved in 35% of patients undergoing LSG 1 year after surgery compared to 33% after LAGB and 66% after RYGB [2,25]. The beneficial effects of bariatric surgery have also been found in longer-term studies. Yang et al. demonstrated improvement in the lipid profile to the point of not requiring lipid-lowering medications in 56% and 53% of patients undergoing LSG and RYGB, respectively, 3 years after surgery [21].

Obstructive sleep apnoea is also one of the comorbidities affecting obese population. A meta-analysis comparing the rate of resolution after bariatric surgery versus non-surgical weight loss demonstrated that both tools had beneficial effects on obstructive sleep apnoea. However, the surgical arm had a greater impact as measured by the apnoea–hypopnea index [26]. Rates of resolution of obstructive sleep apnoea exceed 60% 1 year after LSG and RYGB. However, when compared to LAGB, it only accomplishes it in 38% of the cases [2]. These findings are consistent with those of Carlin et al. who

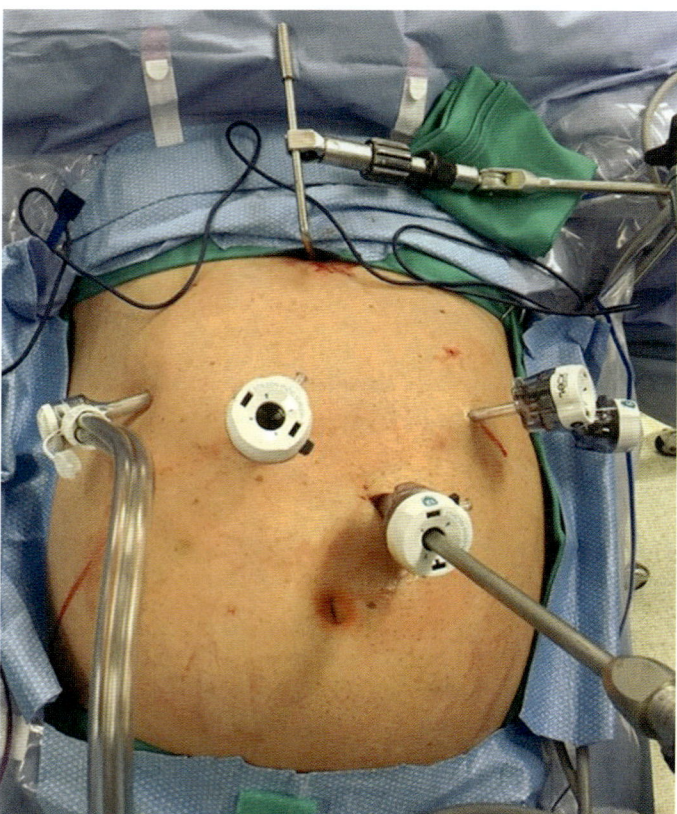

Fig. 16.1 Port placement for laparoscopic sleeve gastrectomy.

found rates of obstructive sleep apnoea resolution of 66%, 57%, and 29% for RYGB, LSG, and LAGB, respectively [21].

It would seem that there is a range of resolution of comorbidities, and this may be related to patient- and procedure-dependent factors. Promising results can be obtained in most patients with regard to diabetes, hypertension, and sleep apnoea (Table 16.1).

CASE REPORT

This case involved a 64-year-old female who presented to clinic after multiple unsuccessful attempts to lose weight by conservative means. The patient had a history of hypertension, rheumatoid arthritis, and a body mass index of 41.9 kg/m². After a thorough discussion, it was decided to perform a LSG. On the day of surgery, after uneventful induction of anaesthesia and intubation, the patient was placed in the supine position and trocars were inserted in the usual manner (Fig. 16.1). The greater curvature was dissected from its attachments to the omentum up to the level of the angle of His. A 36-French bougie was introduced and stapling of the stomach commenced along its trajectory with a 60 mm endostapler. The bougie was easily removed. A leak test was performed with normal saline, which proved negative. Haemostasis at the staple line was confirmed and it was further reinforced with fibrin sealant (Evicel®). A specimen was removed with a polyurethane pouch (Endo Catch™). The fascial defects at the 15 mm and 12 mm port sites were closed intracorporeally. There were no complications and the patient was awakened from anaesthesia. She was started on a clear liquid diet the same day of surgery and discharged home on postoperative day 1. She was seen in the bariatric outpatient clinic 2, 4, 8, and 12 weeks after surgery.

REFERENCES

1. Leslie D, Kellogg T, Ikramuddin S. Laparoscopic Roux-en-Y gastric bypass. In: Soper NJ, Swanstrom LS, Eubanks WS, eds. Mastery of Endoscopic and Laparoscopic Surgery. Philadelphia, PA: Lippincott Williams & Wilkins; 2009:262–71.

2. Hutter MM, Schirmer BD, Jones DB, Ko CY, Cohen ME, Merkow RP, et al. First report from the American College of Surgeons Bariatric Surgery Center Network: laparoscopic sleeve gastrectomy has morbidity and effectiveness positioned between the band and the bypass. Ann Surg. 2011;**254**(3):410–20.

3. Altieri MS, Yang J, Telem DA, Meng Z, Frenkel C, Halbert C, et al. Lap band outcomes from 19,221 patients across centers and over a decade within the state of New York. Surg Endosc. 2015;**30**(5):1725–32.

4. Buchwald H, Oien DM. Metabolic/bariatric surgery worldwide 2011. Obes Surg. 2013;**23**(4):427–36.

5. Allen JW. Laparoscopic gastric band complications. Med Clin North Am. 2007;**91**(3):485–97

6. Ghandhi T, Patterson E. Restrictive procedures for morbid obesity. In: Soper NJ, Swanstrom LS, Eubanks WS, eds. Mastery of Endoscopic and Laparoscopic Surgery. Philadelphia, PA: Lippincott Williams & Wilkins; 2009:249–61.

7. Boza C, Gamboa C, Perez G, Crovari F, Escalona A, Pimentel F, et al. Laparoscopic adjustable gastric banding (LAGB): surgical results and 5-year follow-up. Surg Endosc. 2011;**25**(1):292–97.

8. Al Khalifa K, Violato C, Al Ansari A. Reduction in weight and BMI and changes in co-morbidities following laparoscopic adjustable gastric banding procedure for morbidly obese patients in Bahrain: a five year longitudinal study. Springerplus. 2013;**2**(1):19.

9. Gumbs AA, Gagner M, Dakin G, Pomp A. Sleeve gastrectomy for morbid obesity. Obes Surg. 2007;**17**(7):962–69.

10. Christou NV, Look D, Maclean LD. Weight gain after short- and long-limb gastric bypass in patients followed for longer than 10 years. Ann Surg. 2006;**244**(5):734–40.

11. Shi X, Karmali S, Sharma AM, Birch DW. A review of laparoscopic sleeve gastrectomy for morbid obesity. Obes Surg. 2010;**20**(8):1171–77.

12. Bohdjalian A, Langer FB, Shakeri-Leidenmühler S, Gfrerer L, Ludvik B, Zacherl J, Prager G. Sleeve gastrectomy as sole and definitive bariatric procedure: 5-year results for weight loss and ghrelin. Obes Surg. 2010;**20**(5):535–40.

13. Gagner M. Conversion of adjustable gastric banding to Roux-en-Y gastric bypass: not as optimal as primary gastric bypass? JAMA Surg. 2014;**149**(8):786–87.

14. Inabnet WB 3rd, Belle SH, Bessler M, Courcoulas A, Dellinger P, Garcia L, et al. Comparison of 30-day outcomes after non-LapBand primary and revisional bariatric surgical procedures from the Longitudinal Assessment of Bariatric Surgery study. Surg Obes Relat Dis. 2010;**6**(1):22–30.

15. Courcoulas AP, Christian NJ, Belle SH, Berk PD, Flum DR, Garcia L, et al. Weight change and health outcomes at 3 years after bariatric surgery among individuals with severe obesity. JAMA. 2013 Dec 11;**310**(22):2416–25.

16. Cummings DE, Overduin J, Shannon MH, Foster-Schubert KE; 2004 ABS Consensus Conference. Hormonal mechanisms of weight loss and diabetes resolution after bariatric surgery. Surg Obes Relat Dis. 2005;**1**(3):358–68.

17. Cho JM, Kim HJ, Menzo EL, Park S, Szomstein S, Rosenthal RJ. Effect of sleeve gastrectomy on type 2 diabetes as an alternative treatment modality to Roux-en-Y gastric bypass: systemic review and meta-analysis. Surg Obes Relat Dis. 2015;**11**(6):1273–80.

18. Buchwald H, Avidor Y, Braunwald E, Jensen MD, Pories W, Fahrbach K, et al. Bariatric surgery: a systematic review and meta-analysis. JAMA. 2004;**292**(14):1724–37.

19. Tice JA, Karliner L, Walsh J, Petersen AJ, Feldman MD. Gastric banding or bypass? A systematic review comparing the two most popular bariatric procedures. Am J Med. 2008;**121**(10):885–93.

20. Golomb I, Ben David M, Glass A, Kolitz T, Keidar A. Long-term metabolic effects of laparoscopic sleeve gastrectomy. JAMA Surg. 2015;**150**(11):1051–57.

21. Yang J, Wang C, Cao G, Yang W, Yu S, Zhai H, et al. Long-term effects of laparoscopic sleeve gastrectomy versus Roux-en-Y gastric bypass for the treatment of Chinese type 2 diabetes mellitus patients with body mass index 28–35 kg/m(2). BMC Surg. 2015;**15**:88.

22. Gagner M. Effect of sleeve gastrectomy on type 2 diabetes as an alternative to Roux-en-Y gastric bypass: a better long-term strategy. Surg Obes Relat Dis. 2015;**11**(6):1280–81.

23. Gagner M. Laparoscopic jejunal sleeve: a simple and ideal new technique for revision of Roux-en-Y gastric bypass after weight regains technical aspects. Surg Technol Int. 2010;**20**:147–52.

24. Iannelli A, Schneck AS, Topart P, Carles M, Hébuterne X, Gugenheim J. Laparoscopic sleeve gastrectomy followed by duodenal switch in selected patients versus single-stage duodenal switch for superobesity: case-control study. Surg Obes Relat Dis. 2013;**9**(4):531–38.

25. Carlin AM, Zeni TM, English WJ, Hawasli AA, Genaw JA, Krause KR, et al. The comparative effectiveness of sleeve gastrectomy, gastric bypass, and adjustable gastric banding procedures for the treatment of morbid obesity. Ann Surg. 2013;**257**(5):791–97.

26. Ashrafian H, Toma T, Rowland SP, Harling L, Tan A, Efthimiou E, et al. Bariatric surgery or non-surgical weight loss for obstructive sleep apnoea? A systematic review and comparison of meta-analyses. Obes Surg. 2015;**25**(7):1239–50.

SECTION 5
Specific clinical issues

Preoperative evaluation of the morbidly obese patient

Rajeshwari Subramaniam, Hemkumar Pushparaj, and Ajisha Aravindan

Introduction

With a steep increase in the bariatric population throughout the world, including the morbid obese and super-obese in developed countries as well as the economically 'middle class' population in developing countries, anaesthesia for surgical procedures in bariatric patients is set to become routine. This is reflected by the increasing incidence of bariatric surgery, even in children [1].

Bariatric patients usually present with systemic comorbidities. The presence of comorbidities and procedure-related risks has led to bariatric surgery being classified as an intermediate to high-risk non-cardiac procedure. Since bariatric surgery results in significant reversal of hypertension, diabetes mellitus (DM), obstructive sleep apnoea (OSA), and pulmonary hypertension [2], preoperative optimization of these patients with such comorbidities may minimize perioperative risk.

Preoperative cardiac evaluation

Morbidly obese patients are at an increased risk of cardiovascular disease compared to their non-obese counterparts. In the Framingham Heart Study, after 15 years' follow-up, it was determined that there was an increase in risk by 5% for men and 7% for women to develop heart failure for every increase in one unit of BMI over 30 kg/m^2 [3]. Obesity-related cardiovascular morbidities include atherosclerosis, hypertension, cardiomyopathy, pulmonary hypertension, limited exercise capacity, arrhythmias, and deep vein thrombosis (DVT) [4]. Obesity-induced cardiac disease is also associated with sudden death [5]. Laparoscopic bariatric procedures are classified as intermediate risk due to the numerous comorbidities frequently present in these patients. Early diagnosis and therapy for cardiovascular complications may reduce postoperative mortality [6]. In addition, laparoscopic procedures for bariatric patients have been reported to result in significant cardiac remodelling as well as reversal of other comorbidities such as systemic hypertension, glucose intolerance, and pulmonary hypertension [7].

History

History taking in these patients should include questions regarding symptoms of angina, orthopnoea, exercise tolerance, nocturnal dyspnoea, palpitations, coronary medications, and interventions. Symptoms of dyspnoea, chest discomfort, and pedal oedema may occur frequently, unrelated to clinical cardiac disease. Exertional dyspnoea leading to increased ventilatory demands may be due to non-cardiac causes, elevated right ventricular filling pressures, or increased intra-abdominal pressure, despite an increased cardiac output. Diagnosis of coronary artery disease (CAD) is made more difficult if there is associated pulmonary disease, arthritis, and deconditioning. Jugular venous distension may be masked in obesity. The heart sounds may be muffled and/or distant, masking the quality and even the presence of an S3 gallop.

Utility of electrocardiogram and chest X-ray

Physical examination and electrocardiogram (ECG) may underestimate the presence and degree of cardiac pathology and dysfunction in obese patients. A 12-lead ECG and chest X-ray should be routinely considered in patients awaiting bariatric surgery. Nearly 62% of bariatric patients may have ECG changes considered insignificant on cardiac evaluation [8]. However, the presence of a preoperative ECG abnormality has been correlated to the requirement of ICU care for 48 hours or more after Roux-en-Y gastric bypass (RYGB) surgery [9]. ECG abnormalities may indicate the presence of occult CAD warranting further evaluation. The QTc interval should be assessed for abnormalities.

A posteroanterior chest X-ray provides baseline status for postoperative comparison, and may reveal undiagnosed heart failure, cardiac chamber enlargement, or abnormal pulmonary vascularity suggestive of pulmonary hypertension [4,8].

Resting arterial blood gas analysis (ABG) can document severity of hypoxaemia and/or hypercarbia.

Cardiomyopathy

Nearly 31% of individuals with long-standing obesity are at risk of developing 'obesity cardiomyopathy'. Symptoms and signs of obesity cardiomyopathy occur most commonly in patients with a BMI greater than 40 kg/m². The risk of heart failure due to obesity cardiomyopathy rises steeply after 10 years of severe obesity [4]. Prolonged exposure to insulin resistance, increased leptin levels, steatosis, and neurohumoral overactivation exert direct cardiotoxic effects leading to structural remodelling and mechanical impairment. Nocturnal hypoxaemia and hypercarbia associated with repeated airway obstruction lead to irreversible pulmonary vascular changes, pulmonary hypertension, and eventually biventricular heart failure [10]. Increasing BMI is also associated with concentric, rather than eccentric left ventricular (LV) hypertrophy in both morbidly obese and super-obese patients, with increasing LV diastolic dysfunction.

The 'young' or paediatric bariatric patient may appear to have well-preserved cardiac function; however, a case report of mortality due to undiagnosed dilated cardiomyopathy after sleeve gastrectomy in a 19-year-old morbidly obese male indicates that obesity cardiomyopathy does not spare the young [11].

Hypertension

The prevalence of hypertension is 42% in patients with a BMI of more than 30 kg/m². The presence of hypertension is an independent risk factor for CAD, stroke, and end–organ damage. Hypertension can result from an interplay of genetic factors, insulin resistance, sodium retention, activation of the sympathoadrenal system, and the renin–angiotensin–aldosterone axis [3,10]. The use of angiotensin-converting enzyme inhibitors and angiotensin receptor blockers in obesity-induced hypertension may be beneficial due to their effect on increasing insulin sensitivity. Use of beta blockers, such as metoprolol, may lead to further weight gain. Carvedilol has been found to be superior to metoprolol in this manner [12].

Blood pressure should be recorded with an optimal cuff. According to American Heart Association recommendations, for arm circumferences ranging from 35 to 44 cm, a 16 cm width cuff should be used, and for a 45–52 cm arm circumference, a 20 cm width cuff [13].

Coronary artery disease

The prevalence of CAD ranges from 7% to 11.5% in bariatric patients. Increased cardiac complications have been observed in the first 90 days following emergent hip surgery in the morbidly obese [4]. The extent of plaques and ulceration in the coronaries and abdominal aorta has been directly correlated with abdominal fat and BMI. The morbidly obese patient also has numerous risk factors for CAD, in the form of type 2 diabetes mellitus (T2DM), hypertension, dyslipidaemia, and a prothrombotic and inflammatory state [3].

Arrhythmias

Obese patients may develop idiopathic atrial fibrillation (AF), atrial flutter, and ventricular tachycardia, or bradyarrhythmias

due to sinus node dysfunction. Nearly 10% of arrhythmias in the bariatric patient result from atrial/ventricular hypertrophy, electrolyte imbalance due to diuretic therapy, hypoxaemia, and/or hypercarbia resulting from hypoventilation/OSA. Fatty infiltration of the posterior atrial wall has been proposed as a mechanism [14]. Although there is a strong correlation of BMI with postoperative AF (2.3-fold risk with BMI >40 kg/m²), increased mortality due to AF per se has not been established [15]. Preoperative AF has been shown to be associated with increased perioperative mortality compared to CAD in a separate study. Obesity increases the risk of developing AF by 49% and is a pathogenetic factor leading to cardiovascular and cerebrovascular events [16]. In patients with AF it is recommended to control the ventricular rate to 80 bpm or less, or 110 bpm (in patients with preserved LV function), or conversion to sinus. Nearly 8% of obese have QTc greater than 0.44 seconds. QTc greater than 0.42 is associated with mortality in even 'healthy' obese patients [3].

Cardiovascular autonomic dysfunction leads to an increase in the resting heart rate and reduced heart rate variability, which is a risk factor for sudden death after myocardial infarction. Changes in heart rate variability responses are a valuable, early indicator of impairment of cardiovascular health [17].

Indications for further cardiac evaluation

Bariatric surgery still constitutes an intermediate-risk procedure due to the nature of surgery (position, prolonged visceral manipulation, pneumoperitoneum) and significant comorbidities. Lee's Revised Cardiac Risk Index can be used to stratify patients requiring further cardiac testing. Patients with a score of 3 or higher or documented congestive heart failure must proceed for further evaluation [4].

Functional status in the morbid and super-morbid bariatric patient, body habitus, and lifestyle cannot be reported reliably. It is important to distinguish between expected deconditioning due to obesity from significant cardiac disease. Most bariatric patients have low functional capacity, making cardiac risk assessment imperative [18]. Stress ECG and myocardial perfusion studies and are the two frequently used non-invasive techniques.

Transthoracic dobutamine stress echocardiography

Stress testing is recommended if three or more of Lee's Revised Cardiac Risk Index factors are present and functional capacity less than 4 metabolic equivalent tasks (METs). Factors that hamper stress testing include non-availability of equipment which can bear excess weight, inability of the patient to exercise and poor-quality echocardiographic images. Echocontrast can improve visualization of cardiac borders [19]. Inducible ischaemia, along with an ejection fraction less than 50%, is a reliable predictor of long-term outcome [20]. The advantages of stress echocardiography are its high negative predictive value and lack of torso diameter limitation.

In a series of 611 bariatric patients undergoing transthoracic dobutamine stress echocardiography (DSE), 1.2% of patients had positive DSE findings. Of these, only one in seven had significant CAD confirmed by angiography [21]. Another study in 87 morbidly obese patients undergoing bariatric surgery, revealed prevalence of LV hypertrophy (in 12.6%) and LV end-diastolic diameter index indicating diastolic dysfunction (in 32.7%) [22]. These studies are in contrast with an older study covering 30 bariatric patients which reported that echocardiograms in asymptomatic severely obese patients could detect abnormalities typical of obesity cardiomyopathy (enlarged chambers, diastolic dysfunction, LV hypertrophy), which pointed to greater cardiovascular risk [23].

Transoesophageal DSE has been shown to be a useful alternative for preoperative screening in the morbidly obese with poor echocardiographic window providing superior image quality. However, the number of studies using the technique is low.

Myocardial perfusion imaging

This can be performed by exercise/dobutamine technetium-99m tetrofosmin single-photon emission computed tomography (SPECT) in obese patients with cardiac symptoms or risk factors. Since obesity affects the accuracy of SPECT, a new software termed 'attenuation correction' may improve specificity of SPECT for CAD detection. Positron emission tomography scans have better specificity in diagnosing CAD, especially the right coronary artery territory. Bariatric patients may exceed the weight limit of nuclear imaging tables, and the consoles may not be able to accommodate the obese torso [18].

Computed tomographic coronary angiography

Multidetector spiral computed tomography, although with higher sensitivity and specificity compared to conventional angiography, may offer less spatial resolution in the morbidly obese. Further, computed tomography scanner tables may have weight limitations.

Cardiac catheterization remains the gold standard of evaluation. It is well tolerated by the obese, and the complication rate appears to be lower than in the general population. It may reveal pulmonary hypertension and cor pulmonale secondary to obesity hypoventilation/OSA earlier than clinical or ECG signs [4].

In a series of 193 morbidly obese patients, routine preoperative testing revealed abnormalities in 15% by ECG, and 4% by chest X-ray, none of which required preoperative intervention. It may be prudent to limit pulmonary function and cardiac stress testing to symptomatic individuals [24].

Pulmonary embolism and deep vein thrombosis

The incidence of pulmonary embolism in the morbidly obese is 0.1–2% in the postoperative period, being the commonest cause of death during this time. Preoperative thromboprophylaxis is especially indicated with pre-existing AF or patients with non-bioprosthetic valves.

Low-molecular-weight heparin should ideally be dosed twice daily [4]. For preoperative anticoagulation in patients with AF, the CHA$_2$DS$_2$VASc [8] score can be used. Patients with a score greater than 2, with AF, should receive anticoagulant therapy (Table 17.1).

Other investigations

Brain natriuretic peptide (BNP) is a useful marker in predicting short- and long-term cardiovascular events in patients undergoing non-cardiac surgery. Although it can be considered as a routine,

Table 17.1 The CHA$_2$DS$_2$-VASc score

Parameter	Score
Congestive heart failure	1
Hypertension	1
Age ≥75	2
Age 65–74	1
Diabetes mellitus	1
Stroke, transient ischaemic attack	2
Vascular disease (prior myocardial infarction, peripheral vascular disease, aortic plaque)	1
Sex category (female)	1

Reproduced with permission from Lip, G. Y. H., Nieuwlaat, R., Pisters, R., et al. Refining Clinical Risk Stratification for Predicting Stroke and Thromboembolism in Atrial Fibrillation Using a Novel Risk Factor-Based Approach. The Euro Heart Survey on Atrial Fibrillation, CHEST, 137(2): 263–272. Copyright © 2010 with permission from Elsevier. doi: 10.1378/chest.09-1584

inexpensive, and accurate first-line preoperative parameter for cardiac risk assessment [12] the levels of both BNP and N-terminal pro-BNP have been seen to be inversely related to BMI, bringing into question its utility in the obese [25]. The levels of these humoral factors appear to increase after gastric bypass surgery. An Obesity Surgery Mortality Risk Score (OS-MRS) has been validated using five comorbidity variables [4] (**Box 17.1**).

Box 17.1 Obesity Surgery Mortality Risk Score for gastric bypass

- BMI greater than 50 kg/m²
- Age greater than 45 years.
- Hypertension.
- Risk factors for pulmonary embolism:
  - Previous venous thromboembolism.
  - Vena cava filter.
  - Hypoventilation (sleep-disordered breathing).
  - Pulmonary hypertension.
- Male gender.

Reproduced with permission from Poirier, P., Alpert, M. A., Fleisher, L. A. et al., Cardiovascular Evaluation and Management of Severely Obese Patients Undergoing Surgery, Circulation, 120(1):86–95. Copyright © 2009 Wolters Kluwer Health, Inc. https://doi.org/10.1161/CIRCULATIONAHA.109.192575

- Class A (low risk): patients with none or one comorbidity
- Class B (intermediate risk): patients with two or three comorbidities
- Class C (high risk): patients with four or five comorbidities.

Mortality has been reported as 0.2–0.3% for class A, 1.1–1.5% for class B, and 2.4–3% for class C patients [4]. An algorithm for cardiac and pulmonary evaluation of the severely obese patient undergoing elective non-cardiac surgery has been proposed by Poirier and co-authors [4] (**Fig. 17.1**). Comprehensive medical history, physical examination, and blood chemistry are as clinically indicated.

In summary, history and clinical evaluation of the morbidly obese patient may lead to indicators requiring further cardiac evaluation. The OS-MRS and Revised Cardiac Risk Index can be used to define the population requiring cardiac stress testing.

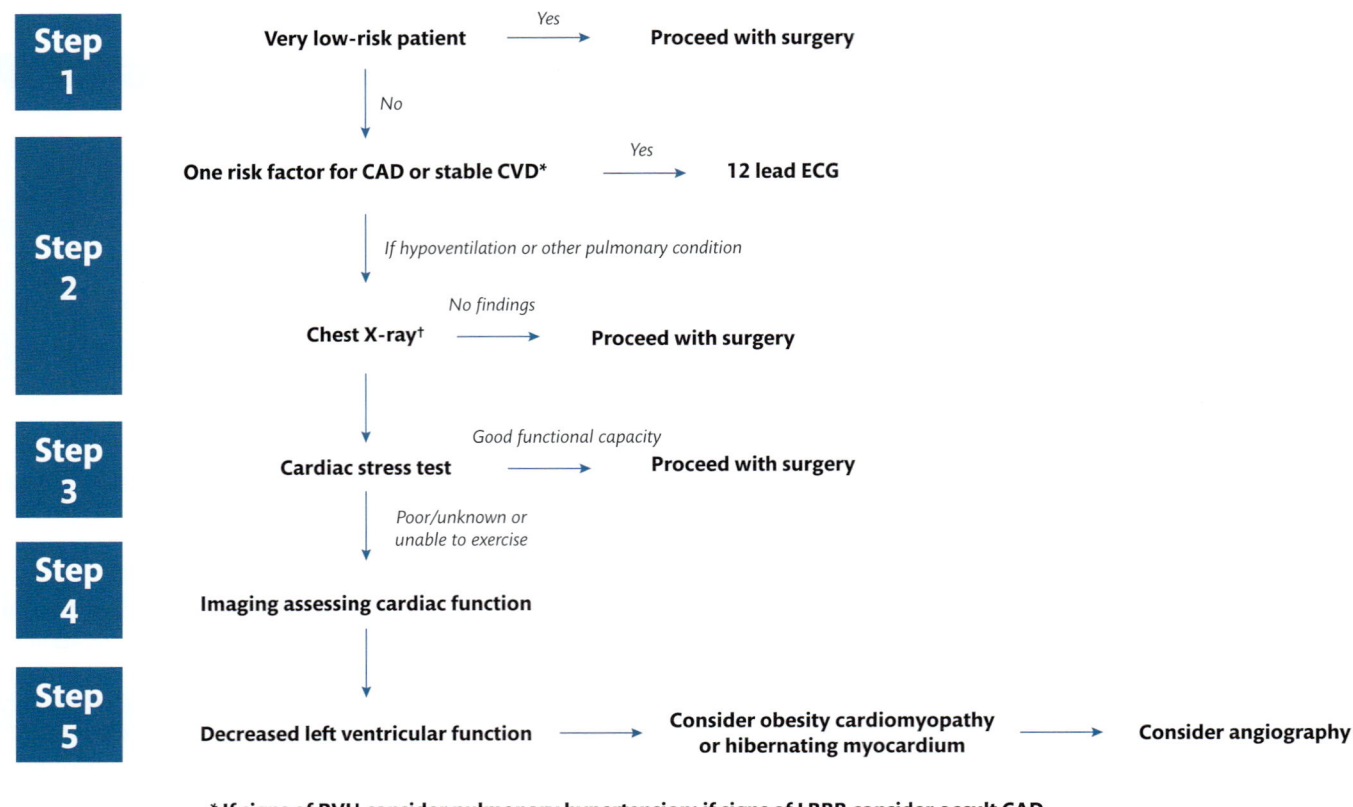

Fig. 17.1 Cardiac and pulmonary algorithm assessment for elective non-cardiac surgery in severely obese patients.

Respiratory system

Lung physiology and anatomy are considerably altered in obese individuals. There is a reduction in compliance of the respiratory system due to reduced compliance of both the lungs and chest wall. This significant decline is thought to be because of fat deposition over the chest, abdomen, and diaphragm [26] and excess pulmonary blood volume [27]. The increased oxygen consumption, lower tidal volume breathing, and increased respiratory rate compensating for minute ventilation [28] cause a subjective feeling of breathlessness.

Lung capacities

Most of the lung capacities are maintained until the range of morbid obesity is reached. Fat loading causes a decrease in total lung capacity, vital capacity, and more notably in the expiratory reserve volume. The residual volume is maintained in ratio with total lung capacity, so the decrease in expiratory reserve volume is mainly seen in functional residual capacity [26,29,30]. A further increase in BMI causes a steeper fall in functional residual capacity, further decreasing the residual volume and closing capacity, further impairing gas exchange [28,29]. In severe forms of morbid obesity, there is a decrease in tidal volume causing a rapid shallow breathing pattern to maintain minute ventilation [26].

Asthma and obesity

Airway hyper-responsiveness in obesity could be due to decreased airway calibre, impaired airway smooth muscle contractility, or chronic inflammation [31]. Adipose tissue may produce proinflammatory cytokines leading to asthma. Airway collapse occurs as a result of closing capacity being lower than the functional residual capacity which may cause expiratory flow limitation in morbid obesity especially in the supine position [27]. The opening and closing of these smaller airways with a turbulent airflow through narrowed calibre might mimic a wheeze [30,32] and most obese 'asthmatics' improve after weight loss [33]. Spirometry shows a decrease in both forced expiratory volume in 1 second (FEV_1) and forced vital capacity (28,29,32). The decline occurs in both concurrently so that the ratio FEV_1/forced vital capacity is maintained. Spirometry after bronchodilator might differentiate the two entities. Asthma, in the obese is more severe and not amenable to standard treatment [29]. A correct diagnosis is imperative as corticosteroid use for treatment of asthma might further worsen the obesity.

Pulmonary hypertension is often seen in morbid obesity due to OSA, obesity hypoventilation syndrome (OHS), pulmonary thromboembolism, and increased pulmonary blood volume [8]. A pulmonary artery systolic pressure of greater than 30 mmHg is seen in two-thirds of obese individuals [29]. Morbidly obese patients with pulmonary hypertension have a higher risk for postoperative morbidity and mortality compared to the morbidly obese without pulmonary hypertension [34]. A preoperative ECG, chest X-ray, and an echocardiogram are imperative for diagnosis. Right heart catheterization is recommended for patients with documented pulmonary hypertension, to assess reactivity to vasodilators and any effect on cardiac output [35]. Although atelectasis may cause decreased ventilation, some patients might show an increase in ventilation/perfusion ratio and alveolar–arterial oxygen pressure gradient widening due to the increase in pulmonary blood volume [36].

Obesity hypoventilation (Pickwickian) syndrome

Popularized by the 'fat boy' (Joe) from Charles Dickens' *The Pickwick Papers* and thus the name, OHS is a clinical entity increasingly recognized in morbid obesity. OHS is characterized by obesity, sleep-disordered breathing, and hypercapnia [28]. The definition of OHS requires a BMI of at least 30 kg/m², daytime awake $PaCO_2$ of at least 45 mmHg, and PaO_2 no higher than 70 mmHg while breathing room air, with a diagnosis of sleep-disordered breathing and other causes of hypoventilation being excluded [37]. The usual presenting feature will be a plethoric morbid obesity with collapsing oropharynx, large neck circumference, and prominent second heart sound [38].

The pathophysiology of OHS relates to obesity, poor respiratory mechanics, OSA with increased upper airway resistance, and poor response to hypercapnia and leptin resistance [30,38,39]. These patients tend to have more severe upper airway collapse, poor lung mechanics, pulmonary hypertension, angina pectoris, and cor pulmonale. On a 50-month follow-up, if left untreated, they exhibited a higher mortality rate [39]. Chronic hypoxaemia and hypercapnia enhance the sensitivity of these patients to anaesthetic agents and opioids. In the postoperative period, these patients are more likely to hypoventilate, require ventilatory support, and more frequently develop postoperative pulmonary complications [28]. The OS-MRS shows that OHS and pulmonary artery hypertension are associated with an increased chance of pulmonary thromboembolism and postoperative mortality as seen in **Box 17.1**.

The mainstay of treatment includes positive airway pressure therapy and weight reduction, by either surgery or pharmacotherapy [39]. Supplemental oxygen therapy is required in almost 50% of the patients with OHS. Reversal of hypoventilation usually reverses erythrocytosis and phlebotomy is rarely required. Tracheostomy may be the option in patients intolerant to positive airway pressure therapy [38]. Hypoxaemia in room air (SpO_2 <90%) or serum bicarbonate levels greater than 27 mEq/L has shown a sensitivity of 92% for screening for OHS and warrants blood gas analysis [40].

Is spirometry required in all morbidly obese patients undergoing surgery?

Abnormal ABG measurements or spirometry values might indicate the patient to be at high risk of perioperative pulmonary complications but fail to stratify them [41]. Spirometry, being non-invasive, easy to perform, quick, and inexpensive, should be performed in all morbidly obese patients undergoing surgery.

Obstructive sleep apnoea

OSA is characterized by the recurrent partial or complete collapse of the pharyngeal airway in sleep. Sleep induces marked blunting of the reflex pharyngeal dilator response to negative pressure. In addition, obese patients' adipose deposition may lead to airway collapse, mostly at the retro-palatal or retro-glossal area. Apnoea is defined as the complete cessation of airflow for more than 10 seconds and hypopnea greater than a 50% reduction in airflow for more than 10 seconds— associated with a 4% drop in saturation. The apnoea–hypopnea index (AHI) is the total number of apnoea and hypopnea episodes per hour. An AHI greater than 5 along with the presence of daytime somnolence is diagnostic of OSA [42]. The prevalence of OSA in middle-aged women and men is 2–3% and 4–5%, respectively [43]. Among obese patients, the prevalence exceeds 30% [44,45], while in morbid obesity it reaches as high as 50–98% (46,47).

A BMI of at least 30 kg/m² is the most important risk factor for OSA which is proven by the remarkable improvement in OSA seen after weight reduction [42]. Other predisposing conditions include age greater than 50 years, male sex, neck circumference greater than 40 cm in females and 43 cm in males, nasal/pharyngeal/laryngeal obstruction, craniofacial anomalies (more in the paediatric age group), use of alcohol, and sedatives.

The obstruction and hypoxaemia associated with sleep apnoea results in increased inspiratory effort, seen as progressively louder snoring, sudden arousal with hyperventilation, and relief of obstruction with wakefulness. This causes sleep fragmentation, excessive daytime somnolence, morning headaches, fatigue, and irritability making patients prone to motor vehicle accidents. Blood gas analysis classically shows arterial hypoxaemia, hypercarbia, and polycythemia. Sympathetic nervous system activation in response to hypoxia can cause systemic and pulmonary hypertension, arrhythmias, and right heart failure.

Obese patients with OSA are more sensitive to depressant effects of hypnotics and opioids which deserve stricter monitoring and judicious use of the same in the perioperative period. Airway difficulties are discussed in a later section. The risk of perioperative cardiorespiratory events increases in proportion to the severity of OSA.

Preoperative evaluation should begin with detailed history taking. Observed loud snoring, sudden arousals from sleep with choking sensation and witnessed apnoea by a partner or parent, presence of daytime somnolence, morning headaches, irritability, and systemic hypertension are very characteristic of OSA. Enquiring about the use of a continuous positive airway pressure (CPAP) or bi-level positive airway pressure (BiPAP) device and assessing the patient's compliance is essential. Patients who are status post uvulopalatopharyngoplasty should be considered still at risk of OSA and its complications.

Many questionnaires have been developed to screen for OSA such as the ASA Checklist, Berlin Questionnaire, Epworth Sleepiness Scale, Flemons Criteria, and others. The most convenient screening tool that has been validated for surgical patients is the STOP-Bang questionnaire [48]:

S Do you **S**nore loudly, enough to be heard through closed doors?

T Do you feel **T**ired or fatigued during the daytime almost every day?

O Has anyone **O**bserved that you stop breathing during sleep?

P Do you have a history of high blood **P**ressure, with or without treatment?

B **B**ody mass index (BMI) greater than 35 kg/m²

A **A**ge over 50 years

N   Neck circumference greater than 40 cm
G   Male Gender.[1]

A score of 0–3 indicates a low risk of OSA, a score of 4–5, an intermediate risk of OSA, and a score of 6–8, a high risk of OSA. At a cut-off score of 3 or higher, it has 93% sensitivity and 47% specificity for an AHI of greater than 15. For an AHI level greater than 30, the STOP-Bang sensitivity is 100% and its specificity is 37% [49]. It implies that a higher score indicates higher probability of OSA, as well as an increased likelihood of a more severe disease.

A majority (80%) of the patients remain undiagnosed preoperatively due to the poor sensitivity and specificity (50–60%) of clinical diagnosis [34]. Presence or severity cannot be reliably predicted by BMI, neck circumference, pulmonary function tests, daytime room air ABGs, or questionnaires aimed to detect sleep-disordered breathing. Overnight oximetry may be used as a screening tool in places where a detailed sleep study is not available.

A polysomnogram is the gold standard to diagnose OSA. Routine polysomnography alone prior to bariatric surgery demonstrated a 91% prevalence of OSA, compared with 58% when clinical parameters and Epworth Sleepiness Scale scores alone were used to screen for OSA [34]. A formal polysomnogram should be performed in high-risk patients, if it is feasible in the given clinical situation.

Polysomnography includes overnight monitoring of ECG, electroencephalogram, electromyogram, chest movements (plethysmography), oro-nasal airflow, and pulse oximetry. The AHI is then used to stratify the level of OSA: AHI 5–15, mild OSA; 15–30, moderate OSA; greater than 30, severe OSA. Peppard et al. demonstrated that a 10% change in body weight was associated with a parallel change of approximately 30% in the AHI [50].

AHI is also used to titrate the optimal CPAP required for a patient to ameliorate the symptoms of OSA. Preoperative initiation of CPAP or BiPAP can effectively reduce hypercarbia, hypoxaemia, and hypertension although the optimal duration of therapy to achieve these benefits is still being debated. Patients should be asked to bring their CPAP devices to the hospital for better compliance in the perioperative period secondary to their familiarity with the device and its mask.

Patients with OSA often have systemic and pulmonary hypertension due to the sympathetic overdrive in response to chronic hypoxaemia and hypercarbia. A supine daytime SpO₂ less than 96% is suggestive of pulmonary hypertension and should prompt a detailed pulmonary evaluation in the form of pulmonary function tests, ABGs, chest X-ray, and echocardiography [34]. In the absence of characteristic symptoms and pulmonary disease, morbid obesity or OSA are not per se indications for pulmonary function testing and ABG analysis [51,52].

OSA increases the risk of CAD, cardiac arrhythmias, and congestive heart failure, all of which show improvement after 4 weeks of CPAP therapy [53]. The presence of cerebral vascular disease, stroke, and gastro-oesophageal reflux disease (GORD) should also be examined.

---

[1] Reproduced courtesy of Dr Frances Chung and UHN. Copyright of University Health Network. Accurate at time of press. For up-to-date information and permission licensing, please access www.stopbang.ca.

Airway of the bariatric patient

The airway of the obese patient is often intuitively considered as difficult. This is partly because external markers of difficult bag-mask ventilation (DBMV), for example, short, thick neck, thick tongue, buffalo hump, and excess fat under the mandible ('double chin') are very obvious in most obese patients (**Fig. 17.2**). Further, more than 50% (up to 95% in patients with BMI ≥60 kg/m²) [54] of morbidly obese patients have OSA, with its attendant effects on airway mechanics, pulmonary vasculature, right ventricular function, and central control of breathing, all of which can contribute to rapid development of hypoxaemia during induction and airway obstruction after extubation. Airway management in the obese is intimidating primarily because of the rapidity of desaturation when bag-mask ventilation and/or intubation fail. The aetiology of the difficult airway in the obese/morbidly obese patient is multifactorial. Accurate prediction of the possible 'difficult airway' in the bariatric patient, followed by meticulous management, remains the cornerstone of safe bariatric anaesthesia practice. The incidence of difficult intubation in the bariatric population has been mentioned as 10–15%. However, these data were obtained from series where the 'sniffing' position was used for intubation. Since the use of the 'ramped' [55–57] and the 'beach chair' [58] positions this incidence is now reduced to as low as 1%.

Assessment of the airway: history

Obtaining history pertaining to the airway not only highlights the possibility of airway difficulty, but also makes for decisive planning. A history of previous failed intubation/surgical access would warrant further airway evaluation by imaging, and the consideration of awake intubation. Patient consent, preparation, and arrangement for the availability of skilled assistance, and equipments (including

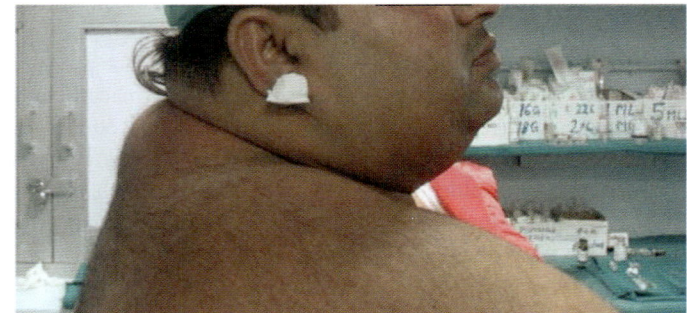
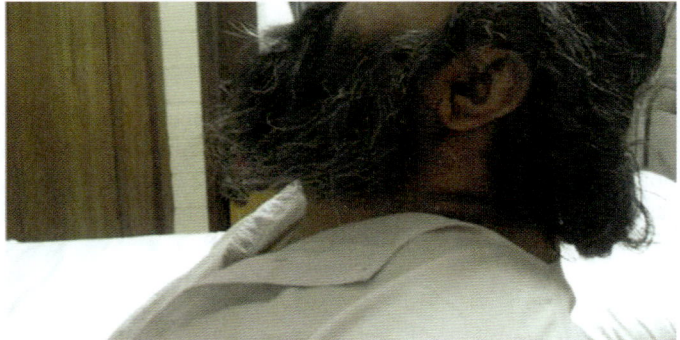

Fig. 17.2 Profile of airway in a morbidly obese patient: (a) buffalo hump and (b) restriction of neck extension.

surgical access), and so on are all important factors for the proper management of obese patients. Recent weight gain, pregnancy in an obese female patient, and recent radiotherapy to the head and neck would point to increased difficulty in accessing the airway. A history of snoring, if elicited, should be followed up by evaluation for OSA, as mentioned in detail previously. Previous anaesthetic records, if available, should be analysed for prior approaches to this airway and the failure or success achieved by various modes of intubation.

Body mass index and a difficult airway

BMI has been found to predict a 'difficult airway' by various investigations, though there is conflicting evidence as to whether obesity in itself is associated with difficult intubation. A BMI greater than 29 kg/m² has been recognized as one of five independent criteria for DBMV, along with age older than 55 years, beard, lack of teeth, and a history of snoring. The presence of any two factors indicate a high likelihood of DBMV— sensitivity, 0.72; specificity, 0.73 [59]. In a cohort of 91,332 patients from the Danish Anesthesia Registry who underwent tracheal intubation, it was found that a BMI of at least 35 kg/m² was a weak, but statistically significant predictor of difficult and failed intubation [60].

Incidence of intubation difficulty using the Intubation Difficulty Scale score has been shown to be significantly higher in obese (BMI >35 kg/m²) compared to non-obese patients (BMI <30 kg/m²) [61,62]. In a recent review of 4303 patients undergoing abdominal surgery with tracheal intubation, of whom 1673 were morbidly obese (BMI 29.7 ± 8.2 kg/m²), BMI reliably predicted potential intubation difficulty, predominantly in the male patients [63]. Two studies, described in the following paragraphs, refute this relationship of increasing BMI to difficult and/or failed intubation.

A study by Ezri et al. found that increased BMI per se was not a predictor of difficult intubation, but that its association with abnormal dentition increased difficulty with tracheal intubation. Similarly, in 915 patients undergoing laparoscopic Roux-en-Y gastric bypass, factors that predicted difficult intubation (6.3% in this series), were Mallampati class, abnormal thyromental distance, jaw mobility, and a history of difficult intubation [64,65].

BMI is often associated with difficult intubation in the ICU, hypoxaemia being one of the factors leading to perceived airway difficulty and morbidity. Major airway complications occurring in ICU and OR have involved obese patients in 47% and 40% of cases, respectively [66]. Suboptimal airway management with consequent risk of hypoxaemia can significantly contribute to the morbidity and mortality associated with anaesthesia in obese patients. In a recent closed claims analyses involving difficult airways, obese patients constituted 42% of all claims [67].

Obstructive sleep apnoea and airway difficulty

It has been recorded by magnetic resonance imaging studies that non-obese subjects with OSA and obese subjects with OSA have 30% and 44% greater amount of total body fat, and 10% and 28% greater neck tissue volume, respectively, when compared to their non-snoring counterparts [68]. The relationship between OSA and incidence of difficult intubation is also not linear.

In a series of 180 bariatric patients with a mean BMI of 49.4 kg/m², 68% of whom had polysomnography-proven OSA, no correlation between the presence and severity of OSA was found with difficult laryngoscopy and/or intubation. The incidence of difficult

intubation was only 8.3%. All patients were intubated in the 'ramped' position. Similar results were observed in a smaller series where Mallampati scores in patients with OSA were more predictive of difficult intubation [69,70].

However, a larger number of studies have found a positive correlation of OSA with difficult intubation. Patients with OSA and difficult airways, were likely to have an AHI greater than 50, with neck circumference greater than 40 cm [71,72]. A high STOP-Bang score is associated with, and can predict, difficult intubations in obese patients [73–75]. Preoperative OSA screening has been recommended to predict airway access.

Anatomical changes associated with morbid obesity, leading to difficult airways, are restricted neck flexion and extension of the neck and atlanto-occipital joint, low cervical and upper thoracic fat pads, large breasts, limited mouth opening, increased pharyngeal fat, and a high anterior and infantile laryngeal position. Mallampati scoring, modified by Samsoon and Yoong, is easy to perform and is done by asking the subject to open the mouth wide and protrude the tongue maximally without phonation. The view of the faucial pillars, tongue, soft palate, and uvula is graded from I to IV in increasing order of potential difficulty for laryngoscopy (**Fig. 17.3**).

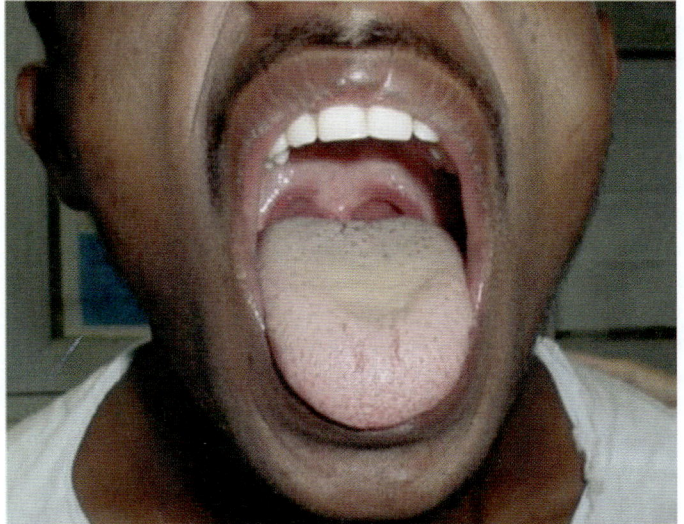

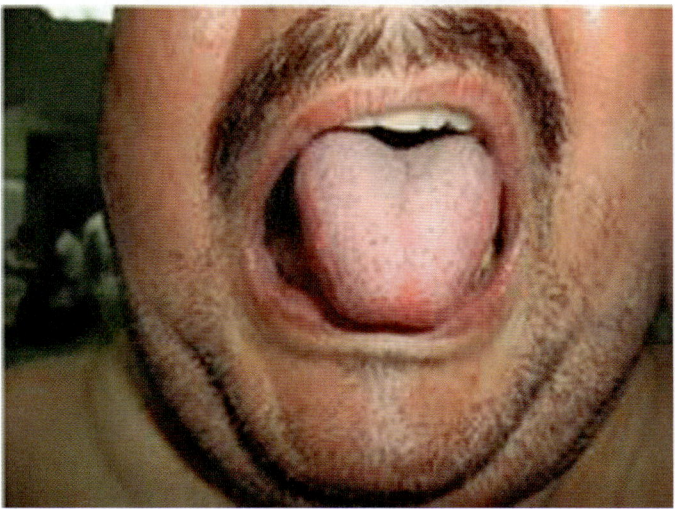

Fig. 17.3 Mallampati class I (a) and Mallampati class IV (b).

The modified Mallampati score has been extensively assessed in obese subjects. Very consistently, most series agree to the sensitivity and predictive value of modified Mallampati scores of classes III and IV to predict difficult intubation. However, in spite of modified Mallampati class III/IV being an independent risk factor for difficult intubation, the scale's specificity has been quoted at 62% and positive predictive value at 29% [61]. According to Brodsky, although morbid obesity on its own may not be a risk factor for difficult airway, its association with modified Mallampati class III/IV significantly increase the incidence of difficult intubation [76]. Interestingly, even after the advent of the 'ramped' position for laryngoscopy, modified Mallampati class III/IV predicted difficult intubation [69]. If the modified Mallampati class is III or greater, neck circumference greater than 40 cm, and AHI greater than 50, the likelihood of a difficult airway is high [72].

Neck circumference is measured with a standard tape measure at the level of the thyroid cartilage (Fig. 17.4). A circumference of greater than 40 cm is associated with snoring and increased difficulty in ventilation and intubation.

Neck circumference as a predictor of difficult intubation has been evaluated in many studies. Both obese and non-obese snorers have increased neck circumference and an increased amount of soft tissue anterior to the larynx, which is largely composed of fat [68,77]. Airway and pharyngeal aperture narrowing in OSA also occur due to a relative increase in amount of the soft tissue within the rigid craniofacial bony enclosure available for the airway and, consequently, a narrowing of the airway [78]. The neck circumference is a useful predictor of difficult intubation in the obese and has a sensitivity of 92% when using a measurement greater than 43 cm as a marker for difficulty, and a specificity of 92% when combined with the Mallampati score [78]. This study was, however, appropriately criticized for the disproportionate number of female patients. Similarly, a neck circumference greater than 44 cm combined with severe OSA has been seen to predict difficult airway in the obese with great sensitivity [71,72]. A neck circumference-to-thyromental distance greater than 5 has been shown to have the highest sensitivity, the highest negative predictive value, and the largest area under a ROC curve, in a study involving 125 morbidly obese patients [79]. The thyromental and sternomental distances, along with assessment of temporomandibular joint function and neck mobility, complete the clinical airway assessment.

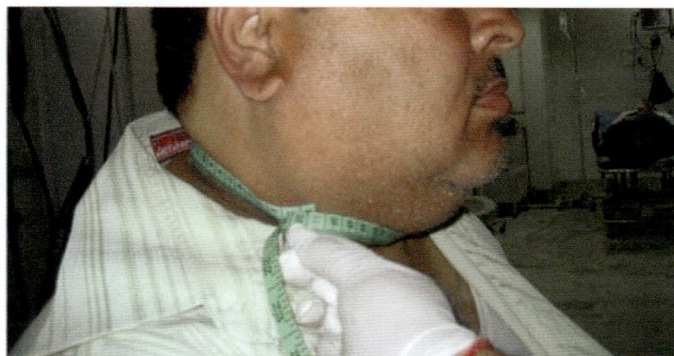

Fig. 17.4 Neck circumference at the level of thyroid cartilage (51 cm in this patient).

Value of combined indices

There are numerous studies which have assessed the accuracy of a group of anatomical variables in the obese patient in predicting DBMV and/or difficult intubation. Age greater than 49 years, short neck, and neck circumference greater than 43 cm have been seen to have a high correlation with DBMV in the obese population. Again, small mouth opening, increasing age, male sex, and temporomandibular joint pathology are all independent predictors of difficult intubation in the obese. A combination of neck circumference greater than 35 cm, sternomental distance less than 12.5 cm, and reduced neck mobility are associated with a high Intubation Difficulty Scale score [77,80]. Obese patients are seen to have a higher Intubation Difficulty Scale score compared to their lean counterparts [80].

Imaging of the airway

Ultrasound

Anterior neck soft tissue thicknesses measured by ultrasound at the hyoid bone, thyrohyoid membrane, and anterior commissure levels, when decreased, have been found to be independent predictors of difficult laryngoscopy, and may be used as additional information. The added benefit of ultrasound examination is to assess the difficulty of a surgical airway in the morbidly obese, and to accurately map the cricothyroid membrane [81,82].

X-ray of the neck

Lateral view X-rays may reveal the thickness of the tongue, epiglottis, and the position of the larynx relative to the cervical spine. If the hyoid, which should normally be at the level of C2 is displaced caudally to C4 or below, it indicates caudal displacement of the larynx and subsequent potentially difficult direct laryngoscopy (Fig. 17.5).

Mirror indirect laryngoscopy

Indirect laryngoscopy, performed in the sitting position, has been seen to predict difficult intubation in the obese. Mirror laryngoscopy had a tendency towards statistical significance in predicting difficult laryngoscopy in these patients [83].

Preoperative endoscopic airway evaluation

This approach has been used in patients scheduled for endotracheal intubation under anaesthesia. A preliminary endoscopic airway evaluation before anaesthetic induction resulted in a change in airway plan in 26% patients. This appears to be a potentially useful tool for the morbidly obese [84].

A combination of Mallampati score greater or equal to class III, neck circumference greater than 40 cm, neck circumference/thyromental distance greater than 5, and the presence of OSA should be significant pointers towards possible difficulty with mask ventilation and/or tracheal intubation.

Gastrointestinal system

Obesity is associated with all grades of hepatobiliary diseases ranging from asymptomatic transaminitis and gall stones to cirrhosis and liver failure. The most striking hepatic changes seen

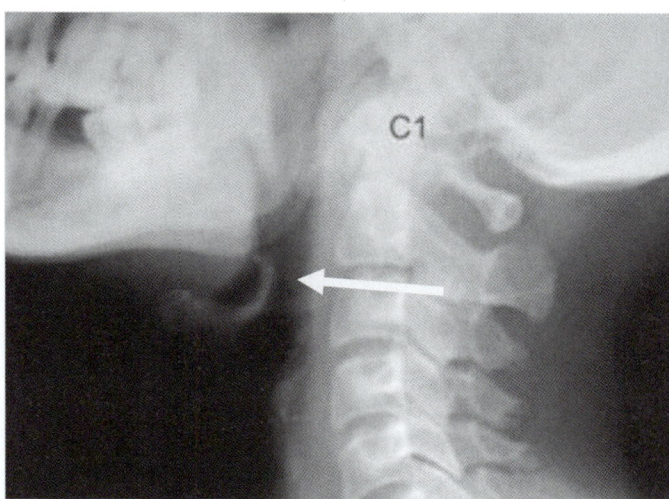

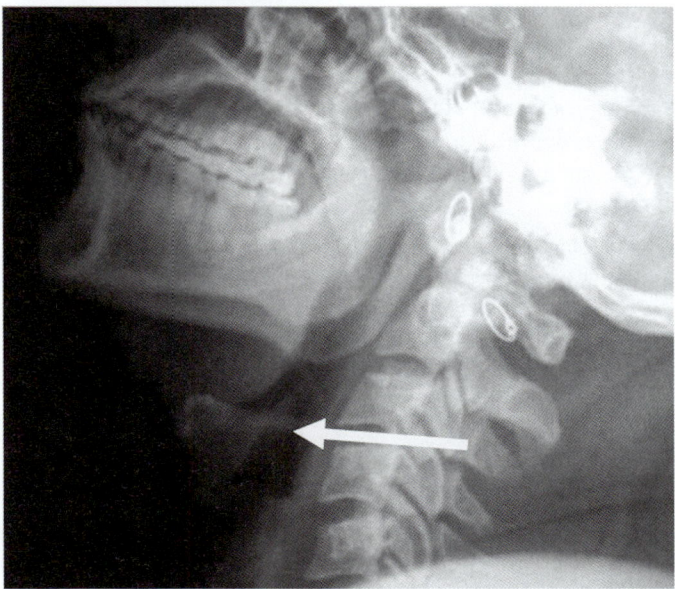

Fig. 17.5 Normal level of larynx (a) and caudad displacement in a morbidly obese patient (b).

are non-alcoholic fatty liver disease (NAFLD) and non-alcoholic steatohepatitis (NASH). NAFLD is the most common liver pathology with a logarithmic growth due to a steady increase in obesity. The histology ranges from mild simple steatosis to advanced fibrosis and cirrhosis. Glucose intolerance and T2DM increase the probability of NASH. The 'two-hit hypothesis' has been postulated which describes initial fat accumulation leading to inflammation and fibrosis [85].

The presenting feature might range from chronic fatigue and elevated liver enzymes to coagulopathy with liver failure. NASH and NAFLD are diagnoses of exclusion and other causes of hepatic dysfunction must be actively looked for. Aspartate aminotransferase and alanine amino transferase levels may be raised along with gamma-glutamyl transferase and alkaline phosphatase, but the prothrombin time and albumin levels remain normal until later stages of the disease [85]. Hepatomegaly might often be missed due to difficult palpation in an obese abdomen. The most common diagnostic method is liver imaging, as an incidental finding [8]. Even though the high prevalence of this disease among the morbidly

obese does not increase the postoperative complications, unless in advanced stages, these patients, however, are prone for kidney injury after surgery [86]. Altered liver metabolism seen in NAFLD might affect drug metabolism and affect postoperative course, but no recommendations exist at present [8].

Gastric emptying time

The gastric emptying may be prolonged in morbid obesity. This might be due to reduced fundal tone, altered stretch receptor sensitivity, gastric distension, and a high-fat diet [87]. Poor fundal and antral tone delays food distribution throughout the stomach and thus its emptying [88]. These alterations might be seen as reasons for increasing 'nothing by mouth' orders in morbid obesity, but recent studies show otherwise. On studies examining gastric emptying in the obese, no delayed gastric motility was detected [89]. So, according to the current scenario, fasting guidelines hold the same in morbid obesity without GORD as in a non-obese patient [90,91].

Risk of aspiration

DM is often seen in these patients as a part of the metabolic syndrome and might cause gastroparesis and impede gastric emptying [92]. Hiatal hernia is seen in almost 50%, with GORD diagnosed in one-third of patients with morbid obesity [93]. This is due to decreased tone of the lower oesophageal sphincter due to anatomical variations of the gastro-oesophageal junction, hormonal factors, and increased intragastric pressure transmitted from increased abdominal pressure [93]. Since morbidly obese individuals may be at a higher risk for GORD and hiatal hernia, they may also have a higher than normal risk for aspiration of gastric contents [94]. Dual prophylaxis with an H_2 blocker or proton pump inhibitor with sodium citrate might be considered appropriate in these individuals. Proton pump inhibitors require two doses for their peak action, while therapeutically active concentrations can be achieved with a single dose of an H_2 blocker [92].

Obesity and endocrine disorders

Obesity has been found to be associated with T2DM, hypothyroidism, and metabolic syndrome [95]. Increased production of adipocytokines by the truncal fat stores, ectopic fat deposition (in liver and skeletal muscle), and mitochondrial dysfunction all have been suggested as possible mechanisms of obesity-induced insulin resistance [96–98]. Diabetes increases the risk of perioperative complications. Hence, management of T2DM is of utmost importance during the perioperative period. Recommendations include to maintain glycated haemoglobin concentration 6.5–7%, fasting blood glucose less than or equal to 110 mg/dL and 2-hour postprandial blood glucose less than or equal to 140 mg/dL. A glycated haemoglobin concentration greater than 8% increases the risk of wound infection and acute kidney injury postoperatively [99]. An elevated glycated haemoglobin concentration in the preoperative setting also increases the likelihood of elevated blood glucose in the postoperative setting and decreases the rate of resolution of T2DM after bariatric surgery [99]. A combination of diet modification, weight loss, and oral hypoglycaemic agents should be initiated in the preoperative period.

Hypothyroidism leads to weight gain, reduced metabolic rate, and thermogenesis. Even subclinical hypothyroidism has been found to be associated with obesity [100]. Serum thyroid-stimulating hormone (TSH) and serum leptin levels positively correlate with BMI [101]. The proposed aetiology is leptin-induced increases in deiodinase enzyme activity, leading to increased conversion of T_4 to T_3 and reduced tissue responsiveness, causing a compensatory increase in thyroid-stimulating hormone levels [102]. This could be an adaptive mechanism to improve energy expenditure in obese individuals. Significant weight loss leads to a return of thyroid-stimulating hormone and free-T_3 to normal level. Most bariatric programmes include a routine thyroid function testing prior to surgery, to rule out an organic cause to the obesity.

Increased abdominal girth or waist-to-hip ratio, is associated with metabolic syndrome, T2DM, and cardiovascular disease [103]. Metabolic syndrome has been defined as the presence of at least three of the following criteria [104], with or without diabetes:

1. Central/truncal obesity (waist circumference in men >102 cm and in women >88 cm)
2. Hypertriglyceridemia ($\geq$150 mg/dL)
3. Low high-density lipoprotein cholesterol (men <40 mg/dL, women <50 mg/dL)
4. Elevated fasting glucose (>110 mg/dL)
5. Hypertension ($\geq$130/85 mmHg).[2]

Obesity predisposes to insulin resistance and is a key predisposing factor for the metabolic syndrome and progressive beta-cell dysfunction. Obese patients with metabolic syndrome have higher risk of CAD, congestive heart failure, OSA, pulmonary dysfunction, hypercoagulability, and deep venous thrombosis [105]. Preoperative evaluation should focus on identifying and managing the individual components and complications of the syndrome.

Preoperative testing, when done appropriately, can mitigate the risk of anaesthetizing morbidly obese individuals and help create a plan for intraoperative and postoperative care for this group of patients.

CASE REPORT Preoperative evaluation of the bariatric patient

Mr IMS was one of the first patients referred for bariatric surgery. He was 65 years old, weighing 115 kg, and 155 cm tall, with a BMI of 47.8 kg/m². As is the practice at our institution, he had his anaesthetic evaluation immediately after the surgical consult. He appeared depressed, and took time to answer questions. He had an extended list of comorbidities:

1. He had had DM for the last 20 years, controlled on combined insulin, metformin, and vildagliptin. He had symptoms and signs of diabetic neuropathy.
2. He had been hypertensive for the last 12 years, on a losartan–hydrochlorothiazide combination, and statins for an abnormal lipid profile.
3. He was diagnosed as having Parkinsonism 7 years ago, and was on pramipexole 3 mg thrice daily, and tianeptine for depression.
4. He had a caregiver accompanying him who put on his shoes, tied his pyjamas, and so on. On questioning Mr IMS, he admitted to very heavy snoring, feeling fatigued and dazed in the morning, being forgetful, and having a headache most of the time.
5. His airway revealed modified Mallampati class IV, with restricted extension of the neck. He was advised about and counselled regarding awake fibreoptic intubation.
6. His SpO_2 on room air was 92%.
7. The following advice was given:
   a. Polysomnography, and to start CPAP 10 cmH$_2$O.
   b. Cardiac evaluation for coronary artery disease. His echocardiogram and stress thallium test were normal.
   c. Endocrine evaluation to rule out hypothyroidism, advise on glycaemic control and help with diet plan.
   d. He was asked to report back to the preoperative testing clinic with these results after 2 weeks.

When he returned for a review 2 weeks later, we had difficulty in recognizing him. He had been tested for OSA and was now on CPAP at night. He strode happily into the clinic. He said he had slept continuously at night after many years, and never felt better. He said the CPAP had changed his life. His evaluations were as follows:

1. The polysomnogram had reported an AHI of 57.
2. Room air ABG showed PaO_2 80 mmHg, $PaCO_2$ 54 mmHg; mild chronic respiratory acidosis.
3. Insulin dosage was adjusted to maintain random blood sugar between 120 and 140 mg/dL.

His room air SpO_2 was 95%. He underwent a laparoscopic sleeve gastrectomy 2 weeks later. The airway was secured using awake fibreoptic intubation. Laryngoscopy after intubation revealed a Cormack–Lehane view of grade IV. Postoperatively he received positive end-expiratory pressure through the endotracheal tube and was extubated the following morning. A dye study ruled out gastric leak, and he was started on oral liquids and ambulation. He was discharged after 3 days. He did not require CPAP any more and was also off insulin and tianeptine. At the end of 1 month he had lost 5 kg.

Discussion

OSA is frequently diagnosed in the morbidly obese and has numerous perioperative implications. A brief period of preoperative optimization with CPAP reduces pulmonary artery pressures, systemic blood pressure, and results in improved patient well-being and compliance with the procedure.

---

[2] Reproduced with permission from Third Report of the National Cholesterol Education Program (NCEP) Expert Panel on Detection, Evaluation, and Treatment of High Blood Cholesterol in Adults (Adult Treatment Panel III) Final Report, Circulation, 106(25): 3143–421. Copyright © 2018 Wolters Kluwer Health, Inc.

REFERENCES

1. Zwintscher NP, Azarow KS, Horton JD, Newton CR, Martin MJ. The increasing incidence of adolescent bariatric surgery. J Pediatr Surg. 2013;**48**(12):2401–407.

2. Buchwald H, Avidor Y, Braunwald E, Jensen MD, Pories W, Fahrbach K, et al. Bariatric surgery. JAMA. 2004;**292**(14):1724–37.

3. Mathew B, Francis L, Kayalar A, Cone J. Obesity: effects on cardiovascular disease and its diagnosis. J Am Board Fam Med. 2008;**21**(6):562–68.

4. Poirier P, Alpert MA, Fleisher LA, Thompson PD, Sugerman HJ, Burke LE, et al. Cardiovascular evaluation and management of severely obese patients undergoing surgery: a science advisory from the American Heart Association. Circulation. 2009;**120**(1):86–95.

5. Duflou J, Virmani R, Rabin I, Burke A, Farb A, Smialek J. Sudden death as a result of heart disease in morbid obesity. Am Heart J. 1995;**130**(2):306–13.

6. Morino M, Toppino M, Forestieri P, Angrisani L, Allaix ME, Scopinaro N. Mortality after bariatric surgery. Ann Surg. 2007;**246**(6):1002–1009.

7. Cavarretta E, Casella G, Calì, B, Dammaro C, Biondi-Zoccai G, Iossa A, et al. Cardiac remodeling in obese patients after laparoscopic sleeve gastrectomy. World J Surg. 2013;**37**(3):565–72.

8. Catheline JM, Bihan H, Le Quang T, Sadoun D, Charniot JC, Onnen I, et al. Preoperative cardiac and pulmonary assessment in bariatric surgery. Obes Surg. 2008;**18**(3):271–77.

9. Gonzalez R, Bowers SP, Venkatesh KR, Lin E, Smith CD. Preoperative factors predictive of complicated postoperative management after Roux-en-Y gastric bypass for morbid obesity. Surg Endosc Other Interv Tech. 2003;**17**(12):1900–1904.

10. Ortiz VE, Kwo J. Obesity: physiologic changes and implications for preoperative management. BMC Anesthesiol. 2015;**15**(1):97.

11. Michalsky M, Teich S, Rana A, Teeple E, Cook S, Schuster D. Surgical risks and lessons learned: mortality following gastric bypass in a severely obese adolescent. J Pediatr Surg Case Rep. 2013;**1**(9):321–24.

12. Katkhouda N, Mason RJ, Wu B, Takla FS, Keenan RM, Zehetner J. Evaluation and treatment of patients with cardiac disease undergoing bariatric surgery. Surg Obes Relat Dis. 2012;**8**(5):634–40.

13. Palatini P, Parati G. Blood pressure measurement in very obese patients: a challenging problem. J Hypertens. 2011;**29**(3):425–29.

14. Hatem SN. Atrial fibrillation and obesity not just a coincidence. J Am Coll Cardiol. 2015;**66**(1):12–13.

15. Magnani JW, Hylek EM, Apovian CM. Obesity begets atrial fibrillation: a contemporary summary. Circulation. 2013;**128**(4):401–405.

16. Wanahita N, Messerli FH, Bangalore S, Gami AS, Somers VK, Steinberg JS. Atrial fibrillation and obesity-results of a meta-analysis. Am Heart J. 2008;**155**(2):310–15.

17. Anna Junior M de S, Carneiro JRI, Carvalhal RF, Torres D de FM, Cruz GG da, Quaresma JC do V, et al. Cardiovascular autonomic dysfunction in patients with morbid obesity. Arq Bras Cardiol. 2015;580–87.

18. Gugliotti D, Grant P, Jaber W, Aboussouan L, Bae C, Sessler D, et al. Challenges in cardiac risk assessment in bariatric surgery patients. Obes Surg. 2008;**18**(1):129–33.

19. Supariwala A, Makani H, Kahan J, Pierce M, Bajwa F, Dukkipati SS, et al. Feasibility and prognostic value of stress echocardiography in obese, morbidly obese, and super obese patients referred for bariatric surgery. Echocardiography. 2014;**31**(7):879–85.

20. Shah BN, Zacharias K, Pabla JS, Karogiannis N, Calicchio F, Balaji G, et al. The clinical impact of contemporary stress echocardiography in morbid obesity for the assessment of coronary artery disease. Heart. 2016;**102**(5):370–75.

21. Lerakis S, Kalogeropoulos AP, El-Chami MF, Georgiopoulou VV, Abraham A, Scott A, et al. Transthoracic dobutamine stress echocardiography in patients undergoing bariatric surgery. Obes Surg. 2007;**17**(11):1475–81.

22. Nuria Vilarrasa TM. Role of echocardiography in bariatric surgery: preoperative assessment of non-cardiopathic morbidly obese patients. J Anesth Clin Res. 2015;**6**(1):1–6.

23. Rocha I, Victor E, Braga M. Echocardiography evaluations for asymptomatic patients with severe obesity. Arq Bras Cardiol. 2007;**88**(1):48–53.

24. Ramaswamy A, Gonzalez R, Smith CD. Extensive preoperative testing is not necessary in morbidly obese patients undergoing gastric bypass. J Gastrointest Surg. 2004;**8**(2):159–65.

25. Vest AR, Schauer PR, Young JB. Failure and fatness. J Am Coll Cardiol. 2016;**67**(8):904–906.

26. Porhomayon J, Papadakos P, Singh a, Nader ND. Alteration in respiratory physiology in obesity for anesthesia-critical care physician. HSR Proc Intensive Care Cardiovasc Anesth. 2011;**3**(2):109–18.

27. Pankow W, Podszus T, Gutheil T, Penzel T, Peter JH, Von Wichert P, et al. Expiratory flow limitation and intrinsic positive end-expiratory pressure in obesity. J Appl Physiol. 1998;**85**(4):1236–43.

28. Nightingale CE, Margarson MP, Shearer E, Redman JW, Lucas DN, Cousins JM, et al. Peri-operative management of the obese surgical patient 2015: Association of Anaesthetists of Great Britain and Ireland Society for Obesity and Bariatric Anaesthesia. Anaesthesia. 2015;**70**(7):859–76.

29. Brazzale DJ, Pretto JJ, Schachter LM. Optimizing respiratory function assessments to elucidate the impact of obesity on respiratory health. Respirology. 2015;**20**(5):715–21.

30. Hodgson LE, Murphy PB, Hart N. Respiratory management of the obese patient undergoing surgery. J Thorac Dis. 2015;**7**(5):943–52.

31. Dixon AE, Holguin F, Sood A, Salome CM, Pratley RE, Beuther DA, et al. An Official American Thoracic Society Workshop Report: obesity and asthma. Proc Am Thorac Soc. 2010;**7**(5):325–35.

32. Schachter LM. Obesity is a risk for asthma and wheeze but not airway hyperresponsiveness. Thorax. 2001;**56**(1):4–8.

33. Sikka N, Wegienka G, Havstad S, Genaw J, Carlin AM, Zoratti E. Respiratory medication prescriptions before and after bariatric surgery. Ann Allergy Asthma Immunol. 2010;**104**(4):326–30.

34. Kaw R, Gali B, Collop N. Perioperative care of patients with obstructive sleep apnea. Curr Treat Options Neurol. 2011;**13**(5):496–507.

35. Minai OA, Yared JP, Kaw R, Subramaniam K, Hill NS. Perioperative risk and management in patients with pulmonary hypertension. Chest. 2013;**144**(1):329–40.

36. Vaughan RW, Cork RC, Hollander D. The effect of massive weight loss on arterial oxygenation and pulmonary function tests. Anesthesiology. 1981;**54**(4):325–28.

37. Mokhlesi B, Kryger MH, Grunstein RR. Assessment and management of patients with obesity hypoventilation syndrome. Proc Am Thorac Soc. 2008;**5**(2):218–25.

38. Mokhlesi B. Obesity hypoventilation syndrome: a state-of-the-art review. Respir Care. 2010;**55**(10):1347–65.

39. Chau EHL, Lam D, Wong J, Mokhlesi B, Chung F. Obesity hypoventilation syndrome: a review of epidemiology, pathophysiology, and perioperative considerations. Anesthesiology. 2012;**117**(1):188–205.

40. Mandal S, Hart N. Respiratory complications of obesity. Clin Med. 2012;**12**(1):75–78.

41. Rock P, Passannante A. Preoperative assessment: pulmonary. Anesthesiol Clin North Am. 2004;**22**(1):77–91.

42. Pillar G, Shehadeh N. Abdominal fat and sleep apnea: the chicken or the egg? Diabetes Care. 2008;31 Suppl:S303–309.

43. Young T, Palta M, Dempsey J, Skatrud J, Weber S, Badr S. The occurrence of sleep-disordered breathing among middle-aged adults. N Engl J Med. 1993;**328**(17):1230–35.

44. Formiguera X, Cantón A. Obesity: epidemiology and clinical aspects. Best Pract Res Clin Gastroenterol. 2004;**18**(6):1125–46.

45. Gami AS, Caples SM, Somers VK. Obesity and obstructive sleep apnea. Endocrinol Metab Clin North Am. 2003;**32**(4):869–94.

46. Resta O, Foschino-Barbaro MP, Legari G, Talamo S, Bonfitto P, Palumbo A, et al. Sleep-related breathing disorders, loud snoring and excessive daytime sleepiness in obese subjects. Int J Obes Relat Metab Disord. 2001;**25**(5):669–75.

47. Valencia-Flores M, Orea A, Castaño VA, Resendiz M, Rosales M, Rebollar V, et al. Prevalence of sleep apnea and electrocardiographic disturbances in morbidly obese patients. Obes Res. 2000;**8**(3):262–69.

48. Nagappa M, Liao P, Wong J, Auckley D, Ramachandran SK, Memtsoudis S, et al. Validation of the STOP-Bang questionnaire as a screening tool for obstructive sleep apnea among different populations: a systematic review and meta-analysis. PLoS One. 2015;**10**(12):e0143697.

49. Chung F, Subramanyam R, Liao P, Sasaki E, Shapiro C, Sun Y. High STOP-Bang score indicates a high probability of obstructive sleep apnoea. Br J Anaesth. 2012;**108**(5):768–75.

50. Peppard PE, Young T, Dempsey J. Longitudinal study of moderate weight change and sleep-disordered breathing. JAMA. 2000;**284**(23):3015–21.

51. Hnatiuk OW, Dillard TA, Torrington KG. Adherence to established guidelines for preoperative pulmonary function testing. Chest. 1995;**107**(5):1294–97.

52. Roche N, Herer B, Roig C, Huchon G. Prospective testing of two models based on clinical and oximetric variables for prediction of obstructive sleep apnea. Chest. 2002;**121**(3 Suppl):747–52.

53. Kaneko Y, Floras JS, Usui K, Plante J, Tkacova R, Kubo T, et al. Cardiovascular effects of continuous positive airway pressure in patients with heart failure and obstructive sleep apnea. N Engl J Med. 2003;**348**(13):1233–41.

54. Lopez PP, Stefan B, Schulman CI, Byers PM. Prevalence of sleep apnea in morbidly obese patients who presented for weight loss surgery evaluation. Am Surg. 2008;**74**(9):834–8.

55. Brodsky JB, Lemmens HJM, Brock-Utne JG, Saidman LJ. Anesthetic considerations for bariatric surgery: proper positioning is important for laryngoscopy. Anesth Analg. 2003;**96**(6):1841–42.

56. Collins JS, Lemmens HJM, Brodsky JB, Brock-Utne JG, Levitan RM. Laryngoscopy and morbid obesity: a comparison of the 'sniff' and 'ramped' positions. Obes Surg. 2004;**14**(9):1171–75.

57. Zvara DA, Calicott RW, Whelan DM. Positioning for intubation in morbidly obese patients. Anesth Analg. 2006;**102**(5):1592.

58. Fox WTA, Harris S, Kennedy NJ. Prevalence of difficult intubation in a bariatric population, using the beach chair position. Anaesthesia. 2008;**63**(12):1339–42.

59. Langeron O, Masso E, Huraux C, Guggiari M, Bianchi A, Coriat P, et al. Prediction of difficult mask ventilation. Anesthesiology. 2000;**92**(5):1229–36.

60. Lundstrøm LH, Møller AM, Rosenstock C, Astrup G, Wetterslev J. High body mass index is a weak predictor for difficult and failed tracheal intubation. Anesthesiology. 2009;**110**(2):266–74.

61. Juvin P, Lavaut E, Dupont H, Lefevre P, Demetriou M, Dumoulin J-L, et al. Difficult tracheal intubation is more common in obese than in lean patients. Anesth Analg. 2003;**97**(2):595–600.

62. Fotopoulou G, Vasileiou I, Dre K, Ntoka P, Lampadariou A, Tsinari K. Can we predict difficult intubation in obese patients? 19AP4–7. Eur J Anaesthesiol. 2011;**24**:234.

63. Uribe AA, Zvara DA, Puente EG, Otey AJ, Zhang J, Bergese SD. BMI as a predictor for potential difficult tracheal intubation in males. Front Med. 2015;**2**(June):38.

64. Ezri T, Medalion B, Szmuk P, Charuzi I. Increased body mass index per se is not a predictor of difficult laryngoscope. Can J Anesth. 2003;**2**(50):179–83.

65. Sheff SR, May MC, Carlisle SE, Kallies KJ, Mathiason MA, Kothari SN. Predictors of a difficult intubation in the bariatric patient: does preoperative body mass index matter? Surg Obes Relat Dis. 2013;**9**(3):344–49.

66. De Jong A, Molinari N, Pouzeratte Y, Verzilli D, Chanques G, Jung B, et al. Difficult intubation in obese patients: incidence, risk factors, and complications in the operating theatre and in intensive care units. Br J Anaesth. 2015;**114**(2):297–306.

67. Peterson GN, Domino KB, Caplan. RA, Posner. KL, Lee. LA, Cheney FW. Management of the difficult airway. A closed claims analysis. Anesthesiology. 2005;(103):33–39.

68. Mortimore IL, Marshall I, Wraith PK, Sellar RJ, Douglas NJ. Neck and total body fat deposition in nonobese and obese patients with sleep apnea compared to that in control subjects. Am J Respir Crit Care Med. 1998;**157**(6):280–83.

69. Neligan PJ, Porter S, Max B, Malhotra G, Greenblatt EP, Ochroch EA. Obstructive sleep apnea is not a risk factor for difficult intubation in morbidly obese patients. Anesth Analg. 2009;**109**(4):1182–86.

70. Vest D, Lee D, Newcome K, Stamper H. A retrospective review of difficult intubations. Clin Nurse Spec. 2013;**27**(3):128–31.

71. Iyer US, Koh KF, Chia NCH, Macachor J, Cheng A. Perioperative risk factors in obese patients for bariatric surgery: a Singapore experience. Singapore Med J. 2011;**52**(2):94–99.

72. Lee SJ, Lee JN, Kim TS, Park YC. The relationship between the predictors of obstructive sleep apnea and difficult intubation. Korean J Anesthesiol. 2011;**60**(3):173–78.

73. Toshniwal G, McKelvey GM, Wang H. STOP-Bang and prediction of difficult airway in obese patients. J Clin Anesth. 2014;**26**(5):360–67.

74. Acar HV, Yarkan Uysal H, Kaya A, Ceyhan A, Dikmen B. Does the STOP-Bang, an obstructive sleep apnea screening tool, predict difficult intubation? Eur Rev Med Pharmacol Sci. 2014;**18**(13):1869–74.

75. Kim JA, Lee JJ. Preoperative predictors of difficult intubation in patients with obstructive sleep apnea syndrome. Can J Anaesth. 2006;**53**(4):393–97.

76. Brodsky JB, Lemmens HJM, Brock-Utne JG, Vierra M, Saidman LJ. Morbid obesity and tracheal intubation. Anesth Analg. 2002;**94**(3):732–36.

77. Magalhaes E, Oliveira Marques F, Sousa Goveia C, Araujo Ladeira LC, Lagares J. Use of simple clinical predictors on preoperative diagnosis of difficult endotracheal intubation in obese patients. Rev Bras Anesthesiol. 2013;**63**(3):262–66.

78. Isono S. Obstructive sleep apnea of obese adults. perioperative airway management. Anesthesiology. 2009;**110**(4):908–21.

79. Kim WH, Ahn HJ, Lee CJ, Shin BS, Ko JS, Choi SJ, et al. Neck circumference to thyromental distance ratio: a new predictor of difficult intubation in obese patients. Br J Anaesth. 2011;**106**(5):743–48.

80. Shailaja S, Nichelle SM, Shetty AK, Hegde BR. Comparing ease of intubation in obese and lean patients using intubation difficulty scale. Anesth Essays Res. 2014;**8**(2):168.

81. Ezri T, Gewurtz G, Sessler DI, Medalion B, Szmuk P, Hagberg C, et al. Prediction of difficult laryngoscopy in obese patients by ultrasound quantification of anterior neck soft tissue. Anaesthesia. 2003;**58**(11):1111–14.

82. Rosero-Britton B, Lopez-Gomez A, Shabsigh M. Ultrasonography of the airway: a bedside predictor of difficult to intubate obese patients. Int J Anesth Res. 2015;**3**(11):172–75.

83. Budde AO, Desciak M, Reddy V, Falcucci OA, Vaida SJ, Pott LM. The prediction of difficult intubation in obese patients using mirror indirect laryngoscopy: a prospective pilot study. J Anaesthesiol Clin Pharmacol. 2013;**29**(2):183–86.

84. Rosenblatt W, Ianus AI, Sukhupragarn W, Fickenscher A, Sasaki C. Preoperative endoscopic airway examination (PEAE) provides superior airway information and may reduce the use of unnecessary awake intubation. Anesth Analg. 2011;**112**(3):602–607.

85. Abd El-Kader SM, El-Den Ashmawy EMS. Non-alcoholic fatty liver disease: the diagnosis and management. World J Hepatol. 2015;**7**(6):846–58.

86. Weingarten TN, Swain JM, Kendrick ML, Charlton MR, Schroeder BJ, Lee REC, et al. Nonalcoholic steatohepatitis (NASH) does not increase complications after laparoscopic bariatric surgery. Obes Surg. 2011;**21**(11):1714–20.

87. Jackson SJ, Leahy FE, Mcgowan AA, Bluck LJC, Coward WA, Jebb SA. Delayed gastric emptying in the obese: an assessment using the non-invasive 13 C-octanoic acid breath test. Obesity. 2004;**6**(4):264–70.

88. Maddox A, Horowitz M, Wishart J, Collins P. Gastric and oesophageal emptying in obesity. Scand J Gastroenterol. 1989;**24**(5):593–98.

89. Buchholz V, Berkenstadt H, Goitein D, Dickman R, Bernstine H, Rubin M. Gastric emptying is not prolonged in obese patients. Surg Obes Relat Dis. 2013;**9**(5):714–17.

90. Brenn BR. Anesthesia for pediatric obesity. Anesthesiol Clin North Am. 2005;**23**(4):745–64.

91. Cartagena R. Preoperative evaluation of patients with obesity and obstructive sleep apnea. Anesthesiol Clin North Am. 2005;**23**(3):463–78.

92. Kalinowski CPH, Kirsch JR. Strategies for prophylaxis and treatment for aspiration. Best Pract Res Clin Anaesthesiol. 2004;**18**(4):719–37.

93. Suter M, Dorta G, Giusti V, Calmes JM. Gastro-esophageal reflux and esophageal motility disorders in morbidly obese patients. Obes Surg. 2004;**14**(7):959–66.

94. Vaughan RW, Bauer S, Wise L. Volume and pH of gastric juice in obese patients. Anesthesiology. 1975;**43**(6):686–89.

95. Jankovic D, Wolf P, Anderwald C-H, Winhofer Y, Promintzer-Schifferl M, Hofer A, et al. Prevalence of endocrine disorders in morbidly obese patients and the effects of bariatric surgery on endocrine and metabolic parameters. Obes Surg. 2012;**22**(1):62–69.

96. Deng Y, Scherer PE. Adipokines as novel biomarkers and regulators of the metabolic syndrome. Ann N Y Acad Sci. 2010;**1212**:E1–19.

97. Bournat JC, Brown CW. Mitochondrial dysfunction in obesity. Curr Opin Endocrinol Diabetes Obes. 2010;**17**(5):446–52.

98. Larson-Meyer DE, Newcomer BR, Ravussin E, Volaufova J, Bennett B, Chalew S, et al. Intrahepatic and intramyocellular lipids are determinants of insulin resistance in prepubertal children. Diabetologia. 2011;**54**(4):869–75.

99. Matharoo GS, Renick E, Afthinos JN, Straker T, Gibbs KE. Preoperative evaluation of bariatric surgery patients, essentials and controversies in bariatric surgery. InTech. 2014;**3**–32.

100. Longhi S, Radetti G. Thyroid function and obesity. J Clin Res Pediatr Endocrinol. 2013;**5**(Suppl 1):40–44.

101. Biondi B. Thyroid and obesity: an intriguing relationship. J Clin Endocrinol Metab. 2010;**95**(8):3614–17.

102. Iacobellis G, Ribaudo MC, Zappaterreno A, Iannucci CV, Leonetti F. Relationship of thyroid function with body mass index, leptin, insulin sensitivity and adiponectin in euthyroid obese women. Clin Endocrinol (Oxf). 2005;**62**(4):487–91.

103. Björntorp P. Metabolic implications of body fat distribution. Diabetes Care. 1991;**14**(12):1132–43.

104. National Cholesterol Education Program (NCEP) Expert Panel on Detection, Evaluation and Treatment of High Blood Cholesterol in Adults (Adult Treatment Panel III). Third Report of the National Cholesterol Education Program (NCEP) Expert Panel on Detection, Evaluation, and Treatment of High Blood Cholesterol in Adults (Adult Treatment Panel III). Circulation. 2002;**106**(25):3143–421.

105. Tung A. Anaesthetic considerations with the metabolic syndrome. Br J Anaesth. 2010;105 Suppl:i24–33.

Perioperative analgesia

Dipty Mangla

Introduction

Pain after surgery is one of the most feared and unpleasant symptoms reported by patients. Despite the prevalence of acute pain teams, specific pain protocols and technological advances in pain management equipment, prevalence of reported pain has been as high as 41% after surgery [1]. Inadequate pain management can lead to increased patient morbidity, slower recovery and increased length of hospital stay, increased healthcare costs, lower patient satisfaction scores, and chronic pain issues. Effective management of pain after surgery involves an interdisciplinary and multimodal approach. Anaesthesiologists, being the leaders of the perioperative team, play an important role in management of pain postoperatively.

Measurement of pain

As pain is a subjective finding, the most effective measure of pain remains patient self-reports. Visual analogue scales and the McGill Pain Questionnaire, the most common tools to measure pain in routine clinical settings, can be used in the perioperative period. However, self-reporting after surgery may be limited by the effects of residual anaesthetics and benzodiazepines. In such a clinical setting, one might look for objective criteria such as hypertension, tachypnoea, and tachycardia with no other obvious cause.

Physiology of surgical pain

Experimental data

It has previously been proven that preclinical models of the response to capsaicin or formalin in rats do not reflect inflammatory mechanisms of surgical pain [2–4]. Brennan et al. observed guarding and increased primary mechanical heat hyperalgesia and mechanical hyperalgesia in rats after hind paw incision [5]. These responses were similar to humans, thus rendering rats to be a plausible animal model for postoperative pain experiments. In experiments on rats, it has also been shown that incision of skin, deep tissues, and muscles evokes a higher nociceptive response than incision of skin alone [6,7]. *In vivo* studies have shown that sensitization of nociceptors

after surgical stimuli can lead to increased spontaneous nociceptor activity, decreased response threshold, increased response to suprathreshold stimulus, increased receptive field, and even an increase in the number of nociceptors responding to noxious stimuli [8]. Surgical stimulus also sensitizes dorsal horn neurons which can be mitigated by injection of bupivacaine at the surgical site [5,9]. Somewhat similar findings have been reported in human studies, where forearm skin incision in healthy volunteers led to mechanical hyperalgesia [10,11]. In a study conducted by Dorr et al. it was shown that minimally invasive hip surgery with minimal deep tissue stimulation produced lesser pain than conventional hip arthroplasties [12].

As can be inferred from experimental data, surgical incision (especially deep tissue and muscle) leads to hypersensitization of peripheral nociceptors. These transmit information through A and C fibres to dorsal horn ganglia. Dorsal horn neurons transmit to the parietal cortex and at the same time receive modulating information from the cerebral cortex (**Fig. 18.1**). Dorsal root neurons also receive modulating information from the cerebral cortex.

Factors affecting perioperative pain

It's not uncommon to see patients undergoing minor surgeries complain of severe pain (defined as morphine consumption of >0.15 mg/kg or its equivalent). Early identification of predictors in patients at risk for postsurgical pain can lead to more effective pain management. The predictors for postoperative pain can be divided into four categories; demographics, psychological factors, preoperative pain, and surgery related.

1. *Demographics*: American Society of Anesthesiologists status of the patient, body mass index, weight, and education level have little bearing on postoperative pain [13–15]. Age has been shown to have a negative correlation with pain after surgery. This means younger patients are more likely to have higher pain scores and thus more narcotic consumption than older patients [16–20]. The effect of male or female sex on pain has been inconclusive.

2. *Psychological factors*: the three major psychological factors include anxiety, psychosocial stress, and coping mechanisms [21]. Anxiety is the most common factor associated with pain

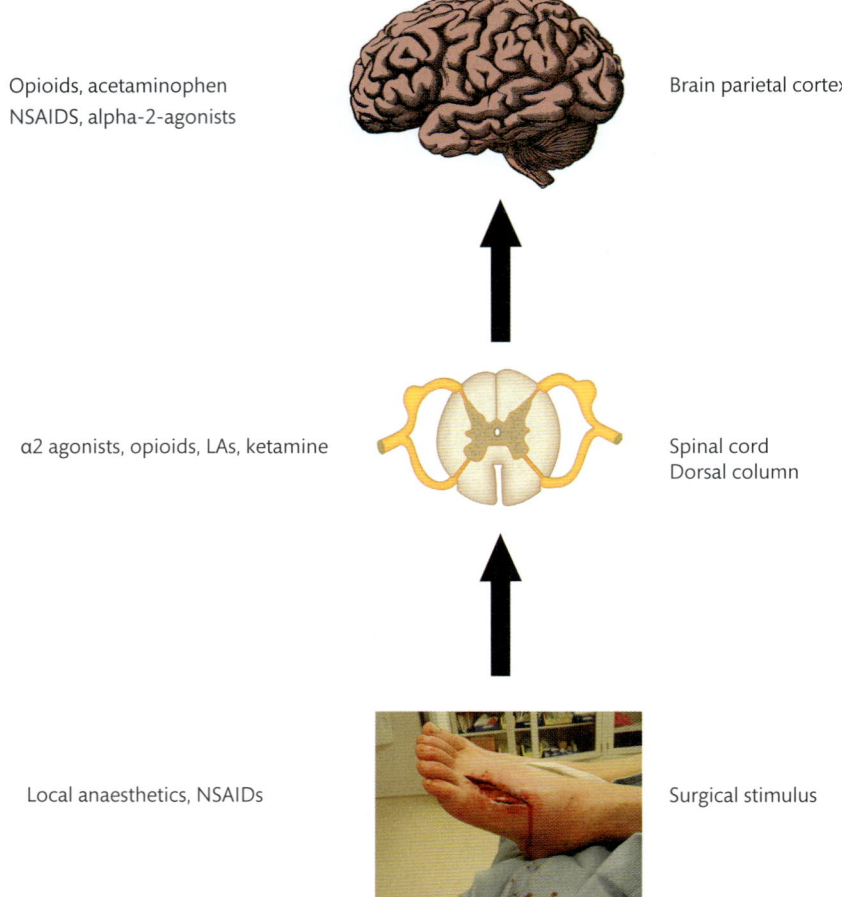

Opioids, acetaminophen
NSAIDS, alpha-2-agonists

Brain parietal cortex

α2 agonists, opioids, LAs, ketamine

Spinal cord
Dorsal column

Local anaesthetics, NSAIDs

Surgical stimulus

Fig. 18.1 Pain pathway following surgical stimulus. NSAIDs, non-steroidal anti-inflammatory drugs.

and is also associated with more consumption of analgesics in the postoperative period [13,14,22–24]. Psychological distress has a positive correlation with pain after surgery [25,26]. Psychological stress can be assessed from patients' mood, affect, and personality traits [27,28]. Coping strategies can also help predict postoperative pain [13,29–31]. Self-distraction and pain catastrophizing were correlated with higher postoperative pain scores [13,32]. It was also seen that patients who sought more information were less likely to suffer from pain [13]. Preoperative pain tolerance is also related to less pain after surgery.

3. *Surgery*: abdominal, thoracic, and orthopaedic procedure are particularly known to be associated with severe pain in the postoperative period [13–15]. Additionally, emergency surgeries, trauma surgeries, cancer-related surgeries, and surgeries lasting longer are known to cause more debilitating pain [33,34].

In summary, the major factors associated with pain include younger age; pre-existing pain; abdominal, thoracic, orthopaedic procedures; emergency or trauma surgeries; and patient anxiety.

Modalities of postoperative pain management

As can be seen from the pathophysiology of postoperative pain, pain pathways can be modulated at various levels to produce pain relief. Narcotics are the mainstay of treatment of pain; however, the dose can be significantly reduced with concomitant use of local anaesthetics. Pain relief in the perioperative period can be in the form of:

1. Intravenous medications: either bolus or in the form of patient-controlled analgesia
2. Local infiltration
3. Peripheral nerve blocks: single shot or continuously infusing catheters
4. Regional anaesthesia: spinal or epidurals
5. Oral medications
6. Transdermal medications.

The medications used in perioperative pain relief include:

1. Mu (μ)-receptor agonists
2. Non-opioid μ-receptor agonists
3. Cyclooxygenase inhibitors
4. Sodium channel antagonists
5. Alpha (α)-2 agonists
6. N-methyl-D-aspartate (NMDA) receptor antagonists
7. Anticonvulsants
8. Transient receptor potential cation channel subfamily V member 1 (TRPV1) agonists.

Drugs for pain relief in the perioperative period

Mu-receptor agonists

Mechanism of action

Opioids are the most common drugs used in the perioperative period to alleviate pain. Opioid drugs such as morphine act on μ, kappa (κ), or delta (δ) receptors on neuronal membranes to produce analgesia. These receptors are distributed throughout the central nervous system including high concentrations in the nuclei of tractus solitarius, periaqueductal grey area, cerebral cortex, thalamus, and substantia gelatinosa of the spinal cord. Opioid receptors are G-protein coupled and their activation produces the following: closing of voltage-sensitive calcium channels, and stimulation of potassium efflux leading to hyperpolarization and reduced cyclic adenosine monophosphate production. The main effect of opioids is on presynaptic neurons leading to decreased neurotransmitter release. However, they do result in a decreased response in postsynaptic neurons. The net result is a reduction in neuronal cell excitability that in turn results in reduced transmission of nociceptive impulses [35].

Depending on their mechanism of action, opioids can be agonists, partial agonists, agonist antagonists, or antagonists:

- Agonists: include morphine, methadone, fentanyl, meperidine, heroin, and hydromorphone
- Partial agonists: include propoxyphene and codeine
- Agonist antagonists: pentazocine, buprenorphine, and nalbuphine
- Antagonists: naloxone and naltrexone.

Opioid μ-receptor agonists

Tapentadol and tramadol are two analgesics which act through opioid receptors. Both tramadol and tapentadol not only act on opioid μ receptors but also inhibit serotonin and norepinephrine reuptake at receptors [36–38].

Tramadol is converted by cytochrome P450 2A6 in liver to its active metabolite which has more affinity for μ receptors than tramadol itself [38]. Pain relief after oral tramadol begins within 1 hour and peaks in 2 hours. Tramadol is indicated for moderate to severe pain relief in adults at a dose of 50–100 mg every 4–6 hours [39].

Tapentadol was approved by the Food and Drug Administration (FDA) in the United States in 2008 for use in moderate to severe pain in adults. Its dosage is 50–100 mg every 4–6 hours, similar to tramadol. Its affinity for μ receptors is 18 times the affinity of morphine. However, its potency is half to a third of the potency of morphine. The oral route of administration of tramadol limits its role as an analgesic in the immediate postoperative period. However, some data show tapentadol to be particularly effective in pain control after bunionectomy and dental surgeries [40,41].

The dual action of these drugs decreases the side effects commonly associated with opioids such as nausea, vomiting, constipation, respiratory depression, euphoria, and tolerance [42–45]. Serotonin uptake inhibition can lead to serotonin syndrome in patients on other serotonergic drugs such as selective serotonin reuptake inhibitor antidepressants. The manifestations of serotonin syndrome include mental status changes such as hallucinations and coma, autonomic instability such as tachycardia and hyperthermia, and neuromuscular abnormalities such as hyperreflexia and incoordination.

Cyclooxygenase inhibition

Non-steroidal anti-inflammatory drugs (NSAIDs) have been used for immediate pain relief after minor surgeries and after 2–3 days following major surgery. Surgery disrupts cell membrane function causing production of prostaglandins which stimulate peripheral nerve endings to produce pain. NSAIDs irreversibly inhibit cyclooxygenase (COX), thus causing decreased production of prostaglandins [46]. The detrimental effects of NSAIDs such as renal damage, gastrointestinal mucosal damage, and platelet inhibition have been attributed to inhibition of the COX-1 enzyme, whereas the pain relief is the result of COX-2 inhibition [47–49]. NSAIDs modulate pain by several mechanisms. By reducing prostaglandin synthesis, they prevent allodynia and hyperalgesia; by decreasing leucocyte response locally, they decrease release of inflammatory mediators; and after crossing the blood–brain barrier they reduce central prostaglandin synthesis. Hence, they reduce the local inflammatory response and possibly decrease central and peripheral sensitization of nociceptors [50]. Traditionally, oral dosing of NSAIDs has been used postoperatively for mild to moderate pain. In more recent times, there is evidence supporting their use pre-emptively for decreasing the hypersensitization of nociceptors. The availability of parenteral ketorolac (Toradol®) and ibuprofen makes them more useful in surgical patients who may not be able to tolerate oral medications. Intravenous Toradol® was approved by the FDA in 1989. It is recommended for moderately severe surgical pain for less than 5 days' duration [51].

Acetaminophen (paracetamol) has been used for decades for alleviation of mild to moderate pain. The action of acetaminophen, at a molecular level, though unclear could be related to the production of reactive metabolites by the peroxidase function of COX-2, which could deplete glutathione, a cofactor of enzymes such as prostaglandin E synthase [52]. In a study by Grocos et al. in patients undergoing elective ambulatory surgeries, intravenous acetaminophen prior to termination of surgery led to higher patient satisfaction when compared to placebo [53]. In a similar study conducted by Salihglu et al. in patients undergoing laparoscopic cholecystectomy, patients who received intravenous acetaminophen were found to have lower visual analogue scale scores, higher patient satisfaction scores, and shorter hospital stays when compared to placebo [54]. Though oral acetaminophen is as effective as an intravenous preparation, favourable pharmacokinetics of the intravenous preparation in the perioperative period may make the intravenous formulation preferred more often in surgical patients. Combinations of acetaminophen and NSAIDs have been shown to be more efficacious in providing pain relief than either drug alone [55,56].

Sodium channel antagonists

Local anaesthetics decrease pain by blocking voltage-dependent sodium channels. At clinical doses they block voltage-dependent potassium channels and calcium channels [57]. The pre-emptive use of local anaesthetics before surgical incision blocks nociceptors, and thus decreases the pain signals transmitted to the central nervous system and improves postoperative pain control [58]. Local infiltration, regional anaesthesia (spinal or epidural), and various nerve blocks using local anaesthetics can alleviate or mitigate pain in a variety of surgeries. Local anaesthetics exert their analgesic effects by acting on nerve roots, dorsal root ganglia, or spinal cord when injected into the epidural space [59]. For local infiltration, a combination of short-acting local anaesthetics (such as lidocaine) are used with long-acting local anaesthetics (such as bupivacaine). Local anaesthetics commonly used for epidurals include ropivacaine and bupivacaine. Liposomal bupivacaine is approved by the FDA for local infiltration in patients undergoing haemorrhoidectomy and bunionectomy. It is a longer-acting preparation of bupivacaine effective as an analgesic for up to 48 hours postoperatively [60–62].

Alpha-2 agonists

The presynaptic and postsynaptic neurons in the central and peripheral nervous systems have α_2 receptors. Activation of presynaptic neurons results in decreased release of norepinephrine. At the same time, stimulation of postsynaptic receptors in the central nervous system inhibits sympathetic activity. α_2 adrenoceptors are present in high concentrations at the locus coeruleus. Locus coeruleus is a major site for neuromodulation at supraspinal level. At the spinal level, stimulation of α_2 receptors in the substantia gelatinosa in the dorsal horn results in the inhibition of nociceptive neurons and in the release of substance P. Clonidine and dexmedetomidine are the two most common drugs used in this class. By activating G-protein-linked potassium channels, they result in hyperpolarization of membranes. They also reduce calcium conductance into cells via G0-protein-coupled N-type voltage-gated calcium channels. Because of these effects, they not only prevent neuronal firing but also prevent the local signal propagation. Intrathecal or epidural α_2 agonists are used as adjuncts to local anaesthetics for postoperative pain. Blaudszun et al. in their systematic review found that systemic clonidine and dexmedetomidine were associated with a moderate decrease in pain intensity, opioid consumption, and early postoperative nausea (numbers needed to treat, approximately 9). They were not associated with prolonged recovery time. Other opioid effects such as respiratory depression, delirium, and effect on immune system were not reported [63].

NMDA receptor antagonists

Recently, there has been an increasing interest in the use of NMDA receptor antagonists as adjuncts in multimodality management of postoperative pain. NMDA receptors are involved in central processing of pain. Ketamine, an NMDA receptor antagonist, has been of particular interest, being touted as both as an analgesic alone and as an adjunct to other drugs for postoperative pain. Anaesthesia from ketamine is attributed to its interaction with NMDA receptors in the brain. Brain concentrations of ketamine are directly related to analgesia when using an ischaemic pain model. Pain activation in the secondary somatosensory cortex, insula, thalamus, and anterior cingulate cortex were all decreased. Pacheco et al. found that central analgesic effects of ketamine were also because of activation of μ and κ opioid receptors [64]. Himmelseher et al. recommended 0.5 mg/kg slow bolus injection of ketamine before or after induction of general anaesthesia, but before incision in very painful procedures, followed by repeated injections of 0.25 mg/kg ketamine at 30-minute time intervals or a continuous infusion of 0.1–0.2 mg/kg/h. For procedures lasting longer than 2 hours, drug administration should be

terminated at least 60 minutes before surgery ends to prevent prolonged recovery from anaesthesia. In procedures expected to be less painful, a 0.25 mg/kg ketamine bolus before incision followed by every 30-minute injections of 0.125 mg/kg ketamine or an infusion of 2 mcg/kg/min was recommended [65]. Intraoperative use of ketamine has been shown to decrease pain in the postoperative period following lumbar surgeries, orofacial surgeries [66], and thoracic [67], orthopaedic [68], and gynaecological studies [69]. Ketamine in these doses is safe and usually well tolerated. However, adverse effects have been reported after its use. They include inebriation, nausea, psychotomimetic effects, and headaches with long-term use, possibly resulting in impaired cognition, memory, and mood [70]. The psychotomimetic effects of ketamine are usually temporary and last up to 60 minutes post administration [71] and can be mitigated by administration of benzodiazepine before ketamine. Other side effects attributed to ketamine are uropathy [72], hepatotoxicity, and central nervous system side effects such as diplopia, hallucinations, lightheadedness, and psychosis.

Anticonvulsants

Gabapentin and pregabalin inhibit calcium currents via high-voltage-activated channels containing the $\alpha_2\delta_1$ subunit, reducing neurotransmitter release and attenuating the postsynaptic excitability. These anticonvulsants have been used for chronic pain relief. Gabapentin has been particularly efficacious in preventing mechanical hyperalgesia following noxious stimuli as compared to morphine alone [73]. Gabapentin when used in a dose of 1200 mg was found to reduce hyperalgesia due to burns in inflamed skin [74] and the heat capsaicin model [75]. Gabapentin was also shown to decrease tolerance to analgesic effects of morphine in rat models [76,77]. A recent review by Dahl et al. included seven studies of reasonable quality. Following oral gabapentin, there was a significant reduction in postoperative analgesic requirements 24 hours after surgery in six of the included studies (abdominal hysterectomy, spinal surgery, vaginal hysterectomy, radical mastectomy, and laparoscopic cholecystectomy) [78–83]. Similar analgesic effects were seen in a study, however the effects lasted longer, that is, 48 hours post mastectomy [84]. Gabapentin 1200 mg, given 1 hour before rhinoplasty or endoscopic sinus surgery under regional anaesthesia and propofol sedation, was associated with reduced postoperative pain scores and analgesic consumption [85]. Gilron et al. suggested that the combination of rofecoxib and gabapentin was more effective than placebo and either single agent in a patient undergoing abdominal hysterectomy [86].

In a study by Menigaux et al., in patients undergoing knee surgery, gabapentin was given orally 2 hours before surgery [87]. Pre-induction visual analogue scale anxiety scores were impressively lower in the gabapentin group (28 vs 68 mm; $P < 0.0001$); postoperative pain control and early knee mobility were also significantly better.

Pregabalin was FDA approved for the treatment of peripheral neuropathic pain in 2007. Its mechanism of action is the same as gabapentin but it has a superior pharmacokinetic profile in terms of better bioavailability and faster absorption [88]. Pregabalin in a dose of 150 mg preoperatively, in patients undergoing laparoscopic cholecystectomy, was found to be associated with lower pain scores and narcotic use postoperatively [89]. Buvanendra et al.

compared pregabalin (300 mg preoperatively with a tapering dose postoperatively for 14 days) to placebo in 240 patients undergoing total knee arthroplasty. They observed decreased epidural drug consumption and increased sedation and confusion on postoperative day 0 and 1 in the pregabalin group. Long-term outcomes included reduced neuropathic pain at 3 and 6 months postoperatively [90]. Similar results were found by Zhang et al. where they demonstrated decreased morphine consumption with use of pregabalin [91]. The use of pregabalin and gabapentin in the perioperative period can be associated with dizziness. There are insufficient data for their interaction with other drugs used in the perioperative period. It seems that gabapentin, and possibly pregabalin, may have a significant role in the treatment of postoperative pain.

TRPV1 agonists

Capsaicin, an active component of chili peppers, is a peripheral TRPV1 agonist. It selectively stimulates unmyelinated C fibre afferent neurons thus causing release of substance P. The continued release of substance P following administration of capsaicin leads to its depletion from unmyelinated C fibres. It can either be used as a cream or injected. It can be used as an adjunct to other analgesic drugs in cases of mild to moderate pain. Injectable capsaicin can be used for the control of postoperative pain, such as after total knee replacement, total hip replacement, hernia repair [92], shoulder arthroscopy, and bunionectomy. It can also be used to decrease neuropathic pain occurring after surgery or trauma. Pre-administration of neural blockade before injection of capsaicin may greatly decrease the burning discomfort.

Capsaicin is a relatively safe drug with the only absolute contraindication being patient hypersensitivity. Relative contraindications include age less than 2 years, elevated liver enzymes, patients on angiotensin-converting enzyme inhibitors, and patients showing signs of septic arthritis and joint infections [93].

Modalities for perioperative pain relief

Intravenous medications

Limited tolerance to oral medications in the perioperative period renders the intravenous route as the most favoured and commonly used method for administration of drugs for pain relief after surgery. Despite undesirable side effects such as respiratory depression, nausea and vomiting, and urine retention, narcotics are the main class of drugs used for pain relief perioperatively. Narcotics can be used as bolus intravenous medications, slow controlled infusions, or in the form of patient-controlled analgesia (PCA).

Narcotics

The most commonly used intravenous opioids for postoperative pain are morphine, hydromorphone (Dilaudid®), and fentanyl (Table 18.1) [94–97]. Morphine is widely used for moderate to severe postoperative pain and the use of small intravenous doses allows titration to adequate pain relief. It has a rapid onset of action with peak effect occurring in 1–2 hours. Fentanyl and hydromorphone are synthetic derivatives of morphine and are more potent, have a shorter onset of action, and shorter half-lives when compared with morphine.

Opioids are commonly used in postoperative period for PCA. PCA is a delivery system in which patients self-administer

Table 18.1 Recommended dose of commonly used narcotics for postoperative pain relief

Drug	Recommended dose every 5–10 minutes until adequate pain relief
Morphine	0.025–0.05 mg/kg [94]
Hydromorphone	0.0075–0.015 mg/kg [95]
Fentanyl	0.25–0.5 mcg/kg [96]
Meperidine	One-time dose of 1–1.5 mg/kg [97]

predetermined doses of analgesic medication to relieve their pain (Table 18.2). PCA results in better pain control, greater patient satisfaction, less sedation, and fewer postoperative complications. All PCA modes contain the following variables: initial loading dose, demand dose, lockout interval, background infusion rate, and 1-hour or 4-hour limits. In opioid-naive patients and some other patients such as those with sleep apnoea, using a basal dose is not recommended. Morphine is the most commonly used drug for PCA in the postoperative period. The adverse side effects of opioid PCA include sedation, respiratory depression, nausea and vomiting, pruritus, and urinary retention.

Meperidine was previously used for PCA, but is not recommended any more, especially in elderly, patients with kidney problems, and patients on MAO inhibitors or selective serotonin reuptake inhibitors. When using intravenous narcotics for postoperative pain, patients should be assessed for pain, sedation, and cardiorespiratory status before and after administration of drugs.

NSAIDs

Toradol® (ketorolac) and Caldolor® (ibuprofen) are two NSAIDs that can be injected via the intravenous routes for perioperative pain relief. These drugs are recommended for mild to moderate pain or as adjuncts to opioids in severe pain. Toradol® is an anti-inflammatory drug with potency comparable to morphine and meperidine; however, it does have a ceiling effect. It is 99% plasma protein bound and Toradol® and its active metabolites are eliminated by the renal system. The recommended dose of Toradol® is 30 mg intravenously every 8 hours, for a maximum of 2 days. Adverse effects include dyspepsia, renal dysfunction, and platelet dysfunction. A double-blind randomized trial on patients undergoing orthopaedic surgery found that the use of Caldolor® had opioid-sparing effect as compared to placebo [98]. The recommended dosage for Caldolor® is 400–600 mg every 6 hours, as needed, with a maximum of 4200 mg/day. The most common adverse effects include nausea, anaemia, vomiting, flatulence, bacteraemia, hypoproteinaemia, and headache. Caldolor® is contraindicated in patients undergoing open heart surgery, asthmatics, and patient with known hypersensitivity to NSAIDs.

Acetaminophen (paracetamol)

Intravenous acetaminophen has faster onset and better absorption than oral or rectal formulations [99,100]. The intravenous route also appears to avoid hepatic first-pass metabolism [101]. Intravenous acetaminophen can be given as single or multiple doses. The recommended dosing for intravenous acetaminophen for an adult is 1000 mg every 6 hours. Recommended dosing for paediatric patients older than 2 years is 15 mg/kg. Acetaminophen is contraindicated

Table 18.2 Recommended doses for patient-controlled analgesia

Drug	Initial bolus	Demand dose	Lockout period	Maximum dose per 4-hour period
Morphine	1–5 mg	0.5–3 mg	6–8 minutes	30 mg
Hydromorphone	0.1–0.5 mg	0.05–0.5 mg	6–8 minutes	6 mg
Fentanyl	25–50 mcg	10–50 mcg	6–8 minutes	300 mcg

in patients with severe hepatic injury or failure. Caution must be used when administering acetaminophen to patients with liver dysfunction or active liver disease, alcoholism, chronic malnutrition, severe hypovolaemia (e.g. due to dehydration or blood loss), or severe kidney dysfunction (i.e. creatinine clearance ≤30 mL/min). The common adverse effects reported are nausea, headaches, and insomnia [101,102].

Local infiltration

Local anaesthetic infiltration is injection of local anaesthetic around the surgical incision site before or after the actual incision. The addition of epinephrine to the local anaesthetic prolongs the duration of analgesia and also allows increased volumes of local anaesthetics to be used for infiltration. The technique has been adopted for use for postoperative analgesia following a range of surgical procedures (orthopaedic, general, gynaecological, and breast surgeries). Local anaesthetics, when infiltrated, bind to fast sodium channels at the nociceptive afferents. This prevents propagation of action potentials and hence inhibits directly the transmission of pain. Local anaesthetics also inhibit the inflammatory response to injury. This is a simple and cost-effective technique of pain relief. Local anaesthetic infiltration is particularly useful in procedures with less visceral components such as hernia repair and other minor procedures [103]. However, it has one major drawback: the duration of analgesia is limited to the duration of action of the local anaesthetic. This tends to be 4–8 hours for bupivacaine and ropivacaine. The availability of liposomal bupivacaine (with duration of about 72 hours) has created a renewed interest in this method of pain relief. Liposomal bupivacaine has been FDA approved for single-dose wound infiltration in postoperative pain relief among patients undergoing haemorrhoidectomy and bunionectomy. Bupivacaine, if used in large doses, can have life-threatening side effects. The most common side effects involve the cardiovascular and central nervous systems [104]. It is more cardiotoxic than lidocaine, and it produces its toxicity by producing cardiac conduction block. The neurological side effects include headache, dizziness, perioral tingling, and numbness. Other than symptomatic treatment, specific treatment of bupivacaine toxicity is 20% Intralipid® (2–4 mL/kg bolus followed by 0.25 to 0.5 mL/kg/min infusion). This formulation should not be co-administered with any other local anaesthetic as it may increase the release of bupivacaine from the liposomes. It should not be allowed to come into contact with antiseptics such as chlorhexidine or povidone iodine as they may disrupt the lipid layers leading to uncontrolled release of bupivacaine.

Peripheral nerve blocks

Selective peripheral nerve blocks offer a prolonged duration of analgesia, selective area of action, and fewer collateral effects compared to regional or general anaesthesia [105]. The use of continuous nerve block catheters leads to prolonged duration of analgesia as compared to a single-shot nerve block. In a large, multicentre prospective study, it was seen that continuous blocks by trained anaesthesiologists led to high-quality postoperative analgesia along with fewer infectious and neurological complications. Continuous peripheral nerve blocks are methods of choice for knee, foot, and shoulder surgeries [104–109]. The improved analgesia provided by continuous peripheral nerve blocks has been reported to result in faster short-term functional recovery during rehabilitation than that provided by intravenous PCA [108,110]. The nerve block for specific surgeries depends on the anatomical location of surgical stimulus.

The continuous catheters have a few technical challenges associated with them. These include difficulty in catheter insertion, catheter migration after placement, and dislodgement of catheter. Serious side effects include nerve injury, acute respiratory failure and recurrent laryngeal nerve block (interscalene block), local anaesthetic toxicity, seizures, abscess formation, and severe hypotension.

Neuraxial block

Central neuraxial blocks alone or in combination with other techniques are performed in various surgical interventions in order to decrease surgically induced stress and inflammation, improve pulmonary functions, and reduce the period for restarting ambulation with better pain control. Central neuraxial techniques include spinal anaesthesia, epidural, combined spinal epidural, and a caudal epidural. The role of subarachnoid block for postoperative pain relief is limited because of shorter duration (up to 4 hours) and side effects such as hypotension and intense motor block. Epidural catheters offer the advantages of longer duration, relatively selective block, and the opportunity to provide patient-controlled epidural analgesia. Epidural analgesia has an added advantage of improved patient mobility, thus decreasing risk of thromboembolic events [111,112]. Epidural analgesia offers better quality of analgesia, earlier return of bowel movements, and better maintenance of cardiac and pulmonary functions than opioids, following abdominal and colorectal surgeries. Local anaesthetics when administered in the epidural space can lead to hypotension; addition of opioids can allow for more

Table 18.3 Surgery and indicated nerve block

Surgery site location	Nerve block
Shoulder	Interscalene
Elbow	Axillary
Hand	Axillary
Hip	Femoral
Knee	Femoral
Foot	Popliteal

Table 18.4 Recommended dosing for epidural anaesthesia

Drug	Volume (mL/h)
Bupivacaine 0.125%	4–12
Bupivacaine 0.0625% and fentanyl 5 mcg/mL	4–12
Ropivacaine 0.2%	6–14
Ropivacaine 0.1% and fentanyl 5 mcg/mL	6–14

dilute solutions and less volume of local anaesthetics. Opioids, however, when given in the epidural space can lead to pruritus, sedation, respiratory depression, and urine retention [113]. Epidural catheters can also be used for patient-controlled epidural analgesia in compliant and cooperative patients. Moawad et al. found that both fentanyl PCA and epidural PCA were effective for pain management after major abdominal surgeries; however, epidural analgesia is less sedating and leads to better patient satisfaction [114]. Epidural analgesia can also be associated with side effects such as hypotension and respiratory depression, so it is recommended that the patient's cardiorespiratory status be monitored at least every 4 hours.

Ropivacaine is advocated for routine use for epidural continuous infusion since it is less cardiotoxic than bupivacaine; however, it is more expensive and less efficacious than bupivacaine. Epidural used to be the modality of choice; more recently, regional techniques with fewer complications are preferred over epidural for postoperative pain relief.

Oral medications

Oral medications such as acetaminophen, NSAIDs, opioids, α_2 agonists, and anticonvulsants are used as sole agents in mild to moderate pain. They are also used as adjuncts in severe pain. There is evidence that starting the oral medications before the surgery pre-emptively helped decrease the severity of pain postoperatively. These medications were discussed earlier in this chapter.

Transdermal medications

Transdermal medications use non-invasive iontophoretic technology—based on the electrotransport principle that similar charges repel each other to deliver medications. The drug most commonly used as a transdermal patch is fentanyl. The relative inaccuracy of this method to predict the effect limits its use for acute pain. However, transdermal fentanyl can be used for acute pain relief in chronic pain patients [115].

Conclusion

Postoperative pain is one of the most feared complications after surgery. As far as pain is concerned, proper communication between surgeons, anaesthesiologists, perioperative nurses, and patients can lead to better outcomes. The use of oral pre-medications such as acetaminophen and NSAIDs before surgery, pre-emptive local anaesthetic infiltration before surgical incision, use of nerve block, and epidural drug delivery via catheter placement leads to improved patient satisfaction and improved pain scores postoperatively. Obese patients can specifically benefit from non-opioid-based pain management regimens.

CASE REPORT

1. A 35-year-old male patient, 189 cm tall, weighing 150 kg, comes to same-day surgery for a right knee arthroscopy. On further questioning, the patient admits to having chronic pain in his knee and lower back. He is on Percocet® (5,125) (oxycodone/acetaminophen), two tablets every 6 hours for his pain. Along with that, he takes 600 mg ibuprofen every 8 hours for his pain. He is really concerned about pain. Formulate a perioperative pain management regimen for him.

    Given his chronic pain, he is more likely to have opioid tolerance. I would give him his regular dose of ibuprofen and 650 mg acetaminophen orally before going back to surgery. Since this procedure is usually associated with mild to moderate pain, I will treat his intraoperative pain with short-acting opioids such as fentanyl. I would also ask the surgeon to use long-acting liposomal bupivacaine for the incision. Before discharging the patient home, I would also recommend to use his Percocet®.

2. A 50-year-female, 152 cm tall, weighing 185 kg, comes for laparoscopic cholecystectomy. She has a history of obstructive sleep apnoea. She denies any history of chronic pain; however, she does have a history of hypertension and diabetes. How will you manage pain in this patient?

    The obese patient with a history of obstructive sleep apnoea, a common problem in this group, is a challenging patient. Apart from other anaesthesia issues, sensitivity to opioids makes pain management difficult in the postoperative period. Operating on a morbidly obese patient can be associated with a higher chance of bleeding postoperatively. As much as possible, preoperative NSAIDs should be avoided. However, if the surgery is not associated with increased bleeding, I would give intravenous Toradol®. Also, I would give intravenous acetaminophen, and fentanyl intraoperatively. I would also arrange for continuous positive airway pressure and bi-level positive airway pressure postoperatively if she is sedated after receiving opioids. Additionally, I would recommend admitting her overnight to observe her respiration and ventilation, given her history of sleep apnoea.

3. A 55-year-old, 189 cm tall patient, weighing 150 kg, is scheduled for total knee arthroplasty. Apart from obesity there is no significant medical history. The surgeon asks you to help manage his postoperative pain.

    This patient is a candidate for femoral nerve block. I would explain to the patient and perform a femoral nerve block preoperatively and use the continuous catheter for continuous nerve block postoperatively.

REFERENCES

1. Mwaka G, Thikra S, Mung'ayi V. The prevalence of postoperative pain in the first 48 hours following day surgery at a tertiary hospital in Nairobi. Afr Health Sci. 2013;**13**(3):768–76.
2. Honore P, Wade CL, Zhong C, Harris RR, Wu C, Ghayur T, et al. Interleukin-1alphabeta gene-deficient mice show reduced nociceptive sensitivity in models of inflammatory and

neuropathic pain but not post-operative pain. Behav Brain Res. 2006;**167**(2):355–64.

3. Zahn PK, Brennan TJ. Primary and secondary hyperalgesia in a rat model for human postoperative pain. Anesthesiology. 1999;**90**(3):863–72.

4. Zahn PK, Pogatzki-Zahn EM, Brennan TJ. Spinal administration of MK-801 and NBQX demonstrates NMDA-independent dorsal horn sensitization in incisional pain. Pain. 2005;**114**(3):499–505.

5. Brennan TJ. Pathophysiology of postoperative pain. Pain. 2011;**152**(3 Suppl):S33–40.

6. Xu J, Brennan TJ. Comparison of skin incision vs. skin plus deep tissue incision on ongoing pain and spontaneous activity in dorsal horn neurons. Pain. 2009;**144**(3):329–39.

7. Xu J, Brennan TJ. Guarding pain and spontaneous activity of nociceptors after skin versus skin plus deep tissue incision. Anesthesiology. 2010;**112**(1):153–64.

8. Meyer RA, Ringkamp M, Campbell JN, Raja SN. Peripheral mechanisms of cutaneous nociception. In: McMahon SB, Koltzenburg M, eds. Wall and Melzack's Textbook of Pain. Amsterdam: Elsevier/Churchill Livingstone; 2006:3–34.

9. Xu J, Richebe P, Brennan TJ. Separate groups of dorsal horn neurons transmit spontaneous activity and mechanosensitivity one day after plantar incision. Eur J Pain. 2009;**13**(8):820–28.

10. Kawamata M, Takahashi T, Kozuka Y, Nawa Y, Nishikawa K, Narimatsu E, et al. Experimental incision-induced pain in human skin: effects of systemic lidocaine on flare formation and hyperalgesia. Pain. 2002;**100**(1–2):77–89.

11. Kawamata M, Watanabe H, Nishikawa K, Takahashi T, Kozuka Y, Kawamata T, et al. Different mechanisms of development and maintenance of experimental incision-induced hyperalgesia in human skin. Anesthesiology. 2002;**97**(3):550–59.

12. Dorr LD, Maheshwari AV, Long WT, Wan Z, Sirianni LE. Early pain relief and function after posterior minimally invasive and conventional total hip arthroplasty. A prospective, randomized, blinded study. J Bone Joint Surg Am. 2007;**89**(6):1153–60.

13. Kalkman CJ, Visser K, Moen J, Bonsel GJ, Grobbee DE, Moons KG. Preoperative prediction of severe postoperative pain. Pain. 2003;**105**(3):415–23.

14. Mamie C, Bernstein M, Morabia A, Klopfenstein CE, Sloutskis D, Forster A. Are there reliable predictors of postoperative pain? Acta Anaesthesiol Scand. 2004;**48**(2):234–42.

15. Caumo W, Schmidt AP, Schneider CN, Bergmann J, Iwamoto CW, Adamatti LC, et al. Preoperative predictors of moderate to intense acute postoperative pain in patients undergoing abdominal surgery. Acta Anaesthesiol Scand. 2002;**46**(10):1265–71.

16. Cohen L, Fouladi RT, Katz J. Preoperative coping strategies and distress predict postoperative pain and morphine consumption in women undergoing abdominal gynecologic surgery. J Psychosom Res. 2005;**58**(2):201–209.

17. Chang KY, Tsou MY, Chiou CS, Chan KH. Correlations between patient-controlled epidural analgesia requirements and individual characteristics among gynecologic patients. Acta Anaesthesiol Taiwan. 2006;**44**(3):135–40.

18. Coulbault L, Beaussier M, Verstuyft C, et al. Environmental and genetic factors associated with morphine response in the postoperative period. Clin Pharmacol Ther. 2006;**79**:316–24.

19. Gagliese L, Gauthier LR, Macpherson AK, Jovellanos M, Chan VW. Correlates of postoperative pain and intravenous patient-controlled analgesia use in younger and older surgical patients. Pain Med. 2008;**9**(3):299–314.

20. Taenzer P, Melzack R, Jeans ME. Influence of psychological factors on postoperative pain, mood and analgesic requirements. Pain. 1986;**24**(3):331–42.

21. Ip HY, Abrishami A, Peng PW, Wong J, Chung F. Predictors of postoperative pain and analgesic consumption: a qualitative systematic review. Anesthesiology. 2009;**111**(3):657–77.

22. Hsu YW, Somma J, Hung YC, Tsai PS, Yang CH, Chen CC. Predicting postoperative pain by preoperative pressure pain assessment. Anesthesiology. 2005;**103**(3):613–18.

23. Kain ZN, Sevarino F, Alexander GM, Pincus S, Mayes LC. Preoperative anxiety and postoperative pain in women undergoing hysterectomy. A repeated-measures design. J Psychosom Res. 2000;**49**(6):417–22.

24. Pud D, Amit A. Anxiety as a predictor of pain magnitude following termination of first-trimester pregnancy. Pain Med. 2005;**6**(2):143–48.

25. Coulbault L, Beaussier M, Verstuyft C, Weickmans H, Dubert L, Trégouet D, et al. Environmental and genetic factors associated with morphine response in the postoperative period. Clin Pharmacol Ther. 2006;**79**(4):316–24.

26. Taenzer P, Melzack R, Jeans ME. Influence of psychological factors on postoperative pain, mood and analgesic requirements. Pain. 1986;**24**(3):331–42.

27. Jamison RN, Taft K, O'Hara JP, Ferrante FM. Psychosocial and pharmacologic predictors of satisfaction with intravenous patient-controlled analgesia. Anesth Analg. 1993;**77**(1):121–25.

28. Bachiocco V, Rucci P, Carli G. Request of analgesics in post-surgical pain. Relationships to psychological factors and pain-related variables. Pain Clinic. 1996;**9**:169–79.

29. Cohen L, Fouladi RT, Katz J. Preoperative coping strategies and distress predict postoperative pain and morphine consumption in women undergoing abdominal gynecologic surgery. J Psychosom Res. 2005;**58**:201–09.

30. Granot M, Ferber SG. The roles of pain catastrophizing and anxiety in the prediction of postoperative pain intensity: a prospective study. Clin J Pain. 2005;**21**(5):439–45.

31. Strulov L, Zimmer EZ, Granot M, Tamir A, Jakobi P, Lowenstein L. Pain catastrophizing, response to experimental heat stimuli, and post-cesarean section pain. J Pain. 2007;**8**(3):273–79.

32. Cohen L, Fouladi RT, Katz J. Preoperative coping strategies and distress predict postoperative pain and morphine consumption in women undergoing abdominal gynecologic surgery. J Psychosom Res. 2005;**58**(2):201–209.

33. Dahmani S, Dupont H, Mantz J, Desmonts JM, Keita H. Predictive factors of early morphine requirements in the post-anaesthesia care unit (PACU). Br J Anaesth. 2001;**87**(3):385–89.

34. Chang KY, Tsou MY, Chan KH, Sung CS, Chang WK. Factors affecting patient-controlled analgesia requirements. J Formos Med Assoc. 2006;**105**(11):918–25.

35. Bovill JG. Mechanisms of actions of opioids and non-steroidal anti-inflammatory drugs. Eur J Anaesthesiol Suppl. 1997;15:9–15.

36. Vanderah TW. Pathophysiology of pain. Med Clin North Am. 2007;**91**(1):1–12.

37. Tzschentke TM, Christoph T, Kögel B, Schiene K, Hennies HH, Englberger W, et al. (-)-(1R,2R)-3-(3-dimethylamino-1-ethyl-2-methyl-propyl)-phenol hydrochloride (tapentadol HCl): a novel mu-opioid receptor agonist/norepinephrine reuptake inhibitor with broad-spectrum analgesic properties. J Pharmacol Exp Ther. 2007;**323**(1):265–76.

38. Lewis KS, Han NH. Tramadol: a new centrally acting analgesic. Am J Health Syst Pharm. 1997;**54**(6):643–52.

39. Charlton JE. Tramadol hydrochloride. Prescr J. 1999;**39**(2):109–12.

40. Daniels S, Upmalis D, Okamoto A, Lange C, Häeussler J. A randomized, double-blind, phase III study comparing multiple doses of tapentadol IR, oxycodone IR, and placebo for postoperative (bunionectomy) pain. Curr Med Res Opin. 2009;**25**(3):765–76.

41. Kleinert R, Lange C, Steup A, Black P, Goldberg J, Desjardins P. Single dose analgesic efficacy of tapentadol in postsurgical dental pain: the results of a randomized, double-blind, placebo-controlled study. Anesth Analg. 2008;**107**(6):2048–55.

42. Hartrick C, Van Hove I, Stegmann JU, Oh C, Upmalis D. Efficacy and tolerability of tapentadol immediate release and oxycodone HCl immediate release in patients awaiting primary joint replacement surgery for end-stage joint disease: a 10-day, phase III, randomized, double-blind, active- and placebo-controlled study. Clin Ther. 2009;**31**(2):260–71.

43. Hale M, Upmalis D, Okamoto A, Lange C, Rauschkolb C. Tolerability of tapentadol immediate release in patients with lower back pain or osteoarthritis of the hip or knee over 90 days: a randomized, double-blind study. Curr Med Res Opin. 2009;**25**(5):1095–104.

44. Wilder-Smith CH, Schimke J, Osterwalder B, Senn HJ. Oral tramadol, a mu-opioid agonist and monoamine reuptake-blocker, and morphine for strong cancer-related pain. Ann Oncol. 1994;**5**(2):141–46.

45. Osipova NA, Novikoy GA, Beresnev VA. Analgesic effect of tramadol in cancer patients with chronic pain: a comparison with prolonged-action morphine sulphate. Curr Ther Res. 1991;**50**:812–21.

46. Cashman J, McAnulty G. Nonsteroidal anti-inflammatory drugs in perisurgical pain management. Mechanisms of action and rationale for optimum use. Drugs. 1995;**49**(1):51–70.

47. Vane JR, Botting RM. Mechanism of action of nonsteroidal anti-inflammatory drugs. Am J Med. 1998;**104**(3A):2S–8S.

48. Warner TD, Giuliano F, Vojnovic I, Bukasa A, Mitchell JA, Vane JR. Nonsteroid drug selectivities for cyclo-oxygenase-1 rather than cyclo-oxygenase-2 are associated with human gastrointestinal toxicity: a full in vitro analysis. Proc Natl Acad Sci U S A. 1999;**96**(13):7563–68.

49. Vardeh D, Wang D, Costigan M, Lazarus M, Saper CB, Woolf CJ, et al. Cox 2in CNS neural cells mediates mechanical inflammatory pain hypersensitivity in mice. J Clin Invest. 2009;**119**(2):287–94.

50. Golan DE. Principles of Pharmacology: The Pathophysiologic Basis of Drug Therapy. 2nd ed. Baltimore, MD: Lippincott Williams & Wilkins; 2008.

51. Drugs.com. Toradol prescribing information. 2015. https://www.drugs.com/pro/ketorolac-tromethamine.html

52. Graham GG, Scott KF. Mechanism of action of paracetamol. Am J Ther. 2005;**12**(1):46–55.

53. Göröcs TS, Lambert M, Rinne T, Krekler M, Modell S. Efficacy and tolerability of ready-to-use intravenous paracetamol solution as monotherapy or as an adjunct analgesic therapy for postoperative pain in patients undergoing elective ambulatory surgery: open, prospective study. Int J Clin Pract. 2009;**63**(1):112–20.

54. Salihoglu Z, Yildirim M, Demiroluk S, Kaya G, Karatas A, Ertem M, et al. Evaluation of intravenous paracetamol administration on postoperative pain and recovery characteristics in patients undergoing laparoscopic cholecystectomy. Surg Laparosc Endosc Percutan Tech. 2009;**19**(4):321–23.

55. Hong JY, Won Han S, Kim WO, Kil HK. Fentanyl sparing effects of combined ketorolac and acetaminophen for outpatient inguinal hernia repair in children. J Urol. 2010;**183**(4):1551–55.

56. Ong CK, Seymour RA, Lirk P, Merry AF. Combining paracetamol (acetaminophen) with nonsteroidal antiinflammatory drugs: a qualitative systematic review of analgesic efficacy for acute postoperative pain. Anesth Analg. 2010;**110**(4):1170–79.

57. Scholz A. Mechanisms of (local) anaesthetics on voltage-gated sodium and other ion channels. Br J Anaesth. 2002;**89**(1):52–61.

58. Ke RW, Portera SG, Bagous W, Lincoln SR. A randomized, double-blinded trial of preemptive analgesia in laparoscopy. Obstet Gynecol. 1998;**92**(6):972–75.

59. Liu SS, Bernards CM. Exploring the epidural trail. Reg Anesth Pain Med. 2002;**27**(2):122–24.

60. Gorfine SR, Onel E, Patou G, Krivokapic ZV. Bupivacaine extended-release liposome injection for prolonged postsurgical analgesia in patients undergoing hemorrhoidectomy: a multicenter, randomized, double-blind, placebo-controlled trial. Dis Colon Rectum. 2011;**54**(12):1552–59.

61. Golf M, Daniels SE, Onel E. A phase 3, randomized, placebo-controlled trial of DepoFoam®bupivacaine (extended-release bupivacaine local analgesic) in bunionectomy. Adv Ther. 2011;**28**(9):776–88.

62. Smoot JD, Bergese SD, Onel E, Williams HT, Hedden W. The efficacy and safety of DepoFoam bupivacaine in patients undergoing bilateral, cosmetic, submuscular augmentation mammaplasty: a randomized, double-blind, active-control study. Aesthet Surg J. 2012;**32**(1):69–76.

63. Blaudszun G, Lysakowski C, Elia N, Tramèr MR. Effect of perioperative systemic α2 agonists on postoperative morphine consumption and pain intensity: systematic review and meta-analysis of randomized controlled trials. Anesthesiology. 2012;**116**(6):1312–22.

64. da Fonseca Pacheco D, Romero TR, Duarte ID. Central antinociception induced by ketamine is mediated by endogenous opioids and μ- and δ-opioid receptors. Brain Res. 2014;**1562**:69–75.

65. Himmelseher S, Durieux ME. Ketamine for perioperative pain management. Anesthesiology. 2005;**102**(1):211–20.

66. Jha AK, Bhardwaj N, Yaddanapudi S, Sharma RK, Mahajan JK. A randomized study of surgical site infiltration with bupivacaine or ketamine for pain relief in children following cleft palate repair. Paediatr Anaesth. 2013;**23**(5):401–406.

67. D'Alonzo RC, Bennett-Guerrero E, Podgoreanu M, D'Amico TA, Harpole DH, Shaw AD. A randomized, double blind, placebo controlled clinical trial of the preoperative use of ketamine for reducing inflammation and pain after thoracic surgery. J Anesth. 2011;**25**(5):672–78.

68. Cengiz P, Gokcinar D, Karabeyoglu I, Topcu H, Cicek GS, Gogus N. Intraoperative low-dose ketamine infusion reduces acute postoperative pain following total knee replacement surgery: a prospective, randomized double-blind placebo-controlled trial. J Coll Phys Surg Pak. 2014;**24**(5):299–303.

69. Thomas M, Tennant I, Augier R, Gordon-Strachan G, Harding H. The role of pre-induction ketamine in the management of postoperative pain in patients undergoing elective gynaecological surgery at the University Hospital of the West Indies. West Indian Med J. 2012;**61**(3):224–29.

70. Azari P, Lindsay DR, Briones D, Clarke C, Buchheit T, Pyati S. Efficacy and safety of ketamine in patients with complex regional pain syndrome: a systematic review. CNS Drugs. 2012;**26**(3):215–28.

71. Katalinic N, Lai R, Somogyi A, Mitchell PB, Glue P, Loo CK. Ketamine as a new treatment for depression: a review of its efficacy and adverse effects. Aust N Z J Psychiatry. 2013;**47**(8):710–27.

72. Subramaniam K, Subramaniam B, Steinbrook RA. Ketamine as adjuvant analgesic to opioids: a quantitative and qualitative systematic review. Anesth Analg. 2004;**99**(2):482–95.

73. Eckhardt K, Ammon S, Hofmann U, Riebe A, Gugeler N, Mikus G. Gabapentin enhances the analgesic effect of morphine in healthy volunteers. Anesth Analg. 2000;**91**(1):185–91.

74. Werner MU, Perkins FM, Holte K, Pedersen JL, Kehlet H. Effects of gabapentin in acute inflammatory pain in humans. Reg Anesth Pain Med. 2001;**26**(4):322–28.

75. Dirks J, Petersen KL, Rowbotham MC, Dahl JB. Gabapentin suppresses cutaneous hyperalgesia following heat-capsaicin sensitization. Anesthesiology. 2002;**97**(1):102–107.

76. Gilron I, Biederman J, Jhamandas K, Hong M. Gabapentin blocks and reverses antinociceptive morphine tolerance in the rat paw-pressure and tail-flick tests. Anesthesiology. 2003;**98**(5):1288–92.

77. Hansen C, Gilron I, Hong M. The effects of intrathecal gabapentin on spinal morphine tolerance in the rat tail-flick and paw pressure tests. Anesth Analg. 2004;**99**(4):1180–84.

78. Turan A, Karamanlioğlu B, Memiş D, et al. Analgesic effects of gabapentin after spinal surgery. Anesthesiology. 2004;**100**(4):935–38.

79. Turan A, Karamanlioğlu B, Memiş D, Usar P, Pamukçu Z, Türe M. The analgesic effects of gabapentin after total abdominal hysterectomy. Anesth Analg. 2004;**98**(5):1370–73.

80. Dierking G, Duedahl TH, Rasmussen ML, et al. Effects of gabapentin on postoperative morphine consumption and pain after abdominal hysterectomy: a randomized, double-blind trial. Acta Anaesthesiol Scand. 2004;**48**(3):322–27.

81. Dirks J, Fredensborg BB, Christensen D, Fomsgaard JS, Flyger H, Dahl JB. A randomized study of the effects of single-dose gabapentin versus placebo on postoperative pain and morphine consumption after mastectomy. Anesthesiology. 2002;**97**(3):560–64.

82. Pandey CK, Priye S, Singh S, Singh U, Singh RB, Singh PK. Preemptive use of gabapentin significantly decreases postoperative pain and rescue analgesic requirements in laparoscopic cholecystectomy. Can J Anesth. 2004;**51**(4):358–63.

83. Rorarius MGF, Mennander S, Suominen P, Rintala S, Puura A, Pirhonen R, et al. Gabapentin for the prevention of postoperative pain after vaginal hysterectomy. Pain. 2004;**110**(1–2):175–81.

84. Fassoulaki A, Patris K, Sarantopoulos C, Hogan Q. The analgesic effect of gabapentin and mexiletine after breast surgery for cancer. Anesth Analg. 2002;**95**(4):985–91.

85. Turan A, Memiş D, Karamanlioğlu B, Yağiz R, Pamukçu Z, Yavuz E. The analgesic effects of gabapentin in monitored anesthesia care for ear-nose-throat surgery. Anesth Analg. 2004;**99**(2):375–78.

86. Gilron I, Orr E, Tu DS, O'Neill JP, Zamora JE, Bell AC. A placebo-controlled randomized clinical trial of perioperative administration of gabapentin, rofecoxib and their combination for spontaneous and movement-evoked pain after abdominal hysterectomy. Pain. 2005;**113**(1–2):191–200.

87. Ménigaux C, Adam F, Guignard B, Sessler DI, Chauvin M. Preoperative gabapentin decreases anxiety and improves early functional recovery from knee surgery. Anesth Analg. 2005;**100**(5):1394–99.

88. Ben-Menachem E. Pregabalin pharmacology and its relevance to clinical practice. Epilepsia. 2004;**45** (Suppl 6):13–18.

89. Agarwal A, Gautam S, Gupta D, Agarwal S, Singh PK, Singh U. Evaluation of a single preoperative dose of pregabalin for attenuation of postoperative pain after laparoscopic cholecystectomy. Br J Anaesth. 2008;**101**(5):700–704.

90. Buvanendran A, Kroin JS, Della Valle CJ, Kari M, Moric M, Tuman KJ. Perioperative oral pregabalin reduces chronic pain after total knee arthroplasty: a prospective, randomized, controlled trial. Anesth Analg. 2010;**110**(1):199–207.

91. Zhang J, Ho KY, Wang Y. Efficacy of pregabalin in acute postoperative pain: a meta-analysis. Br J Anaesth. 2011;**106**(4):454–62.

92. Aasvang EK, Hansen JB, Malmstrøm J, Asmussen T, Gennevois D, Struys MM, et al. The effect of wound instillation of a novel purified capsaicin formulation on post herniotomy pain: a double-blind, randomized, placebo-controlled study. Anesth Analg. 2008;**107**(1):282–91.

93. Vadivelu N, Mitra S, Narayan D. Recent advances in postoperative pain management. Yale J Biol Med. 2010;**83**(1):11–25.

94. Lvovschi V, Aubrun F, Bonnet P, et al. Intravenous morphine titration to treat severe pain in the ED. Am J Emerg Med. 2008;**26**:676–82.

95. Chang AK, Bijur PE, Baccelieri A, Gallagher EJ. Efficacy and safety profile of a single dose of hydromorphone compared with morphine in older adults with acute, severe pain: a prospective, randomized, double-blind clinical trial. Am J Geriatr Pharmacother. 2009;**7**(1):1–10.

96. Kurihara Y, Kagawa T, Suzuki T, Ohnishi H, Ikeshima N. Efficacy and complications of fentanyl intravenous infusions in postoperative pediatric patients. Masui. 2008;**57**(11):1414–20.

97. Clark RF, Wei EM, Anderson PO. Meperidine: therapeutic use and toxicity. J Emerg Med. 1995;**13**:797–802.

98. Southworth S, Peters J, Rock A, Pavliv L. A multicenter, randomized, double-blind, placebo-controlled trial of intravenous ibuprofen 400 and 800 mg every 6 hours in the management of postoperative pain. Clin Ther. 2009;**31**(9):1922–35.

99. Bertolini A, Ferrari A, Ottani A, Guerzoni S, Tacchi R, Leone S. Paracetamol: new vistas of an old drug. CNS Drug Rev. 2006;**12**(3–4):250–75.

100. Singla NK, Parulan C, Samson R, Hutchinson JL, Bushnell R, Beja EG, et al. Plasma and cerebrospinal fluid pharmacokinetic parameters after single-dose administration of intravenous, oral or rectal acetaminophen. Presented at the 10th Annual American Society of Regional Anesthesia Pain Medicine Meeting and Workshops, 17–20 November, 2011.

101. Jahr JS, Lee VK. Intravenous acetaminophen. Anesthesiol Clin. 2010;**28**(4):619–45.

102. Food and Drug Administration. Cadence Pharmaceuticals. Ofirmev (acetaminophen) injection. 2010. https://www.accessdata.fda.gov/drugsatfda_docs/label/2010/022450lbl.pdf

103. Moiniche S, Mikkelsen S, Wetterslev J, Dahl JB. A qualitative systematic review of incisional local anaesthesia for post-operative pain relief after abdominal operations. Br J Anaesth. 1998;**81**:377–83.

104. Tucker GT, Mather LE. Clinical pharmacokinetics of local anaesthetics. Clin Pharmacokinet. 1979;**4**(4):241–78.

105. Grossi P, Urmey WF. Peripheral nerve blocks for anaesthesia and postoperative analgesia. Curr Opin Anaesthesiol. 2003;**16**(5):493–501.

106. Borgeat A, Tewes E, Biasca N, Gerber C. Patient-controlled interscalene analgesia with ropivacaine after major shoulder surgery: PCIA vs PCA. Br J Anaesth. 1998;**81**(4):603–605.

107. Borgeat A, Schäppi B, Biasca N, Gerber C. Patient-controlled analgesia after major shoulder surgery: patient-controlled interscalene analgesia versus patient-controlled analgesia. Anesthesiology. 1997;**87**(6):1343–47.

108. Capdevila X, Barthelet Y, Biboulet P, Ryckwaert Y, Rubenovitch J, d'Athis F. Effects of perioperative analgesic technique on the surgical outcome and duration of rehabilitation after major knee surgery. Anesthesiology. 1999;**91**(1):8–15.

109. Grant SA, Nielsen KC, Greengrass RA, Steele SM, Klein SM. Continuous peripheral nerve block for ambulatory surgery. Reg Anesth Pain Med. 2001;**26**(3):209–14.

110. Capdevila X, Barthelet Y, Biboulet P, Ryckwaert Y, Rubenovitch J, d'Athis F. Effects of perioperative analgesic technique on the surgical outcome and duration of rehabilitation after major knee surgery. Anesthesiology. 1999;**91**(1):8–15.

111. Singelyn FJ, Deyaert M, Joris D, Pendeville E, Gouverneur JM. Effects of intravenous patient-controlled analgesia with morphine, continuous epidural analgesia, and continuous three-in-one block on postoperative pain and knee rehabilitation after unilateral total knee arthroplasty. Anesth Analg. 1998;**87**(1):88–92.

112. Rodgers A, Walker N, Shug S, McKee A, Kehlet H, van Zundert A, et al. Reduction of postoperative mortality and morbidity with epidural and spinal anaesthesia: results from overview of randomized trials. Br Med J. 2002;**321**:1493–96.

113. Rigg JR, Jamrozik K, Myles PS, Silbert BS, Peyton PJ, Parsons RW, et al. Epidural anaesthesia and analgesia and outcome of major surgery: a randomised trial. Lancet. 2002;**359**(9314):1276–82.

114. Staren ED, Cullen ML. Epidural catheter analgesia for the management of postoperative pain. Surg Gynecol Obstet. 1986;**162**(4):389–404.

115. Moawad HS, Mokbel EM. Postoperative analgesia after major abdominal surgery: fentanyl–bupivacaine patient controlled epidural analgesia versus fentanyl patient controlled intravenous analgesia. Eur J Anaesth. 2014;**30**(4):393–97.

116. Sathyan G, Jaskowiak J, Evashenk M, Gupta S. Characterisation of the pharmacokinetics of the fentanyl HCl patient-controlled transdermal system (PCTS): effect of current magnitude and multiple-day dosing and comparison with IV fentanyl administration. Clin Pharmacokinet. 2005;**44** (Suppl 1):7–15.

Postoperative complications in the obese patient and their management

Sara Bowman and S. R. Moonesinghe

Introduction

This chapter discusses surgical, medical, and management challenges faced by the clinicians involved in the care of obese or bariatric surgical patients in the postoperative period. Obesity itself is an independent risk factor for postoperative morbidity and mortality. This is, in part, due to the direct impact of obesity and also to the increased prevalence of comorbidities in obese patients, including cardiovascular, respiratory, and endocrine disease, all of which may also be independently associated with adverse outcomes. More specifically, with the worldwide increase in obesity and increasing evidence of their benefits, greater numbers of weight loss operations are being undertaken, most commonly, laparoscopic gastric bypass or sleeve gastrectomy procedures. Surgery is commonly undertaken in specialist centres and length of stay is generally short; therefore, these patients may present with late complications at non-specialist hospitals, where general surgeons, anaesthetists, or physicians may not be familiar with the techniques of bariatric surgery. Thus, generalists may be faced with the management of acute or chronic complications of weight reduction surgery in an emergency setting and therefore an understanding of the surgery and the care of the obese patient is important for subsequent management.

Complications after surgery may be considered surgical (i.e. directly related to the operative procedure) or medical (physiological deterioration indirectly related to the procedure). These will be discussed in turn.

Surgical complications

Wound infection

Obesity is a risk factor for surgical site infections (SSIs). Postoperative SSIs occur in approximately 8–15% of bariatric surgical patients, prolonging length of stay from 5 to 20 days [1,2]. Infections occur less frequently after laparoscopic procedures, with rates of 1–4% being reported. Surgical wounds have been classified by the Centers for Disease Control and Prevention in the United States as superficial

incisional, deep incisional, and peritoneal infections [1]. Organisms include skin commensals such as *Staphylococcus aureus* and *Streptococcus* species (including methicillin-resistant pathogens). *Streptococcus*, most commonly, followed by Enterobacteriaceae and Gram-negative anaerobes are implicated in more severe infections originating from an intra-abdominal source perhaps secondary to an anastomotic leak [2].

Several explanations for the increased rate of SSIs in obese patients have been hypothesized. Adipose tissue is relatively avascular, resulting in tissue hypoperfusion and decreased oxygen partial pressure. Oxidative killing by neutrophils is the first line of attack against surgical infection and increases as oxygen partial pressure rises. This is particularly important in the immediate period after bacterial contamination, as this is the time when infections are established. Infection rates are affected by factors that decrease tissue oxygenation not only during surgery but in the postoperative period. Many of these patients suffer from obstructive sleep apnoea (OSA) with an associated desaturation during sleep which is exacerbated by opioid analgesics [1]. Supplemental oxygen in the perioperative period has been shown to reduce the incidence of wound infections in some randomized studies but not in others [1].

Postoperative surgical infections should be treated with broad-spectrum antibiotics including Gram-positive and Gram-negative aerobic and anaerobic cover. Antibiotic treatment should be adjusted as per microbiology advice based on culture and susceptibility testing. A delay, both in appropriate antibiotic treatment and surgical intervention, increases mortality [2]; however, the Centers for Disease Control and Prevention endorses the use of antibiotics only where there is evidence of cellulitis or systemic infection [3]. Where more severe infection is evident, the surviving sepsis guidelines should be followed (https://www.sccm.org/SurvivingSepsisCampaign/Guidelines). A number of surgical strategies have been recommended for both the prevention and management of SSIs. Primary closure is preferred to delayed closure unless the wound is contaminated. Incision and drainage are required for abscesses, seromas, or haematomas. Enzymatic wound debridement and negative pressure wound therapy have been tested but there is little high-quality evidence for their use [3,4].

Bleeding

Postoperative haemorrhage is a potentially life-threatening complication after any surgery in the obese patient. After bariatric surgery, bleeding is relatively uncommon, with the incidence after laparoscopic Roux-en-Y gastric bypass (RYGB) reaching 4.4% and 3.5% after laparoscopic sleeve gastrectomy [5,6]. Bleeding after insertion of an adjustable gastric band is rare. In obesity surgery, early bleeding (within 30 days of operation), which usually originates from a staple or suture line, can be divided into intra- or extraluminal [7]. Late bleeding is rare after laparoscopic RYGB and typically results from marginal or stomal ulceration [7,8]. A systematic review revealed that rates of postoperative bleeding were lower in open RYGB (around 0.5%) than after a laparoscopic approach [5,9,10]. The reason for this is thought to be the reinforcement of the gastric staple line by over-sewing [10].

Signs and symptoms suggestive of bleeding include hypotension, tachycardia, bloody drain effluent, a decrease in the haemoglobin concentration, haematemesis, melena, fresh blood per rectum and, rarely, small bowel obstruction [5–7]. External influences which predispose to perioperative bleeding include patient factors such as underlying clotting abnormalities (either congenital or drug induced), infection, or ulceration, and surgical factors such as inadequate intraoperative haemostasis, and more complex and prolonged procedures [5].

Management of these patients is initially with prompt effective resuscitation including monitoring of vital signs, good intravenous access, fluid administration, cessation and reversal of anticoagulants, serial blood tests, and blood and blood products if indicated [7]. If the patient is haemodynamically stable, contrast computed tomography (CT) may be indicated to detect the source of intraluminal, extraluminal, or abdominal wall bleeding [6]. Definitive treatment is influenced by the site of the bleeding. Extraluminal bleeding can be managed conservatively if the patient is stable. Intraluminal bleeding may be managed by endoscopy and the bleeding controlled by adrenaline (epinephrine) injection, electrocoagulation, or endoclips [5,7,8]. If endoscopy proves difficult or the patient is unstable in an extraluminal bleed, laparoscopic exploration or laparotomy is indicated [5].

Anastomotic leak

Anastomotic leaks are generally more common after laparoscopic bariatric surgery than after the corresponding open procedure but this is levelling out as surgeons become more experienced with laparoscopic techniques [11]. A leak is defined as 'the leak of luminal contents from a surgical joint between two hollow viscera' [12]. The incidence of an anastomotic leak after laparoscopic sleeve gastrectomy varies between 0.7% and 7% and most commonly occurs at the gastro-oesophageal junction [12,13]. After an open or laparoscopic gastric bypass, leaks occur in up to 6.1% of cases, usually at the gastrojejunostomy anastomosis, the gastric remnant, or the gastric pouch [10,14]. Most patients present acutely in the 7–10 days after surgery but presentation can be late, very late, or chronic [10,15].

On obtaining the history, details on the type of surgery and when it was performed should be ascertained. Sepsis and peritonitis can present as the final stage of an anastomotic leak [7]. Patient signs and symptoms play a key role in the diagnosis [16]. Symptoms that should alert the treating physician to a diagnosis of anastomotic leak include

a tachycardia greater than 120 beats per minute (may be the earliest sign), abdominal pain resistant to treatment with simple analgesics, fever, hypotension, tachypnoea, decreased urine output, left pleural effusion, and hypoxia [6,12,13,17–19]. Abdominal examination is of limited value and the patient may show no signs of peritonitis [10]. Blood tests may reveal an elevated C-reactive protein concentration and leucocytosis (white blood cell count >11,000/mm³) [20]. Fluid resuscitation should be commenced with non-glucose-containing solutions. There may be a coexisting thiamine deficiency and this should be replaced before infusing glucose solutions to avoid precipitating Wernicke's encephalopathy [7]. Input from a bariatric surgeon is desirable. Abdominal X-ray is unlikely to aid diagnosis and contrast-enhanced CT scan and oral Gastrografin tests give significant false-negative rates [6,15,19,21,22]; however, combining both tests improves the detection rate to approximately 70%.

In the case of an early leak or multiple leaks with a diffuse fluid collection, emergency laparoscopy or laparotomy should be performed to washout the abdominal cavity, repair the defect in the rare circumstances that the tissue condition is satisfactory, place drains around the leakage site, and to establish a feeding route [12,13,20,22]. In the more stable patient, conservative treatment may be considered, including resting the upper gastrointestinal tract, fluid resuscitation, broad-spectrum antibiotics, insertion of a nasojejunal tube to provide enteral nutritional support, and analgesia [5,12]. Enteral feeding has been recommended by one study as a 40% rate of central venous line infection was observed in obese patients requiring prolonged total parenteral nutrition [21]. Endoscopic stent insertion is a recognized treatment for a post-laparoscopic sleeve gastrectomy leak but there can be issues with distal migration of the stent [6,7,10,12]. Those presenting with late leaks may, in addition to supportive measures, be managed with percutaneous drainage under CT or ultrasound guidance [12,23]. The later the leak occurs, the more receptive to treatment and the better the outcome [14].

Medical complications

Cardiac complications

Obesity is a risk factor for postoperative cardiac complications such as myocardial infarction, heart failure, and arrhythmias [24]. The increase in blood volume in the obese patient causes structural changes in the heart as a consequence of the increase in stroke volume that is required to perfuse the excess body fat. The result is systemic and pulmonary hypertension causing left and right ventricular dilatation, leading to left and right ventricular hypertrophy, and ultimately bilateral cardiomyopathy. OSA exacerbates pulmonary hypertension and right-sided changes to the heart causing possible right-sided heart failure [25,26]. Patients with central obesity are more at risk of cardiac complications. Perioperative invasive monitoring should be used in those who were identified in the preoperative period as having a high cardiac risk [24].

Atrial fibrillation is the most common arrhythmia after cardiac and non-cardiac surgery with an incidence of around 4%. Developing atrial fibrillation is associated with longer hospital stay, and increased morbidity and mortality [25,27]. Arrhythmias that occur less commonly include atrial flutter and ventricular tachycardia. Causes of postoperative cardiac arrhythmias in the obese include hypercapnia, electrolyte imbalance, excess production of catecholamines, fatty in-filtration or perioperative inflammation affecting the cardiac conducting system, left atrial hypertrophy secondary to left ventricular hypertrophy, and chronic hypoxia. The latter is exacerbated in patients with OSA and can be alleviated by using non-invasive continuous positive pressure ventilation (CPAP) [17,26].

Treatment of new-onset postoperative atrial fibrillation involves initial correction of haemodynamic or electrolyte imbalance. If the patient is unstable, advanced life support algorithms should be followed and electrical cardioversion should be attempted immediately. More often, in the stable patient, or unstable patient resistant to electrical cardioversion, chemical cardioversion using drugs such as amiodarone or digoxin is indicated. In general, treating arrhythmias in the obese patient is more difficult as they are more resistant to treatment. Patients are at high risk of thromboembolism and stroke. Anticoagulation should be weighed against the risk of bleeding when postoperative atrial fibrillation has been present for more than 48 hours.

Respiratory complications

In the obese patient, changes in respiratory physiology favour the development of pulmonary postoperative complications. The 1992 National Bariatric Surgery Registry study for obesity found that the most common type of postoperative complication was respiratory, occurring in 5% of patients [28]. Postoperative pulmonary complications include aspiration, atelectasis, pneumonia, prolonged intubation, and reintubation [28,29]. Changes in the respiratory physiology of the obese (see Chapter 8 and Chapter 9) should be considered when planning a strategy for the prevention and management of postoperative pulmonary complications. These patients have a fatty chest wall with reduced compliance causing a restriction of lung volumes. Functional residual capacity (FRC) is reduced due to a decrease in expiratory reserve volume [24–27,30]. These changes are exaggerated as body mass index (BMI) increases.

Optimal intraoperative management is the first step towards achieving good postoperative respiratory management. General anaesthesia causes postoperative atelectasis and hypoxaemia, particularly in the morbidly obese [26]. This is exacerbated with the patient supine when the FRC decreases further. If possible, maintaining the patient in the reverse Trendelenburg position perioperatively will increase oxygenation by encouraging the diaphragm to fall away from the lungs and FRC to increase. Currently, the optimum ventilator strategy involves an adequate positive end-expiratory pressure level after a recruitment manoeuvre which should help prevent atelectasis. During extubation and the postoperative period, the patient should be sat up to optimize the FRC until early ambulation can be commenced [19,24]. Atelectasis has been shown to persist for a minimum of 24 hours in the morbidly obese patient whereas it resolves within a few hours in non-obese patients [24,25,30].

Early extubation is desired when muscle relaxation is fully reversed. Factors that might exacerbate atelectasis postoperatively are poor pain control affecting respiratory effort or the use of intraoperative drugs with residual respiratory depressant effects [24]. Multimodal analgesia should be employed to avoid such side effects particularly in the patient with OSA. An epidural technique will address both of these concerns and may reduce the risk of postoperative atelectasis, reintubation, and pneumonia [30]. All of these factors together reduce hospital length of stay [25].

Supplemental oxygen should be continued postoperatively until hypoxaemia is no longer present [29]. Preoperatively, morbidly obese patients using CPAP should restart treatment as soon as possible after surgery [26]. However, Jensen et al. [30] showed that CPAP was not necessary postoperatively if other respiratory strategies were instituted such as chest physiotherapy or early mobilization. Ahmad et al. [30] showed that CPAP support required in the postoperative period is greater than that required at home, and therefore, may not be as effective. Essentially CPAP improves oxygenation and decreases respiratory work but its use should be carefully monitored [30].

In the event that an obese patient develops pneumonia postoperatively, management is supportive. Appropriately selected and dosed antibiotics are imperative for successful treatment. Many of the strategies already mentioned are still applicable as well as rigorous chest physiotherapy. Non-invasive ventilation and ultimately reintubation might be necessary. A meta-analysis by Wie Nie et al. [31] revealed an 'obesity survival paradox' in pneumonia which might be partly explained by their greater nutritional reserve.

Thrombotic disorders

Obesity and surgery of any type are independently associated with postoperative thrombotic events [9,19,24,32,33]. Venous thromboembolism (VTE) includes both deep vein thrombosis and pulmonary embolism and has an incidence varying from 0.3% to 3% in the obese patient [5,6,15,23,32]. Pulmonary embolism is a leading cause of death in this group with up to 50% being fatal [15]. Patients are most at risk in the immediate postoperative period but VTE can still occur up to 2 months after surgery [2,11].

The physiological basis behind the increased risk of VTE in the obese patient relates to increased blood volume and relative polycythaemia [26]. Other contributing factors include decreased circulating antithrombin 3 and decreased fibrinolytic activity [24].

VTE prophylaxis strategies include early mobilization, hydration, graduated compression stockings, intermittent pneumatic calf compression, and subcutaneous unfractionated or low-molecular-weight heparin [2,15,19,24,29,33]. Opinions on the dose or type of heparin, the commencement, and the duration of treatment vary [2,4]. Some studies suggest that standard doses for dalteparin and enoxaparin are sufficient and there is no need for weight adjustment [33]. In high-risk cases, deep vein thrombosis prophylaxis should be started in the preoperative period and continued past the immediate postoperative period, although there is no consensus on for how long [15,24,32,33].

Placement of an inferior vena cava filter before surgery is considered an option in high-risk patients. Indications would include patients with a previous history of deep vein thrombosis/pulmonary embolism, BMI greater than 55–60 kg/m², confirmed venous stasis disease, contraindication to adequate anticoagulation, and expected prolonged immobilization [19,23,24,26]. However, recent studies report an increased incidence of complications without any benefit from insertion of a prophylactic inferior vena cava filter [2,23].

Pulmonary embolism most commonly presents as tachycardia and respiratory difficulties. However, anastomotic leaks may present with similar symptoms and should be considered as a differential diagnosis, alongside atelectasis and pneumonia [11,15,26]. The management of VTE is unchanged in the obese postoperative patient [11]. Where there is high suspicion of a pulmonary embolism,

CT pulmonary angiography is the investigation of choice. The ability to scan such patients may be impeded by the size of the patient relative to the scanner [15]. VTE is treated pharmacologically but there is no agreement on the dose or duration of therapy [2,34]. Patients on formal anticoagulation therapy postoperatively are at risk of bleeding and vigilance should remain high [15].

Nutritional consequences

Pre-existing nutritional deficiencies are common in the morbidly obese patient [35,36]. These deficiencies are exacerbated by the anatomical and physiological changes to digestion and absorption as a result of obesity surgery and can be life-threatening. Pre- and postoperative nutritional monitoring and supplementation where indicated is essential [35].

The aetiology behind these nutrient deficiencies is complex. The resultant small pouch, in the restrictive component of the RYGB, makes sufficient consumption of fluids, calories, protein, and nutrients difficult [10]. This is exacerbated by food intolerance causing nausea, vomiting, or regurgitation in approximately 35–65% of patients [36]. Thiamine deficiency is most commonly associated with persistence of such symptoms [35]. Vitamin and mineral deficiencies result from the malabsorptive component of the RYGB, in that the main body of the stomach and duodenum have now been bypassed. Those micronutrients particularly implicated include iron, vitamin B_{12}, folate, vitamin D, and less so, fat-soluble vitamins, calcium, potassium, magnesium, and thiamine [10,36]. Other contributing factors include changes in pancreatic and biliary function secondary to surgery, a decrease in intestinal transport time as a result of short bowel syndrome, decreased gastric acid production [35,37], and postoperatively, despite dietary advice to the contrary, patients may opt for foods with high calorific content and poor protein or micronutrient value [35–37].

Small intestinal bacterial overgrowth may also develop in the bypassed portion of the stomach in 25–40% of subjects. The patient may be asymptomatic or typically develop symptoms including diarrhoea, nausea, vomiting, abdominal pain, dyspepsia, weight loss, and malabsorption which are caused by a number of mechanisms. The diagnosis of bacterial overgrowth is made by a number of techniques, with the gold standard measuring the bacterial concentration of the jejunum aspirate. The treatment is an elemental diet and antibiotics, although an optimal regimen for the latter has not been established [35]. In terms of macronutrients, protein malnutrition most commonly occurs in malabsorptive procedures such as biliopancreatic diversion (4–18%) or distal gastric bypass (1–5%) [10,35,37]. The aim of obesity surgery is to reduce body fat mass [35]. If average daily protein intake is insufficient there will be a greater loss of lean tissue mass resulting in protein malnutrition. Muscle mass decreases over time and clinical symptoms include hair loss and oedema [35]. Annually, 1% of these severe cases are hospitalized and may require parenteral nutrition for at least 3–4 weeks [37].

Symptoms of micronutrient deficiencies include hair loss, dry skin, muscle pain, and fatigue. The prevalence, for all types of bariatric surgery, has been found to be between 28% and 59% within the first year after surgery [37]. Mineral and multivitamin supplements are recommended after surgery although there are currently no guidelines for the dosage and duration of treatment. Treatments for specific deficiencies also lack an evidence base. Vitamin B_{12} deficiency should be treated with oral replacement therapy of 350–1000 mcg daily, in severe cases intramuscular or subcutaneous injections may be necessary [35,37]. Vitamin D supplementation ranges from 800 to 150,000 IU daily. Severe cases of thiamine (vitamin B_1) deficiency may manifest as Wernicke's encephalopathy and require inpatient therapy with intravenous thiamine. Individual micronutrient deficiencies such as zinc, vitamin C, vitamin A, selenium, and copper should be identified and supplemented with close monitoring [35,37].

Neurological complications

In all types of surgery, the risk of complications to the peripheral nervous system is increased in the obese patient. The incidence overall ranges from 4.6% to 8.6% and includes mononeuropathies (most commonly carpal tunnel syndrome), peripheral neuropathies, plexopathies, and myopathy [11]. Mechanical causes result from prolonged surgery and immobilization of the affected limb, causing increased pressure from excessive adipose tissue on the peripheral nerve in question. Alternatively, excessive abduction of the upper or lower limb can lead to stretch injuries of the brachial or lumbosacral plexus. Peripheral nerves that are prone to injury include particularly the ulnar nerve at the elbow, the brachial plexus, the peroneal nerve at the knee, the sciatic nerve, and the lateral femoral cutaneous nerve [17,24,32,33]. The high incidence of diabetes in these patients is a further risk factor for developing neurological complications.

Prevention involves careful positioning of the patient, avoiding over-abduction of the limbs, and padding exposed pressure areas such as the ulnar nerve at the elbow [24,33,38]. When such injuries occur, a full neurological examination should be documented and expert neurological input obtained as soon as possible. Nerve conduction studies may be indicated. Generally, most peripheral nerve injuries of this type resolve in time without intervention.

Should the patient present with a polyneuropathy, a systemic process as opposed to a mechanical one should be considered a more likely cause. In the bariatric patient who describes protracted vomiting postoperatively, a nutrient deficiency, usually thiamine (vitamin B_1), would be implicated. Bariatric patients can experience neurological complications anywhere from 3 to 20 months postoperatively and this includes Wernicke's encephalopathy [11,17].

Rhabdomyolysis

Postoperative rhabdomyolysis (RML) is a rare but life-threatening complication in morbidly obese surgical patients. It results from compression to the skeletal muscle during prolonged surgery. This results in ischaemic necrosis and release of intracellular myoglobin and creatine phosphokinase into the systemic circulation. When the amount of myoglobin that can be filtered by the kidneys is exceeded, acute kidney injury develops [19,26,39].

Risk factors include prolonged surgical time, super-obesity (BMI >50 kg/m²), male sex, and comorbidities such as hypertension, diabetes, or peripheral vascular disease. Case reports mention involvement of the shoulder girdle and upper arm muscles or the gluteal, hip, or lumbar region. Postoperatively there should be a high index of suspicion in any patient with muscular pain and numbness. Weakness, swelling, and bruising of the limb are other symptoms that have been described. Prevention includes padding of pressure points and careful positioning of the patient intraoperatively, reducing the surgical time with experienced surgeons, and sufficient perioperative fluid therapy [19,26,39].

In the postoperative period, any patient presenting with symptoms suggestive of RML should have their creatine phosphokinase measured. A level greater than 5000 IU/L is indicative of RML and acute kidney injury is more likely at levels above 16,000 IU/L. Early and aggressive treatment will minimize the risk of developing acute kidney injury. Myoglobinuria causing brown urine is also diagnostic of RML in the absence of haemoglobinaemia and haematuria. Electrolyte abnormalities such as hyperkalaemia develop as a result of disruption to the skeletal muscle membrane [19,26,39].

Treatment includes aggressive fluid therapy and diuretics such as mannitol or frusemide to a target urine output of greater than 1.5 mL/kg/h. Alkalization of the urine using sodium bicarbonate increases the solubility of myoglobin and aids treatment. Dialysis may be indicated in cases of severe acute kidney injury, hyperkalaemia, or acidosis. Management of RML should take place in an intensive care unit setting [19,26,39].

Management challenges

Analgesia

Postoperative analgesia is challenging in the obese patient with or without OSA. More operations are being performed laparoscopically, which has led to a reduction in postoperative analgesic requirements and hence a decrease in the length of hospital stay [2,40]. Despite other analgesics being available, opioids still play a large part in the treatment of postoperative pain [2]. The difficulty is achieving good pain relief without excessive sedation. Postoperatively, the morbidly obese patient in pain will hypoventilate leading to hypoxaemia, hypercapnia, and possibly atelectasis. Any analgesic that depresses ventilation will induce a similar effect particularly in the patient with OSA [26]. Opioids cause central sleep apnoea in both obese and non-obese subjects. In OSA, opioids increase deep sleep-induced apnoeas on starting treatment, and furthermore, after stopping opioids, natural deep rapid eye movement sleep rebounds causing further apnoeas [40,41]. One should consider using a combination of analgesics that act by different mechanisms, reducing the need for opioid analgesics and their side effects in the postoperative period (see Chapter 5). Good pain relief, in addition to reducing pulmonary complications, also promotes early ambulation which is paramount in a population prone to thromboembolism [29,32,40].

Simple analgesics such as paracetamol and non-steroidal anti-inflammatory drugs have opioid-sparing effects and are widely employed in general surgery. In bariatric surgery, the general consensus is to avoid non-steroidal anti-inflammatory drugs because of the increased risk of anastomotic ulcerations and perforations. Systemic adjuvants include pre-induction low-dose ketamine which acts synergistically with opioids without causing respiratory depression. Studies have shown that intraoperative dexmedetomidine infusion, lidocaine infusion, or magnesium supplementation reduces both intraoperative and postoperative opioid requirements [2,26,40,42]. Pregabalin as a single-dose premedication has so far been shown to reduce analgesic requirements in the first 24 hours [40,42].

Central neuraxial blocks will technically be more challenging and have a higher failure rate than in non-obese patients, but they are the gold standard postoperative analgesic therapy in open abdominal and thoracic operations alongside a general anaesthetic technique [26,29,43,44]. When used as a sole technique it avoids the risks of the difficult airway and pulmonary complications. Peripheral nerve blocks are again more difficult and likely to fail but they substantially reduce the use of opioids in the postoperative period [40].

Intravenous opioid patient-controlled analgesia can be used in the postoperative period using ideal body weight to guide dosing requirements [26,33]. Large doses should be avoided for the reasons already mentioned and so a background infusion should be used with extreme care [26,43]. However, the amount of opioid to control pain in these patients may vary widely and increased amounts of opioid may be needed. Close monitoring is warranted to prevent respiratory compromise. Promising techniques that may reduce opioid usage include giving a long-acting local anaesthetic infusion either at the surgical wound site or directly into the peritoneum [32,40].

After laparoscopic procedures the residual carbon dioxide used for insufflation causes pain from irritation or stretching of the peritoneum. Whether warming and humidifying the carbon dioxide reduces postoperative pain and analgesic requirements is not clear. However, giving more opioids in this situation provides little relief from the pain but may instead depress ventilation [26,42].

Imaging

There are several challenges faced by the radiology department when it comes to imaging obese patients. Firstly, the technical issues involved, as each imaging modality has its own weight and size limits. Typical restrictions include a width limit of 70 cm and a weight limit of 200 kg in CT, a width limit of 60 cm and a weight limit of 200 kg in magnetic resonance imaging, and a weight limit of 200 kg in interventional radiology. In a hospital delivering a bariatric service, these weight restrictions should be made available in a policy document and all appropriate staff made aware [24,45]. Secondly, the images produced may be of poor quality because of the abundance of adipose tissue and this makes the ability of radiologists to provide an accurate diagnosis more challenging [24].

Radiologists also need appropriate training in the changes in the anatomy they will expect to see after bariatric surgery and which treatment modalities are appropriate for which suspected complication. There will be an expected increase in the use of imaging modalities in these patients especially as their symptoms are so non-specific [24].

Conclusion

Obese patients undergoing surgery are at substantial risk of some postoperative complications, and present significant challenges for perioperative clinicians and cost to healthcare providers. There are gaps in the evidence base with regard to some important therapies, including those aimed at preventing thromboembolism and respiratory complications. High-quality data from randomized trials of perioperative interventions in this rapidly expanding cohort of patients would help to address these areas of need.

CASE REPORT

The patient, aged 44 years, presented to hospital with diarrhoea and vomiting, progressive weakness, upper and lower limb pitting oedema, and a tremor of the right upper limb. Her weight was 80 kg but prior to bariatric surgery she was 130 kg with a height of 170 cm and therefore her BMI was 44.9 kg/m².

Previous surgery to address her weight included a gastric bypass 10 years ago followed a year later by a laparoscopy and omentoplasty for a duodenal perforation and repair of an anastomotic leak. She had a duodenal switch procedure 6 years after her initial bariatric surgery to assist with further weight loss. She had an oesophagogastroduodenoscopy 2 weeks ago which revealed oesophagitis and an ulcer.

She has Charcot–Marie–Tooth disease and as a consequence had a pre-existing weakness in her upper and lower limbs prior to bariatric surgery. She suffers with chronic back pain and takes regular pregabalin and tramadol.

She had been building up her diet until 4 months ago when she started to struggle eating solid food. She was also taking protein, copper, and thiamine supplements.

The impression was malnutrition and bloods confirmed this with a low total protein of 43 g/L, a profoundly low albumin of 14 g/L, a low ionized calcium of 1.11 mmol/L, low copper (4.8 µmol/L), selenium (49.9 µg/L), zinc (4.1 µmol/L), and vitamin D (53 nmol/L) levels. A normocytic normochromic anaemic (94 g/L) was detected but her iron profile could not be interpreted due to the coexisting hypoalbuminaemia and significantly low transferrin.

In view of her low calcium, an electrocardiogram was done which was normal. She had a dose of 10 mL of 10% calcium gluconate in 5% glucose. This was repeated that evening. The tetany in her right upper limb resolved the following day.

A nasojejunal tube was inserted. Refeeding was initiated with a protein-rich regimen via the nasojejunal tube. Oral protein supplements were taken as tolerated. Nasojejunal feeding was poorly tolerated and a peripherally inserted central catheter line was inserted in order to commence total parenteral nutrition. Once her full protein and fluid requirements were met via the total parenteral nutrition, the nasojejunal feed and intravenous fluids were stopped.

Surgery was planned for 2 weeks after her admission. Prior to surgery an attempt was made to optimize her electrolytes. Magnesium was replaced as necessary particularly as high doses of vitamin D supplementation deplete body magnesium stores. Copper and zinc infusions were administered just prior to surgery. She was transfused 2 units of blood because of a further haemoglobin drop to 72 g/L, possibly due to fluid haemodilution. Her albumin level just prior to surgery was still only 10 g/L.

Surgery was uneventful and a laparoscopic revision of her duodenal switch procedure was performed to address her malabsorption. Ascites was noted during the procedure.

While she was re-established on a soft diet which she tolerated well, she was weaned off total parenteral nutrition. Her diarrhoea started to reduce in frequency and her pitting oedema improved. On discharge, her albumin level had increased to 14 g/L and 2 months after her initial presentation had improved to 20 g/L.

Discussion

This case demonstrates the possible complex metabolic sequelae of having bariatric surgery that require lifelong monitoring [35,37].

This was a patient who required multidisciplinary input not only to optimize her preoperatively but also to discuss the correct timing for surgery. The multidisciplinary team specifically specializing in bariatrics consisted of the surgical team, dietician, physiotherapist, nurses, enteral nurse, chemical pathologist, bariatric and lipid specialist, and the anaesthetist once surgery was decided. All are integral in the management of such patients.

A delay in surgery was contemplated to allow the albumin to improve to a more satisfactory level. Hypoalbuminaemia preoperatively can be associated with postoperative complications including infections which can be further augmented by depleted levels of copper and zinc [37]. On balance, it was deemed that surgery was the only definitive management that would resolve her malnutrition issues and she could have deteriorated further had we waited.

REFERENCES

1. Wadhwa A, Kabon B, Fleischmann E, Kurz A, Sessler DI. Supplemental postoperative oxygen does not reduce surgical site infection and major healing-related complications from bariatric surgery in morbidly obese patients: a randomized, blinded trial. Anesth Analg. 2014;**119**(2):357–65.
2. Quidley AM, Bland CM, Bookstaver PB, Kuper K. Perioperative management of bariatric surgery patients. Am J Health Syst Pharm. 2014;**71**(15):1253–64.
3. Tipton AM, Cohen SA, Chelmow D. Wound infection in the obese pregnant woman. Semin Perinatol. 2011;**35**(6):345–49.
4. Matthews KJ, Brock E, Cohen SA, Chelmow D. Hysterectomy in obese patients: special considerations. Clin Obstet Gynecol. 2014;**57**(1):106–14.
5. Hussain A, EL-Hasani S. Bariatric emergencies: current evidence and strategies of management. World J Emerg Surg. 2013;**8**(1):58.
6. Weiner RA, El-Sayes IA, Theodoridou S, Weiner SR, Scheffel O. Early post-operative complications: incidence, management, and impact on length of hospital stay. A retrospective comparison between laparoscopic gastric bypass and sleeve gastrectomy. Obes Surg. 2013;**23**(12):2004–12.
7. Campanile FC, Boru CE, Rizzello M, Puzziello A, Copaescu C, Cavallaro G, et al. Acute complications after laparoscopic bariatric procedures: update for the General Surgeon. Langenbecks Arch Surg. 2013;**398**(5):669–86.
8. Hamdan K, Somers S, Chand M. Management of late postoperative complications of bariatric surgery. Br J Surg. 2011;**98**(10):1345–55.
9. Mourelo R, Kaidar-Person O, Fajnwaks P, Roa PE, Pinto D, Szomstein S, et al. Hemorrhagic and thromboembolic complications after bariatric surgery in patients receiving chronic anticoagulation therapy. Obes Surg. 2008;**18**(2):167–70.
10. Ellison SR, Ellison SD. Bariatric surgery: a review of the available procedures and complications for the emergency physician. J Emerg Med. 2008;**34**(1):21–32.
11. Luber SD, Fischer DR, Venkat A. Care of the bariatric surgery patient in the emergency department. J Emerg Med. 2008;**34**(1):13–20.

12. de Aretxabala X, Leon J, Wiedmaier G, Turu I, Ovalle C, Maluenda F, et al. Gastric leak after sleeve gastrectomy: analysis of its management. Obes Surg. 2011;**21**(8):1232–37.

13. Sakran N, Goitein D, Raziel A, Keidar A, Beglaibter N, Grinbaum R et al. Gastric leaks after sleeve gastrectomy: a multicenter experience with 2,834 patients. Surg Endosc. 2013;**27**(1):240–45.

14. Csendes A, Burgos AM, Braghetto I. Classification and management of leaks after gastric bypass for patients with morbid obesity: a prospective study of 60 patients. Obes Surg. 2012;**22**(6):855–62.

15. Monkhouse SJW, Morgan JDT, Norton SA. Complications of bariatric surgery: presentation and emergency management—a review. Ann R Coll Surg Engl. 2009;**91**(4):280–86.

16. Lehnert B, Moshiri M, Osman S, Khandelwal S, Elojeimy S, Bhargava P, et al. Imaging of complications of common bariatric surgical procedures. Radiol Clin North Am. 2014;**52**(5):1071–86.

17. McGlinch BP, Que FG, Nelson JL, Wrobleski DM, Grant JE, Collazo-Clavell ML. Perioperative care of patients undergoing bariatric surgery. Mayo Clin Proc. 2006;**81**(10 Suppl):S25–33.

18. Jacobsen HJ, Nergard BJ, Leifsson BG, Frederiksen SG, Agajahni E, Ekelund M, et al. Management of suspected anastomotic leak after bariatric laparoscopic Roux-en-Y gastric bypass. Br J Surg. 2014;**101**(4):417–23.

19. Pieracci FM, Barie PS, Pomp A. Critical care of the bariatric patient. Crit Care Med. 2006;**34**(6):1796–804.

20. Lacy A, Ibarzabal A, Pando E, Adelsdorfer C, Delitala A, Corcelles R et al. Revisional surgery after sleeve gastrectomy. Surg Laparosc Endosc Percutan Tech. 2010;**20**(5):351–56.

21. Moszkowicz D, Arienzo R, Khettab I, Rahmi G, Zinzindohoué F, Berger A, et al. Sleeve gastrectomy severe complications: is it always a reasonable surgical option? Obes Surg. 2013;**23**(5):676–86.

22. Tan JT, Kariyawasam S, Wijeratne T, Chandraratna HS. Diagnosis and management of gastric leaks after laparoscopic sleeve gastrectomy for morbid obesity. Obes Surg. 2010;**20**(4):403–409.

23. Corona M, Zini C, Lucatelli P, D'Adamo A, Rosignuolo M, Salvatori FM. Complications of bariatric surgery: what can IR do? OMICS J Rad. 2013;**2**(8):148.

24. Lascano CA, et al. Challenges of laparoscopic colectomy in the obese patient: a review. Am J Surg. 2006;**192**:357–65.

25. Cooper L. Postoperative complications after thoracic surgery in the morbidly obese patient. Anesthesiol Res Pract. 2011;**2011**:865634.

26. Brodsky JB. Post-operative complications following bariatric surgery. Mex Anestesiol. 2008;**31**:93–6.

27. Doyle SL, Lysaght J, Reynolds JV. Obesity and post-operative complications in patients undergoing non-bariatric surgery. Obes Rev. 2010;**11**(12):875–86.

28. Blouw EL, Rudolph AD, Narr BJ, Sarr MG. The frequency of respiratory failure in patients with morbid obesity undergoing gastric bypass. AANA J. 2003;**71**(1):45–50.

29. Tanaka M, Watanabe S, Nishikawa T. Anesthetic management in obese parturients. J Anesth. 1999;**13**:217–29.

30. Rovira Soriano L, Belda Nácher J. Postoperative respiratory management of morbidly obese patient. Trends Anaesth Crit Care. 2013;**3**(1):49–54.

31. Nie W, et al. Obesity survival paradox in pneumonia: a meta-analysis. BMC Medicine. 2014;**12**:61.

32. Abir F, Bell R. Assessment and management of the obese patient. Crit Care Med. 2004;**32**(4 Suppl):S87–91.

33. Guss D, Bhattacharyya T. Perioperative management of the obese orthopaedic patient. J Am Acad Orthop Surg. 2006;**14**(7):425–32.

34. Kebede S, Prakasa KR, Shermock K, Shihab HM, Brotman DJ, Sharma R et al. A systematic review of venous thromboembolism prophylaxis strategies in patients with renal insufficiency, obesity, or on antiplatelet agents. J Hosp Med. 2013;**8**(7):394–401.

35. Stein J, Stier C, Raab H, Weiner R. Review article: the nutritional and pharmacological consequences of obesity surgery. Aliment Pharmacol Ther. 2014;**40**(6):582–609.

36. Moizé VL, Pi-Sunyer X, Mochari H, Vidal J. Nutritional pyramid for post-gastric bypass patients. Obes Surg. 2010;**20**(8):1133–41.

37. Strohmayer E, Via MA, Yanagisawa R. Metabolic management following bariatric surgery. Mt Sinai J Med. 2010;**77**(5):431–45.

38. Bamgbade OA, Rutter TW, Nafiu OO, Dorje P. Postoperative complications in obese and nonobese patients. World J Surg. 2007;**31**(3):556–60.

39. Ankichetty S, Angle P, Margarido C, Halpern SH. Case report: rhabdomyolysis in morbidly obese patients: anesthetic considerations. Can J Anaesth. 2013;**60**(3):290–93.

40. Singh PM, Wadhwa A. Multimodal analgesia in patients with morbid obesity. Bariatric Times. 26 November 2013. http://bariatrictimes.com/multimodal-analgesia-in-patients-with-morbid-obesity/

41. Porhomayon J, Leissner KB, El-Solh AA, Nader ND. Strategies in postoperative analgesia in the obese obstructive sleep apnea patient. Clin J Pain. 2013;**29**(11):998–1005.

42. Lloret-Linares C, Lopes A, Declèves X, Serrie A, Mouly S, Bergmann JF, et al. Challenges in the optimisation of post-operative pain management with opioids in obese patients: a literature review. Obes Surg. 2013;**23**(9):1458–75.

43. Schumann R, Jones SB, Ortiz VE, Connor K, Pulai I, Ozawa ET, et al. Best practice recommendations for anesthetic perioperative care and pain management in weight loss surgery. Obes Res. 2005;**13**(2):254–66.

44. Gaszynski T. Anesthetic complications of gross obesity. Curr Opin Anaesthesiol. 2004;**17**(3):271–76.

45. Shah S, Shah V, Ahmed AR, Blunt DM. Imaging in bariatric surgery: service set-up, post-operative anatomy and complications. Br J Rad. 2011;**84**(998):101–11.

Ventilatory strategies in obesity and obesity hypoventilation syndrome

Ranjani Venkataramani, Scott R. Coleman, and Ashish C. Sinha

Introduction

Key aspects to ventilating an obese patient after induction include:

- Low tidal volume ventilation (6–8 mL/kg ideal body weight)
- Recruitment manoeuvres with positive end-expiratory pressure (PEEP) with optimal PEEP titration using transpulmonary pressure (P_{tp}) estimation where possible
- Inspired oxygen concentration of less than 80% to minimize absorption atelectasis
- Optimize positioning in the form of reverse Trendelenburg position to improve functional residual capacity (FRC) when possible (which helps counteract effects of weight of abdominal contents and surgical retractors).

As obesity continues to be a more prominent medical comorbidity, the physiological sequelae it has on the body are of more interest. The changes that occur in the respiratory system have been widely studied. In this chapter, we will discuss how obesity affects pulmonary function, how anaesthesia may alter the clinical scenario, and techniques to help improve outcomes in the perioperative period and the intensive care unit for patients with obesity.

Physiological changes

Lung volumes

Obesity affects respiratory function in many ways. The most well-accepted change is a decrease in the expiratory reserve volume (ERV) and the FRC as body mass index (BMI) increases [1–7]. Increased abdominal visceral fat can displace the diaphragm further into the thorax, limiting lung expansion and affecting these lung volumes [2]. A basic understanding of lung volumes and capacities is important to appreciate these concepts. The FRC is comprised of the ERV and residual volume. The ERV is the volume able to be exhaled beyond passive expiration. The residual volume is the volume left in the lungs after maximal expiration. The decrease in FRC in obesity is due to decreased ERV as the residual volume remains unchanged

or slightly increases [3,4]. The importance of this is related to closing volume and closing capacity. Closing volume is the volume beyond residual volume at which airways begin to close. The closing capacity is the sum of the residual and closing volumes [8]. Therefore, if the closing volume is greater than the expiratory reserve volume, airways will close during normal tidal breathing. Hence, the threshold for airway closure is lowered in the obese population. The closing of distal airways at lower lung volumes will not only decrease the amount of gas exchange due to air trapping and increased dead space, but it also will decrease airway compliance [1]. This leads to a decreased arterial pressure of oxygen (PaO_2) and increased work of breathing.

Lung and chest wall compliance

Compliance refers to the ability of the lungs to stretch and expand with increased volumes. Decreases in both airway and chest wall compliance also lead to hypoventilation and decreased PaO_2. The decrease in FRC, which was previously mentioned, results in decreased airway compliance. Obese patients also have increased pulmonary blood volume, which limits airway compliance [7]. Decreased chest wall compliance also plays a role in hypoventilation. Deposition of fat on the ribcage limits the ability for the chest to expand normally. In obese patients, the increased loading overwhelms the efforts of the respiratory muscles to expand the chest wall. As a result, work of breathing increases, oxygen consumption increases, and hypoventilation occurs [9].

Distribution of adipose tissue

Studies have also shown that the distribution of adipose deposition is important [1,2]. Those with increased waist-to-hip ratio and bicep skinfold thickness, which are indicative of greater upper body mass, are affected more. In fact, the location of adipose deposition appears more important in predicting decreased respiratory function than BMI [2].

Airway resistance

Obesity is also associated with increased airway resistance. The mechanism for this, however, has not been fully elucidated. The traditional cause was thought to be a decrease in diameter of the airway due to decreased lung volumes [10]. However, Littleton [3] points out that a few studies have indicated that airway resistance is only partly decreased by low lung volumes. Therefore, multiple additional elements are likely contributing to increased resistance. Other proposed factors include smooth muscle dysfunction secondary to long-standing changes in airway diameter, hyper-allergenic responses unique to obesity, and proinflammatory processes associated with adipose tissue [1]. In fact, increased interleukin-6 and cyclooxygenase-2 activity have been linked with adipose cells [5]. The proinflammatory molecules create airway remodelling and increase airway responsiveness. Although evidence clearly shows airway resistance is increased in obesity, the dynamics of why this happens are still to be determined.

Ventilation/perfusion mismatch

Three different zones can be distinguished in the lungs based upon their relative alveolar, venous, and arterial pressures. In zone one, alveolar pressure is greater than arterial and venous pressures. In this zone, ventilation occurs without perfusion. In zone two, alveolar pressure is between that of arterial and venous pressures, and the perfusion pressure will depend upon the gradient between the arterial and alveolar pressures. In zone 3, alveolar pressure is less than venous pressure and perfusion pressure is determined by the difference between arterial and venous pressures [8]. This means the majority of blood flow to the lungs is in the dependent regions. Unfortunately, in obese patients, it has been noted that ventilation tends to shift upward [1,11]. The implication is that less ventilation occurs at the dependent lung portions, which receive the most perfusion. Therefore, generation of a ventilation/perfusion (V/Q) mismatch will occur leading to a widened A–a gradient and lower PaO_2.

Oxygen consumption

All the physiological changes previously mentioned affect the ability of oxygen to reach the bloodstream, resulting in a decreased PaO_2. Making the situation worse, oxygen consumption and demand is increased in obese patients. Intuitively, obese patients have a higher basal metabolic rate, as more energy is required to supply a larger habitus. They also require more energy for their work of breathing. Muscles of respiration are often weaker and yet need to move more mass for adequate ventilation [6]. This leads to greater oxygen demand and patients often feeling dyspnoeic [3].

Obesity hypoventilation syndrome

Obesity hypoventilation syndrome (OHS) is vaguely defined by a partial pressure of arterial carbon dioxide ($PaCO_2$) greater than 45 mmHg and a BMI greater than 30 kg/m² with no other cause for hypoventilation [12,13]. Patients experience daytime hypoxaemia and hypercapnia, which can lead to pulmonary hypertension and right heart failure [12,13]. Several factors have been identified in OHS patients, which differ from patients of similar weight without OHS. OHS patients have thicker necks, higher central-to-peripheral ratio of fat, and decreased lung compliance [13]. The pathophysiology of OHS is not clearly understood, however, and multiple physiological changes appear to contribute. OHS follows the same pathway as described previously in obese patients, only the effects

are more exaggerated. Greater restriction of the airway occurs, compliance decreases further, and intrapulmonary shunt increases as small airways close more easily. This increases the work of breathing leading to more oxygen consumption and carbon dioxide (CO_2) production [14].

A theory regarding the involvement of leptin is also gaining support. Leptin is produced by adipose cells and is known to both decrease appetite and stimulate respiration by acting centrally on the hypothalamus [14]. OHS patients have increased levels of leptin compared to similar weight, non-OHS patients. Therefore, it is believed that resistance to leptin has developed and OHS patients have ineffective leptin [15].

In addition to this, obstructive sleep apnoea (OSA) is thought to increase the risk of OHS. In fact, when comparing patients with OSA and OHS versus those with OHS only, patients with both diagnoses had increased $PaCO_2$ even though minute ventilation and dead space changes were similar. This is an indication that OSA contributes to production of CO_2 in addition to the CO_2 retention from hypoventilation [13]. A likely explanation is that during nocturnal respiration, OSA patients will stimulate their kidneys to retain bicarbonate in response to elevated $PaCO_2$ from apnoea and hypopnea. Increased levels of bicarbonate ions will help to compensate for the acid–base disturbance generated during this time. Then, during the day, the hyperventilatory response to hypercapnia is diminished because the body has already created compensation by retained bicarbonate [14].

Ventilation in obesity

Obesity has traditionally been a clinical scenario of high tidal volume ventilation [16]. The size of the lungs does not increase in relation to body weight and hence the need for delivery of tidal volumes appropriate to predicted body weight (PBW) to prevent atelectrauma and barotrauma.

Using actual body weight tends to overestimate ventilatory volumes the patient should receive, as opposed to using ideal body weight.

It is important to use predicted body weight for calculation of estimated tidal volume as shown:

$$\text{Male: PBW (kg)} = 50 + 2.3(\text{height (in)} - 60)$$

$$\text{Female: PBW (kg)} = 45.5 + 2.3(\text{height (in)} - 60)$$

An association between higher tidal volumes and acute respiratory distress syndrome (ARDS)/increased inflammation has been seen in subjects without pre-existing pulmonary disease [17]. Recent findings reveal improved clinical outcomes (lower incidence of ARDS, mortality) when low tidal volume ventilation is used in mechanically ventilated patients without ARDS [18].

Recent literature in the general population has yielded mixed results. The IMPROVE trial [19] showed improved pulmonary outcomes (pneumonia, acute respiratory failure, atelectasis) and shortened hospital stays in patients ventilated for elective major abdominal surgery with a protective ventilation management approach (tidal volume 6–8 mL/kg PBW, PEEP 6–8 cmH₂O, and protocolized recruitment manoeuvres) compared to a non-protective strategy (tidal volume 10–12 mL/kg PBW, PEEP 0 cmH$_2$O, no recruitment manoeuvres).

However, the PROVHILO trial [20] showed no difference in a composite of varied pulmonary complications (including hypoxaemia or ARDS but also pneumothorax or cardiogenic pulmonary oedema) during the first 5 postoperative days in patients undergoing open abdominal surgery under general anaesthesia and ventilation at tidal volumes of 8 mL/kg PBW. In this study, one group received high PEEP (12 cmH$_2$O and recruitment manoeuvres) and another received low PEEP (2 cmH$_2$O and no recruitment manoeuvres). Intraoperatively, the PROVHILO low-PEEP group required more interventions for desaturation and the high-PEEP group required more interventions for hypotension.

While the benefit of low tidal volume is reasonable in ventilating obese individuals, conclusive evidence is lacking at the present time. The PROBESE study examined the benefits of high PEEP with recruitment manoeuvres versus low PEEP with no recruitment manoeuvres. The study found no statistically significant difference in pulmonary complications between the two groups [21].

Bariatric laparoscopic procedures imply a rapid change in lung compliance given external factors including pneumoperitoneum and Trendelenburg positions. This, in addition to low lung compliance and increased resistance in the supine position, can make ventilation challenging.

Traditional modes such as pressure-controlled ventilation (PCV) and volume-controlled ventilation (VCV) have been used equally well with no clear advantage discernible in studies [22].

Common sense dictates that while PCV aids in reducing barotrauma due to increased plateau pressures, hypoventilation and atelectasis formation due to low tidal volumes may ensue. VCV, while ensuring tidal volume delivery, may induce barotrauma.

No differences in intraoperative tidal volume, mean airway pressure, or oxygenation were noted in a systematic review comparing PCV and VCV in obese patients.

PCV–volume guarantee (VG) is a time-cycled, pressure-regulated mode with a variable inspiratory flow to achieve a preset tidal volume. PCV-VG or similar modes utilize the advantages of pressure control while ensuring the delivery of a target tidal volume with lower peak inspiratory pressures thereby avoiding hypoventilation.

In a study performed on adolescents undergoing bariatric laparoscopic procedures, no difference in oxygenation, ventilation, or haemodynamic variables was noted between these three modes of ventilation. However, lower peak inspiratory pressures were observed in the PCV-VG and PCV modes [23].

PEEP settings

Having dealt with basic intubation and ventilation under anaesthesia, one should focus on preventing the derecruitment of alveoli, which would lead to a reduction in compliance and oxygenation. Unlike the non-obese population, the threshold for inhomogeneous ventilation is higher in the obese population. Addition of PEEP preceded by a recruitment manoeuvre helps improve lung volumes and diminish atelectasis, an important issue in helping reduce derecruitment and reduction in FRC after extubation of the patient. This phenomenon of the 'open lung concept' is important in preventing the development of ventilator-induced lung injury by stabilizing open alveoli, especially in patients undergoing major surgery. Additionally, the application of PEEP may also efficiently offset airflow limitation in the supine position and eliminate auto-PEEP without raising plateau pressure [24].

PEEP titration

Traditionally, a plateau pressure of 30–35 cmH$_2$O has been used as an upper limit to ventilating obese individuals. This, however, may represent underventilation of obese lungs as the P$_{tp}$ is much lower in this population because of the increased chest wall pressures:

$$P_{tp} = P_{alv} - P_{ip}$$

where P$_{alv}$ is alveolar pressure, and P$_{ip}$ is intrapleural pressure.

A focus on P$_{tp}$ is key in understanding respiratory mechanics with reference to this population in particular. P$_{tp}$ has been shown to be better at targeted tidal volume and PEEP delivery in non-obese patients. Given the altered non-compliant chest wall, this may serve as a tool to ventilate obese patients using a lung protective strategy.

Oesophageal pressure, or P$_{es}$, is usually measured via an oesophageal catheter with an air-filled thin-walled latex balloon inserted nasally or orally and is used as a surrogate of pleural pressure. P$_{alv}$ is either the plateau pressure or the PEEP as seen on the pressure waveform.

Aiming for a P$_{tp}$ above 0 cmH$_2$O using P$_{es}$ is useful in preventing cyclic collapse and reopening of alveoli. Limiting the P$_{tp}$ to less than 20 cmH$_2$O may serve as an upper limit of lung distension.

Pirrone et al. studied the use of P$_{tp}$-guided PEEP with and without recruitment manoeuvres in 14 critically ill patients with a BMI greater than 35 kg/m^2. Recruitment manoeuvres followed by titrated PEEP were effective at increasing end-expiratory lung volumes while decreasing end-inspiratory P$_{tp}$, suggesting an improved distribution of lung aeration and reduction of overdistension [25].

Detailed studies of oesophageal balloons in obese patients and in patients with acute lung injury have demonstrated oesophageal pressure values consistent with physiological expectations and predictions of pleural pressure [26].

Recruitment manoeuvres

Small airway opening in the form of recruitment manoeuvres can be achieved by applying intermittent hyperinflation of the lung [27]. Some common techniques have been reported as follows [28].

A study by Almarakbi et al. [29] compared four different intraoperative ventilation strategies (PEEP alone, single recruitment manoeuvre, single recruitment manoeuvre plus PEEP, and recruitment manoeuvre plus PEEP with recruitment manoeuvre performed every 10 minutes) in obese patients undergoing laparoscopic surgery. The study revealed that recruitment manoeuvre every 10 minutes with PEEP of 10 cmH$_2$O was associated with the best intraoperative oxygenation and respiratory compliance.

Talab et al. [30] determined the optimum PEEP to be 10 cmH$_2$O after a vital capacity manoeuvre performed by maintaining a pressure of 40 cmH$_2$O for 7–8 seconds. The results revealed that the patients in the group undergoing an alveolar recruitment manoeuvre and PEEP maintained at 10 cmH$_2$O after the manoeuvre exhibited a better oxygenation, shorter post-anaesthesia care unit stay, and fewer pulmonary complications in the postoperative period in obese patients undergoing laparoscopic bariatric surgery.

Recruitment manoeuvres have also shown to be useful when performed prior to extubation. Using a single manual inflation of lungs post pneumoperitoneum release, Cakmakkaya et al. [31] showed an improvement in pulmonary compliance after a recruitment manoeuvre was performed as a single manual inflation of the lungs to 40 cmH$_2$O, maintained for 10 seconds, in laparoscopic radical nephrectomies.

A transient drop in mean arterial pressure is a distinct possibility to be prepared for while performing recruitment manoeuvres. The timing and duration of ideal recruitment manoeuvres are still topics of ongoing research.

Patient positioning

Positioning obese patients in a manner so as to improve FRC and oxygenation is vital when possible. Beach chair position [32], reverse Trendelenburg [33], and lateral decubitus [34] positions help offload the abdominal contents and pannus away from the thorax, improving lung compliance.

Absorption atelectasis

While it is again important to maintain adequate oxygenation and prepare for hypoxaemic events peri-extubation, it is prudent to consider the possibility of absorption atelectasis. Some studies recommend maintaining a fraction of inspired oxygen (FiO$_2$) of less than 0.8 intraoperatively [35] while a meta-analysis by Hovaguimian et al. [36] failed to find statistical evidence to support this recommendation.

Postoperatively

Given the propensity of having OSH or OSA that worsens with narcotics, an analgesic plan with an opioid-sparing strategy is not just prudent but recommended (see Chapter 5 for details). Incentive spirometry and use of non-invasive ventilation (NIV)/continuous positive airway pressure (CPAP) must be considered where feasible.

Non-invasive ventilation

During the early postoperative period and spontaneous breathing, obese surgical patients experience more severe alveolar collapse and impairment of gas exchange than their normal-weight counterparts. CPAP provides ventilatory support to restore and maintain the lung volumes by recruiting atelectatic lung which, in turn, improves oxygenation and reduces work of breathing.

Use of NIV in the post-extubation period, specifically post abdominal surgery, has been shown to reduce post-pulmonary complications, atelectasis, and pneumonia. This benefit is better obtained when initiated immediately post extubation and has been shown to enhance pulmonary function for at least the following 24 hours. See **Fig. 20.1** for an algorithm in treating acute hypercapnic respiratory failure in obese patients.

Pressure support settings between 5 and 10 cmH$_2$O, PEEP of 10 cmH$_2$O, at an adjusted FiO$_2$ of 0.5 with each patient in a 30-degree head-up position led to improved spirometry and oxygenation for 24 hours post surgery [37].

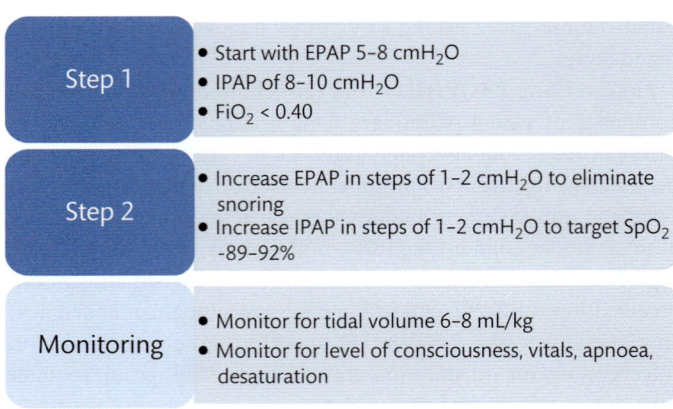

Fig. 20.1 Algorithm for hypercapnic respiratory failure. EPAP, expiratory positive airway pressure; IPAP, inspiratory positive airway pressure.

Adapted with permission from Sequeira, T. C., BaHammam, A. S., Esquinas, A. M., Noninvasive Ventilation in the Critically Ill Patient With Obesity Hypoventilation Syndrome: A Review, *Journal of Intensive Care Medicine*, 32(7):421–428. Copyright © 2017 SAGE. doi: 10.1177/0885066616663179

Additionally, the adoption of a sitting position has been shown to lower the PEEP requirements for the reversal of expiratory flow limitation and the restoration of FRC [32].

Intensive care unit ventilation

With the open lung concept extendable to the obese population from studies on non-obese critically ill patients needing mechanical ventilation, a focus on setting appropriate tidal volumes to prevent lung injury is pertinent. Obese patients are more likely to develop postoperative acute respiratory failure and/or acute hypercapnic respiratory failure that necessitate NIV or intubation and mechanical ventilation. The duration of mechanical ventilation surprisingly has been shown to be equivalent to the non-obese counterparts. Rates of tracheostomy, secondary to failure to wean from ventilator, however, have been shown to be higher [38].

Key aspects to ventilating an obese individual in the intensive care unit include:

- Lung protective ventilation with PBW-targeted tidal volumes[1] to prevent barotrauma/atelectrauma
- Using P$_{tp}$ and optimal/targeted PEEP to guide homogeneous lung expansion, as opposed to preset values of plateau/peak pressures
- Head-up sitting position, encouragement of deep breathing, extubation while awake, and non-opioid analgesic regimens
- NIV as a bridge to extubation.

In the non-obese population, limiting plateau pressures to a preset limit of 35 cmH$_2$O [39] has been used as the upper limit to prevent barotrauma, making this number suboptimal given the previously mentioned changes in respiratory mechanics in the obese population. Using lower than required PEEP is a common occurrence

---

[1] Tidal volume to be based on PBW with 6–8 mL/kg of ideal body weight. A tidal volume calculated according to total body weight is likely to result in excessively high airway pressures, alveolar overdistension, and baro/atelectrauma.

in this population, which leads to cyclic collapse and reopening of alveoli.

The use of oesophageal balloons helps determine the pleural pressure as a surrogate of P_{tp} in ventilated patients. Optimal PEEP may then be determined following a recruitment manoeuvre targeting a P_{tp} greater than 0 cmH$_2$O.

Head-end elevation helps physically offload the abdominal contents and increases end-expiratory lung volumes, thereby minimizing the need for high PEEP settings [25].

Non-invasive ventilation as a bridge to extubation

NIV in patients with a BMI greater than 35 kg/m^2 showed a reduced length of intensive care unit stay and a 16% absolute risk reduction in post-extubation acute respiratory failure [40].

Early application of NIV may be effective in averting respiratory failure before the development of respiratory distress and may be responsible for decreasing mortality in selected patients with chronic hypercapnia.

Oronasal masks are better tolerated and preferred in the acute setting, as they are associated with less air leakage to deliver optimal tidal volumes and minimize hypoventilation. This is also a method to circumvent the mouth-breathing pattern noted in most of these patients. Alternatives such as a helmet have been devised to serve as a better interface to improving patient acceptance and leaks from the oronasal devices.

CASE REPORT

A 50-year-old female with morbid obesity presents for a laparoscopic hysterectomy. She is 165 cm tall and weighs 120 kg (BMI 44 kg/m^2, ideal body weight 57 kg). Her preoperative evaluation is positive for hypertension and OSA. She uses a CPAP machine at home, but does not know her settings. She has limited exercise tolerance due to knee and back pain. On examination, her lungs are clear to auscultation. Mallampati score is II with adequate mouth opening, normal thyromental distance, and appropriate neck extension.

1. How does the surgical technique and positioning affect her respiratory physiology?

   - Laparoscopic hysterectomies require both insufflation of the abdomen with CO$_2$ and the Trendelenburg position. Insufflation of the abdomen increases intra-abdominal pressure, which pushes the diaphragm cephalad. This reduces the patient's FRC and increases airway pressures during positive pressure ventilation. The use of CO$_2$ for insufflation places the patient at risk for hypercapnia. This can be magnified in a patient with OHS or OSA, where CO$_2$ retention is already a concern.
   - The Trendelenburg position also shifts the abdominal contents towards the thoracic cavity. This mimics restrictive lung physiology. Airway pressures will rise and achieving adequate ventilation while avoiding barotrauma from high airway pressures can become difficult.

2. What ventilatory strategies may be used after induction of anaesthesia to minimize decruitment and atelectasis? What can be done to combat elevated peak airway pressures?

   - Atelectasis commonly occurs during intubation as alveoli collapse during this period of apnoea. Performing a lung

recruitment manoeuvre can help reopen the collapse alveoli. Such a manoeuvre can be done by using a CPAP of 30 cmH$_2$O/vital capacity breath for 30 seconds. Additionally, adjusting the PEEP to 10 cmH$_2$O can help recruit atelectatic alveoli as well.

   - Atelectasis can also be due to high inspired oxygen concentrations. After induction of anaesthesia, using the lowest tolerated FiO$_2$ (40–60%) is beneficial to reduce absorptive atelectasis.
   - Consistently reassessing driving pressures, the pressure–volume loop, and static compliance should occur. A low static compliance and high driving pressures (plateau pressure minus PEEP) greater than 14 cmH$_2$O suggests the need for repeating a recruitment and up-titrating PEEP to 15–20 cmH$_2$O.
   - Limited ventilation secondary to elevated airway pressures is commonplace for such patients in this scenario. Ventilating using the VCV with inspiratory:expiratory ratios of 1:1 to 1:1.5 helps deliver the flow at lower inspiratory pressures and can both improve ventilation and reduce the risk of barotrauma.

3. What strategies can be used to optimize the patient for extubation and the immediate post-extubation time period?

   - Any hypercapnia that has occurred in this patient due to insufflation or decreased ventilation should be corrected. Hypercapnia can result in somnolence and delayed awakening from anaesthesia.
   - Positioning the patient in the sitting/reverse Trendelenburg position helps improve respiratory mechanics.
   - Use of CPAP post extubation with nasal or oronasal masks helps re-establish adequate lung reinflation.

REFERENCES

1. Porhomayon J, Papadakos P, Singh A, Nader ND. Alteration in respiratory physiology in obesity for anesthesia-critical care physician. HSR Proc Intensive Care Cardiovasc Anesth. 2011;**3**(2):109–18.
2. Sue D. Obesity and pulmonary function. Chest. 1997;**111**(4):844–45.
3. Littleton S. Impact of obesity on respiratory function. Respirology. 2011;**17**(1):43–49.
4. Jones R, Nzekwu M. The effects of body mass index on lung volumes. Chest. 2006;**130**(3):827–33.
5. Jubber A. Respiratory complications of obesity. Int J Clin Pract. 2004;**58**(6):573–80.
6. Luce J. Respiratory complications of obesity. Chest. 1980;**78**(4):626–31.
7. Ray C, Sue D, Bray G, Hansen J, Wasserman K. Effects of obesity on respiratory function. Am Rev Resp Dis. 1983(3);**128**:501–506.
8. Miller RD. Respiratory physiology. In: Miller's Anesthesia. 7th ed. Philadelphia, PA: Elsevier; 2010:**368**, 371–72.
9. Lourenço R. Diaphragm activity in obesity. J Clin Invest. 1969;**48**(9):1609–14.
10. Rubinstein I, Zamel N, Dubarry L, Hoffstein V. Airflow limitation in morbidly obese, nonsmoking men. Ann Intern Med. 1990;**112**(11):828–32.
11. Holley H, Milic-Emili J, Becklake M, Bates D. Regional distribution of pulmonary ventilation and perfusion in obesity. J Clin Invest. 1967;**46**(4):475–81.

12. Sequeira T, BaHammam A, Esquinas A. Noninvasive ventilation in the critically ill patient with obesity hypoventilation syndrome: a review. J Intensive Care Med. 2016;**32**(7):421–28.

13. Javaheri S, Simbartl L. Respiratory determinants of diurnal hypercapnia in obesity hypoventilation syndrome. What does weight have to do with it? Ann Am Thorac Soc. 2014;**11**(6):945–50.

14. Pierce A, Brown L. Obesity hypoventilation syndrome. Curr Opin Pulm Med. 2015;**21**(6):557–62.

15. Phipps P. Association of serum leptin with hypoventilation in human obesity. Thorax. 2002;**57**(1):75–76.

16. Fernandez-Bustamante A, Wood CL, Tran ZV, Moine P. Intraoperative ventilation: incidence and risk factors for receiving large tidal volumes during general anesthesia. BMC Anesthesiol. 2011;**11**(1):22.

17. Gajic O, Frutos-Vivar F, Esteban A, Hubmayr RD, Anzueto A. Ventilator settings as a risk factor for acute respiratory distress syndrome in mechanically ventilated patients. Intensive Care Med. 2005;**31**(7):922–26.

18. Serpa Neto A, Cardoso SO, Manetta JA, et al. Association between use of lung-protective ventilation with lower tidal volumes and clinical outcomes among patients without acute respiratory distress syndrome: a meta-analysis. JAMA. 2012;**308**(16):1651–59.

19. Futier E, Constantin JM, Paugam-Burtz C, et al. A trial of intraoperative low-tidal-volume ventilation in abdominal surgery. N Engl J Med. 2013;**369**(5):428–37.

20. Hemmes SN, Gama de Abreu M, Pelosi P, Schultz MJ, PROVE Network Investigators for the Clinical Trial Network of the European Society of Anaesthesiology. High versus low positive end-expiratory pressure during general anaesthesia for open abdominal surgery (PROVHILO trial): a multicentre randomised controlled trial. Lancet. 2014;**384**(9942):495–503.

21. Writing Committee for the PROBESE Collaborative Group of the PROtective VEntilation Network (PROVEnet) for the Clinical Trial Network of the European Society of Anaesthesiology. Effect of intraoperative high positive end-expiratory pressure (PEEP) with recruitment maneuvers vs low PEEP on postoperative pulmonary complications in obese patients: a randomized clinical trial. JAMA. 2019;**321**(23):2292–305.

22. Aldenkortt M, Lysakowski C, Elia N, Brochard L, Tramèr MR. Ventilation strategies in obese patients undergoing surgery: a quantitative systematic review and meta-analysis. Br J Anaesth. 2012;**109**(4):493–502.

23. Dion JM, McKee C, Tobias JD, et al. Ventilation during laparoscopic-assisted bariatric surgery: volume-controlled, pressure-controlled or volume-guaranteed pressure-regulated modes. Int J Clin Exp Med. 2014;**7**(8):2242–47.

24. Lemyze M, Mallat J, Duhamel A, et al. Effects of sitting position and applied positive end-expiratory pressure on respiratory mechanics of critically ill obese patients receiving mechanical ventilation. Crit Care Med. 2013;**41**(11):2592–99.

25. Pirrone M, Fisher D, Chipman D, et al. Recruitment maneuvers and positive end-expiratory pressure titration in morbidly obese ICU patients. Crit Care Med. 2016;**44**(2):300–307.

26. Owens RL, Campana LM, Hess L, Eckert DJ, Loring SH, Malhotra A. Sitting and supine esophageal pressures in overweight and obese subjects. Obesity. 2012;**20**(12):2354–60.

27. Reinius H, Jonsson L, Gustafsson S, et al. Prevention of atelectasis in morbidly obese patients during general anesthesia and paralysis: a computerized tomography study. Anesthesiology. 2009;**111**(5):979–87.

28. Forgiarini Júnior LA, Rezende JC, Forgiarini SG. Alveolar recruitment maneuver and perioperative ventilatory support in obese patients undergoing abdominal surgery. Rev Bras Ter Intensiva. 2013;**25**(4):312–18.

29. Almarakbi WA, Fawzi HM, Alhashemi JA. Effects of four intraoperative ventilatory strategies on respiratory compliance and gas exchange during laparoscopic gastric banding in obese patients. Br J Anaesth. 2009;**102**(6):862–68.

30. Talab HF, Zabani IA, Abdelrahman HS, et al. Intraoperative ventilatory strategies for prevention of pulmonary atelectasis in obese patients undergoing laparoscopic bariatric surgery. Anesth Analg. 2009;**109**(5):1511–16.

31. Cakmakkaya OS, Kaya G, Altintas F, Hayirlioglu M, Ekici B. Restoration of pulmonary compliance after laparoscopic surgery using a simple alveolar recruitment maneuver. J Clin Anesth. 2009;**21**(6):422–26.

32. Valenza F, Vagginelli F, Tiby A, et al. Effects of the beach chair position, positive end-expiratory pressure, and pneumoperitoneum on respiratory function in morbidly obese patients during anesthesia and paralysis. Anesthesiology. 2007;**107**(5):725–32.

33. Perilli V, Sollazzi L, Bozza P, et al. The effects of the reverse Trendelenburg position on respiratory mechanics and blood gases in morbidly obese patients during bariatric surgery. Anesth Analg. 2000;**91**(6):1520–25.

34. Brodsky JB, Wyner J, Ehrenwerth J, Merrell RC, Cohn RB. One-lung anesthesia in morbidly obese patients. Anesthesiology. 1982;**57**(2):132–34.

35. Pelosi P, Gregoretti C. Perioperative management of obese patients. Best Pract Res Clin Anaesthesiol. 2010;**24**(2):211–25.

36. Hovaguimian F, Lysakowski C, Elia N, Tramèr MR. Effect of intraoperative high inspired oxygen fraction on surgical site infection, postoperative nausea and vomiting, and pulmonary function: systematic review and meta-analysis of randomized controlled trials. Anesthesiology. 2013;**119**(2):303–16.

37. Zoremba M, Kalmus G, Begemann D, et al. Short term non-invasive ventilation post-surgery improves arterial blood-gases in obese subjects compared to supplemental oxygen delivery—a randomized controlled trial. BMC Anesthesiol. 2011;**11**:10.

38. Lee CK, Tefera E, Colice G. The effect of obesity on outcomes in mechanically ventilated patients in a medical intensive care unit. Respiration. 2014;**87**(3):219–26.

39. El-Solh AA. Clinical approach to the critically ill, morbidly obese patient. Am J Respir Crit Care Med. 2004;**169**(5):557–61.

40. El-Solh AA, Aquilina A, Pineda L, Dhanvantri V, Grant B, Bouquin P. Noninvasive ventilation for prevention of post-extubation respiratory failure in obese patients. Eur Respir J. 2006;**28**(3):588–95.

Difficult airway management

Jeremy Collins and Brita M. Mittal

Introduction

As the worldwide epidemic of morbid obesity grows, anaesthesiologists are increasingly likely to encounter such patients. Morbid obesity is associated with several other conditions including hypertension, diabetes, ischaemic heart disease, heart failure, peripheral vascular disease, obstructive sleep apnoea (OSA), cancer, and osteoarthritis. These increase the need for inpatient medical care and surgical intervention. In the postoperative setting, morbidly obese patients are also at higher risk for complications including cardiac arrest, venous thromboembolism, acute kidney injury, rhabdomyolysis, and wound infections, increasing their chances of needing additional procedures and invasive respiratory support [1]. As such, the anaesthesiologist must be prepared to manage morbidly obese patients not only in the operating room, but also in remote locations and in the emergency setting, often with less equipment and with greater concern for gastric aspiration.

The airway in the morbidly obese patient must be approached with caution. According to the American Society of Anesthesiologists (ASA) Closed Claims Database, obese patients were involved in 37% of all adverse airway events occurring upon induction of anaesthesia and 58% of those occurring following airway extubation [2]. Alterations in airway anatomy and respiratory physiology lead to rapid desaturation during apnoea, limiting the time available for securing the airway. At baseline, obese patients have higher oxygen consumption, reduced functional residual capacity (FRC) and total lung capacity, increased minute ventilation, and decreased pulmonary compliance when compared to their lean counterparts [3]. Following anaesthetic induction, marked decreases in FRC occur as abdominal contents move cephalad against the relaxed diaphragmatic tone. This leads to a large intrapulmonary shunt, which frequently results in hypoxia when combined with increased metabolic rate. The consequences of this are limited time for rescue of failed oxygenation and increased potential for hypoxic brain injury [4].

Despite numerous published reports, there is still no clear agreement about the relationship between an elevated body mass index (BMI) and the risk of a 'difficult' airway, probably because excess adipose tissue has a variable distribution among obese patients. However, it is possible to stratify this risk using predictive features to identify the subset of morbidly obese patients where significant difficulty is expected. In these patients, airway anatomy is more greatly affected by an uneven distribution of upper body adipose tissue. When dealing with such patients, strategies to optimize oxygenation during anaesthetic induction should be a priority. How to achieve this will be discussed, as well as intubation techniques that minimize time and maximize success.

Identifying risk factors for a difficult airway in morbid obesity

The ASA Task Force on the management of the difficult airway defines it as 'the clinical situation in which a conventionally trained anaesthesiologist experiences problems with face mask ventilation of the upper airway or tracheal intubation, or both' [5]. This is purposefully vague because for both of these skills, difficulty is hard to measure. In this section, we will review risk factors for both difficult mask ventilation and difficult direct laryngoscopy specific to morbidly obese patients.

Difficult mask ventilation

It is reassuring to note that the incidences of difficult (1.4%) and impossible (0.15%) mask ventilation remain rare [6,7]. That being said, a study by Kheterpal et al. identified obesity (BMI >30 kg/m²) as one of the five independent risk factors for difficult mask ventilation as defined by instability, inadequacy, or requirement for two providers [6]. In addition, in a subsequent study by the same authors, OSA was found to be an independent risk factor for *impossible* mask ventilation [7]. Although only a small percentage of morbidly obese patients may have a formal diagnosis of OSA, it is very likely that many remain undiagnosed given the high prevalence of snoring among morbidly obese patients. Therefore, many morbidly obese patients have more than one risk factor for difficult or impossible face mask ventilation.

It is also important to note that the data available probably underestimates the incidence of problematic ventilation and the contribution of very extreme obesity. Patients predicted to be especially difficult are often excluded from studies when clinical judgement suggests the safest approach would be to secure the airway with the patient awake. The study of difficult airways will always be compromised by the responsibility to deliver safe clinical care over the scientific merit of the patient's inclusion in a study. Over a 9-year period, Hagberg et al. found that as many as 4.2% of obese patients were managed in this way, and were likely to be male, those with Mallampati scores of 3 or 4, and those with extreme obesity (BMI >60 kg/m²) [8].

Difficult mask ventilation occurs when there is failure to establish a seal between mask and face, when the airway partially or completely collapses, and/or when the resultant gas exchange cannot maintain adequate oxygenation. The association between morbid obesity and difficult ventilation is consistent with the anatomical changes and pathophysiology that occur in obese patients. Problems in maintaining a seal occur because excess adipose tissue in the face and cheeks dampen the applied pressure from the mask, cushioning it from the more stable foundation of the bony skeleton.

Maintaining airway patency may also be more challenging. There is an inverse relationship between pharyngeal area and obesity. Pharyngeal airway size is determined by a balance between the soft tissues through which it is formed and the bony craniofacial skeleton that supports it. A greater tendency to collapse exists when the mass of soft tissue increases. Magnetic resonance imaging shows deposition of excess adipose tissue into nearly all pharyngeal structures in obesity including the uvula, tonsils, tonsillar pillars, tongue, aryepiglottic folds, and, most predominantly, the lateral pharyngeal walls [9]. Airway narrowing from these depositions can be further exaggerated by external compression from superficial depositions in the neck, especially seen in android patterns of obesity. This localized effect is further compromised by a 'distant' consequence of reduced lung volumes following anaesthetic induction as abdominal contents move upward. The trachea moves in a cephalad direction along with the mediastinum during this lung deflation, reducing the longitudinal tension that is normally applied to the upper airway and causing the pharyngeal mucosa to possibly unfold [10].

Difficult direct laryngoscopy

The anatomical changes that lead to difficulties with mask ventilation may also produce difficulties securing a definitive airway. Large breasts in both male and female patients encroach into the submandibular area and restrict access for external laryngeal manipulation, laryngoscope handles, and other intubation devices. Fat deposition also occurs at the occiput and posterior aspect of the neck. When severe, this reduces craniocervical mobility and interferes with optimal head positioning for intubation and reduces maximal mouth opening. Head extension can also be restricted by deposition of glycosylated collagen in cervical joints of morbidly obese patients who develop diabetes. Deposition of adipose tissue within laryngeal structures can change the normal appearance at laryngoscopy so much that it may be hard to recognize glottic anatomy. Other factors that have been shown to increase the risk of difficult laryngoscopy in obese patients include high Mallampati score (3 or 4), increased neck circumference (>43 cm), and excessive pre-tracheal adipose tissue [11,12].

Although not all studies show an association between morbid obesity and difficult intubation, it is possible that the strength of this relationship has been underestimated for three reasons [13]. First, as previously mentioned, some patients are channelled into an awake intubation strategy that precludes their inclusion in research studies. Second, a large proportion of patients recruited for airway studies in the morbidly obese are recruited for bariatric surgical populations, which typically consist of a preponderance of female patients. Male fat deposition usually exhibits a more visceral and truncal pattern than the peripheral deposition seen in female patients. Higher rates of OSA are seen in men due to a greater accumulation of fat around the airway. It is therefore possible that studies of the airway in the morbidly obese select greater numbers of patients where the anatomical impact of obesity is reduced. Third, there is a lack of consensus about how to measure obesity as a risk factor for a difficult airway. The clinical cut-off value defining morbid obesity as a BMI greater than 35 kg/m² and not BMI greater than 40 kg/m² has been applied in many studies. However, this may not be appropriate and may diminish the full impact of excess weight on airway anatomy and management. For example, for a male patient of average weight, an additional 16 kg will change the BMI from 35 to 40 kg/m² and this modest change can contribute to further airway difficulties, especially if the additional fat is distributed in the upper body.

It should be noted, however, that the negative predictive value of the previously discussed risk factors is high. Therefore, when the Mallampati score is 1 or 2, the neck is not short or thick and has normal range of motion, and thyromental distance is normal, one should expect no difficulties with direct laryngoscopy in a patient with a high BMI. Because of differences seen in male and female patterns of adipose distribution, this clinical pattern is frequently seen in morbidly obese female patients. In the authors' experience, no difficulty has been encountered in these patients when the airway examination is otherwise favourable.

Optimizing modifiable factors

An important part of any airway management strategy is optimization of modifiable risk factors such as preoxygenation, patient positioning, and apnoeic oxygenation prior to commencing induction of general anaesthesia. This will increase the time available before hypoxia ensues and is described as the 'safe apnoea period' (SAP).

Preoxygenation

SAP is reduced in morbidly obese patients chiefly due to decreases in FRC but also due to increased oxygen consumption and pulmonary shunting. Therefore, it is important to adequately preoxygenate morbidly obese patients in order to increase the SAP as much as possible. For patients with a mean BMI of 43 kg/m² the SAP was 2.7 minutes compared to 6.1 minutes in lean controls [14]. Although reduced FRC will allow for faster wash-in of oxygen, vital capacity is also reduced and rapid techniques of four deep breaths in 30 seconds are not recommended over a traditional approach of tidal breathing for 3 minutes. Despite similar values of arterial oxygenation that are achieved in the two techniques, the traditional approach produces a greater SAP [15]. This is because the tissue and venous compartments need more than 30 seconds to fill with oxygen; these compartments have the capability of holding a significant amount of additional oxygen above that contained while breathing room air.

The facemask should provide a tight seal with the patient's face in order to prevent the entrainment of room air. One hundred per cent oxygen should be administered during preoxygenation. The application of continuous positive end-expiratory pressure of up to

10 cmH$_2$O helps to splint alveoli open and offset the effect of high concentrations of inspired oxygen that promote atelectasis.

Patient positioning

The impact of optimizing patient positioning on successful airway management cannot be overstated. Proper patient positioning has a significant impact on both adequacy of preoxygenation and success of direct laryngoscopy. In one study, preoxygenated obese patients could sustain SAP for 46 seconds longer in a 25-degree head-up position than when supine, presumably due to increased FRC [16].

In addition to being placed in the head-up position, morbidly obese patients should be 'ramped' with blankets placed under their upper body, head, and neck so that the external auditory meatus is aligned horizontally with the sternal notch. This position improves laryngeal exposure and the view obtained during direct laryngoscopy as compared to the 'sniff' position [17]. Alternatively, some operating tables can also be configured into the shape of a ramp to facilitate proper positioning.

Apnoeic oxygenation

Recent data have shown that use of transnasal high-flow oxygen administration prolongs apnoeic time in patients with difficult airways [18]. During apnoea, oxygen is absorbed from alveoli, but only replaced by a much smaller volume of carbon dioxide due to the high efficiency of blood buffering systems. If oxygen is delivered it will replenish stores absorbed from alveoli and maintain oxygenation even if no ventilation is occurring as long as upper airway patency is maintained. Using transnasal high-flow oxygenation at a rate of 70 L/min, Patel and Nouraei demonstrated average apnoeic times of 17 minutes without desaturation below 90% in 25 patients with difficult airways undergoing general anaesthesia [18]. High-flow oxygen is also thought to create a continuous positive airway pressure that helps splint open the upper airway. In morbidly obese patients, transnasal high-flow oxygenation is unlikely to extend the SAP as dramatically but should be considered as a strategy to extend the apnoeic time. Patel and Nouraei's series included patients with BMIs as high as 52 kg/m^2.

Airway management strategies

An evidence-based approach when planning anaesthetic induction must take into account those factors that were identified as independent predictors of both failed ventilation and difficult intubation. This suggests that obese OSA patients with thick necks and limited mandibular protrusion are in the highest risk group for potentially serious airway complications. Advancement of the mandible is a key manoeuvre for airway maintenance during mask ventilation as well as tracheal intubation with direct laryngoscopy. An awake intubation should therefore be considered when all elements of the triple airway manoeuvre, including mandible advancement, neck extension, and mouth opening, are disturbed in obese patients with severe OSA.

If there is uncertainty whether to proceed with an awake intubation versus anaesthetic induction, a flexible nasal endoscopy with the flexible fibreoptic bronchoscopy (FOB) may be performed by the anaesthesiologist to obtain more information about the patient's airway anatomy. This preoperative endoscopic airway examination can be quickly performed in the awake patient after topicalization of the nares and is generally well tolerated. Preoperative endoscopic airway examination provides critical information about the airway that may not be obvious from standard preoperative airway assessment. Specifically, it can be used to determine the optical path to the larynx, the presence of mass lesions or distortions that may prevent effective placement of a supraglottic airway (SGA), and airway lesions that may be traumatized by direct laryngoscopy or video laryngoscopy [19]. In a study by Rosenblatt et al., preoperative endoscopic airway examination findings resulted in a change in airway management plan in 26% of patients presenting for elective airway procedures and reduced the number of unnecessary awake intubations [19].

A robust airway strategy should include an alternative means of securing the endotracheal tube when direct laryngoscopy fails. An alternative to Macintosh and Miller laryngoscope blades is also necessary when asleep intubation is planned. Traditional teaching has focused on FOB, but the airways of morbidly obese patients may not be well suited to this particular technique. FOB can be difficult in morbidly obese patients because of the reduced pharyngeal space and redundant tissues, which may severely restrict the field of view. This is particularly true when the patient is anaesthetized and tone is lost in the pharyngeal dilator muscles. It is often necessary to use an adjunct technique such as a SGA to provide a conduit, which splints the tissues open and improves visualization [20]. Even in experienced hands, FOB can be time-consuming compared to other techniques and without a means of ventilation during intubation attempts, oxyhaemoglobin desaturation may occur. This often precludes the use of FOB as a rescue technique. In the awake setting, breathing may be restricted once the fibreoptics cord enters the glottis as the cross-sectional area of the available airway is diminished. As it is desirable in these patients to choose a tracheal tube of adequate internal diameter, there is a greater chance of tube impingement on glottic structures as the tube is railroaded into the trachea blindly.

The many video and optical laryngoscopes currently available may provide a better alternative to FOB in the morbidly obese patient. The 2013 ASA Practice Guidelines for Management of the Difficult Airway and the updated Difficult Airway Algorithm now suggest video-assisted laryngoscopy as an initial approach to a predicted difficult intubation [5]. Video laryngoscopes have been shown to significantly improve laryngeal view and intubating conditions in the morbidly obese and published reports suggest high success rates after direct laryngoscopy has failed [21–23]. The curved blades of video laryngoscopes allow for better visualization of the glottis without having to align the oral, pharyngeal, and tracheal axes which also makes them useful in patients with limited neck mobility [24]. A study of the Airtraq™ (Prodol Meditec S.A., Spain) showed that learning curves are steep and successful intubation is generally fast, even when compared to conventional laryngoscopy [22], although this may not be the case for Glidescope® (Verathon Inc., USA) intubation [24]. Video laryngoscopes can also be used for awake intubations because they facilitate glottic visualization with much less force than direct laryngoscopy. In such cases, the rigidity of the device allows rapid control of the tip and easy navigation through soft tissues. The moveable screen of the Pentax-AWS® (Pentax Corporation, Japan) is designed for awake intubation where the operator faces a patient in the sitting position [25]. As with all video laryngoscopes, the passage of the tube is under direct visual control.

SGAs have also been shown to be effective for ventilation prior to intubation and as rescue devices in the morbidly obese. In particular, second-generation or newer devices are preferred in the obese population because they are capable of providing higher leak pressures, better airway seal, and separation of the gastrointestinal tract and the airway to minimize aspiration risk. A study of the laryngeal mask airway Proseal™ (Teleflex Medical Europe Ltd., Ireland) for temporary ventilation in morbidly obese patients showed effective placement within 15 seconds in 90% of patients, a mean oropharyngeal leak pressure of 32 cmH₂O, and positive pressure ventilation with 8 mL/kg tidal volume was possible in more than 95% of patients [26]. Studies have also shown that the intubating laryngeal mask airway has a 96% success rate for blind tracheal intubation on the first attempt and can be safely used in morbidly obese patients for safe and effective ventilation prior to intubation [27,28]. Furthermore, fewer adjustment manoeuvres were required in morbidly obese patients when compared to lean patients, which may be explained by reduced pharyngeal space leading to more successful initial placement and better stabilization of the device [28].

As previously mentioned, SGAs can also be used as a conduit for FOB-guided intubation. Multiple case reports have documented the safety and effectiveness of FOB–airway exchange catheter (AEC)-assisted airway exchange through SGAs in patients with history of difficult direct laryngoscopy. In this method, a FOB is loaded with an AEC and then advanced though a properly positioned SGA into the trachea. The FOB is removed while the AEC is left in place. The SGA is then exchanged for an endotracheal tube over the AEC. A retrospective review of 128 patients undergoing this technique for difficult airway management demonstrated that 93% were successfully intubated without complications [29].

For the reasons listed, the authors' preference would always be to have a video laryngoscope and a SGA available for rescue rather than a FOB if direct laryngoscopy fails in a morbidly obese patient.

Extubation

Formulating a safe extubation strategy is increasingly recognized as a critical component and the final step of difficult airway management [30,31]. According to data from the Report of the Fourth National Audit Project of the Royal College of Anaesthetists and the Difficult Airway Society, one-third of serious airway complications occurred during or in the immediate post-extubation period and were noted to be associated with poor anticipation and planning [31,32]. Morbidly obese patients and patients with OSA in particular are at high risk for respiratory depression, upper airway collapse, and airway obstruction after receiving anaesthetics and opioids and therefore are at higher risk for respiratory complications upon extubation [31,33]. Before proceeding with extubation, it is important to ensure that the morbidly obese patient is fully awake and following commands and that the necessary equipment for reintubation is readily available. Care should be taken to reposition the patient in the 'ramped' position to both optimize pulmonary function and to facilitate reintubation if needed. If tracheal reintubation is anticipated to be difficult, extubation over an AEC should be strongly considered. AECs are generally well tolerated by patients and provide a guide

to facilitate reintubation. The AEC should be inserted to the same depth as the endotracheal tube and the use of a semirigid, hollow AEC is recommended in order to minimize risk of trauma and allow for oxygen insufflation if necessary [31]. Finally, all morbidly obese patients should be closely monitored after extubation for respiratory decompensation.

Conclusion

Airway management in morbidly obese patients can be challenging because of the increased likelihood of difficulty and rapid development of hypoxia. It is important to be able to identify the subset of morbidly obese patients who are at high risk for difficult mask ventilation and direct laryngoscopy in order to carefully formulate an appropriate airway management plan. Modifiable factors such as positioning, preoxygenation, and apnoeic oxygenation should be optimized in order to maximize apnoeic time and chances for successful tracheal intubation. Alternatives to direct laryngoscopy such as video laryngoscopy may be considered as a primary strategy and should also be available for back-up along with other techniques such as FOB and SGAs. Once the airway is successfully secured, care should be taken to formulate a safe extubation strategy.

REFERENCES

1. Tsai A, Schumann R. Morbid obesity and perioperative complications. Curr Opin Anesthesiol. 2016;**29**(1):103–108.
2. Peterson GN, Domino KB, Caplan RA, Posner KL, Lee LA, Cheney FW. Management of the difficult airway: a closed claims analysis. Anesthesiology. 2005;**103**(1):33–39.
3. Littleton SW. Impact of obesity on respiratory function. Respirology. 2012;**17**(1):43–49.
4. Wadhwa A, Singh PM, Sinha AC. Airway management in patients with morbid obesity. Int Anesthesiol Clin. 2013;**51**(3):26–40.
5. Apfelbaum JL, Hagberg CA, Caplan RA, Blitt CD, Connis RT, Nickinovich DG, et al. Practice guidelines for management of the difficult airway: an updated report by the American Society of Anesthesiologists Task Force on Management of the Difficult Airway. Anesthesiology. 2013;**118**(2):251–70.
6. Kheterpal S, Han R, Tremper KK, Shanks A, Tait AR, O'Reilly M, et al. Incidence and predictors of difficult and impossible mask ventilation. Anesthesiology. 2006;**105**(5):885–91.
7. Kheterpal S, Martin L, Shanks AM, Tremper KK. Prediction and outcomes of impossible mask ventilation: a review of 50,000 anesthetics. Anesthesiology. 2009;**110**(4):891–97.
8. Hagberg CA, Vogt-Harenkamp C, Kamal J. A retrospective analysis of airway management in obese patients at a teaching institution. J Clin Anesth. 2009;**21**(5):348–51.
9. Horner R, Mohiaddin R, Lowell D, Shea S, Burman E, Longmore D, et al. Sites and sizes of fat deposits around the pharynx in obese patients with obstructive sleep apnoea and weight matched controls. Eur Respir J. 1989;**2**(7):613–22.
10. Tagaito Y, Isono S, Remmers JE, Tanaka A, Nishino T. Lung volume and collapsibility of the passive pharynx in patients with sleep-disordered breathing. J Appl Physiol. 2007;**103**(4):1379–85.
11. Gonzalez H, Minville V, Delanoue K, Mazerolles M, Concina D, Fourcade O. The importance of increased neck circumference

to intubation difficulties in obese patients. Anesthes Analg. 2008;**106**(4):1132–36.

12. Ezri T, Gewürtz G, Sessler D, Medalion B, Szmuk P, Hagberg C, et al. Prediction of difficult laryngoscopy in obese patients by ultrasound quantification of anterior neck soft tissue. Anaesthesia. 2003;**58**(11):1111–14.

13. Brodsky JB, Lemmens HJ, Brock-Utne JG, Vierra M, Saidman LJ. Morbid obesity and tracheal intubation. Anesthes Analg. 2002;**94**(3):732–36.

14. Jense HG, Dubin SA, Silverstein PI, O'Leary-Escolas U. Effect of obesity on safe duration of apnea in anesthetized humans. Anesthes Analg. 1991;**72**(1):89–93.

15. Gambee AM, Hertzka RE, Fisher DM. Preoxygenation techniques: comparison of three minutes and four breaths. Anesthes Analg. 1987;**66**(5):468–70.

16. Dixon BJ, Dixon JB, Carden JR, Burn AJ, Schachter LM, Playfair JM, et al. Preoxygenation is more effective in the 25° head-up position than in the supine position in severely obese patients: a randomized controlled study. Anesthesiology. 2005;**102**(6):1110–15.

17. Collins JS, Lemmens HJ, Brodsky JB, Brock-Utne JG, Levitan RM. Laryngoscopy and morbid obesity: a comparison of the "sniff" and "ramped" positions. Obes Surg. 2004;**14**(9):1171–75.

18. Patel A, Nouraei S. Transnasal Humidified Rapid-Insufflation Ventilatory Exchange (THRIVE): a physiological method of increasing apnoea time in patients with difficult airways. Anaesthesia. 2015;**70**(3):323–29.

19. Rosenblatt W, Ianus AI, Sukhupragarn W, Fickenscher A, Sasaki C. Preoperative endoscopic airway examination (PEAE) provides superior airway information and may reduce the use of unnecessary awake intubation. Anesthes Analg. 2011;**112**(3):602–607.

20. Doyle DJ, Zura A, Ramachandran M, Lin J, Cywinski JB, Parker B, et al. Airway management in a 980-lb patient: use of the Aintree intubation catheter. J Clin Anesth. 2007;**19**(5):367–69.

21. Dhonneur G, Ndoko S, Amathieu R, el Housseini L, Poncelet C, Tual L. Tracheal intubation using the Airtraq® in morbid obese patients undergoing emergency cesarean delivery. J Am Soc Anesthesiol. 2007;**106**(3):629–30.

22. Ndoko S, Amathieu R, Tual L, Polliand C, Kamoun W, El Housseini L, et al. Tracheal intubation of morbidly obese patients: a randomized trial comparing performance of Macintosh and Airtraq™ laryngoscopes. Br J Anaesth. 2008;**100**(2):263–68.

23. Marrel J, Blanc C, Frascarolo P, Magnusson L. Videolaryngoscopy improves intubation condition in morbidly obese patients. Eur J Anaesthesiol. 2007;**24**(12):1045–49.

24. Sun D, Warriner C, Parsons DG, Klein R, Umedaly H, Moult M. The GlideScope® video laryngoscope: randomized clinical trial in 200 patients. Br J Anaesth. 2004;**94**(3):381–84.

25. Suzuki A, Terao M, Aizawa K, Sasakawa T, Henderson JJ, Iwasaki H. Pentax-AWS airway Scope as an alternative for awake flexible fiberoptic intubation of a morbidly obese patient in the semi-sitting position. J Anesth. 2009;**23**(1):162–63.

26. Keller C, Brimacombe J, Kleinsasser A, Brimacombe L. The laryngeal mask airway ProSeal™ as a temporary ventilatory device in grossly and morbidly obese patients before laryngoscope-guided tracheal intubation. Anesth Analg. 2002;**94**(3):737–40.

27. Frappier J, Guenoun T, Journois D, Philippe H, Aka E, Cadi P, et al. Airway management using the intubating laryngeal mask airway for the morbidly obese patient. Anesth Analg. 2003;**96**(5):1510–15.

28. Combes X, Sauvat S, Leroux B, Dumerat M, Sherrer E, Motamed C, et al. Intubating laryngeal mask airway in morbidly obese and lean patients: a comparative study. Anesthesiology. 2005;**102**(6):1106–109.

29. Berkow LC, Schwartz JM, Kan K, Corridore M, Heitmiller ES. Use of the laryngeal mask airway-Aintree intubating catheter-fiberoptic bronchoscope technique for difficult intubation. J Clin Anesth. 2011;**23**(7):534–39.

30. Langeron O, Amour J, Vivien B, Aubrun F. Clinical review: management of difficult airways. Crit Care. 2006;**10**(6):243.

31. Cavallone LF, Vannucci A. Extubation of the difficult airway and extubation failure. Anesth Analg. 2013;**116**(2):368–83.

32. Cook T, Woodall N, Frerk C, Project FNA. Major complications of airway management in the UK: results of the Fourth National Audit Project of the Royal College of Anaesthetists and the Difficult Airway Society. Part 1: anaesthesia. Br J Anaesth. 2011;**106**(5):617–31.

33. Benumof J. Obesity, sleep apnea, the airway and anesthesia. Curr Opin Anaesthesiol. **2004**(17):21–30.

Healthy obese

A paradox?

Anupama Wadhwa and Detlef Obal

Introduction

At least 30% of the surgical population consists of 'obese' patients, mirroring the obesity epidemic in the general population in the United States [1–3]. Nearly 74% of participants in the American College of Surgery's National Surgical Quality Improvement Program had an abnormally high body mass index (BMI) [4], including 17% of patients under the age of 18 years [5]. This development is particularly concerning as obesity is associated with increased risk of metabolic syndrome, hypertension, coronary artery disease, and diabetes mellitus. However, physicians, nutritionists, and the general public struggle with definitions of obesity based only on total body weight proportionate to height and, therefore, BMI. This leads to the question of whether BMI is adequate to describe the physical condition and potential risk of our patients.

Body mass index: an outdated measurement?

According to the World Health Organization, obesity is a 'condition in which percentage body fat is increased to an extent in which health and well-being are impaired'. Based on BMI (i.e. body weight in kilograms divided by the square of the height in metres (kg/m^2)), patients are considered to be obese if the total body weight reaches 20% above ideal body weight. However, the usefulness of BMI, or Quetelet index, first described by Belgian Statistician Adolphe Quetelet, has been questioned in recent years as this almost 200-year-old classification is based solely on an arithmetic approximation. It ignores the complex interaction of genetic life style, dietary habits, energy exposure, nutritional and metabolic factors, as well as adipocyte metabolism resulting in different body compositions (e.g. body frame and muscularity, fluid retention, sarcopenia in ageing or disease, spinal deformities) and relative quantities of body fat and muscle. Percentage and type of distribution of adipose tissue and the duration of obesity may play a major role in determining metabolic abnormalities, leading to a higher cardiovascular risk and higher mortality in some subsets of patients [6,7]. Waist circumference has been used to predict the extent of visceral fat which is associated with

increased insulin resistance (consequently, type 2 diabetes mellitus), hepatic steatosis, hypertension, hyperlipidaemia, and an increased risk of thrombosis and inflammation, leading to higher mortality rates [8]. However, none of these reflect the metabolic and inflammatory profile of patients. Therefore, a new definition of obesity was introduced emphasizing the term adiposopathy and acknowledging individuals' body fat composition and functionality [9]. According to the definition of this term, four different types of phenotypes are distinguished: normal-weight obese (NWO), metabolically obese with normal weight (MONW), metabolically healthy obese (MHO), and metabolically unhealthy obese (MUO) or 'at-risk' obese patients suffering from complications directly related to obesity.

Characterization of metabolically healthy obese patients

MHO patients were first described in the 1980s as a subgroup of obese patients without the presence of hypertension, hyperlipidaemia, or type 2 diabetes mellitus characterized by insulin resistance [10,11]. The incidence of MHO is estimated to be between 25% and 40% [6,8]. A preserved insulin sensitivity is the hallmark of these patients [8]. Insulin resistance can be calculated by the homeostatic model assessment of insulin resistance (HOMA-IR). It is the product of fasting glucose and fasting insulin levels. A HOMA-IR value less than 3.16 is categorized as MHO and a value of 3.16 or greater is classified as MUO [12]. On the basis of healthy white adipose tissue expansion, MHO individuals are relatively immune to the pathological consequences associated with obesity and associated lipotoxic side effects [13,14]. They have lower C-reactive protein and high adiponectin levels [15–17]. Furthermore, these patients are characterized by a higher level of fitness, defined as maximal exercise capacity on a treadmill [18]. Ortega and colleagues [18] extracted data out of the Aerobics Center Longitudinal Study (ACLS) including 43,265, mainly male, white adults with a BMI of at least 18.5 kg/m^2. After adjustment for BMI, body fat percentage, and fitness level, MHO individuals had a 38% lower risk of all-cause mortality than their MUO counterparts did. Interestingly, there was no difference between MHO and metabolically healthy normal weight participants. Furthermore, fat distribution in the trunk, chest, abdomen, and subcutaneous regions in the upper body (android phenotype) had stronger association with diabetes, coronary artery disease, gout, and uric acid renal stones [19] while reduced peri-hepatic and visceral fat accumulation occurred more frequent in MHO participants. Other characteristics of MHO are the absence of hypertension; a reduced intima-to-media thickness ratio of the carotid artery; and a favourable lipid, inflammation, hormonal, and liver enzyme profile [18,20]. After adjusting for fitness and several confounders, MHO participants had a lower risk (30–50%, estimated by hazard ratios (HRs)) of all-cause mortality, non-fatal and fatal cardiovascular disease, and cancer mortality than their MUO peers [21].

The incidence of MHO is estimated between 6% and 19% in children and adolescents [12], and 10% of the population in the United States has a normal BMI but increased body fat content [22,23].

Recently, the idea that MHO patients might have a better survival following catastrophic illness has been in favour. However, the concept of MHO patients having a similar cardiovascular risk profile as normal-weight patients and having a survival benefit, over the underweight ('obesity paradox') has been questioned by several investigators. In a recent population-based prospective cohort study, including a total of 6299 men and women without evidence of cardiovascular disease at baseline, MHO individuals were not at an increased risk of acute myocardial infarction compared with normal-weight individuals, but at an increased risk of developing heart failure [24]. Prado and colleagues have criticized the concept of the obesity paradox, because less than 10% of studies looking at the obesity paradox actually used a direct measure of body composition. They suggested that loss of lean tissue or muscle mass actually removes the protective advantage of high BMI and having low muscle mass is associated with poor prognosis [25,26]. Banack et al. identified four major flaws in studies postulating an 'obesity paradox': (1) incorrect reference values were used (i.e. a lower overall BMI reference range); (2) a stratification bias, a type of selection bias, can often be observed by which variables affected by exposure share common causes with the proposed outcome; (3) the majority of data originated from observational and cross-sectional study designs and randomized, prospective controlled trials are missing in the literature; and (4) as stated in our introduction, BMI rather than body fat composition and lean mass tissue is used in most studies suggesting the existence of an obesity paradox [27].

According to current data, the obesity paradox seems to be an 'underlying disease'-specific phenomenon, in which patients having disease conditions dominated by a 'catabolic' metabolic state seem to have a survival advantage if they belong to the 'slightly' obese cohort. For example, Lee and colleagues found that obese Chinese nursing home residents (BMI >25kg/m², using Asia Pacific cut-off) had the lowest mortality compared with normal-weight residents [28]. Nursing home residents who were underweight had a significantly higher mortality (HR 1.53, 95% confidence interval 1.33–1.76) [28]. Similar findings are observed in elderly patients [29], either admitted for exacerbation of chronic obstructive pulmonary disease [30] or suffering from dementia [31], patients with pulmonary artery hypertension [32], patients with exacerbation of coronary artery disease or congestive heart failure [33–36], or patients requiring intensive care in the perioperative setting [37].

In contrast, patients with non-catabolic medical conditions do not benefit from obesity or an additional energy support. For example, Galesanu studied the impact of obesity on survival in patients attending a rehabilitation programme for chronic obstructive pulmonary disease [38]. After controlling for their lung function, a previous observed benefit from obesity disappeared. Similar results were found by Zafrir when investigating the significance of BMI in patients with heart failure on their first visit to the heart failure clinic, that is, at an early stage of the disease. The authors did not find an advantage in obese patients after they adjusted for patients' age [39]. Even in patients suffering from organ ischaemia for the first time (e.g. myocardial infarction or stroke), obesity does not improve patient outcomes or prognosis and the 'obesity paradox' was not observed in several studies [40–44].

These overall findings reflect a broad mixture of studies investigating survival and mortality benefits in different types of medical specialties. Surgical procedures pose a significant stress to patients and their metabolic profile during elective surgery and particularly during urgent/emergent procedures. Therefore, it is of particular interest to discuss whether the 'obesity paradox' exists under these conditions and whether being obese provides a survival benefit for patients undergoing surgical procedures.

The obesity paradox—fat as a survival factor after general surgery?

It is an interesting and appealing concept that obesity might provide potential additional energy reserves during acute catabolic illness which might result in decreased mortality of surgical patients [45]. Jorgen and colleagues observed in a small study that the basal rate of lipolysis was doubled and there was a 50% increase in the lipolytic effects of catecholamines. The effect of surgical trauma on the regulation of lipolysis was studied in isolated fat cells obtained before and 24 hours after elective cholecystectomy in 12 patients who were not obese and otherwise healthy. The actions of various agents that selectively stimulate lipolysis at different early or late steps in the cyclic adenosine monophosphate system beyond the adrenoceptors were also increased about 50% after surgery (P <0.01). These changes occurred without altering β-adrenergic receptor density, suggesting that patients with additional fat reserve might be more able to mobilize additional energy than can normal-weight individuals in the absence of obesity-induced side effects, which may in turn result in a beneficial outcome after surgery [46].

Surgical stress leads to increased circulating catecholamine levels resulting in increased lipolysis in fat cells in order to meet rising energy demands [47]. However, catecholamines activate both β and α2-receptors meaning that the net effect of stress is dependent on the balance between both receptor systems. Under normal conditions, β-receptor-mediated lipolysis predominates [46]. Interestingly, in patients undergoing cholecystectomy, the properties of the β-adrenoceptors were not altered as determined by radioligand binding and isoprenaline sensitivity. In comparison to untreated control participants, the antilipolytic properties of catecholamines were also not changed when given the same type of postoperative nutrition as surgical patients [46]. Therefore, it seems that the recognized increased lipolytic activity of adipocytes might be caused by modification at more distal steps in the cyclic adenosine monophosphate system after moderate surgical trauma (e.g. cholecystectomy), which may involve the protein kinase/hormone sensitive lipase complex.

Another question arising is whether the location of the adipose tissue plays a role in this issue. Patel and Abate suggested that location of adipose tissue (subcutaneous versus visceral) may be a major contributor to free fatty acid flux. An increased level of circulating free fatty acids blocks the glucose uptake to the skeletal muscle resulting in insulin resistance [48,49]. Furthermore, for each mole of ATP produced, free fatty acid oxidation consumes more oxygen than needed by carbohydrates, leading to a disturbed energy balance. By contrast, accumulation of fat in the subcutaneous depot is an independent predictor of lower cardiovascular and diabetes-related mortality and protects against impaired glucose metabolism [50,51]. Interestingly, removal of visceral fat depots (e.g. omentum) resulted in improvements in oral glucose tolerance, insulin sensitivity, and fasting plasma glucose with insulin levels doubling or tripling [52]. Similar data were observed by McLaughlin and colleagues [53] who found that increased visceral adipose tissue results in insulin resistance while increased subcutaneous fat tissue seems to protect against insulin resistance. Wang and colleagues [54] proposed that the differences between visceral and subcutaneous fat tissue in terms of lipotoxicity and insulin resistance are based on a disturbed expansion and storage of lipids within the adipocytes. Expansion can occur either by an increase in volume of pre-existing adipocytes (hypertrophy) or by hyperplasia through recruitment of new preadipocytes. Data in rodents suggest that visceral fat expands predominantly by adipocyte hypertrophy while subcutaneous depots undergo adipocyte hyperplasia. The difference is important as hyperplasia leads to small adipocytes, which are more insulin sensitive and provide enhanced lipid storage capacity [54]. Interestingly, preliminary data suggest that the distribution might be determined by the expression of oestrogens, which direct fat increase towards subcutaneous hyperplasia by increasing adipocyte progenitor cells [55]. The vascular supply of subcutaneous adipose tissue consists of a higher capillary density and angiogenesis compared with visceral fat depots [56], which prevents tissue hypoxia during expansion and, subsequently, alters hypoxia-inducible factor activation of adipokine expression, proinflammatory macrophage recruitment, and insulin resistance.

Oestrogens not only influence the distribution and mass of adipose tissue, but also influence the metabolic activity of adipose tissue by selective neural modulation leading to 'browning,' that is, higher light reflection caused by an increased number of mitochondria [55]. Brown adipose tissue is metabolically more active due to an increased number of mitochondria. These observations are important as women accumulate energy reserves in the subcutaneous areas to prepare for adipose tissue mobilization required for lactation. Thus, one could speculate that these mechanisms provide additional energy for patients undergoing surgical procedures and increased perioperative stress. It might be advisable, therefore, to measure the activity of subcutaneous fat reservoirs in future studies to predict patients' individual ability to cope with surgical stress. Our classical view on adipocytes has been extended towards its important role in lipid and glucose metabolism, in which it releases bioactive proteins (e.g. adipokines and myokines) [57] and modulates cardiovascular risk factors related to obesity [58]. At this point, however, it is unclear to what extent different adipose tissue components (i.e.

brown or white adipose tissue, subcutaneous and visceral fat depots) contribute to an improved outcome after surgical procedures. Early studies investigating the effect of overfeeding in the perioperative period by total parenteral nutrition suggest that both lipogenesis as well as lipolysis occur simultaneously [47]; however, experimental evidence from the same author suggests that surgically stressed individuals provided with additional energy activate a futile cycle of lipogenesis and lipolysis involving primarily brown adipose tissue instead of visceral, white adipose tissue [59].

Current studies and concepts (e.g. enhanced recovery after surgery) try to determine whether preoperative high-carbohydrate-based caloric intake in combination with adequate perioperative pain management results in improved postoperative outcome. Therefore, an 'endogenous' energy 'backpack' carried by MHO individuals might be necessary for recovery during perioperative stress/catabolism.

Obesity paradox in surgical populations

Is insulin sensitivity changed by anaesthetics?

Previous animal studies suggest that volatile anaesthetics might inhibit basal and glucose-stimulated insulin secretion, increasing perioperative insulin resistance [60]. These changes are dose dependent and rapidly reversible, but it remains questionable whether these changes will affect patient outcomes after surgery. Yasuda and colleagues studied propofol-anaesthetized rats in which insulin sensitivity, insulin-stimulated glucose uptake, and hepatic glucose output were determined by a hyperinsulinaemic euglycaemic clamp [61]. Compared with awake rats, propofol decreased insulin-stimulated glucose uptake in skeletal muscle and the heart, but not in liver or adipose tissue, suggesting that fat tissue might not be affected by propofol during general anaesthesia. Interestingly, glucose output from the liver was significantly increased in the anaesthetized animals suggesting that anaesthesia with propofol induces systemic insulin resistance.

Surgical outcomes in metabolically healthy obese patients

Criteria for bariatric surgery are based on weight, BMI, and presence of metabolic syndrome. There are no specific criteria to perform bariatric surgery in metabolically healthy patients. As their fat mass is increased and they develop a high body fat percentage, many patients are counselled to have bariatric surgery. There are emerging data on the prognosis and outcomes of patients after bariatric and non-bariatric surgery and how they differ in patients with different metabolic profiles. MHO patients have lower neck circumference, lower fasting blood glucose, lower insulin and triglycerides levels, and higher high-density lipoprotein levels [62]. A retrospective analysis of the metabolically healthy group among 710 patients revealed about 150 patients with no hypertension and diabetes. However, almost 89% of these patients had developed hepatic steatosis, 20% had liver fibrosis, and 7% had non-alcoholic steatohepatitis. This challenges the notion of MHO as being truly metabolically healthy. Bariatric surgery is now considered as one of the best options to achieve significant weight loss and significant metabolic alterations leading to cure type 2 diabetes mellitus and other comorbidities [3,4]. Bariatric surgery is recommended for adults with a BMI of 40 kg/m² or more and in those with a BMI of 35 kg/m² with comorbidities [18]. It is considered the most effective treatment for morbid obesity and its associated metabolic abnormalities and sleep-disordered breathing. Bariatric surgery also improves the histological and biochemical parameters of non-alcoholic fatty liver disease such as insulin resistance, altered glucose metabolism, hypertension, plasma free fatty acids, transaminases, and steatohepatitis and fibrosis of the liver [63]. Bariatric surgery effectively reduces neck and waist circumference, increases maximum ventilator pressures, enhances sleep architecture, and reduces obstructive sleep apnoea in patients with severe obesity [64].

Pelascini et al. retrospectively studied patients with gastric bypass outcomes in MHO versus MUMO patients, looking at whether obesity phenotype influences the results of bariatric surgery. Their goal was to determine if surgical management could be based on stratification of obese individuals according to their metabolic health phenotype [65]. MHMO patients were generally female patients with a history of previous bariatric surgery. The most common metabolic disorder in the MHMO group was low-grade inflammation. The authors found a favourable effect on glycaemia and an improvement of HOMA-IR in MHMO patients compared with the MUMO patients. Weight loss with the Roux-en-Y procedure had beneficial effects on the metabolic alterations encompassed by the metabolic syndrome, but the effects were more prominent in the MHO group even 24 months after surgery. The authors argue that these two phenotypes are just different stages of disease evolution.

Ethnic differences have been noted between white populations of European ancestry and Asians, indicating that the latter have higher metabolic risk at the same BMI, with higher body fat and central fat, higher fasting blood sugar, and lower high-density lipoprotein levels [66–68].

There is an increase in obesity-related disorders that require non-bariatric surgery [69,70]. While increased body mass is associated with an increased cardiac risk, it would be expected to carry a higher rate of perioperative complications. Some studies have demonstrated an increase in hospital length of stay, postoperative surgical site infections, and reoperations. [4]. Despite this, a paradoxical phenomenon of a survival benefit has been observed in the surgical obese population, both for cardiac [34,49,71–74] and non-cardiac surgery [42,75–81] and in different ethnic populations [82,83]. Thus, although higher fat mass exhibited survival benefits, this advantage disappeared after adjustment for lean body mass, suggesting that non-fat tissue bears the primary role in conferring greater survival [84].

Obesity paradox in cardiac and renal disease

In the adult heart, the major pathway for ATP production is fatty acid oxidation while the relative contribution of glucose increases during stress or injury, such as exercise or ischaemia [85,86]. Indeed, under pathological conditions, the heart exhibits a severe malfunction of different metabolic pathways, such as the tricarboxylic acid cycle and beta-oxidation [87,88]. Benedetto et al. performed a retrospective analysis in patients undergoing coronary artery bypass graft (CABG) surgery and found that long-term survival in obese and severely obese patients was worse than in normal-weight patients, suggesting that an obesity paradox does not exist in patients suffering from coronary artery disease with poor cardiovascular health [73].

These data are in clear contrast to Davenport's observation that patients undergoing vascular surgery have a lower 30-day mortality rate if their BMI ranges between 25 and 30 kg/m², even compared to normal-weight control patients [89]. In addition, Takagi's data suggests that overweight but not obesity is associated with a 10% reduction in mid-to-long term mortality after CABG surgery [90].

Why do we have these types of differences between several studies? Recent observations from Lopez-Delgado et al. suggested that overweight patients have a better 1-year survival than normal patients. In a prospective study, 2499 patients were divided into four groups based on BMI. Although patients with a higher BMI presented with worse oxygenation and a higher risk of perioperative myocardial infarction, the authors could not find any difference of in-hospital mortality between the BMI groups and therefore questioned whether obesity protects patients undergoing cardiac surgery [91]. Similar results were presented by Ho and colleagues who did not find any survival benefit in patients with higher BMIs [92]. However, the Australian group of Ho described a strong correlation between BMI and new-onset atrial fibrillation with BMI being the second most important predictor after age [93]. In contrast, Johnson and colleagues found that in 78,762 patients undergoing first-time CABG or combined CABG/aortic valve replacement surgery, overweight and obese patients had a lower mortality and adverse perioperative outcome compared to normal-weight, underweight, and morbidly obese patients [74]. In an attempt to explain their findings, the authors suggested that malnourished or cachectic patients were older with a higher prevalence of comorbidities [18,93,94] and that patients with a higher BMI seemed to be treated sooner [95,96].

Conclusion

Current data are inconclusive regarding the benefit of mild obesity on perioperative outcome. Several studies suggest that there might be an obesity paradox in which mildly obese patients will have a better outcome after surgery than patients with normal or 'reduced' BMIs. However, these positive results achieved in studies performed in patient populations suffering from catabolism, might not sustain the normal patient population with a regular metabolic profile. In fact, current concepts of enhanced recovery after surgery providing high-caloric intake preoperatively raise the question of whether an 'endogenous' energy pack might be necessary to provide a beneficial outcome bias. Anaesthesia providers do not have a good way to measure the metabolic profile with point-of-care detection devices and, therefore, it might be more harmful than beneficial to suggest that obesity provides any advantage in perioperative medicine as it is known to cause definite harm by increasing complication rates caused by increased comorbidities seen in obese patients. Although the obesity paradox appears to be an attractive concept, its translation into modern perioperative medicine remains questionable.

REFERENCES

1. Myles PS, et al. The safety of addition of nitrous oxide to general anaesthesia in at-risk patients having major non-cardiac surgery (ENIGMA-II): a randomised, single-blind trial. Lancet. 2014;**384**(9952):1446–54.

2. Devereaux PJ, et al. Clonidine in patients undergoing noncardiac surgery. N Engl J Med. 2014;**370**(16):1504–13.

3. Devereaux PJ, et al. Aspirin in patients undergoing noncardiac surgery. N Engl J Med. 2014;**370**(16):1494–503.

4. Sood A, et al. The effect of body mass index on perioperative outcomes after major surgery: Results from the National Surgical Quality Improvement Program (ACS-NSQIP) 2005-2011. World J Surg. 2015;**39**(10): 2376–85.

5. Ogden CL, et al. Prevalence of obesity in the United States, 2009-2010. NCHS Data Brief. 2012;**82**:1–8.

6. Wallenius V, et al. Interleukin-6-deficient mice develop mature-onset obesity. Nat Med. 2002;**8**(1):75–79.

7. Janssen I, Katzmarzyk PT, Ross R. Waist circumference and not body mass index explains obesity-related health risk. Am J Clin Nutr. 2004;**79**(3):379–84.

8. Ni Y, et al. Circulating unsaturated fatty acids delineate the metabolic status of obese individuals. EBioMedicine. 2015;**2**(10):1513–22.

9. De Lorenzo A, et al. New obesity classification criteria as a tool for bariatric surgery indication. World J Gastroenterol. 2016;**22**(2):681–703.

10. Ruderman NB, Schneider SH, Berchtold P. The 'metabolically-obese,' normal-weight individual. Am J Clin Nutr. 1981;**34**(8):1617–21.

11. Ruderman NB, et al. The metabolically obese, normal-weight individual revisited. Diabetes. 1998;**47**(5):699–713.

12. Bervoets L. Massa G. Classification and clinical characterization of metabolically 'healthy' obese children and adolescents. J Pediatr Endocrinol Metab. 2016;**29**(5):553–60.

13. Unger RH, Scherer PE. Gluttony, sloth and the metabolic syndrome: a roadmap to lipotoxicity. Trends Endocrinol Metab. 2010;**21**(6):345–52.

14. Rayner JJ, Neubauer S, Rider OJ. The paradox of obesity cardiomyopathy and the potential for weight loss as a therapy. Obes Rev. 2015;**16**(8):679–90.

15. Karelis AD, et al. Clinical markers for the identification of metabolically healthy but obese individuals. Diabetes Obes Metab. 2004;**6**(6):456–57.

16. Stefan N, et al. Identification and characterization of metabolically benign obesity in humans. Arch Intern Med. 2008;**168**(15):1609–16.

17. Stefan N, et al. Metabolically healthy obesity: epidemiology, mechanisms, and clinical implications. Lancet Diabetes Endocrinol. 2013;**1**(2):152–62.

18. Ortega FB, et al. The intriguing metabolically healthy but obese phenotype: cardiovascular prognosis and role of fitness. Eur Heart J. 2013;**34**(5):389–97.

19. Garg A. Regional adiposity and insulin resistance. J Clin Endocrinol Metab. 2004;**89**(9): 4206–10.

20. Bluher M. Are metabolically healthy obese individuals really healthy? Eur J Endocrinol. 2014;**171**(6):209–19.

21. Guo F. Garvey WT. Cardiometabolic disease risk in metabolically healthy and unhealthy obesity: Stability of metabolic health status in adults. Obesity. 2016;**24**(2):516–25.

22. Romero-Corral A, et al. Normal weight obesity: a risk factor for cardiometabolic dysregulation and cardiovascular mortality. Eur Heart J. 2010;**31**(6):737–46.

23. Main ML, Rao SC, O'Keefe JH. Trends in obesity and extreme obesity among US adults. JAMA. 2010;**303**(17):1695–96.

24. Morkedal B, et al. Risk of myocardial infarction and heart failure among metabolically healthy but obese individuals: HUNT (Nord-Trondelag Health Study) Norway. J Am Coll Cardiol. 2014;**63**(11):1071–78.

25. Prado CM, Gonzalez MC, Heymsfield SB. Body composition phenotypes and obesity paradox. Curr Opin Clin Nutr Metab Care. 2015;**18**(6):535–51.

26. Despres JP. Obesity and cardiovascular disease: weight loss is not the only target. Can J Cardiol. 2015;**31**(2):216–22.

27. Banack HR, Kaufman JS. Does selection bias explain the obesity paradox among individuals with cardiovascular disease? Ann Epidemiol. 2015;**25**(5):342–49.

28. Lee JS, et al. Obesity can benefit survival-a 9-year prospective study in 1614 Chinese nursing home residents. J Am Med Dir Assoc. 2014;**15**(5):342–48.

29. Perna S, et al. Association between muscle mass and adipo-metabolic profile: a cross-sectional study in older subjects. Clin Interv Aging. 2015;**10**:499–504.

30. Yamauchi Y, et al. Paradoxical association between body mass index and in-hospital mortality in elderly patients with chronic obstructive pulmonary disease in Japan. Int J Chron Obstruct Pulmon Dis. 2014;**9**:1337–46.

31. Garcia-Ptacek S, et al. Body-mass index and mortality in incident dementia: a cohort study on 11,398 patients from SveDem, the Swedish Dementia Registry. J Am Med Dir Assoc. 2014;**15**(6):447.

32. Hu EC, et al. Survival advantages of excess body mass index in patients with idiopathic pulmonary arterial hypertension. Acta Cardiol. 2014;**69**(6):673–78.

33. Khalid U, et al. Pre-morbid body mass index and mortality after incident heart failure: the ARIC Study. J Am Coll Cardiol. 2014;**64**(25):2743–49.

34. Konigstein M, et al. The obesity paradox in patients undergoing transcatheter aortic valve implantation. Clin Cardiol. 2015;**38**(2):76–81.

35. Littnerova S, et al. Positive influence of being overweight/obese on long term survival in patients hospitalised due to acute heart failure. **PLoS One.** 2015;**10**(2): e0117142.

36. Wang J, et al. Obesity paradox in patients with atrial fibrillation and heart failure. Int J Cardiol. 2014;**176**(3):1356–58.

37. Utzolino S, et al. The obesity paradox in surgical intensive care patients with peritonitis. J Crit Care. 2014;**29**(5):887.

38. Galesanu RG, et al. Obesity in chronic obstructive pulmonary disease: is fatter really better? Can Respir J. 2014;**21**(5):297–301.

39. Zafrir B, et al. Comparison of body mass index and body surface area as outcome predictors in patients with systolic heart failure. Cardiol J. 2015;**22**(4):375–81.

40. Witassek F, et al. Impact of body mass index on mortality in Swiss hospital patients with ST-elevation myocardial infarction: does an obesity paradox exist? Swiss Med Wkly. 2014;**144**:w13986.

41. Wohlfahrt P, et al. The obesity paradox and survivors of ischemic stroke. J Stroke Cerebrovasc Dis. 2015;**24**(6):1443–50.

42. Tawk RG, et al. Influence of body mass index and age on functional outcomes in patients with subarachnoid hemorrhage. Neurosurgery. 2015;**76**(2):136–41.

43. Kim Y, et al. Obesity-stroke paradox and initial neurological severity. J Neurol Neurosurg Psychiatry. 2015;**86**(7):743–47.

44. Dehlendorff C, Andersen KK, Olsen TS. Body mass index and death by stroke: no obesity paradox. JAMA Neurol. 2014;**71**(8):978–84.

45. Clark DO, et al. Obesity and 10-year mortality in very old African Americans and Yoruba-Nigerians: exploring the obesity paradox. J Gerontol A Biol Sci Med Sci. 2014;**69**(9):1162–69.

46. Jorgen N, et al. Catecholamine regulation of adipocyte lipolysis after surgery. Surgery. 1991;**109**(4):488–96.

47. Nordenström J, et al. Free fatty acid mobilization and oxidation during total parenteral nutrition in trauma and infection. Ann Surg. 1983;**198**(6):725–35.

48. McNulty PH, et al. Cardiovascular implications of insulin resistance and non-insulin-dependent diabetes mellitus. J Cardiothorac Vasc Anesth. 2001;**15**(6):768–77.

49. Patel P, Abate N. Body fat distribution and insulin resistance. Nutrients. 2013;**5**(6):2019–27.

50. Van Pelt RE, et al. Contributions of total and regional fat mass to risk for cardiovascular disease in older women. Am J Physiol Endocrinol Metab. 2002;**282**(5):1023–28.

51. Tanko LB, et al. Central and peripheral fat mass have contrasting effect on the progression of aortic calcification in postmenopausal women. Eur Heart J. 2003;**24**(16):1531–37.

52. Thorne A, et al. A pilot study of long-term effects of a novel obesity treatment: omentectomy in connection with adjustable gastric banding. Int J Obes Relat Metab Disord. 2002;**26**(2):193–99.

53. McLaughlin T, et al. Preferential fat deposition in subcutaneous versus visceral depots is associated with insulin sensitivity. J Clin Endocrinol Metab. 2011;**96**(11):1756–60.

54. Wang QA, et al. Tracking adipogenesis during white adipose tissue development, expansion and regeneration. Nat Med. 2013;**19**(10):1338–44.

55. Palmer BF, Clegg DJ. The sexual dimorphism of obesity. Mol Cell Endocrinol. 2015;**402**:113–19.

56. Gealekman O, et al. Depot-specific differences and insufficient subcutaneous adipose tissue angiogenesis in human obesity. Circulation. 2011;**123**(2):186–94.

57. Hajer GR, van Haeften TW, Visseren FL. Adipose tissue dysfunction in obesity, diabetes, and vascular diseases. Eur Heart J. 2008;**29**(24):2959–71.

58. Shah A, Mehta N, Reilly MP. Adipose inflammation, insulin resistance, and cardiovascular disease. J Parenter Enteral Nutr. 2008;**32**(6):638–44.

59. Felländer G, et al. Lipolysis during abdominal surgery. J Clin Endocrinol Metab. 1994;**78**(1):150–55.

60. Saho S, et al. The effects of sevoflurane anesthesia on insulin secretion and glucose metabolism in pigs. Anesth Analg. 1997;**84**(6):1359–65.

61. Yasuda Y, et al. Anesthesia with propofol induces insulin resistance systemically in skeletal and cardiac muscles and liver of rats. Biochem Biophys Res Commun. 2013;**431**(1):81–85.

62. Bachmayer C, et al. Healthy obese and post bariatric patients—metabolic and vascular patterns. Exp Clin Endocrinol Diabetes. 2013;**121**(8):483–87.

63. Aguilar-Olivos NE, et al. The role of bariatric surgery in the management of nonalcoholic fatty liver disease and metabolic syndrome. Metabolism. 2016;**65**(8):1196–207.

64. Aguiar IC, et al. Obstructive sleep apnea and pulmonary function in patients with severe obesity before and after bariatric surgery: a randomized clinical trial. Multidiscip Respir Med. 2014;**9**(1):43.

65. Pelascini E, et al. Should we wait for metabolic complications before operating on obese patients? Gastric bypass outcomes in metabolically healthy obese individuals. Surg Obes Relat Dis. 2016;**12**(1):49–56.

66. Consultation, WHOE. Appropriate body-mass index for Asian populations and its implications for policy and intervention strategies. Lancet. 2004;**363**(9403):157–63.

67. Deurenberg P, Deurenberg-Yap M, Guricci S. Asians are different from Caucasians and from each other in their body mass index/body fat per cent relationship. Obes Rev. 2002;**3**(3):141–46.

68. Wang D, et al. Ethnic differences in body composition and obesity related risk factors: study in Chinese and white males living in China. PLoS One. 2011;**6**(5):e19835.

69. Flegal KM, et al. Association of all-cause mortality with overweight and obesity using standard body mass index categories: a systematic review and meta-analysis. JAMA. 2013;**309**(1):71–82.

70. Hawn MT, et al. Impact of obesity on resource utilization for general surgical procedures. Ann Surg. 2005;**241**(5):821–26.

71. Vaduganathan M, et al. Relation of body mass index to late survival after valvular heart surgery. Am J Cardiol. 2012;**110**(11):1667–78.

72. Benedetto U, Danese C, Codispoti M. Obesity paradox in coronary artery bypass grafting: myth or reality? J Thorac Cardiovasc Surg. 2014;**147**(5):1517–23.

73. Gruberg L, et al. Impact of body mass index on the outcome of patients with multivessel disease randomized to either coronary artery bypass grafting or stenting in the ARTS trial: The obesity paradox II? Am J Cardiol. 2005;**95**(4):439–44.

74. Johnson AP, et al. Body mass index, outcomes, and mortality following cardiac surgery in Ontario, Canada. J Am Heart Assoc. 2015;**4**(7):e002140.

75. Whiting PS, et al. Body mass index predicts perioperative complications following orthopaedic trauma surgery: an ACS-NSQIP analysis. Eur J Trauma Emerg Surg. 2017;**43**(2):255–264.

76. Valentijn TM, et al. Impact of obesity on postoperative and long-term outcomes in a general surgery population: a retrospective cohort study. World J Surg. 2013;**37**(11):2561–68.

77. Valentijn TM, et al. The obesity paradox in the surgical population. Surgeon. 2013;**11**(3):169–76.

78. Platz J, et al. The impact of the body mass index on outcome after subarachnoid hemorrhage: is there an obesity paradox in SAH? A retrospective analysis. Neurosurgery. 2013;**73**(2):201–8.

79. Jackson RS, et al. Class I obesity is paradoxically associated with decreased risk of postoperative stroke after carotid endarterectomy. J Vasc Surg. 2012;**55**(5):1306–12.

80. Mullen JT, Moorman DW, Davenport DL. The obesity paradox: body mass index and outcomes in patients undergoing nonbariatric general surgery. Ann Surg. 2009;**250**(1):166–72.

81. Morgan MA, et al. Prognostic significance of body mass indices for patients undergoing esophagectomy for cancer. Dis Esophagus. 2007;**20**(1):29–35.

82. Aasheim ET, et al. Effect of bariatric surgery on sulphur amino acids and glutamate. Br J Nutr. 2011;**106**(3):432–40.

83. Andrews TG, et al. Cardiac assessment in pediatric mice: strain analysis as a diagnostic measurement. Echocardiography. 2014;**31**(3):375–84.

84. De Schutter A, Lavie CJ, Milani RV. The impact of obesity on risk factors and prevalence and prognosis of coronary heart disease—the obesity paradox. Prog Cardiovasc Dis. 2014;**56**(4):401–8.

85. Wisneski JA, et al. Myocardial metabolism of free fatty acids. Studies with 14C-labeled substrates in humans. J Clin Invest. 1987;**79**(2):359–66.

86. Bing RJ, et al. Metabolism of the human heart. II. Studies on fat, ketone and amino acid metabolism. Am J Med. 1954;**16**(4):504–15.

87. Neubauer S. The failing heart—an engine out of fuel. N Engl J Med. 2007;**356**(11):1140–51.

88. Stanley WC, Recchia FA, Lopaschuk GD. Myocardial substrate metabolism in the normal and failing heart. Physiol Rev. 2005;**85**(3):1093–129.

89. Davenport DL, et al. The influence of body mass index obesity status on vascular surgery 30-day morbidity and mortality. J Vasc Surg. 2009;**49**(1):140–7.

90. Takagi H, Umemoto T, ALICE (All-Literature Investigation of Cardiovascular Evidence) Group. Overweight, but not obesity, paradox on mortality following coronary artery bypass grafting. J Cardiol. 2016;**68**(3):215–21.

91. Lopez-Delgado JC, et al. The influence of body mass index on outcomes in patients undergoing cardiac surgery: does the obesity paradox really exist? PLoS One. 2015;10(3):e0118858.

92. Klattenhoff CA, et al. Braveheart, a long noncoding RNA required for cardiovascular lineage commitment. Cell. 2013;**152**(3):570–83.

93. Janssen I. Heart disease risk among metabolically healthy obese men and metabolically unhealthy lean men. CMAJ. 2005;**172**(10):1315–16.

94. Kramer CK, Zinman B, Retnakaran R. Are metabolically healthy overweight and obesity benign conditions?: A systematic review and meta-analysis. Ann Intern Med. 2013;**159**(11):758–69.

95. Hastie CE, et al. Obesity paradox in a cohort of 4880 consecutive patients undergoing percutaneous coronary intervention. Eur Heart J. 2010;**31**(2):222–26.

96. Diercks DB, et al. The obesity paradox in non-ST-segment elevation acute coronary syndromes: results from the Can Rapid risk stratification of Unstable angina patients Suppress ADverse outcomes with Early implementation of the American College of Cardiology/American Heart Association Guidelines Quality Improvement Initiative. Am Heart J. 2006;**152**(1):140–48.

Peripheral nerve blocks in the morbidly obese patient

Ammar Mahmoud, Mansoor M. Aman, and Fahad Aman

Introduction

The incidence of morbid obesity has seen an exponential rise when compared to being overweight or obese [1,2]. Clinically, the body mass index is commonly utilized when quantifying weight classification. It serves as a surrogate for the more precise measurement of body fat content. Excess adipose tissue is associated with increased risk of cardiovascular disease, diabetes, cancer, and premature degenerative joint disease [3–6]. As these patients present for surgical intervention, it is prudent to be cognizant of their physiological differences when compared to lean patients. Morbidly obese patients have an increased tendency for anatomical airway obstruction, increased oxygen consumption, and reduced functional residual capacity. All of these factors contribute to their propensity to rapidly become hypoxaemic. The synergistic effects of commonly used anxiolytics and opioids also play an important role in respiratory depression [7,8]. The utility of multimodal analgesia including regional techniques can help minimize the untoward effects of opioids and benzodiazepines while optimizing pain control [9,10]. This chapter will provide a detailed review of special considerations of regional anaesthesia in morbid obesity and various upper extremity and lower extremity blocks that are utilized for surgical anaesthesia or postoperative pain control.

Special considerations for regional anaesthetics in the obese

Before initiating any regional anaesthetic, standard American Society of Anesthesiologists monitoring guidelines including oxygenation, circulation, and heart rate monitoring must be satisfied. Emergency rescue equipment and medications should readily be available in anticipation of any potential complications. A safety checklist or time-out sheet is recommended, which should at minimum include the regional block performed, the surgical site, and indicated surgical procedure [11]. A successfully performed regional block can be utilized as the sole surgical anaesthetic or may be combined with a general anaesthetic or sedation. The decision to deliver sedation for patient comfort should be individualized based on the anticipated tolerance of procedure, patient comorbidities, and the provider's experience.

Basics in regional anaesthesia

Local anaesthetics should be dosed based on standardized weight-based guidelines. For large-volume blocks such as fascia iliaca compartment block, a mixture of maximum dose of local anaesthetic can be diluted with part normal saline to achieve the desired volume. Several techniques including ultrasound guidance, frequent negative aspiration, addition of intravascular markers, and intermittent dosing should be utilized to minimize the risk of intravascular injection [12]. Should intravascular administration occur, presenting symptoms may be subtle and can range from perioral numbness and tinnitus, to seizure activity, electrocardiogram changes, and cardiovascular collapse [13]. Local anaesthetic systemic toxicity can have devastating consequences if not recognized and treated promptly. In addition to emergency rescue equipment availability and knowledge of both basic and advanced cardiac life support, intralipid should be readily accessible to the regional anaesthesia team whenever large doses of local anaesthetics are delivered. The detailed management of local anaesthetic systemic toxicity is beyond the scope of this chapter; an in-depth practice advisory and checklist for the management of local anaesthetic systemic toxicity is made available by the American Society of Regional Anesthesia and Pain Medicine [14,15].

Prior to starting any interventional procedure, the site should be prepped with an antiseptic solution such as chlorhexidine or betadine to minimize the risk of infection. Any pre-existing infection on the overlying skin is an absolute contraindication to performing a peripheral nerve block as the needle could theoretically transfer the infection into deeper tissue [16]. Caution is advised when there is concern for post-surgical compartment syndrome or the extent of traumatic injury is unknown. A pre-procedure conversation with the surgical team, addressing these concerns, is prudent in such situations.

Although exceedingly rare, nerve injury following peripheral nerve blockade may occur [17]. Fortunately, this devastating complication is often transient with recovery expected within weeks to months [18]. However, permanent neuropathy following peripheral nerve blockade has been reported. Proposed mechanisms include injury from direct needle trauma, intraneural injection of local anaesthetic, high injection pressures, and the use of vasoconstrictive adjuvants [19]. Patient risk factors for injury include a history of previous nerve injury and pre-existing peripheral neuropathy [20]. A comprehensive approach to evaluating such injuries is necessary and should not be limited to the details of the performed peripheral nerve block. Other factors such as intraoperative patient positioning, prolonged tourniquet use, excessive intraoperative nerve manipulation by the surgeon, or nerve compression from postoperative casting should be considered [20].

Peripheral nerve stimulation can be utilized to enhance safety, and ensure adequate target nerve distribution. The needle is simply connected to the nerve stimulator and a grounding pad placed on any extremity to complete the circuit. A 'seeking' current of 0.8–1 mA is applied as the needle is advanced towards the target nerve until twitches in the desired innervated distribution are noted. When the needle is in an appropriate location for injection, the current is slowly reduced to 0.2–0.4 mA and the twitches should disappear. If the twitches persist at this low current, the needle is likely to be intraneural with risk of nerve palsy/injury. The needle is retracted until the twitch disappears and only then is local anaesthetic deposited.

Finally, block-specific risks should be assessed prior to performing any regional procedure. For example, a patient with severe pulmonary compromise disease presenting for shoulder surgery may not tolerate the resultant hemidiaphragmatic paresis from phrenic nerve blockade. Individual risk factors for upper and lower extremity blocks will be discussed.

Upper extremity

Effective anaesthesia/analgesia of the upper extremities requires a thorough understanding of the anatomy of the brachial plexus. Moreover, proficiency with the attempted block technique (nerve stimulator, ultrasound, or combined) is essential to ensure block success. Finally, accommodation for individual variation regarding adipose accumulation in various tissue compartments should be accounted for, as they may render identification of important landmarks more difficult [21].

The brachial plexus provides sensory and motor innervation to the upper extremity. As the nerve roots of C5–T1 exit the intervertebral foramina they converge to create trunks, divisions, cords, and branches of terminal nerves. Upper extremity anaesthesia can be accomplished by the deposition of local anaesthetic at any point along the brachial plexus (**Table 23.1**). In addition to single-injection nerve blocks, percutaneous catheter placement allows for intraoperative redosing to prolong nerve blocks and offers a route for postoperative analgesia. There are four main upper extremity blocks: interscalene, supraclavicular, infraclavicular, and axillary.

Interscalene block

Indications for interscalene brachial plexus block include shoulder and proximal arm surgery. The patient is placed in the semi-Fowler position, described as lying in bed supine with the head of the bed

Table 23.1 Upper extremity blocks

Nerve block	Location
Interscalene	Roots/trunks
Supraclavicular	Divisions
Infraclavicular	Cords
Axillary	Terminal nerves

elevated approximately between 30 and 45 degrees. The head should also be turned towards the non-operative side. Traditionally, the cricoid cartilage (at the level of C6) is used as a surface landmark for ultrasound probe placement and needle insertion. If identifying the cricoid cartilage proves difficult, placement of the ultrasound probe more distally (at the level of supraclavicular block) and moving cephalad to obtain an image of the C5–C6 nerve roots between the anterior and middle scalene muscles can be helpful. Under direct visualization, the block needle is advanced from lateral to medial through the middle scalene towards these target nerve roots where local anaesthetic is deposited (**Fig. 23.1**).

An obvious concern regarding a successful block is ipsilateral hemidiaphragmatic paresis secondary to associated phrenic nerve paralysis. This is of particular importance in the morbidly obese patient population with underlying obstructive sleep apnoea where consequent dyspnoea, hypercapnia, and hypoxaemia can increase patient morbidity. When compared to ultrasound-guided interscalene brachial plexus block, the nerve stimulator technique has been associated with a higher incidence of hemidiaphragmatic paresis [22]. Efforts to reduce the incidence of phrenic nerve paralysis have been extensively studied. While a direct relationship between total volume of anaesthetic injected and degree of phrenic nerve paralysis has been demonstrated, phrenic nerve paralysis can occur with as little as 5 mL of local anaesthetic [23]. It is therefore pivotal to understand the anatomical relationship of the phrenic nerve with the C5 nerve root and its path as it continues to travel caudally. Under ultrasound guidance the phrenic nerve can be identified and

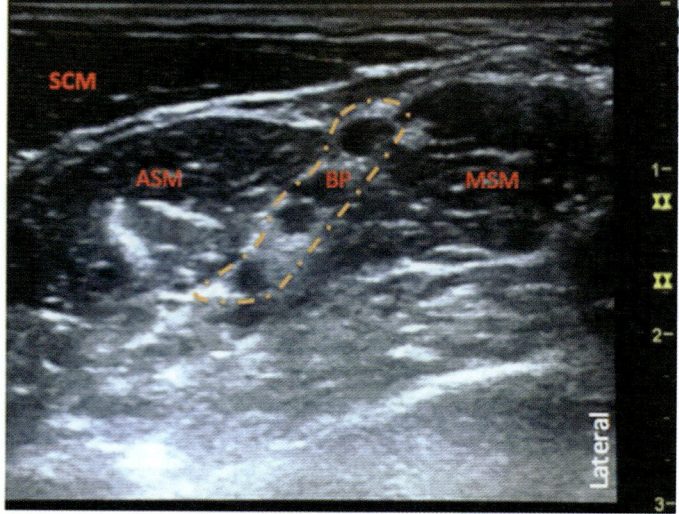

Fig. 23.1 Interscalene brachial plexus (BP) position between the middle scalene muscle (MSM) and anterior scalene muscle (ASM). The sternocleidomastoid muscle (SCM) is seen overlying the ASM.

is located within 2 mm of the brachial plexus at the cricoid cartilage level, with additional 3 mm separation for every centimetre more caudal in the neck [24]. With this in mind, a modified interscalene brachial plexus block, termed superior trunk block, has been described. It involves tracing the C5–C6 nerve roots caudally to where they coalesce into the superior trunk where local anaesthetic is injected lateral to the superior trunk but proximal to the take-off of the suprascapular nerve [25].

In addition to single-injection techniques, continuous catheter infusions should be considered when severe pain and the requirement for postoperative opioid therapy are anticipated (open rotator cuff repair, as opposed to shoulder arthroscopy). Theoretically, as the catheter is placed at the level of the nerve roots/trunks, less volume is required to achieve comparable analgesia as opposed to catheters placed distally along the brachial plexus. Additionally, catheter infusions improve pain control, decrease opioid consumption, shorten length of stay in the post-anaesthesia care unit, and increase patient satisfaction [26]. Decreasing opioid consumption is of striking benefit in the early postoperative period where the undesired respiratory effects of opioid therapy can be compounded with the effects of residual anaesthetic medications. Interestingly, placement of a continuous catheter does not significantly prolong phrenic paresis and demonstrates a limited pulmonary impact [27].

Supraclavicular block

Commonly referred to as 'the spinal of the upper extremity', a successful supraclavicular block (SCB) consistently provides reliable, dense upper extremity surgical anaesthesia. It is indicated for surgical procedures of the upper extremity distal to the shoulder joint. The patient is placed in the semi-Fowler position with the head turned towards the non-operative side with the ipsilateral shoulder displaced inferiorly. The ultrasound probe is initially placed parallel to the clavicle at the insertion site of the sternocleidomastoid muscle. Following the identification of the pleural dome, the probe is moved laterally towards the brachial plexus located superficial and lateral to the subclavian artery. If identifying the pleura proves difficult, observing the pleural movement with breathing helps distinguish the pleura from other surrounding structures. Adjusting image depth is often necessary and allows for the identification of the four critical components (brachial plexus, subclavian artery, first rib, and pleura) of the supraclavicular block.

Under direct visualization, the block needle is advanced from lateral to medial with the goal of reaching the 'corner pocket' formed between the first rib and subclavian artery. Depositing local anaesthetic at this location utilizes pulsations of the subclavian artery against the first rib to spread the local anaesthetic to the more superficial plexus. To reach this location safely, it is necessary to obtain an ultrasound image where the first rib lies below the subclavian artery thereby protecting the underlying pleura (Fig. 23.2). If the first rib does not lie under the subclavian artery, the pleura is no longer protected, increasing the possibility of inadvertent pleural injury at that location.

Prior to the emergence of ultrasound-guided regional anaesthesia, the most worrisome complication associated with the SCB was an ipsilateral iatrogenic pneumothorax. At that time, the reported incidence rates ranged between 0.2% and 6.1% [28]. Even more alarming were reports of a 'delayed pneumothorax' that occurred days following a successful block [29]. For these reasons,

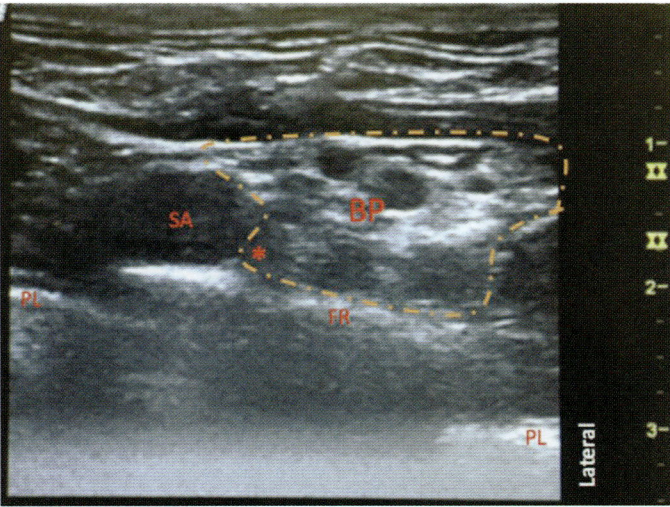

Fig. 23.2 Supraclavicular brachial plexus (BP) is seen superficially and lateral to the subclavian artery (SA). Lateral and medial to the first rib (FR) the deeper pleura (PL) is seen. middle scalene muscle (MSM). * denotes the 'corner pocket' between the FR and SA.

anaesthesiologists have avoided this block in the morbidly obese population in hopes of preserving pulmonary function.

In the era of ultrasound-guided regional anaesthesia, interest in the SCB has been revived. The SCB has been re-demonstrated as an effective block that can be performed safely. The incidence of iatrogenic pneumothorax with ultrasound-guided SCB has been studied extensively. Large observational studies have reported pneumothorax incidence rates between zero and 0.04–0.06% [30,31].

Although the risk of pneumothorax is markedly reduced with ultrasound guidance, SCBs in the morbidly obese are technically challenging and require special consideration. Obesity has been found to increase the difficulty and decrease the success rate of a SCB [31]. Among the contributing factors is the necessary increase in ultrasound image depth required to visualize deeper structures, consequently producing a poor-quality ultrasound image. This makes identification of key structures and the entire block needle more challenging, potentially explaining the increased difficulty and decreased success rate. Interestingly, there are no differences in the acute post-block complication rates in the morbidly obese [31].

Infraclavicular block

Indications for the infraclavicular block (ICB) are similar to that of the SCB, namely surgical procedures of the upper extremity distal to the shoulder joint. The ICB is performed at the level of the brachial plexus cords that surround the axillary artery deep to the pectoral muscles. The patient is placed in the semi-Fowler position with the head turned towards the non-operative side. The ipsilateral arm is slightly abducted at 30 degrees. This slight abduction (30 degrees) moves the underlying plexus to a more superficial position as it is stretched towards the anterior wall. Greater abduction (110 degrees) has been shown to decrease the incidence of associated pneumothorax [32]. The ultrasound probe is placed in a parasagittal orientation below the clavicle and medial to the coracoid process. A curved, low-frequency ultrasound probe is recommended for obese patients as it will provide a wide field of view and superior visualization of deep structures [33]. The block needle is inserted cephalad to the

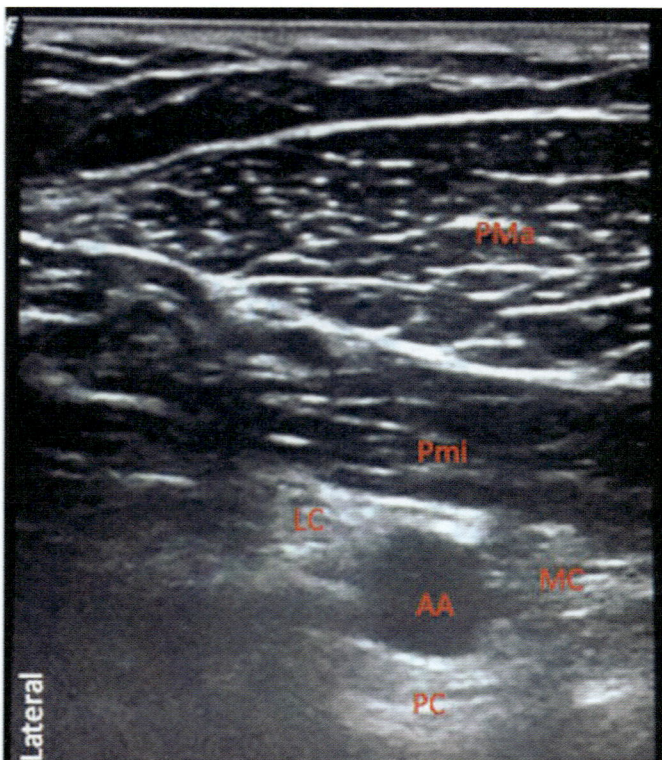

Fig. 23.3 Infraclavicular block, the axillary artery (AA) is seen with the surrounding brachial plexus cords: lateral cord (LC), posterior cord (PC), and medial cord (MC). The pectoralis minor (Pmi) and pectoralis major (PMa) are seen superficially.

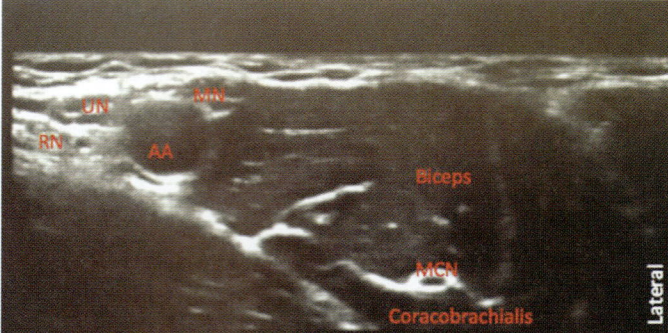

Fig. 23.4 The axillary block demonstrating the relation of the radial nerve (RN), ulnar nerve (UN), median nerve (MN) to the axillary artery (AA). The musculocutaneous nerve is seen between the biceps and coracobrachialis muscles.

ultrasound probe in the direction of the brachial plexus cords (lateral, posterior, and medial) surrounding the axillary artery (**Fig. 23.3**).

Even in patients with a normal body mass index the ICB is a relatively deep block with the target cords approximately 3–5 cm deep. In the morbidly obese, identification of these structures can become technically challenging given the added subcutaneous tissue. Simply identifying the axillary artery and performing this block by assumption of cord location is ineffective and, more importantly, dangerous. Additionally, procedural discomfort as the needle transverses the pectoral muscles is a common issue faced when performing an ICB. This discomfort can often be overcome by light anaesthetic premedication. Judicious titration of premedication is warranted as morbidly obese patients are more susceptible to the adverse effects, primarily respiratory depression. Keeping this in mind, if safely performing an ICB on a morbidly obese patient proves to be difficult, the anaesthesiologist should substitute the ICB for another upper extremity block at a different location.

Due to its deep location, the ICB is the best site throughout the brachial plexus for catheter placement. The structural support provided by pectoral muscles minimizes catheter migration and dislodgment. Infraclavicular catheters have been shown to provide superior postoperative analgesia when compared to supraclavicular catheters for upper extremity surgery [34].

Axillary block

Indications of axillary block (AB) include surgical procedures of the upper extremity distal to the elbow joint. The AB is performed at

the level of the terminal branches of the brachial plexus. While a single injection may be sufficient, more commonly, multiple injections are required to block all terminal branches (radial, ulnar, median, and musculocutaneous nerves) and provide a complete upper extremity block.

The patient is placed in the semi-Fowler position with the head turned towards the non-operative side. The ipsilateral arm is abducted (90 degrees) and flexed at the elbow. The ultrasound probe is placed perpendicular to the underlying nerve structures at the insertion of the pectoralis major muscle onto the humerus. The axillary artery can be easily identified at this location. Three of the four terminal branches surround the axillary artery. Commonly, the median nerve is located superficial and lateral, the ulnar nerve is located superficial and medial, and the radial nerve is located posterior and lateral to the artery. The fourth terminal branch of the brachial plexus, the musculocutaneous nerve, is located in the fascial layer between the biceps and coracobrachialis muscles (**Fig. 23.4**). Scanning distally, along the long axis of the arm is often required to clearly identify this nerve. Following distal identification, rescanning the nerve path proximally allows the performance of this block with a single injection site. Under direct visualization, the block needle is inserted cephalad and directed towards the target terminal branches as they surround the axillary artery.

In the obese population, considerable individual anatomical variation regarding nerve location in relation to the axillary artery can exist. Prior to ultrasound guidance, performance of the AB on obese patients required multiple injection sites and was associated with increased failure rates, greater immediate complications, and overall patient dissatisfaction [35]. Since then, sonographic studies examining these obesity-associated changes have emerged. In obese patients, the axillary artery and the radial nerve are located deeper. The distance between the median and ulnar nerves and the axillary artery are similar to that of a non-obese patient. Additionally, the musculocutaneous nerve is located further from the axillary artery suggesting that a longer block needle may be necessary in obese patients [36]. These changes help explain the issues surrounding the performance of the AB in obese patients prior to ultrasound guidance.

The AB is of particular benefit to morbidly obese patients with underlying pulmonary disease requiring upper extremity anaesthesia. Due to its distal location, pleural integrity and phrenic nerve function are maintained following a successful AB. In addition, the axillary artery can be directly compressed in the case of inadvertent puncture.

Lower extremity

Obesity is recognized as an independent risk factor for osteoarthritis due to the elevated weight burden on the axial skeleton [37]. As a result, these patients commonly present for total hip and total knee arthroplasty, which are associated with significant postoperative pain. Regional anaesthetic techniques aim to reduce opioid consumption and provide adequate analgesia, while minimally affecting functional recovery. The common regional blocks performed that will be discussed in this section are femoral, fascia iliaca, adductor canal, and sciatic–popliteal approach.

Femoral nerve block

Indications for femoral nerve block include surgeries of the anterior thigh, and knee arthroplasty [38]. It is effective as an intraoperative regional anaesthetic and for postoperative pain control and is associated with higher patient satisfaction when compared to epidural and oral analgesics [39,40]. Historically, femoral and sciatic nerve blocks have been utilized to provide coverage of both the anteromedial and posterolateral knee capsule respectively [40,41]. While this provides extensive coverage of the affected joint, a femoral nerve block reduces quadriceps strength by greater than 80% [42]. This side effect has a profound impact on the patient's surgical recovery as it delays rehabilitation and elevates the risk of falls and immobility-related complications.

The femoral nerve is the largest branch arising from the lumbar plexus and receives contributions from L2–L4. It traverses through the psoas muscle, emerging between the psoas and iliacus muscles, before passing below the inguinal ligament. At the level below the inguinal ligament, the femoral nerve is positioned lateral and deep to the femoral artery (**Fig. 23.5**). The femoral nerve gives rise to numerous motor and sensory branches. The anterior division gives rise to the middle cutaneous, medial cutaneous, and muscular branch to the sartorius. The posterior division gives branches that supply the quadriceps muscle, the hip, and the knee, and terminates as the saphenous nerve. Adequate blockade results in anaesthesia of the skin and muscles of the anterior thigh, a significant portion of the femur and knee joint, and the medial aspect of the leg below the knee.

Needle insertion should be at the level of the femoral crease, a few centimetres below the inguinal ligament and lateral to the femoral arterial pulse. In obese patients, redundant abdominal fat should be retracted as it can make it difficult to palpate the femoral pulse and obscures the needle entry point. Although it is acceptable to perform the block with ultrasound guidance alone, a peripheral nerve stimulator may be concomitantly utilized. When using stimulation, it should be noted that the branch to the sartorius muscle arises from the anteromedial aspect of the femoral nerve. A sartorial twitch may be the result of stimulation of this branch and not the femoral nerve. The needle should be redirected laterally and advanced deeper by a few millimetres. A quadriceps twitch should then be noted, as it results in a more reliable blockade. Sufficient blockade is achieved with 15–20 mL of local anaesthetic. Due to elevated fall risk, it is advisable to not use catheters for postoperative pain control [43,44]. Obesity and advanced age are independent risk factors for falls with femoral catheters [45].

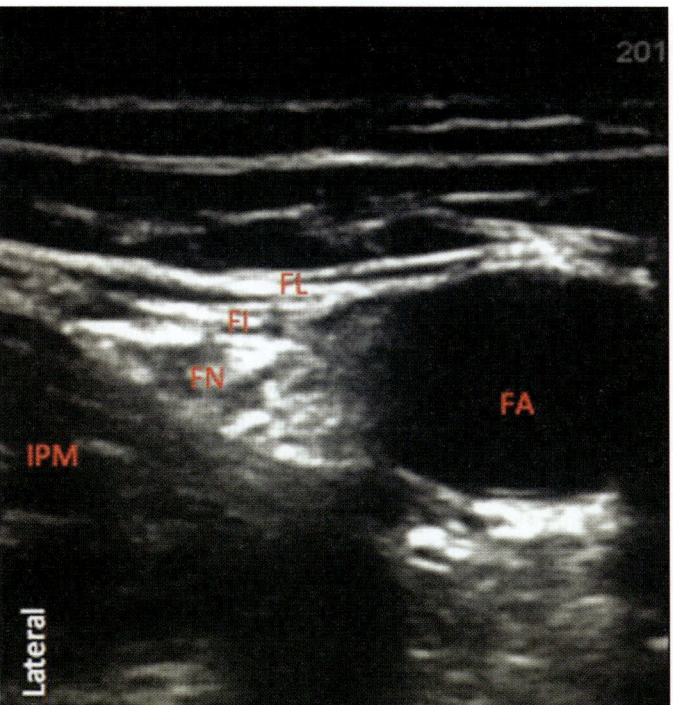

Fig. 23.5 The femoral nerve (FN) is seen lateral to the femoral artery (FA) with the overlying fascia iliaca (FI) and fascia lata (FL) superficially. The iliopsoas muscle lies posterolateral to the FN.

Fascia iliaca compartment block

The fascia iliaca compartment block is indicated for surgeries of the anterolateral thigh and knee, and for postoperative pain control following hip and knee arthroplasty [46,47]. It is an alternative to a femoral nerve block with similar efficacy to analgesia [48]. This compartment block requires a relatively larger volume of local anaesthetic (30 mL) when compared to femoral nerve block as the local anaesthetic is deposited within a fascial plane where the nerves lie. Successful blockade will anaesthetize the femoral and lateral femoral cutaneous nerves reliably. Coverage of the obturator nerve is less reliable clinically, and recent magnetic resonance imaging-based data failed to show its involvement [49].

The fascia iliaca is anterior to the iliacus muscle, bordered medially by the fascia covering the psoas muscle, and superolaterally by the iliac crest.

Using the landmark approach, a line can be drawn from the anterior superior iliac spine to the femoral artery and divided in thirds. When the needle is introduced in the lateral third of this line, it will traverse the skin, subcutaneous fat, the fascia lata (first 'pop'), and then the fascia iliaca (second 'pop'). This blind 'double-pop' technique is described in the literature but produces varying results because of a high incidence of false positives due to local anaesthetic likely being instilled within the incorrect location [50].

The probe should be positioned laterally from the anterior superior iliac spine towards the pubic tubercle. The femoral artery is then identified and the probe moved laterally to bring the sartorius muscle (lateral) and iliopsoas muscle (medial) in view. After a skin wheal of local anaesthetic, the needle is directed in-plane and should traverse the layers described previously until it passes the fascia iliaca. A 30–40 mL volume of local anaesthetic is deposited in between the fascia iliaca and iliacus muscle.

Adductor canal block

The adductor canal block offers the advantage of quadriceps sparing due to its distal injection point while still providing adequate coverage of the anteromedial knee capsule, the predominant site of incisional pain [51]. The adductor canal block is useful for surgeries of the knee, below-knee amputations, and medial ankle incisions [52]. Effective blockade is dependent on provider proficiency in ultrasonography, and understanding of various injection points along with their limitations, anatomy, and nerve root contributions.

The adductor canal (Hunter's canal) extends from the apex of the femoral triangle to the adductor hiatus of the adductor magnus. It can be divided into thirds, with the middle third approximately halfway between the anterior superior iliac spine and base of the patella. The sartorius muscle forms the anterior border of the canal, the vastus medialis occupies the lateral border, and the adductor longus and adductor magnus muscles form the posterior border (Fig. 23.6). A thick aponeurosis named the vastoadductor membrane also lies anterior to the adductor canal. The canal extends approximately 15 cm and serves as a passageway to the superficial femoral artery and vein as they transition from the anterior thigh to the posterior leg. After exiting the canal, they are known as the popliteal artery and vein. The saphenous nerve, and nerve to the vastus medialis (NVM) also traverse the adductor canal. A cadaveric study examining the course of all nerves that traverse the adductor canal to innervate the knee highlighted the importance of blocking the NVM. It was found that the NVM entered lateral to the femoral artery in all specimens at the apex of the femoral triangle and coursed through the belly of the vastus medialis to supply the anterior and medial knee capsule [53]. Furthermore, the deep nerve plexus formed by contributions from both the saphenous nerve

and NVM was found in 90% of the specimens. It lies between the femoral artery and femur, giving rise to the anterior and medial genicular nerves. The final innervation of the genicular nerve was found to be the deep anteromedial joint capsule [53].

Relative to the femoral nerve block, the adductor canal block requires a greater comfort with ultrasonography. The success of blockade is dependent on the optimal site of local anaesthetic deposition within the canal. The middle third is the preferred location within the canal to include all branches of the NVM, and saphenous nerve. An in-plane short-axis view allows for the needle to be visualized as it traverses various structures. Position the leg slightly abducted and externally rotated allowing for placement of the probe on the medial aspect of the middle third of the adductor canal as detailed previously. The belly of the sartorius muscle should be visualized forming the anterior border of the canal with the superficial femoral artery below. After negative aspiration, approximately 15–20 mL of local anaesthetic should be deposited for adequate spread. A catheter may be placed for continuous infusion or administration of intermittent boluses. Aspiration of the catheter agitates echogenic bubbles making it easier to visualize the catheter using ultrasound. When larger volumes are deposited, it is conceivable that unintentional spread to nerves outside the canal may occur. These large volumes may provide superior analgesia; however, it is at the expense of quadriceps weakness secondary to blockage of vastus intermedius, vastus lateralis, and rectus femoris. Injection in the proximal third of the canal is no longer encouraged as it has also been associated with significant quadriceps weakness.

Popliteal–sciatic nerve block

Indications for sciatic nerve block at the popliteal fossa include surgical procedures of the foot and ankle. When combined with a saphenous nerve block, complete lower extremity anaesthesia can be achieved.

The superomedial boundary of the popliteal fossa is formed by the semimembranosus muscle, and superolaterally by the biceps femoris muscle. The large gastrocnemius muscle occupies the inferomedial and inferolateral aspects of the popliteal fossa. Contents of the popliteal fossa include the tibial nerve (TN), popliteal vein, popliteal artery, and the common peroneal nerve (CPN).

The PB can be performed in both the supine and prone positions. In morbidly obese patients, the supine approach is beneficial as prone positioning can be difficult to achieve and is often uncomfortable. In addition, maintenance of this position throughout the block duration is poorly tolerated in obese patients given the changes in respiratory mechanics associated with lying prone. A reliable image can be obtained in the supine position, negating the theoretical benefit of improved image quality in the prone position. Finally, performing this block supine allows anaesthesiologists easier access to the patient's airway should an emergency requiring airway control occur.

With the patient positioned in the supine position, a pillow is used to raise the affected limb. A curved, low-frequency ultrasound probe may be necessary in larger patients. Traditionally, the ultrasound probe is placed at the popliteal crease where the popliteal artery, popliteal vein, and TN can be identified (Fig. 23.7). Starting at the popliteal crease is particularly beneficial in obese patients given the superficial location that these nerves assume at this location [54]. Following identification of these structures, the probe is moved superiorly bringing the CPN (located lateral) into the ultrasound

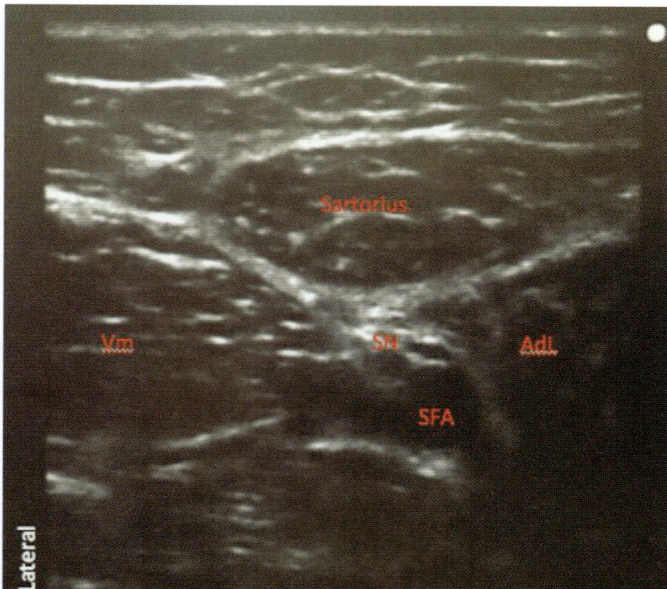

Fig. 23.6 The adductor canal is seen with the sartorius, vastus medialis (Vm), and adductor longus (AdL) muscles forming its superior, lateral, and medial borders respectively. The pulsations of the superficial femoral artery (SFA) are identified and the saphenous nerve (SN) is seen superior to the artery.

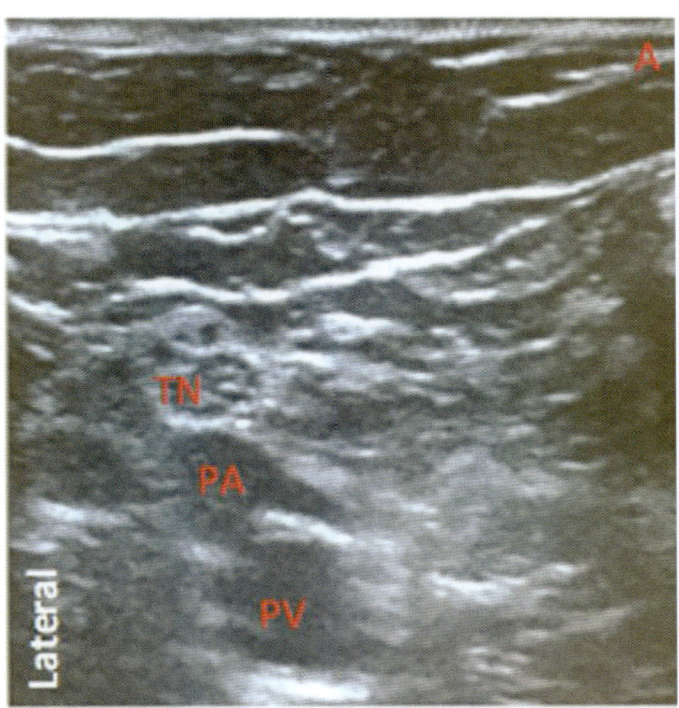

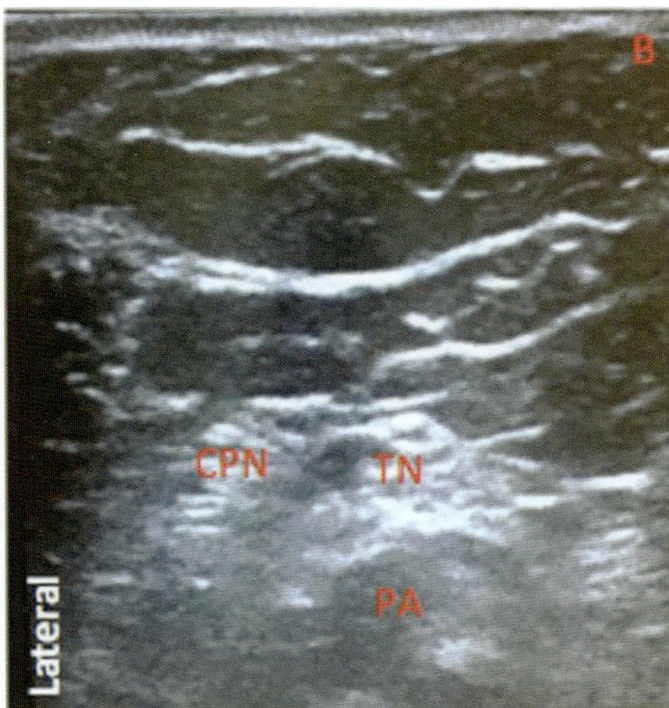

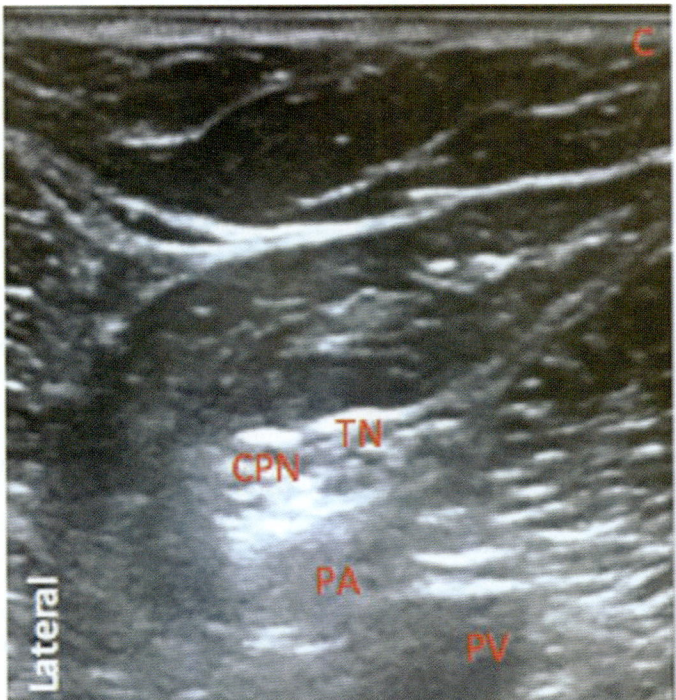

Fig. 23.7 Popliteal block of the sciatic nerve. (a) The popliteal vein (PV) and popliteal artery (PA) are visualized at the popliteal crease. The tibial nerve (TN) is seen superficial to the PA. (b) The probe is then moved laterally to bring the common peroneal nerve (CPN) into view. (c) The probe is the moved proximal to as the TN and CPN join to form the sciatic nerve.

image. By tracing the TN and CPN proximally, the sciatic nerve can be identified at its bifurcation (approximately 7–10 cm proximally).

Attempting a block at this proximal location can be challenging in obese patients. Adipose tissue accumulation will increase the skin-to-nerve distance. To accommodate these changes, increasing ultrasound image depth is often necessary. This will result in a poor-quality ultrasound image making this approach technically challenging. To avoid this, a distal popliteal block has been described in

morbidly obese patients. Given the superficial location of the TN and CPN at the popliteal crease, the distal approach results in better visualization, making this block less challenging. The TN and CPN are blocked at the popliteal crease separately. This distal approach to the popliteal block is not more time-consuming and provides a faster onset of surgical sensorimotor blockade, a lower incidence of repeat blockade or need for local anaesthetic supplementation, and lower pain scores in the post-anaesthesia care unit [55].

REFERENCES

1. Ogden CL, Carroll MD, Kit BK, Flegal KM. Prevalence of obesity among adults: United States, 2011–2012. NCHS Data Brief. 2013;**131**:1–8.
2. Sturm R, Hattori A. Morbid obesity rates continue to rise rapidly in the United States. International Journal of Obesity (2005). 2013;**37**(6):889–91.
3. Lakka HM, Laaksonen DE, Lakka TA, Niskanen LK, Kumpusalo E, Tuomilehto J, et al. The metabolic syndrome and total and cardiovascular disease mortality in middle-aged men. JAMA. 2002;**288**(21):2709–16.
4. Kopelman P. Health risks associated with overweight and obesity. Obesity Reviews. 2007;**8**(Suppl 1):13–17.
5. Lau DC, Dhillon B, Yan H, Szmitko PE, Verma S. Adipokines: molecular links between obesity and atheroslcerosis. American Journal of Physiology. Heart and Circulatory Physiology. 2005;**288**(5):H2031–41.
6. Neligan PJ. Metabolic syndrome: anesthesia for morbid obesity. Current Opinion in Anaesthesiology. 2010;**23**(3):375–83.
7. Hitt HC, McMillen RC, Thornton-Neaves T, Koch K, Cosby AG. Comorbidity of obesity and pain in a general population: results from the Southern Pain Prevalence Study. Journal of Pain. 2007;**8**(5):430–36.
8. Janke EA, Collins A, Kozak AT. Overview of the relationship between pain and obesity: what do we know? Where do we go next? Journal of Rehabilitation Research and Development. 2007;**44**(2):245–62.
9. Chou R, Gordon DB, de Leon-Casasola OA, Rosenberg JM, Bickler S, Brennan T, et al. Management of postoperative pain: a clinical practice guideline from the American Pain Society, the American Society of Regional Anesthesia and Pain Medicine, and the American Society of Anesthesiologists' Committee on Regional Anesthesia, Executive Committee, and Administrative Council. Journal of Pain. 2016;**17**(2):131–57.
10. Elkassabany N, Cai LF, Mehta S, Ahn J, Pieczynski L, Polomano RC, et al. Does regional anesthesia improve the quality of postoperative pain management and the quality of recovery in patients undergoing operative repair of tibia and ankle fractures? Journal of Orthopaedic Trauma. 2015;**29**(9):404–409.
11. Mulroy MF, Weller RS, Liguori GA. A checklist for performing regional nerve blocks. Regional Anesthesia and Pain Medicine. 2014;**39**(3):195–99.
12. Barrington MJ, Kluger R. Ultrasound guidance reduces the risk of local anesthetic systemic toxicity following peripheral nerve blockade. Regional Anesthesia and Pain Medicine. 2013;**38**(4):289–99.
13. Di Gregorio G, Neal JM, Rosenquist RW, Weinberg GL. Clinical presentation of local anesthetic systemic toxicity: a review of published cases, 1979 to 2009. Regional Anesthesia and Pain Medicine. 2010;**35**(2):181–87.
14. Neal JM, Hsiung RL, Mulroy MF, Halpern BB, Dragnich AD, Slee AE. ASRA checklist improves trainee performance during a simulated episode of local anesthetic systemic toxicity. Regional Anesthesia and Pain Medicine. 2012;**37**(1):8–15.
15. Neal JM, Bernards CM, Butterworth JF 4th, Di Gregorio G, Drasner K, Hejtmanek MR, et al. ASRA practice advisory on local anesthetic systemic toxicity. Regional Anesthesia and Pain Medicine. 2010;**35**(2):152–61.
16. Hebl JR, Neal JM. Infectious complications: a new practice advisory. Regional Anesthesia and Pain Medicine. 2006;**31**(4):289–90.
17. Sites BD, Taenzer AH, Herrick MD, Gilloon C, Antonakakis J, Richins J, et al. Incidence of local anesthetic systemic toxicity and postoperative neurologic symptoms associated with 12,668 ultrasound-guided nerve blocks: an analysis from a prospective clinical registry. Regional Anesthesia and Pain Medicine. 2012;**37**(5):478–82.
18. Brull R, McCartney CJ, Chan VW, El-Beheiry H. Neurological complications after regional anesthesia: contemporary estimates of risk. Anesthesia and Analgesia. 2007;**104**(4):965–74.
19. Hogan QH. Pathophysiology of peripheral nerve injury during regional anesthesia. Regional Anesthesia and Pain Medicine. 2008;**33**(5):435–41.
20. Neal JM, Bernards CM, Hadzic A, Hebl JR, Hogan QH, Horlocker TT, et al. ASRA Practice Advisory on Neurologic Complications in Regional Anesthesia and Pain Medicine. Regional Anesthesia and Pain Medicine. 2008;**33**(5):404–15.
21. Adams JP, Murphy PG. Obesity in anaesthesia and intensive care. British Journal of Anaesthesia. 2000;**85**(1):91–108.
22. Ghodki PS, Singh ND. Incidence of hemidiaphragmatic paresis after peripheral nerve stimulator versus ultrasound guided interscalene brachial plexus block. Journal of Anaesthesiology, Clinical Pharmacology. 2016;**32**(2):177–81.
23. Riazi S, Carmichael N, Awad I, Holtby RM, McCartney CJ. Effect of local anaesthetic volume (20 vs 5 ml) on the efficacy and respiratory consequences of ultrasound-guided interscalene brachial plexus block. British Journal of Anaesthesia. 2008;**101**(4):549–56.
24. Kessler J, Schafhalter-Zoppoth I, Gray AT. An ultrasound study of the phrenic nerve in the posterior cervical triangle: implications for the interscalene brachial plexus block. Regional Anesthesia and Pain Medicine. 2008;**33**(6):545–50.
25. Burckett-St Laurent D, Chan V, Chin KJ. Refining the ultrasound-guided interscalene brachial plexus block: the superior trunk approach. Canadian Journal of Anaesthesia. 2014;**61**(12):1098–102.
26. Bingham AE, Fu R, Horn JL, Abrahams MS. Continuous peripheral nerve block compared with single-injection peripheral nerve block: a systematic review and meta-analysis of randomized controlled trials. Regional Anesthesia and Pain Medicine. 2012;**37**(6):583–94.
27. Cuvillon P, Le Sache F, Demattei C, Lidzborski L, Zoric L, Riou B, et al. Continuous interscalene brachial plexus nerve block prolongs unilateral diaphragmatic dysfunction. Anaesthesia, Critical Care & Pain Medicine. 2016;**35**(6):383–90.
28. Brand L, Papper E. A comparison of supraclavicular and axillary techniques for brachial plexus blocks. Anesthesiology. 1961;**22**:226–29.
29. Kumari A, Gupta R, Bhardwaj A, Madan D. Delayed pneumothorax after supraclavicular block. Journal of Anaesthesiology, Clinical Pharmacology. 2011;**27**(1):121–22.
30. Gauss A, Tugtekin I, Georgieff M, Dinse-Lambracht A, Keipke D, Gorsewski G. Incidence of clinically symptomatic pneumothorax in ultrasound-guided infraclavicular and supraclavicular brachial plexus block. Anaesthesia. 2014;**69**(4):327–36.
31. Franco CD, Gloss FJ, Voronov G, Tyler SG, Stojiljkovic LS. Supraclavicular block in the obese population: an analysis of 2020 blocks. Anesthesia and Analgesia. 2006;**102**(4):1252–54.
32. Bigeleisen P, Wilson M. A comparison of two techniques for ultrasound guided infraclavicular block. British Journal of Anaesthesia. 2006;**96**(4):502–507.

33. Ihnatsenka B, Boezaart AP. Ultrasound: basic understanding and learning the language. International Journal of Shoulder Surgery. 2010;**4**(3):55–62.

34. Mariano ER, Sandhu NS, Loland VJ, Bishop ML, Madison SJ, Abrams RA, et al. A randomized comparison of infraclavicular and supraclavicular continuous peripheral nerve blocks for postoperative analgesia. Regional Anesthesia and Pain Medicine. 2011;**36**(1):26–31.

35. Hanouz JL, Grandin W, Lesage A, Oriot G, Bonnieux D, Gerard JL. Multiple injection axillary brachial plexus block: influence of obesity on failure rate and incidence of acute complications. Anesthesia and Analgesia. 2010;**111**(1):230–33.

36. Daccache G, Jouini R, Hanouz J-L, Fellahi J-L. Axillary block in obese and non-obese patients: a comparative sono-anatomic study: 8AP2-4. European Journal of Anaesthesiology. 2012;**29**:119–20.

37. Lementowski PW, Zelicof SB. Obesity and osteoarthritis. American Journal of Orthopedics (Belle Mead, NJ). 2008;**37**(3):148–51.

38. Fischer HB, Simanski CJ, Sharp C, Bonnet F, Camu F, Neugebauer EA, et al. A procedure-specific systematic review and consensus recommendations for postoperative analgesia following total knee arthroplasty. Anaesthesia. 2008;**63**(10):1105–23.

39. Fowler SJ, Symons J, Sabato S, Myles PS. Epidural analgesia compared with peripheral nerve blockade after major knee surgery: a systematic review and meta-analysis of randomized trials. British Journal of Anaesthesia. 2008;**100**(2):154–64.

40. Paul JE, Arya A, Hurlburt L, Cheng J, Thabane L, Tidy A, et al. Femoral nerve block improves analgesia outcomes after total knee arthroplasty: a meta-analysis of randomized controlled trials. Anesthesiology. 2010;**113**(5):1144–62.

41. Morin AM, Kratz CD, Eberhart LH, Dinges G, Heider E, Schwarz N, et al. Postoperative analgesia and functional recovery after total-knee replacement: comparison of a continuous posterior lumbar plexus (psoas compartment) block, a continuous femoral nerve block, and the combination of a continuous femoral and sciatic nerve block. Regional Anesthesia and Pain Medicine. 2005;**30**(5):434–45.

42. Charous MT, Madison SJ, Suresh PJ, Sandhu NS, Loland VJ, Mariano ER, et al. Continuous femoral nerve blocks: varying local anesthetic delivery method (bolus versus basal) to minimize quadriceps motor block while maintaining sensory block. Anesthesiology. 2011;**115**(4):774–81.

43. Ilfeld BM, Duke KB, Donohue MC. The association between lower extremity continuous peripheral nerve blocks and patient falls after knee and hip arthroplasty. Anesthesia and Analgesia. 2010;**111**(6):1552–54.

44. Muraskin SI, Conrad B, Zheng N, Morey TE, Enneking FK. Falls associated with lower-extremity-nerve blocks: a pilot investigation of mechanisms. Regional Anesthesia and Pain Medicine. 2007;**32**(1):67–72.

45. Wasserstein D, Farlinger C, Brull R, Mahomed N, Gandhi R. Advanced age, obesity and continuous femoral nerve blockade are independent risk factors for inpatient falls after primary total knee arthroplasty. Journal of Arthroplasty. 2013;**28**(7):1121–24.

46. Nie H, Yang YX, Wang Y, Liu Y, Zhao B, Luan B. Effects of continuous fascia iliaca compartment blocks for postoperative analgesia in hip fracture patients. Pain Research & Management. 2015;**20**(4):210–12.

47. Foss NB, Kristensen BB, Bundgaard M, Bak M, Heiring C, Virkelyst C, et al. Fascia iliaca compartment blockade for acute pain control in hip fracture patients: a randomized, placebo-controlled trial. Anesthesiology. 2007;**106**(4):773–78.

48. Williams H, Paringe V, Shenoy S, Michaels P, Ramesh B. Standard preoperative analgesia with or without fascia iliaca compartment block for femoral neck fractures. Journal of Orthopaedic Surgery (Hong Kong). 2016;**24**(1):31–35.

49. Swenson JD, Davis JJ, Stream JO, Crim JR, Burks RT, Greis PE. Local anesthetic injection deep to the fascia iliaca at the level of the inguinal ligament: the pattern of distribution and effects on the obturator nerve. Journal of Clinical Anesthesia. 2015;**27**(8):652–57.

50. Dolan J, Williams A, Murney E, Smith M, Kenny GN. Ultrasound guided fascia iliaca block: a comparison with the loss of resistance technique. Regional Anesthesia and Pain Medicine. 2008;**33**(6):526–31.

51. Jaeger P, Zaric D, Fomsgaard JS, Hilsted KL, Bjerregaard J, Gyrn J, et al. Adductor canal block versus femoral nerve block for analgesia after total knee arthroplasty: a randomized, double-blind study. Regional Anesthesia and Pain Medicine. 2013;**38**(6):526–32.

52. Jenstrup MT, Jaeger P, Lund J, Fomsgaard JS, Bache S, Mathiesen O, et al. Effects of adductor-canal-blockade on pain and ambulation after total knee arthroplasty: a randomized study. Acta Anaesthesiologica Scandinavica. 2012;**56**(3):357–64.

53. Burckett-St Laurant D, Peng P, Giron Arango L, Niazi AU, Chan VW, Agur A, et al. The nerves of the adductor canal and the innervation of the knee: an anatomic study. Regional Anesthesia and Pain Medicine. 2016;**41**(3):321–27.

54. Bruhn J, Van Geffen GJ, Gielen MJ, Scheffer GJ. Visualization of the course of the sciatic nerve in adult volunteers by ultrasonography. Acta Anaesthesiologica Scandinavica. 2008;**52**(9):1298–302.

55. Soberon JR, McInnis C, Bland KS, Egger AL, Patterson ME, Elliott CE, et al. Ultrasound-guided popliteal sciatic nerve blockade in the severely and morbidly obese: a prospective and randomized study. Journal of Anesthesia. 2016;**30**(3):397–404.

Cardiopulmonary resuscitation in the obese patient

Eric Stander

Airway considerations

Obese patients do not tolerate apnoea well due to overall lower base-line natural resting oxygen saturations [1] and also tend to desaturate more rapidly [2] due to high metabolic demand and low functional residual capacity. In addition, it is more difficult to ventilate obese patients with bag-valve masks as a result of altered anatomy and physiology, including decreased chest wall compliance, and eleva-tion of the diaphragm [2]. With these factors in mind, there may be only enough time for one attempt at tracheal intubation before crit-ical oxygen desaturation occurs [3]. Obesity has also been demon-strated to predict difficult mask ventilation [4]. In a prospective study of more than 1500 individuals undergoing elective surgery, a body mass index greater than 26 kg/m^2 predicted difficulty in maintaining oxygen saturations above 92% with mask ventilation during general anaesthesia [5]. Thus, all clinicians who may be required to provide CPR, which is almost always in an acute and unexpected setting, need to remain proficient in the ability to mask ventilate the obese patient as physicians traditionally rely on this rescue technique fol-lowing failed attempts at tracheal intubation [5].

Though a factor in difficult mask ventilation, there is little evi-dence to discern obesity as an independent predictor for diffi-cult intubation; obesity alone does not seem to affect the ability to directly visualize airway structures [6]. Mallampati score and diabetes mellitus have been demonstrated to be more predictive of difficult tracheal intubation [2]. Other considerations for diffi-culty intubation include small jaw, limitations in mouth opening, and limitations in ability to extend the neck [7]. Additionally, in a study reviewing traumatic intubations, obese patients were actu-ally found to be no more difficult than lean patients [8]. However, proper positioning utilizing a modified procedure has been found to facilitate intubation in the obese. Considering a non-traditional positioning has been demonstrated to help in endotracheal intub-ation. The classic sniffing position may be detrimental in the obese patient [9–12]. Therefore, considering a manoeuvre called stacking using towels or blankets folded and placed under the shoulders will lift the chin above the chest. The auditory canal is placed at the level of the sternal notch. This position is also referred to as the 'HELP' or 'head-elevated laryngoscopy position'. This positioning adjusts for posterior cervical fat, which generates an increased flexion of the neck [13].

Another consideration is to utilize nasotracheal intubation. In patients whose pre-intubation assessment suggests a likely difficult oral intubation, blind nasotracheal intubation by an experienced physician is a valid first choice. Two reports place the success rate of blind nasotracheal intubation at 79% and 95% respectively in an experienced physician's hands [14,15].

Other considerations must be given to oesophageal-tracheal intubating devices as direct visualization is not necessary, and sev-eral types of commercially available oesophageal obturator tubes have been shown to be successful in the obese. In addition, video laryngoscopy and fibreoptic-guided intubation also have been shown to be acceptable alternatives [16–19]. Fibreoptic intubation, expectedly but unfortunately, requires set up and preparation along with a cooperative and conscious patient, factors not always met in the situation of an emergent intubation.

A final option and the most invasive approach to a definitive airway is the surgical airway. The least invasive approaches among these include transtracheal needle jet ventilation and retrograde wire intubation. In obese patients, loss of anatomical landmarks and redundant tissue can interfere with the needle placement, making these procedures more difficult [20]; however, it has been dem-onstrated that needle and surgical cricothyroidotomy can be per-formed effectively [21].

Ventilatory considerations

During resuscitation, ventilation also may be more difficult. Several factors play into this difficulty. As mentioned earlier, obese pa-tients will desaturate more rapidly and bag-valve mask ventilation is more difficult. Increased chest wall resistance, decreased lung compliance, and an elevated diaphragm also interfere with ven-tilation [22]. Additionally, increased airway pressures, secondary

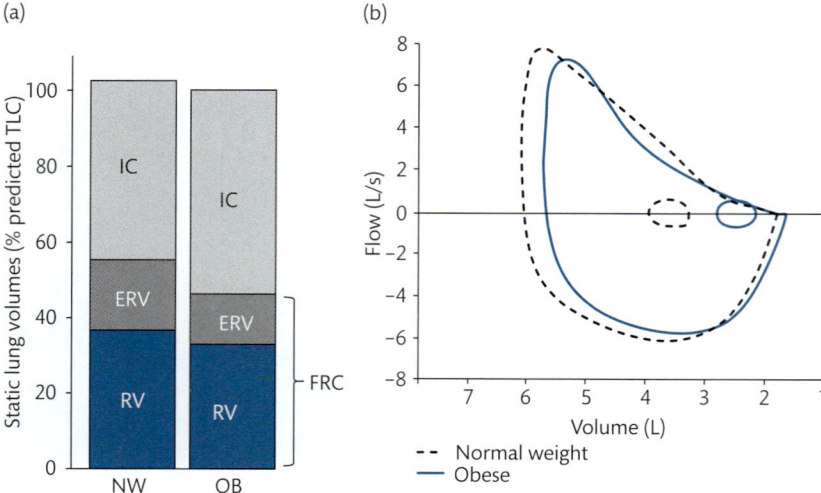

(a) Static lung volumes measured by body plethysmography are shown at rest: expiratory reserve volume (ERV) and functional residual capacity (FRC) are decreased, and inspiratory capacity (IC) is increased in the obese (OB) group compared with the normal weight (NW) group of healthy adults. (b) Maximal and tidal flow-volume loops are shown at rest in normal weight (dashed lines) and obese (solid lines) subjects. In obesity, tidal flow-volume loops are shifted rightwards and maximal midexpiratory flow rates may be reduced resulting in greater expiratory flow limitation during resting breathing. RV: residual volume.

Fig. 24.1 Change of chest wall compliance due to obesity.

Reproduced with permission from O'Donnell, D. E., Webb, K. A., and Guenette, J. A., Respiratory Consequences of Mild-to-Moderate Obesity: Impact on Exercise Performance in Health and in Chronic Obstructive Pulmonary Disease, *Pulmonary Medicine.* Copyright © 2012 Denis E. O'Donnell et al. Distributed under the Creative Commons Attribution 3.0 Unported (CC BY 3.0). https://creativecommons.org/licenses/by/3.0/

to these factors mentioned previously, will cause added stomach distention and higher risk of aspiration. Intubation early in resuscitation is a safer consideration than continued bag-valve masks, which get progressively harder and less effective as the time of bag-mask ventilation increases. Tolerance of higher than normal peak expiratory pressures as well as acceptance of increased ventilator rates (smaller lung capacity, increased oxygen demands, and increased carbon dioxide production) may be needed to maintain oxygenation [21]. This added ventilatory effort, in concert with chest compression, may lead to an increased risk of barotrauma to the lung.

The overall effect of obesity can be demonstrated in multiple studies. Airway resistance increases [23], chest wall compliance decreases [24], gas exchange decreases [25], and arterial saturations are negatively affected [26]. There is a direct correlation in all components of lung volume with increasing obesity (**Fig. 24.1**). Overall, as obesity increases, the total lung volumes decrease and pulmonary resistance increases [27].

In addition, ventilator settings are also critical due to all the same factors seen while using the bag-valve mask. This stems from both functional issues (i.e. low end-expiratory volumes, lower tidal volumes, decreased lung wall compliance) and cellular issues (i.e. increased inflammatory processes on distal airways) and requires that the ventilator uses '(1) stepwise recruitment manoeuvre before positive end-expiratory pressure application, which requires titration according to respiratory system dynamic compliance; and (2) tidal volume (VT) titration according to inspiratory capacity' [28].

Cardiopulmonary resuscitation considerations

Performance of CPR in the morbidly obese generates additional challenges. Due to body habitus, external compression devices may not fit around the patient. Proper positioning may be difficult as adipose tissue may roll the patient out of the ideal position, and access to the chest wall may be limited by space constraints. In addition, it may be difficult to access the appropriate depth of compressions, as palpation of peripheral arteries may not be possible.

Because of these issues, standard practice must be followed. First, ensure the patient is on a hard surface such as a spine board or CPR board or table. Second, be sure the patient is best positioned to allow optimum access to the chest area. Third, consider an arterial line, with maintenance of diastolic pressure greater than 25 mmHg [29], or end-tidal capnography to assure adequacy of circulation during compressions. It appears that maintaining an end-tidal carbon dioxide level of 20 mmHg correlates to a higher likelihood of survival, as do sudden increases in end-tidal carbon dioxide indicating spontaneous return of circulation [30].

In addition, consider placing the patient in the lateral tilt position, as this has been suggested in pregnant patients in order to increase venous return by reducing intraabdominal pressure [31]. It has been demonstrated in manikin studies, however, that compressions in the lateral position are inferior to those done in the supine position. If the left lateral tilt position is used, maximizing the tilt to greater than 30 degrees is recommended [32].

With regard to defibrillating, whether monophasic or biphasic energy delivery is used appears to make no real difference to the result, since both deliver adequate energy to the heart and there appears to be no superiority of one type of energy over the other in clinical trials [33]. It is recommended to use whichever defibrillator is most readily available. What appears to be more important is the use of higher energy but less often, as it is possible that multiple shocks damage myocardial tissue more than total energy [34] and high energy does not cause more damage than low energy in a single shock [35].

Another reason to consider higher-energy defibrillation at the outset is that tissue impedance is greater in obesity directly due to excess tissue. There is a direct correlation to body weight and transthoracic impedance, with average impedance ranging from 70 to 80 ohms [36], but impedance in humans can range from 25 to 180 ohms. In one animal model study, it was demonstrated that there was decreased success to defibrillation at lower energies [37]. However, in human studies, there have been no clear advantages to using increased initial energy in the obese [38–40]. Probably the most important factor in energy delivery is the size of and the pressure applied to the defibrillator pad [41]. Commercially available pads, especially those that are of the adhesive type, have optimized that consideration.

Pharmacological considerations

There are many considerations in dosing of medications, not the least of which is volume of distribution. In obese patients, the volume of distribution will increase significantly in fat-soluble drugs, and individual drug dosing change based on body habitus. However, other considerations such as plasma protein binding, albumin concentrations, and alpha-1-acid glycoprotein concentrations do not appear to be affected with any clinical significance [42].

Currently, there are not specific dosing guidelines for most ACLS drugs and it is well recognized that controlled studies are necessary. Until such studies can be performed, medication dosing will continue to follow weight-based models [43–48]. The doses shown in Table 24.1 are guidelines only and should be adjusted based on clinical situations.

Table 24.1 Suggested dosing of some critical drugs

Class	Drug	Recommended dosing weight	Comments
Paralytics	Succinyl choline [49]	TBW	Provides better intubating conditions
	Rocuronium [50]	IBW	Longer durations of action when dosed at TBW
	Vecuronium [50]	IBW	Longer durations of action when dosed at TBW
Sedative-hypnotics	Etomidate [50]	IBW	
	Ketamine [51]		No evidence currently available
	Propofol [50]	LBW	Clearance at steady state increases with TBW
	Fentanyl [50]	LBW	Clearance increases correlate with increased lean body mass
	Lorazepam [52]	Load—IBW, maintenance—TBW	
	Midazolam [53]	Load—TBW, maintenance—IBW	
	Pentobarbital [53]	TBW	Monitor serum blood levels
Pressors	Epinephrine [54]	TBW	No evidence currently available
	Dobutamine [55]	No evidence currently available	
	Dopamine [55]	No evidence currently available	
	Norepinephrine [55]	No evidence currently available	
	Vasopressin [55]	Not dosed by weight	No evidence currently available
Antiarrhythmics	Lidocaine [55]	No evidence currently available	
	Procainamide [56]	IBW	Used for load and maintenance
	Amiodarone [55]	No evidence currently available	
	Diltiazem [55]	Consider loading by adjusted body weight and titrate to effect	
	Verapamil [55]	Consider loading by adjusted body weight and titrate to effect	
	Adenosine [56]	Not dosed by weight	
	Esmolol	TBW	Brand drug monograph
	Propranolol [55]	Initial dose based on IBW with subsequent dosing by effect	
	Labetalol [55]	Initial dose based on IBW with subsequent dosing by effect	
	Metoprolol	No weight-based dosing	Brand drug monograph
	Nifedipine	No weight-based dosing	Brand drug monograph
Inotropes	Isoproterenol [56]	IBW	No evidence currently available

IBW, ideal body weight; LBW, lean body weight; TBW, total body weight.
Note: there is little data to support these guidelines.

Survival considerations

There have been very few studies addressing the probability of obese patients to achieve return of spontaneous circulation following cardiac arrest, and it is well known that obesity places the patient at risk for worsening outcomes with chronic disease, surgery, and traumatic injury [56–63]. To note, one large study on in-hospital cardiac arrest in obese children demonstrated lower survival in the obese patients [64]. In addition, several case studies in adults demonstrate no difference in survivability following cardiac arrest despite multiple authors discussing the obesity paradox which demonstrates better outcomes when surviving cardiovascular events [65–67]. In fact, one study following patients with implantable defibrillators demonstrated better survival when obese [68].

Therapeutic hypothermia has been demonstrated to improve neurological outcomes post cardiac resuscitation. This is a process in which the body is cooled to 32°C immediately following the return of circulation. There are no specific data on the use of therapeutic hypothermia in obese patients, but many logistical issues do arise. Forethought will need to be given, as the patient may not fit commercially available vests used for cooling. Significantly greater quantities of ice may be necessary to achieve the desired temperatures due to the insulating qualities of body fat. Location of and positioning of ice packs may be difficult due to space limitations on beds. There are several commercially available devices to aid in this process, and special considerations have been made by the manufacturer. For instance, in the package insert for the Arctic Sun™ (Medivance, Louisville, CO, USA), it is suggested that in patients weighing greater than 100 kg, additional pads will need to be placed over the thorax to achieve appropriate cooling.

Resuscitation in the obese is best summarized by the American Heart Association guideline for cardiopulmonary resuscitation as 'cardiac arrest in the morbidly obese morbid obesity can provide challenges during the resuscitation attempt. Airway management may be more challenging, and changes to the thorax may make resuscitative efforts more demanding' [32].

REFERENCES

1. Kapur VK, Wilsdon AG, Au D, Avdalovic M, Enright P, Fan VS, et al. Obesity is associated with a lower resting oxygen saturation in the ambulatory elderly: results from the cardiovascular health study. Respir Care. 2013;**58**(5):831–37.
2. Rocke DA, Murray WB, Rout CC, Gouws E. Relative risk analysis of factors associated with difficult intubation in obstetric anesthesia. Anesthesiology. 1977;**77**(1):67–73.
3. Benumof JL, Dagg R, Benumof R. Critical hemoglobin desaturation will occur before return to an unparalyzed state following 1 mg/kg intravenous succinylcholine. Anesthesiology. 1997;**87**(4):979–82.
4. Apfelbaum JL, Hagberg CA, Caplan RA, Blitt CD, Connis RT, Nickinovich DG, et al. Practice guidelines for management of the difficult airway: an updated report by the American Society of Anesthesiologists Task Force on Management of the Difficult Airway. Updated by the Committee on Standards and Practice Parameters. Anesthesiology. 2013;**118**(2):251–70.
5. Langeron O, Masso E, Huraux C, Guggiari M, Bianchi A, Coriat P, et al. Prediction of difficult mask ventilation. Anesthesiology. 2000;**92**(5):1229–36.
6. Ezri T, Warters RD, Szmuk P, Saad-Eddin H, Geva D, Katz J, et al. The incidence of class "zero" airway and the impact of Mallampati score, age, sex, and body mass index on prediction of laryngoscopy grade. Anesth Analg. 2001;**93**(4):1073–75.
7. Mallampati SR, Gatt SP, Gugino LD, Desai SP, Waraksa B, Freiberger D, et al. A clinical sign to predict difficult tracheal intubation: a prospective study. Can Anaesth Soc J. 1985;**32**(4):429–34.
8. Mashour GA, Kheterpal S, Vanaharam V, Shanks A, Wang LY, Sandberg WS, et al. The extended Mallampati score and a diagnosis of diabetes mellitus are predictors of difficult laryngoscopy in the morbidly obese. Anesth Analg. 2008;**107**(6):1919–23.
9. Ogunnaike BO, Whitten CW. Anesthetic management of morbidly obese patients. Semin Anesth Perioperat Med Pain. 2002;**21**(1):46–58.
10. Rao SL, Kunselman AR, Schuler HG, DesHarnais S. Laryngoscopy and tracheal intubation in the head-elevated position in obese. Anesth Analg. 2008;**107**(6):1912–18.
11. Collins JS, Lemmens HJ, Brodsky JB, Brock-Utne JG, Levitan RM. Laryngoscopy and morbid obesity: a comparison of the "sniff" and "ramped" positions. Obes Surg. 2004;**14**(9):1171–75.
12. Lee BJ, Kang JM, Kim DO. Laryngeal exposure during laryngoscopy is better in the 25 degrees back-up position than in the supine position. Br J Anaesth. 2007;**99**(4):581–86.
13. Levitan RM, Mechem CC, Ochroch EA, Shofer FS, Hollander JE. Head-elevated laryngoscopy position: improving laryngeal exposure during laryngoscopy by increasing head elevation. Ann Emerg Med. 2003;**41**(3):322–30.
14. Roppolo LP, Vilke GM, Chan TC, Krishel S, Hayden SR, Rosen P, et al. Nasotracheal intubation in the emergency department, revisited. J Emerg Med. 1999;**17**(5):791–99.
15. Van Elstraete AC, Mamie JC, Mehdaoui H. Nasotracheal intubation in patients with immobilized cervical spine: a comparison of tracheal tube cuff inflation and fiberoptic bronchoscopy. Anesth Analg. 1998;**87**(2):400–402.
16. Rosenblatt WH, Murphy M. The intubating laryngeal mask: use of a new ventilating-intubating device in the emergency department. Ann Emerg Med. 1999;**33**(2):234–38.
17. Reed AP. The unanticipated difficult airway. Anesthesiology Clin North Am. 1996;**14**:443–69.
18. Andersen LH, Rovsing L, Olsen KS. GlideScope videolaryngoscope vs. Macintosh direct laryngoscope for intubation of morbidly obese patients: a randomized trial. Acta Anaesthesiol Scand. 2011;**55**(9):1090–97.
19. Abdelmalak, BB, Bernstein E, Egan C, Abdallah R, You J, Sessler DI, et al. GlideScope vs flexible fibreoptic scope for elective intubation in obese patients. Anaesthesia. 2011;**66**(7):550–55.
20. Patel RG. Percutaneous transtracheal jet ventilation. Chest. 1999;**116**(6):1689–94.
21. Rehm CG, Wanek SM, Gagnon EB, Pearson SK, Mullins RJ. Cricothyroidotomy for elective airway management in critically ill trauma patients with technically challenging neck anatomy. Crit Care. 2002;**6**(6):531–35.
22. Dargin J, Medzon R. Emergency department management of airway in obese adults. Ann Emerg Med. 2010;**56**(2):95–104.
23. Zerah F, Harf A, Perlemuter L, Lorino H, Lorino AM, Atlan G. Effects of obesity on respiratory resistance. Chest. 1993;**103**(5):1470–76.
24. Surratt P, Wilheit S, Hsiao H. Compliance of the chest wall in obese subjects. Appl Physiol. 1984;**57**:403–409.
25. Pelosi P, Croci M, Ravagnan I, Tredici S, Pedoto A, Lissoni A, et al. The effect of body mass on lung volumes, respiratory

mechanics, and gas exchange during general anesthesia. Anesth Analg. 1998;**87**(3):654–60.

26. Pelosi P, Croci M, Ravagnan I, Vicardi P, Gattioni L. Total respiratory system, lung and chest wall mechanics in sedated paralysed postoperative morbidly obese patients. Chest. 1996;**109**(1):144–51.

27. Brazzale DJ, Pretto JJ, Schachter LM. Optimizing respiratory function assessment to elucidate the impact of obesity on respiratory health. Respirology. 2015;**20**(5):715–21.

28. Leme Silva P, Pelosi P, Rocco PR. Mechanical ventilation in obese patients. Minerva Anestesiol. 2012;**78**(10):1136–45.

29. Meaney PA, Bobrow BJ, Mancini ME, Christenson J, de Caen AR, Bhanji F, et al. CPR quality: improving cardiac resuscitation outcomes both inside and outside the hospital. A consensus statement from the American Heart Association. Circulation. 2013;**128**(4):417–35.

30. Shankar Kodali B, Urman RD. Capnography during cardiopulmonary resuscitation: current evidence and future directions. J Emerg Trauma Shock. 2014;**7**(4):332–40.

31. Sugerman H, Windsor A, Bessos M, Wolfe, L. Intra-abdominal pressure, sagittal abdominal diameter and obesity comorbidity. J Intern Med. 1997;**241**(1):71–79.

32. Vanden Hoek TL, Morrison LJ, Shuster M, Donnino M, Sinz E, Lavonas EJ, et al. Part 12: cardiac arrest in special situations. 2010 American Heart Association guidelines for cardiopulmonary resuscitation and emergency cardiovascular care. Circulation. 2010;**122**(18 Suppl 3):S829–61.

33. Morrison LJ, Henry RM, Ku V, Nolan JP, Morley P, Deakin CD. Single-shock defibrillation success in adult cardiac arrest: a systematic review. Resuscitation. 2013;**84**(11):1480–86.

34. Hasdemir C, Shah N, Rao AP, Acosta H, Matsudaira K, Neas BR, Reynolds DW, et al. Analysis of troponin I levels after spontaneous implantable cardioverter defibrillator shocks. J Cardiovasc Electrophysiol. 2002;**13**(2):144–50.

35. Walcott GP, Melnick SB, Killingsworth CR, Ideker RE. Comparison of low-energy versus high-energy biphasic defibrillation shocks following prolonged ventricular fibrillation. Prehosp Emerg Care. 2010;**14**(1):62–70.

36. Link MS, Atkins DL, Passman RS, Halperin HR, Samson RA, White RD, et al. Part 6: electrical therapies; automated external defibrillators, defibrillation, cardioversion, and pacing; 2010 American Heart Association guidelines for cardiopulmonary resuscitation and emergency cardiovascular care. Circulation. 2010;**122**(18 Suppl 3):S706–19.

37. Zhang Y, Clark CB, Davies LR, Davies LR, Karlsson G, Zimmerman MB, et al. Body weight is a predictor of biphasic shock success for low energy transthoracic defibrillation. Resuscitation. 2002;**54**(3):281–87.

38. White RD, Blackwell TH, Russell JK, Jorgenson DB. Body weight does not affect defibrillation, resuscitation, or survival in patients with out-of-hospital cardiac arrest treated with a nonescalating biphasic waveform defibrillator. Crit Care Med. 2004;**32**(9 Suppl):S387–92.

39. Gascho JA, Crampton RS, Sipes JN, Cherwek ML, Hunter FP, O'Brien WM. Energy levels and patient weight in ventricular defibrillation. JAMA. 1979;**242**(13):1380–84.

40. DeSilva RA, Lown B. Energy requirement for defibrillation of a markedly overweight patient. Circulation. 1978;**57**(4):827–30.

41. Kerber RE, Grayzel J, Hoyt R, Marcus M, Kennedy J. Transthoracic resistance in human defibrillation: Influence of body weight, chest size, serial shocks, paddle size and paddle contact pressure. Circulation. 1981;**63**(3):676–82.

42. Wiles MD, Hardman JG, Moppett IK. Pharmacokinetic variation. Anaesth Intensive Care Med. 2008;**9**(8):369–71.

43. Rowe S, Siegel D, Benjamin DK Jr. Gaps in drug dosing for obese children: a systematic review of commonly prescribed emergency care medications. Best Pharmaceuticals for Children Act— Pediatric Trials Network Administrative Core Committee. Clin Ther. 2015;**37**(9):1924–32.

44. Pai MP. Drug dosing based on weight and body surface area: mathematical assumptions and limitations in obese adults. Pharmacotherapy. 2012;**32**(9):856–68.

45. Erstad BL. Dosing of medications in morbidly obese patients in the intensive care unit setting. Intensive Care Med. 2004;**30**(1):18–32.

46. Abernethy DR, Greenblatt DJ. Lidocaine disposition in obesity. Am J Cardiol. 1984;**53**(8):1183–86.

47. Christoff PB, Conti DR, Naylor C, Jusko WJ. Procainamide disposition in obesity. Drug Intell Clin Pharm. 1983;**17**(7–8):516–22.

48. Kowey PR, Marinchak RA, Rials SJ, Bharucha DB. Classification and pharmacology of antiarrhythmic Drugs. Am Heart J. 2000;**140**(1):12–20.

49. Ingrande J, Lemmens HJM. Dose adjustment of anaesthetics in the morbidly obese. Br J Anaesth. 2010;**105**(Suppl 1):i16–23.

50. Gaszynski TM, Jakubiak J, Szewczyk T. Etomidate can be dosed according to ideal body weight in morbidly obese patients. Eur J Anaesthesiol. 2014;**31**(12):713–14.

51. Aantaa R, Tonner P, Conti G, Longrois D, Mantz J, Mulier JP. Sedation options for the morbidly obese intensive care unit patient; a concise survey and an agenda for development. Multidiscip Respir Med. 2015;**10**(1):8.

52. Casati A, Putzu M. Anesthesia in the obese patient: pharmacokinetic considerations. J Clin Anaesthesia. 2005;**27**(2):134–45.

53. Wilkes L, Danziger LH, Rodvold KA. Phenobarbital pharmacokinetics in obesity. A case report. Clin Pharmacokinet. 1992;**22**(6):481–484.

54. Erstad BL. Dosing of medications in morbidly obese patients in the intensive care unit setting. Intensive Care Med. 2004;**30**(1):18–32.

55. Kane-Gill S, Dasta J. High-Risk IV Medications in Special Patient Populations. London: Springer-Verlag; 2011.

56. Lewandowski K, Lewandowski M. Intensive care in the obese. Best Pract Res Clin Anaesthesiol. 2011;**25**(1):95–108.

57. Bamgbade OA, Rutter TW, Nafiu OO, Dorje P. Postoperative complications in obese and nonobese patients. World J Surg. 2007;**31**(3):556–60.

58. Drenick EJ, Fisler JS. Sudden cardiac arrest in morbidly obese surgical patients unexplained after autopsy. Am J Surg. 1988;**155**(6):720–26.

59. Ciesla DJ, Moore EE, Johnson JL, Burch JM, Cothren CC, Sauaia A. Obesity increases risk of organ failure after severe trauma. J Am Coll Surg. 2006;**203**(4):539–45.

60. Byrnes MC, McDaniel MD, Moore MB, Helmer SD, Smith RS. The effect of obesity on outcomes among injured patients. J Trauma. 2005;**58**(2):232–37.

61. Duane TM, Dechert T, Aboutanos MB, Malhotra AK, Ivatury RR. Obesity and outcomes after blunt trauma. J Trauma. 2006;**61**(5):1218–21.

62. Winfield RD, Delano MJ, Lottenberg L, Cendan JC, Moldawer LL, Maier RV, et al. Traditional resuscitative practices fail to resolve metabolic acidosis in morbidly obese patients after severe blunt trauma. J Trauma. 2010;**68**(2):317–30.

63. Calle EE, Thun MJ, Petrelli JM, Rodriguez C, Heath CW Jr. Body-mass index and mortality in a prospective cohort of U.S. adults. N Engl J Med. 1999;**341**(15):1097–105.

64. Srinivasan V, Nadkarni VM, Helfaer MA, Carey SM, Berg RA. Childhood obesity and survival after in-hospital pediatric cardiopulmonary resuscitation. Pediatrics. 2010;**125**(3):e481–88.

65. Testori C, Sterz F, Losert H, Krizanac D, Haugk M, Uray T, et al. Cardiac arrest survivors with moderate elevated body mass index may have a better neurological outcome: a cohort study. Resuscitation. 2011;**82**(7):869–73.

66. Banack HR, Kaufman JS. The obesity paradox: understanding the effect of obesity on mortality among individuals with cardiovascular disease. Prev Med. 2014;**62**:96–10.

67. Greenberg JA. The obesity paradox in the US population. Am J Clin Nutr. 2013;**97**(6):1195–200.

68. Bunch TJ, White RD, Lopez-Jimenez F, Thomas RJ. Association of body weight with total mortality and with ICD shocks among survivors of ventricular fibrillation in out-of-hospital cardiac arrest. Resuscitation. 2008;**77**(3):351–55.

Day care surgery

Adrian Sultana

Overview

Anaesthetists encounter morbidly obese patients in every aspect of their daily practice. It is estimated that at least 36.5% of adults in the United States presenting as day surgery clients are morbidly obese [1]. Of even greater concern to the occasional paediatric anaesthetist, 20% of children presenting for ambulatory surgery are obese [2].

Day surgery endows undoubted benefits to the patient, clinician, and hospital; however, controversy rages about whether morbidly obese patients are suitable for day surgery. Should anaesthetists set limits of weight, body mass index (BMI), or comorbidities that exclude certain patients from the freestanding day surgery environment (Table 25.1) [3–5]?

The majority of anaesthetists are concerned about airway management, sleep-disordered breathing, or obstructive sleep apnoea and the raft of comorbidities that accompany obesity [6].

It is clear that obese patients should not be excluded from the benefits of day surgery if their management for a particular surgical episode would be unaltered had they been treated as an inpatient [7]. Guidelines from the Association of Anaesthetists and the British Association of Day Surgery emphasize that neither obesity nor obstructive sleep apnoea should preclude patients from day surgery [8].

There is also increasing evidence that the less invasive cohort of the bariatric surgical spectrum including laparoscopic gastric banding and sleeve gastrectomy may be performed as an outpatient, in this context defined as discharge within 23 hours of surgery [9].

Preoperative assessment

No morbidly obese patient should present for anaesthesia and surgery unannounced on the day that the procedure is scheduled. These patients should be assessed by the anaesthesia team at least a few days prior to presentation and preferably 1 month prior to allow for planning and optimization of comorbidities.

This evaluation is predominantly clinical and extensive laboratory tests or imaging are not performed unless specifically indicated [10].

Some units take the opportunity to educate and institute a weight loss adjunct such as a very-low-carbohydrate diet [11].

The venue for this visit is generally a dedicated preassessment clinic, or the bariatric multidisciplinary clinic and the seamless transmission of data between the anaesthetists in the clinic and the treating anaesthetist is paramount.

Airway assessment

Obesity is widely feared by anaesthetists and emergency healthcare providers as a portent of difficult airway management (Box 25.1). Difficult bag and mask ventilation [12], difficult intubation [13], and rapid desaturation are entrenched in the literature and rightly so.

Each of these difficulties may be avoided by precise airway assessment, correct preoxygenation in the head-up position with end-tidal oxygraphy [14,15], and skilful airway selection [16].

Every day surgery unit that considers admitting morbidly obese patients should have access to the whole range of sophisticated airway equipment sometimes known as 'the difficult intubation

Table 25.1 Timeline of limits set for obese patients scheduled for day surgery

1992: Royal College of Surgeons of England	BMI <30 kg/m² [3]
2012: Society for Ambulatory Anesthesia guidelines focused on obstructive sleep apnoea and comorbidities	BMI <40 kg/m² [4]
2017	BMI <50 g/m² [5] No BMI limit Day case bariatric

Box 25.1 Difficult airway predictors in the morbidly obese

- Male sex.
- (Facial hair).
- Mallampati score 3 and 4.
- Obstructive sleep apnoea: diagnosed or presumed.
- Poor neck movement.
- Neck circumference greater than 40 cm.
- Previous documented failed/difficult intubation.

trolley' and the services of an 'airway guru' [17] (**Fig. 25.1**) skilled in all modern elective and emergency airway techniques including front-of-neck rescue.

Good clinical practice and avoidance of medicolegal attrition dictate that these predictors should all be carefully examined and documented well in advance of the surgical episode.

Respiratory assessment

The morbidly obese patient presents us with a triple respiratory conundrum:

1. Increasing obesity is accompanied by profound pathophysiological impairment of gas exchange [18]
2. Sleep-disordered breathing is common [19]
3. A mixed obstructive/restrictive lung lesion accompanies obesity [20].

Although preoperative spirometry is not routinely indicated in the morbidly obese patient presenting for day surgery, any evidence of reactive lower airways due to smoking or asthma should be aggressively sought and treated by routine means such as bronchodilators, chest physiotherapy, and smoking cessation.

Many patients will present with a frank diagnosis of sleep apnoea and will own and use a continuous positive airway pressure machine at home; these patients are asked to bring their machine to the centre and generally do well. In contrast, other patients will

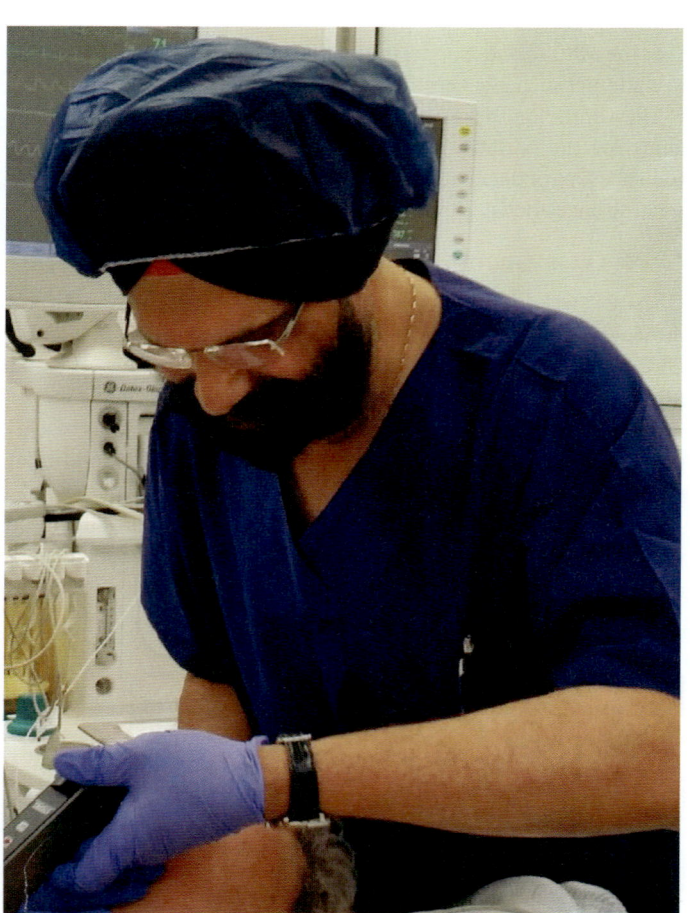

Fig. 25.1 An 'airway guru'.

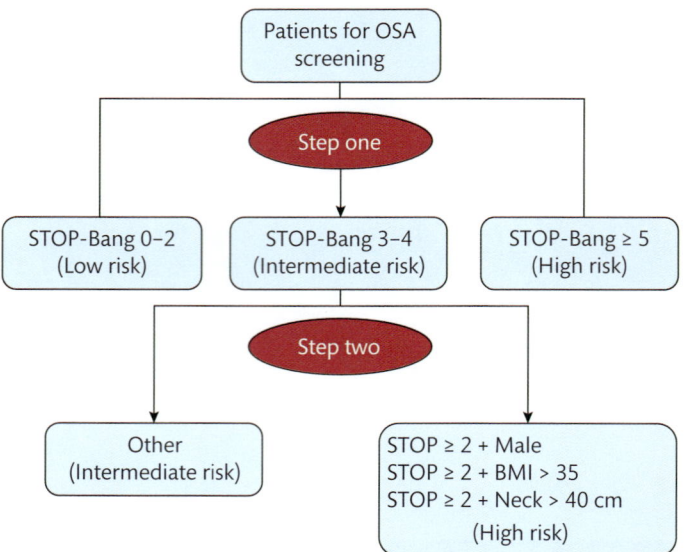

Fig. 25.2 Screening for obstructive sleep apnoea.

Reproduced from Chung, F., Abdullah, H. R., Liao, P., STOP-Bang Questionnaire A Practical Approach to Screen for Obstructive Sleep Apnea, *CHEST*, 149(3):631–638. Copyright (2016) American College of Chest Physicians with permission from Elsevier. DOI: https://doi.org/10.1378/chest.15-0903

have undiagnosed sleep-disordered breathing and need to be carefully evaluated.

In the author's practice, if the 'STOP-Bang' questionnaire [21] renders a score greater than 5 and the surgical procedure is not urgent, patients are referred for polysomnography and titrated continuous positive airway pressure (**Fig. 25.2**).

Cardiovascular assessment

It is every anaesthetist's nightmare to appear on television escorting a critically ill patient out of a free-standing suburban day surgery into a waiting ambulance with flashing lights or worse still to be present at an outcome of death or severe brain injury in the day surgery environment [22,23]. It is therefore imperative that no stone be left unturned or comorbidity left untreated when a morbidly obese patient is proposed for day surgery.

The general public, and indeed the American Heart Association [24], regard ambulatory surgery as low risk but this low risk has been achieved by institutions investing time and money on infrastructure and staffing together with experienced physician anaesthesiologists who have achieved excellence both in the selection of patients and in the delivery of high-quality ambulatory anaesthesia.

An absolute minimum of standard clinical history and examination together with a resting 12-lead electrocardiogram (ECG), chest X-ray, and basic blood tests form the cornerstone of the initial cardiac assessment of any morbidly obese patient presenting for surgery.

The astute clinician will be on the lookout for risk factors of coronary artery disease such as:

- Male sex
- Metabolic syndrome [25]
- Tobacco use
- Arrhythmia

- Deep vein thrombosis
- Cardiovascular medication history.

ECG changes may need to be followed up with further non-invasive testing.

In particular, atrial fibrillation is now known to be independently associated with obesity [26] and must be controlled by pharmacological means or the patient may need to be referred for electrical treatment or ablation.

Patients with atrial fibrillation may also need their anticoagulation suspended prior to surgery; many of these patients will now be on a 'non-vitamin K antagonist oral anticoagulant' (NOAC) and anaesthetists will need to be knowledgeable in managing these drugs around the time of surgery [27].

Application of the Fleisher algorithm [24] allows the day surgery anaesthetist to select obese surgery patients and assess their cardiovascular risk. Patients are rejected if their coronary risk factors are three or more and their perioperative management would have been different as an inpatient.

Selection of surgical procedures and the morbidly obese outpatient

At the turn of this century, approximately 25 procedures were identified as commonly suited for day surgery in the general population; by contrast, up to 200 different procedures are routinely performed as day-only procedures in modern healthcare systems.

The principles of surgical selection for day surgery have been clarified in a recent review [28]:

- Abdominal and thoracic surgery should use minimally invasive techniques.
- The degree of surgical trauma is more important than its duration.
- Postoperative pain should be manageable using local anaesthesia and oral analgesia.
- There is a low risk of postoperative complications.
- No continuing blood loss or need for fluid therapy.
- No specialist postoperative care or observation should be needed.
- Patients should be able to mobilize before discharge.
- The operating surgeon must have sufficient experience and a low complication rate in the procedure.

While body surface procedures and limb surgeries are amenable to local and regional analgesia with minimal sedation, many surgical procedures that are popular such as day surgery may represent further challenges to the anaesthetist.

Upper gastrointestinal endoscopy

Typically, upper gastrointestinal endoscopies imply a brief period of shared airway and effective sedation may prove difficult in the morbidly obese because of profound desaturation with minimal doses. In such cases, the operating proceduralist may have to accept compromises such as a head-up position or lesser level of sedation. Dexmedetomidine may have a specific role in this scenario [29]. Conversely, the anaesthetist may seek to control the airway by tracheal intubation.

We have noted an increase in operative gastroscopic procedures, which may mean a longer shared airway time; these include bariatric endoluminal techniques [30] such as:

- Intragastric balloon
- Endoluminal vertical gastroplasty
- Endoscopic sleeve gastroplasty
- Endoscopic gastrointestinal bypass devices.

The 'Stretta' procedure [31] for intractable reflux may also be included.

These procedures probably mandate tracheal intubation during the early adoption phase, although a recent development of the supraglottic airway may hold forth promise in this area [32].

Head and neck; ear, nose, and throat; and dental procedures

These procedures present similar challenges of the shared airway and poor access for the anaesthetist; early and often conservative decisions will need to be made about airway management and scaling up of equipment and staffing may be required.

Gynaecological laparoscopy

In morbidly obese patients, this procedure may present a triple challenge because of:

- Head-down positioning
- Requests for profound neuromuscular blockade
- Ultra-short surgical times.

We recommend that anaesthetists use all the available technology and pharmacology to overcome these obstacles. They will have a need for up-to-date equipment and disposables to manage the airway including video-laryngoscopy, highly rated operating tables, skill in the use of short-acting anaesthetic agents, effective reversal of neuromuscular blockade [33], and non-sedative non-emetic analgesia regimens to ensure early ambulation.

Is there a place for bariatric procedures in the day surgery?

The bariatric surgical literature promotes laparoscopic gastric banding and sleeve gastrectomy as suitable for day surgery and one group has even tried (and failed) 23-hour laparoscopic gastric bypass [34].

In our practice, check endoscopy, intragastric balloon, laparoscopic removal of gastric band, and primary gastric banding in ultra-fit moderately obese patients are the only frequent day case bariatric procedures.

Anaesthesia techniques

We have shown the role of careful patient selection and skilful airway techniques in managing the morbidly obese day surgery patient; however, challenges will abound for the anaesthetist who accepts these patients in a day-only environment. It may be prudent to schedule morbidly obese patients who are being operated in a day surgery environment early in the day to allow for an extended period of monitoring in the post-anaesthesia care unit prior to discharge home.

Premedication

There is a role for 'medical' premedication, in particular broncho-dilators, gastric acid inhibitors, and thromboprophylaxis should be used wherever indicated and may be organized ahead of the day of surgery.

Within this realm, the correct administration or omission of the patient's regular medication often takes some effort. The need to withhold angiotensin-converting enzyme inhibitors and angio-tensin blockers seems poorly appreciated in the mainstream surgical environment [35].

Locoregional anaesthesia

In suitable patients, a local or regional technique should be the first choice. Traditionally, block failure was common in the obese patient; however, the advent of ultrasound-guided blocks has probably min-imized this problem [36].

In our practice, we are keen to use total intravenous anaesthesia–target-controlled infusion despite the problems of titrating the Schnider and Minto protocols at the upper limits of obesity [37] (**Box 25.2**) More recently, we have adopted the opioid-free tech-niques of Mulier [38,39] in conjunction with either desflurane or target-controlled infusion propofol [40].

We also find that the routine application of processed electro-encephalography techniques [41] improves our patients' early awakening and rapid throughput and would regard these as man-datory for this group.

Dosing scalars for anaesthetic agents in the morbidly obese

The Stanford group reviewed dosing scalars for most anaesthetic drugs and we recommend following the advice elegantly summar-ized in their table (**Table 25.2**) [38,42–53].

One of the most feared complications in day surgery is ana-phylaxis. Efficient resuscitation will achieve survival in between 98.6% and 100% of victims [54] but will require calling in of extra manpower and resources together with a well-rehearsed transfer protocol.

Therefore, the use of common precipitants of anaphylaxis such as neuromuscular blocking agents, antibiotics, and synthetic colloids is carefully assessed on a case-by-case basis.

Airway choices

The Fourth National Audit Project of the Royal College of Anaesthetists in the United Kingdom [55] has enunciated the dangers of supraglottic airways in the morbidly obese, However, Nicholson et al. [56] have also published a Cochrane review showing the following benefits of second-generation supraglottic airway use in morbidly obese populations:

- Significant improvement in oxygenation during and after surgery
- Better pulmonary performance
- Reduced postoperative coughing
- Overall better recovery for patients.

Indeed, our practice has benefited enormously [57] from the ex-pert use of second-generation supraglottic airways with a built-in gastric channel and more recently with the added option of trans-supraglottic airway intubation. We have used the ProSeal™ LMA routinely with a pre-loaded, positively located, gastric tube since 2007 and more recently replaced it with the Supreme™ LMA or the AuraGain™ device for the following day-only procedures in the morbidly obese and occasionally in the super-obese:

- Primary laparoscopic gastric banding
- Laparoscopic removal of gastric band
- Laparoscopic cholecystectomy
- Laparoscopic hernia repairs
- Arthroscopic knee surgery
- Arthroscopic hip surgery
- Arthroscopic shoulder surgery.

Endotracheal intubation is, of course, still required in a propor-tion of cases and our first-choice direct laryngoscope for these is the McCoy [58] levering modification of the Macintosh blade (**Fig. 25.3**). We also insist that all our attending anaesthetists are skilled in the use of a range of video-laryngoscopes including the C-Mac®, Pentax, Glidescope®, and McGrath® devices.

While facilities for elective and/or emergent fibreoptic intubation are made available in our day surgery unit, this choice of airway management would probably sway the client towards an inpatient pathway.

Fluid management

Experts disagree about the optimum fluid regimen for obese pa-tients undergoing surgery; however, with regard to day surgery, the benefits of a fluid preload have been defined [59,60] and most clin-icians are comfortable with a fluid load of about 20–30 mL/kg (lean body mass).

Within the limits of day surgery, anaesthetists are unlikely to re-quire or indeed achieve the sophistication of goal-directed fluid

---

Box 25.2 Ideal anaesthesia technique for the morbidly obese patient undergoing day surgery

- Diligent preoxygenation in the head-up position with added con-tinuous positive airway pressure titrated to an end-tidal oxygen frac-tion of greater than 90%.
- Rapid induction and maintenance with a fast-track technique:
  - Total intravenous anaesthesia–target-controlled infusion.
  - Remifentanil.
  - Short-acting inhalational agents.
  - Rapid-onset and rapid-offset neuromuscular blockade.
- Immediate airway control and intermittent positive pressure ventilation.
- Rapid awakening with good residual analgesia.
- No airway obstruction.

Table 25.2 Weight-based dosing scalar recommendation for commonly used intravenous anaesthetics

Drug	Dosing scalar	Comments
c	Induction: LBW Maintenance: TBW	Simulations showed a 60% decrease in peak plasma concentration in morbidly obese subjects compared with lean subjects after a 250 mg dose [42]. Induction dose adjusted to LBW results in same peak plasma concentration as dose adjusted to CO [38]. Volumes and clearances increase proportionally with TBW [43]
Propofol	Induction: LBW Maintenance: TBW	Morbidly obese subjects given an induction dose based on LBW required similar amounts of propofol and similar times to loss of consciousness compared with lean subjects given propofol based on TBW [44]. Volume of distribution and clearance at steady state increases with increasing TBW [45]
Fentanyl	LBW	Clearance increases linearly with 'PK mass', an arbitrary scalar highly correlated to LBW [46]
Remifentanil	LBW	An infusion based on LBW results in similar plasma concentrations as normal-weight subjects who were given an infusion based on TBW [47]
Succinylcholine	TBW	Administration of 1 mg/kg based on TBW resulted in a more profound block and better intubating conditions compared with doses based on IBW or LBW [48]
Vecuronium	IBW	Doses based on TBW result in a prolonged duration of action in obese vs non-obese subjects [49,50]
Rocuronium	IBW	There is an increased duration of action when the drug is given based on TBW vs IBW [51]
Atracurium, cisatracurium	IBW	The duration of action is prolonged in obese subjects when given on the basis of TBW vs IBW [52,53]

CO, cardiac output; IBW, ideal body weight LBW, lean body weight; TBW, total body weight.
Source: Data from Ingrande, J., Brodsky, J. B. Lemmens, H. J., Lean Body Weight Scalar for the Anesthetic Induction Dose of Propofol in Morbidly Obese Subjects, *Anesthesia & Analgesia*, 113(1):57–62, 2011, International Anesthesia Research Society.

therapy [61]; however, these techniques may have a role in the more complex procedures.

Conclusion

Restrictions on BMI for day surgery appear to have become obsolete [62]. Obese patients who are medically fit do well after day case surgery. Difficulty may still be encountered at the outer limits of BMI because of non-anaesthetic issues such as technical surgical difficulties, equipment limitations, or local patient transfer problems. Although high BMI is not an absolute contraindication, the comorbidities that often accompany obesity must be adequately assessed, pretreated, and accounted for in the anaesthesia technique.

The ideal anaesthetic technique is one which delivers a patient to street fitness and adequate analgesia with a minimum of side effects.

We have achieved new heights of sophistication in what can be achieved for morbidly obese day surgical patients; however, it is only with continued critical review, reflection, and quality improvement that we can maintain these high standards and avoid morbidity and mortality.

In addition to a consummate skill level that embraces both preoperative assessment and technical prowess, anaesthetists who look after morbidly obese patients in a day surgery environment must possess the ability to adopt recent advances in technology and pharmacology for the benefit of these often-complex patients.

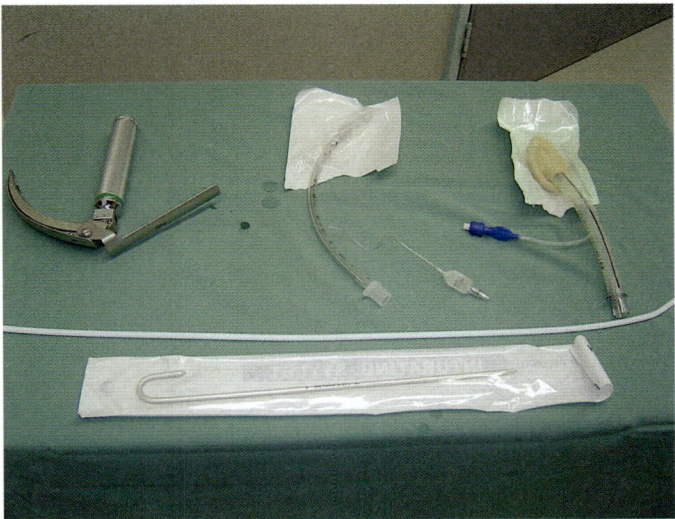

Fig. 25.3 The McCoy levering direct laryngoscope and other aids to airway management.

CASE REPORT

During a busy dental list of surgical extractions, the anaesthetist was informed that a patient who had previously been told that he was rescheduled to the main hospital campus had actually arrived at the venue, fasted, and expecting to be operated for a 'full upper dental clearance'.

On arrival, the patient is a male volunteer fireman aged 56 years, weighing 157 kg, and standing 179 cm tall, thus reaching a BMI of 51.3 kg/m². He is under treatment for hypertension with olmesartan and his wife says that he snores heavily. He denies chest pain and shortness of breath and says he is 'quite active' in his normal employment.

There were no preoperative blood tests or investigations available apart from his dental imaging and a 12-lead ECG which revealed voltage criteria for mild left ventricular hypertrophy. His STOP-Bang [21] score was 6.

A number of options were discussed with management and the patient including funding a ride home and rebooking him into a tertiary hospital. It was emphasized in no uncertain terms that he presented a high-risk situation in the day surgery environment; however, he insisted on having his procedure on the same day.

After discussion with the operating surgeon it was decided to attempt local anaesthesia with minimal sedation, together with full precautions for emergency airway management.

The difficult airway tray was located, checked, and prepared for use; a second attending anaesthetist with special experience in the management of morbidly obese patients was located and agreed to assist on site. Intravenous access was obtained with a 20-gauge cannula and a size no. 6.0 silastic nasopharyngeal cannula was inserted under local anaesthesia to the left nostril. Supplemental oxygen was administered via a split (carbon dioxide-sensing) nasal cannula at 3.0 L/min.

The patient was positioned semi-sitting on the dental operating table and 2.5 mg of intravenous midazolam were administered. In addition, small increments of clonidine 30 mcg every 2–5 minutes were administered to a total of 90 mcg. The surgeon performed bilateral maxillary blocks with a total of 10 mL lidocaine 5% with adrenaline 1:80,000. The surgeon then proceeded to extract 18 very decayed teeth without event.

The patient was able to leave the day surgery accompanied by his wife approximately 2 hours later.

Discussion

A case is presented of a morbidly obese outpatient presenting virtually unheralded to a freestanding day surgery. A range of options were available to the treating team starting with an apology and a referral to tertiary hospital through to providing some form of anaesthesia care.

Clearly, an unplanned general anaesthetic could have led to a disastrous outcome and equally, sending the patient home with a mouthful of decayed teeth was not a desirable outcome.

Conclusion

The management of this case highlights a number of issues for this group of patients:

- BMI limits are not necessarily a contraindication to day surgery per se.
- Wherever possible, a local or regional-based technique is safer than general anaesthesia.
- With extra considerations and meticulous perioperative management, it is possible to accept obese patients for ambulatory surgery.
- The super-obese, however, are at a higher risk for perioperative adverse events [63].
- Sedative drugs may be chosen that are non-opioid in nature and preserve sleep architecture and airway patency [64,65].

REFERENCES

1. Ogden CL, Carroll MD, Fryar CD, Flegal KM. Prevalence of obesity among adults and youth: United States, 2011–2014. NCHS Data Brief. 2015;**219**(219):1–8.
2. Olutoye OA, Watcha MF, Andropoulos DB. Pediatric obesity: observed impact in the ambulatory surgery setting. J Natl Med Assoc. 2011;**103**(1):27–30.
3. Commission on the Provision of Surgical Services. Guidelines for Day Case Surgery. A Report of the Royal College of Surgeons of England (Revised ed.). London: Royal College of Surgeons of England; 1992.
4. Joshi GP, Ankichetty SP, Gan TJ, Chung F. Society for Ambulatory Anesthesia Consensus statement on preoperative selection of adult patients with obstructive sleep apnea scheduled for ambulatory surgery. Anesth Analg. 2012;**115**(5):1060–68.
5. Billing PS, Crouthamel MR, Oling S, Landerholm RW. Outpatient laparoscopic sleeve gastrectomy in a freestanding ambulatory surgery center: first 250 cases. Surg Obes Relat Dis. 2014;**10**(1):101–105.
6. Ogunnaike B. The morbidly obese patient undergoing outpatient surgery. Int Anesthesiol Clin. 2013;**51**(3):113–35.
7. Moon TS, Joshi GP. Are morbidly obese patients suitable for ambulatory surgery? Curr Opin Anaesthesiol. 2016;**29**(1):141–45.
8. Bailey CR, Ahuja M, Bartholomew K, Bew S, Forbes L, Lipp A, et al. Guidelines for day-case surgery 2019: guidelines from the Association of Anaesthetists and the British Association of Day Surgery. Anaesthesia. 2019;**74**(6):778–92.
9. Rebibo L, Dhahri A, Badaoui R, Dupont H, Regimbeau JM. Laparoscopic sleeve gastrectomy as day-case surgery (without overnight hospitalization). Surg Obes Relat Dis. 2015;**11**(2):335–42.
10. Ramaswamy A, Gonzales R, Smith CD. Extensive preoperative testing is not necessary in morbidly obese patients undergoing gastric bypass. J Gastrointest Surg. 2004;**8**(2):159–65.
11. Edholm D, Kullberg J, Haenni A, Karlsson FA, Ahlström A, Hedberg J, et al. Preoperative 4-week low-calorie diet reduces liver volume and intrahepatic fat, and facilitates laparoscopic gastric bypass in morbidly obese. Obes Surg. 2011;**21**(3):345–50.
12. Langeron O, Masso E, Huraux C, Guggiari M, Bianchi A, Coriat P, et al. Prediction of difficult mask ventilation. Anesthesiology. 2000;**92**(5):1229–36.
13. El-Ganzouri AR, McCarthy RJ, Tuman KJ, Tanck EN, Ivankovich AD. Preoperative airway assessment: predictive value of a multivariate risk index. Anesth Analg. 1996;**82**(6):1197–204.
14. Couture EJ, Provencher S, Somma J, Lellouche F, Marceau S, Bussières JS. Effect of position and positive pressure ventilation on functional residual capacity in morbidly obese patients: a randomized trial. Can J Anesth J Can Anesth. 2018;**65**(5):522–28.
15. Nimmagadda U, Salem MR, Crystal GJ. Preoxygenation: physiologic basis, benefits, and potential risks. Anesth Analg. 2017;**124**(2):507–17.
16. Ogunnaike B, Joshi GP. Obesity, sleep apnea, the airway, and anesthesia. In: Hagberg CA. Benumof and Hagberg's Airway Management. 3rd ed. Philadelphia, PA: Elsevier Inc; 2012:892–901.
17. Oxford Online Dictionary. Guru. n.d. https://en.oxforddictionaries.com/definition/guru
18. Parameswaran K, Todd DC, Soth M. Altered respiratory physiology in obesity. Can Respir J. 2006;**13**(4):203–10.
19. van Boxem TJ, de Groot GH. Prevalence and severity of sleep disordered breathing in a group of morbidly obese patients. Neth J Med. 1999;**54**(5):202–206.
20. Biring MS, Lewis MI, Liu JT, Mohsenifar Z. Pulmonary physiologic changes of morbid obesity. Am J Med Sci. 1999;**318**(5):293–97.
21. Chung F, Abdullah HR, Liao P. STOP-Bang questionnaire: a practical approach to screen for obstructive sleep apnea. Chest. 2016;**149**(3):631–38.
22. Christensen J, Rivers J. How a minor elective surgery could end in death. CNN; 7 September, 2014. http://edition.cnn.com/2014/09/05/health/joan-rivers-death/

23. Anderson S. Second patient suffers heart complications at cosmetic surgery clinic. Mamamia.com; 2 September, 2015. http://www.mamamia.com.au/cardiac-arrest-during-breast-enlargement/

24. Fleisher LA, Beckman JA, Brown KA, Calkins H, Chaikof E, Fleischmann KE, et al. ACC/AHA. 2007 Guidelines on perioperative cardiovascular evaluation and care for noncardiac surgery: a report of the American College of Cardiology/American Heart Association Task Force on Practice Guidelines (Writing Committee to Revise the 2002 Guidelines on Perioperative cardiovascular Evaluation for Noncardiac Surgery). Circulation. 2007;**116**(17):e418–99. [Erratum in Circulation 2008;118(9):e143–e144 and Circulation 2008;117(5):e154].

25. Huang PL. A comprehensive definition for metabolic syndrome. Dis Models Mech. 2009;**2**(5–6):231–37.

26. Lavie CJ, Pandey A, Lau DH, Alpert MA, Sanders P. Obesity and atrial fibrillation prevalence, pathogenesis, and prognosis: effects of weight loss and exercise. J Am Coll Cardiol. 2017;**70**(16):2022–35.

27. Clinical Excellence Commission. Non-Vitamin K Antagonist Oral Anticoagulant (NOAC) Guidelines (updated July 2017). Sydney: Clinical Excellence Commission; 2017.

28. Darwin L. Patient selection for day surgery. Anaesth Intensive Care Med. 2016;**17**(3):151–54.

29. Demiraran Y, Korkut E, Tamer A, Yorulmaz I, Kocaman B, Sezen G, et al. The comparison of dexmedetomidine and midazolam used for sedation of patients during upper endoscopy: a prospective, randomized study. Can J Gastroenterol. 2007;**21**(1):25–29.

30. Cohen J, Chuttani R. Endoluminal bariatric procedures. In: Romanelli J, Desilets D, Earle D, eds. NOTES and Endoluminal Surgery: Clinical Gastroenterology. Cham: Springer; 2017;121–42.

31. Stretta TG. A valuable endoscopic treatment modality for gastroesophageal reflux disease. World J Gastroenterol. 2014;**20**(24):7730–38.

32. Skinner MW, Terblanche N, Middleton C. Endoscopic success using LMAGastro™ for upper gastrointestinal endoscopic procedures: preliminary findings, abstract A 3022. The Anesthesiology Annual Meeting. American Society of Anesthesiologists, 22–26 October, Chicago, USA; 2016.

33. Soto R, Jahr JS, Pavlin J, Sabo D, Philip BK, Egan TD, et al. Safety and efficacy of rocuronium with sugammadex reversal versus succinylcholine in outpatient surgery: a multicenter, randomized, safety assessor-blinded trial. Am J Ther. 2016;**23**(6):e1654–62.

34. Morton JM, Winegar D, Blackstone R, Wolfe B. Is ambulatory laparoscopic Roux-en-Y gastric bypass associated with higher adverse events? Ann Surg. 2014;**259**(2):286–92.

35. Roshanov PS, Rochwerg B, Patel A, Salehian O, Duceppe E, Belley-Côté EP et al. Withholding versus continuing angiotensin-converting enzyme inhibitors or angiotensin ii receptor blockers before noncardiac surgery an analysis of the vascular events in noncardiac surgery patients. Anesthesiology. 2017;**126**(1):16–27.

36. Lemmens HJ. Local and regional anesthesia in the obese patients. In: Finucane B, Tsui B, eds. Complications of Regional Anesthesia. Cham: Springer; 2017:319–25.

37. Sepúlveda VPO, Cortínez LI. Intravenous anesthesia in obese patients. In: Absalom A, Mason K, eds. Total Intravenous Anesthesia and Target Controlled Infusions. Cham: Springer; 2017:429–40.

38. Mulier JP. Perioperative opioids aggravate obstructive breathing in sleep apnea syndrome: mechanisms and alternative anesthesia strategies. Curr Opin Anaesthesiol. 2016;**29**(1):129–33.

39. Sultana A, Torres D, Schumann R. Special indications for OFA, patient and procedure related. Best Pract Res Clin Anaesthesiol. 2017;**31**(4):547–60.

40. Ziemann-Gimmel P, Goldfarb AA, Koppman J, Marema RT. Opioid-free total intravenous anaesthesia reduces postoperative nausea and vomiting in bariatric surgery beyond triple prophylaxis. Br J Anaesth. 2014;**112**(5):906–11.

41. Goddard N, Smith D. Unintended awareness and monitoring of depth of anaesthesia. Contin Educ Anaesth Crit Care Pain. 2013;**13**(6):213–17.

42. Wada DR, Björkman S, Ebling WF, Harashima H, Harapat SR, Stanski DR. Computer simulation of the effects of alterations in blood flows and body composition on thiopental pharmacokinetics in humans. Anesthesiology. 1997;**87**(4):884–99.

43. Jung D, Mayersohn M, Perrier D, Calkins J, Saunders R. Thiopental disposition in lean and obese patients undergoing surgery. Anesthesiology. 1982;**56**(4):269–74.

44. Ingrande J, Brodsky JB, Lemmens HJ. Lean body weight scalar for the anesthetic induction dose of propofol in morbidly obese subjects. Anesth Analg. 2011;**113**(1):57–62.

45. Servin F, Farinotti R, Haberer JP, Desmonts JM. Propofol infusion for maintenance of anesthesia in morbidly obese patients receiving nitrous oxide. A clinical and pharmacokinetic study. Anesthesiology. 1993;**78**(4):657–65.

46. Shibutani K, Inchiosa MA Jr, Sawada K, Bairamian M. Pharmacokinetic mass of fentanyl for postoperative analgesia in lean and obese patients. Br J Anaesth. 2005;**95**(3):377–83.

47. Egan TD, Huizinga B, Gupta SK, Jaarsma RL, Sperry RJ, Yee JB, et al. Remifentanil pharmacokinetics in obese versus lean patients. Anesthesiology. 1998;**89**(3):562–73.

48. Lemmens HJ, Brodsky JB. The dose of succinylcholine in morbid obesity. Anesth Analg. 2006;**102**(2):438–42.

49. Weinstein JA, Matteo RS, Ornstein E, Schwartz AE, Goldstoff M, Thal G. Pharmacodynamics of vecuronium and atracurium in the obese surgical patient. Anesth Analg. 1988;**67**(12):1149–53.

50. Schwartz AE, Matteo RS, Ornstein E, Halevy JD, Diaz J. Pharmacokinetics and pharmacodynamics of vecuronium in the obese surgical patient. Anesth Analg. 1992;**74**(4):515–18.

51. Leykin Y, Pellis T, Lucca M, Lomangino G, Marzano B, Gullo A. The pharmacodynamic effects of rocuronium when dosed according to real body weight or ideal body weight in morbidly obese patients. Anesth Analg. 2004;**99**(4):1086–89.

52. Leykin Y, Pellis T, Lucca M, Lomangino G, Marzano B, Gullo A. The effects of cisatracurium on morbidly obese women. Anesth Analg. 2004;**99**(4):1090–94.

53. Kirkegaard-Nielsen H, Helbo-Hansen HS, Lindholm P, Severinsen IK, Pedersen HS. Anthropometric variables as predictors for duration of action of atracurium-induced neuromuscular block. Anesth Analg. 1996;**83**(5):1076–80.

54. Gibbs NM, Sadleir PH, Clarke RC, Platt PR. Survival from perioperative anaphylaxis in Western Australia 2000–2009. Br J Anaesth. 2013;**111**(4):589–93.

55. Cook TM, Woodall N, Frerk C, Fourth National Audit Project. Major complications of airway management in the UK: results of the 4th National Audit Project of the Royal College of Anaesthetists and the Difficult Airway Society. Part 1. Br J Anaesth. 2011;**106**(5):617–31.

56. Nicholson A, Cook TM, Smith AF, Lewis SR, Reed SS. Supraglottic airway devices versus tracheal intubation for airway management during general anaesthesia in obese patients. Cochrane Database Syst Rev. 2013;**9**:CD010105.

57. Sultana A. The ProSeal™ LMA is an ideal airway for gastric banding surgery. Anaesthesiol Intensive Care. 2009;**37**(4):660–61.

58. McCoy EP, Mirakhur RK. The levering laryngoscope. Anaesthesia. 1993;**48**(6):516–19.

59. Lambert KG, Wakim JH, Lambert NE. Preoperative fluid bolus and reduction of postoperative nausea and vomiting in patients undergoing laparoscopic gynecologic surgery. AANA J. 2009;**77**(2):110–14.

60. Holte K, Klarskov B, Christensen DS, Lund C, Nielsen KG, Bie P, et al. Liberal versus restrictive fluid administration to improve recovery after laparoscopic cholecystectomy: a randomized, double-blind study. Ann Surg. 2004;**240**(5):892–99.

61. Miller T, Gan TJ. Goal-directed fluid therapy. In: Hahn RG, ed. Clinical Fluid Therapy in the Perioperative Setting. 1st ed. Cambridge: Cambridge University Press; 2011:91–99.

62. Buckley H, Palmer J. Overview of anaesthesia and patient selection for day surgery. Anaesth Intensive Care Med. 2010;**11**(4):147–52.

63. Rosero EB, Joshi GP. Nationwide use and outcomes of ambulatory surgery in morbidly obese patients in the United States. J Clin Anesth. 2014;**26**(3):191–98.

64. Cheung CW, Ying CL, Chiu WKW, Wong GT, Ng KF, Irwin MG. A comparison of dexmedetomidine and midazolam for sedation in third molar surgery. Anaesthesia. 2007;**62**(11):1132–38.

65. Capasso R, Rosa T, Tsou DY, Nekhendzy V, Drover D, Collins J, et al. Variable findings for drug-induced sleep endoscopy in obstructive sleep apnea with propofol versus dexmedetomidine. Otolaryngol Head Neck Surg. 2016;**154**(4):765–70.

Fluid management in the obese patient

Michelle Cole, David Gilhooly†, and S. R. Moonesinghe

Introduction

Fluid management in the perioperative period plays a pivotal role in the overall pathway of the surgical patient. Particular care is required for the morbidly obese patient, for reasons which shall be described. Fluid therapy has been the topic of debate within the literature and is surrounded by controversy over which fluid compositions, volumes, rates of administration, and clinical settings are associated with improved outcomes. This chapter will discuss the basic physiological principles underlying fluid therapy and how this has been shown to differ in the obese patient. Then approaches will be described to the types of surgery which are most commonly conducted in the obese patient. Finally, an overview will be provided of the current evidence pertaining to preoperative, intraoperative, and postoperative fluid management in the obese surgical patient taking into consideration the types of surgery seen, the comorbidities of the obese patient, and the risks associated with operating on the obese patient.

Fluid compartments, homeostasis, and the glycocalyx model

In the absence of pathology, total body water content is dependent upon three factors: age, sex, and weight. With regard to weight, it is the type of weight that becomes important to determine whether water content is increased or decreased. Lean muscle weight is associated with a higher water content than adipose tissue. Although the mean total body water content expressed in absolute terms is higher in the obese group, if it is expressed as a percentage of body weight it is significantly lower [1]. Thus, the obese patient, despite the clear weight increase, has a disproportionate reduction in total body water content (Fig. 26.1).

The fluid compartment model for non-obese individuals is based on the approximation that total body water accounts for 60% of body weight. This proportion does not apply for the obese patient, because adipose tissue is composed of hydrophobic fat molecules and thus has a lower water content. Biostatistical models of fluid compartments for obese individuals have not yet been published. As a result, the estimation of total body water is on a case-by-case basis.

Nevertheless, the basic principles of how body fluid is distributed between compartments do apply to the obese population. Total body water is composed of intracellular fluid and extracellular fluid in a ratio of approximately two-thirds to one-third [2].

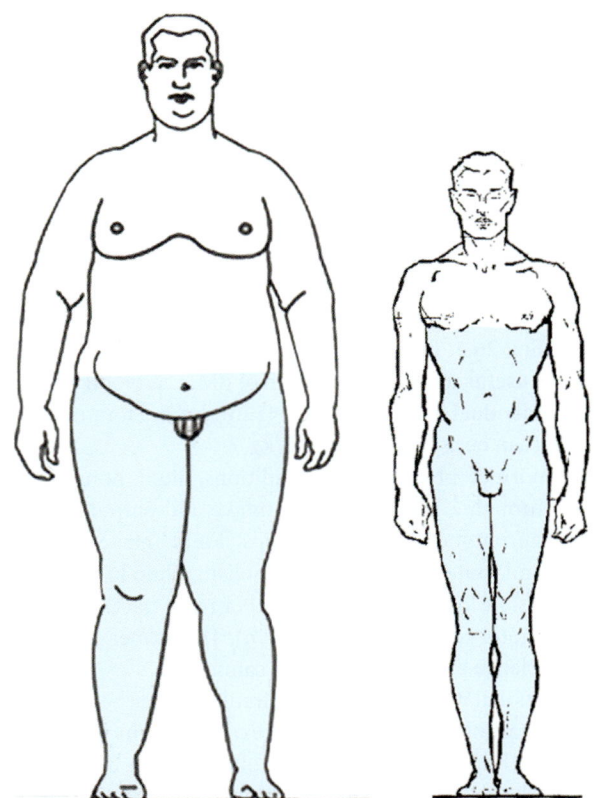

Fig. 26.1 Diagram demonstrating that absolute total body water may be increased but there is a relative decrease in total body water in the obese patient.

---

† It is with great regret that we report the death of David Gilhooly during the production of this textbook.

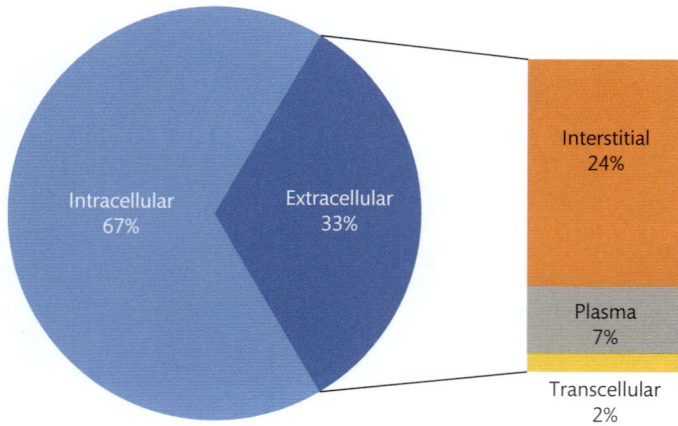

Fig. 26.2 Pie chart to show the distribution of total body water as a percentage of total body weight.

The extracellular compartment is composed of mainly interstitial fluid, plasma fluid, and, to a smaller degree, transcellular fluid such as pleural, ascitic, or pericardial fluid. The compartment distribution is shown in **Fig. 26.2**.

Blood volume is a composite compartment of extracellular fluid and red cell volume. Blood volume can also be related to weight, usually quoted as 70 mL/kg for normal-weight adults. However, in obese individuals, although the absolute volume of blood increases as body mass index (BMI) increases, there is a fall in the blood volume per kilogram gained (i.e. the mean value for indexed blood volume): this is because most of the weight gained is adipose tissue rather than lean mass. This reduction occurs in a non-linear manner with increased weight [3]. This is important, because if the accepted value of 70 mL/kg is applied, it is possible to grossly overestimate the indexed blood volume. Patients may therefore lose significant amounts of blood, with or without haemodynamic changes; however, if the preoperative blood volume is accurately measured, then accurate and timely replacement of the correct fluid may prevent organ under-perfusion. Lemmens et al. [3] derived an equation, as shown in **Fig. 26.3**, to allow this to be more accurately measured; this may be useful across the spectrum of BMIs, as blood volume for an obese individual may be as low as 45 mL/kg and for underweight individuals can be as high as 100 mL/kg.

Under normal physiological conditions, fluid homeostasis is achieved through a balance of fluid intake and output, controlled through neurohumoral feedback loops. Fluid intake is achieved via the enteral route and aerobic metabolism. Fluid loss is achieved through sensible losses (gastrointestinal or renal tract) or insensible losses (respiratory tract or from the skin). The former can be measured with relative ease while the latter cannot.

The traditional model of capillary circulation has been described in terms of Starling's forces. It is these forces upon which many of the debates regarding crystalloids versus colloids as the choice of fluid therapy are based. The modern model of the glycocalyx dismisses many of the shortfalls of the traditional model. The endothelial glycocalyx is a mesh-like, membrane-bound glycoprotein and proteoglycan layer present on the luminal side of capillaries. It serves as an active interface between the capillary wall and the blood or central plasma volume. Within the glycocalyx model exist three intravascular volumes: plasma volume and red cell mass volume, making up the circulating volume, and the glycocalyx layer, comprising the

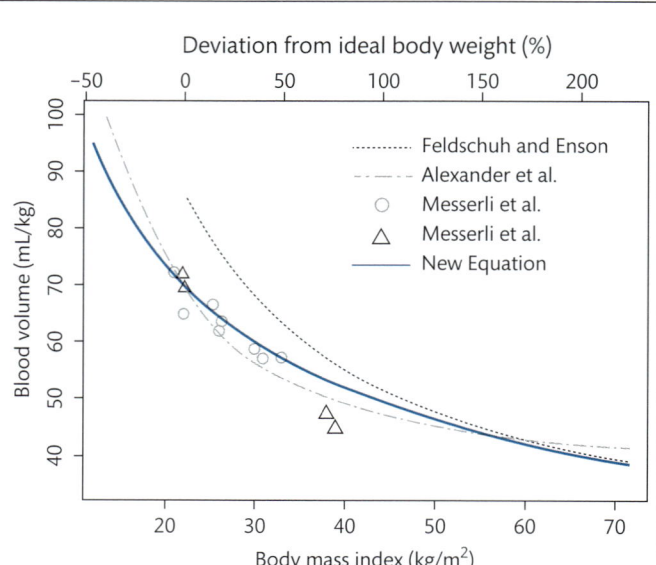

The figure displays the relationship between blood volume (BV) and body mass index (BMI) and the relationship between BV and deviation from ideal body weight (% ΔIBW).

The solid line is BV predicted by the equation:

$$\ln BV = \frac{70}{\sqrt{\dfrac{BMI_P}{22}}}$$

The dashed lines are the BV values predicted by Feldschuh; Enson; and Alexander et al. The open circles and triangles are the BV values measured by Messerli et al. Changes in BV are non-linearly related to both BMI and ΔIBW.

Fig. 26.3 Equation and graphical representation of the relationship between BMI and blood volume.

Reproduced with permission from Lemmens, H.J., Bernstein, D.P. Brodsky, J. B. Estimating blood volume in obese and morbidly obese patients. *Obesity Surgery*, 16(6):773–6. Copyright © 2006, Springer Nature. https://doi.org/10.1381/096089206777346673

non-circulating volume [4]. The modern model suggests that net fluid movement across the capillary wall is much less than that explained using Starling's model, and rather the protein-rich glycocalyx layer provides the oncotic pressure restricting fluid movement out of the capillary. Maintaining the integrity of the glycocalyx layer is crucial for preserving intravascular volume rather than capillary leak. This integrity can be insulted under pathological conditions such as sepsis or iatrogenic hypervolaemia.

Challenges with determining fluid balance

The cardiovascular changes that are associated with obesity need to be understood, as these will affect the manner in which such patients will respond to hypovolaemia or hypervolaemia. We will provide a brief overview of these changes and how they relate to the many challenges posed when attempting to achieve optimal fluid management.

Those who are at the extreme spectrum of obesity may develop functional and structural changes in the heart, a phenomenon known as obesity cardiomyopathy [5,6], features of which may include impaired relaxation and compliance of the left ventricle; thus, targeted fluid therapy could be crucial in more major cases to ensure optimal care of the patient. Systemic hypertension is more prevalent among the obese population and, as such, they are at increased risk of left ventricular dilatation, hypertrophy, and diastolic and systolic failure. Chronic respiratory impairment can also predispose to right-sided heart failure. Obese patients with respiratory compromise, long-standing obstructive sleep apnoea, or obesity hypoventilation syndrome may develop polycythaemia secondary to chronic hypoxaemia; thus, hypovolaemia or dehydration may further increase viscosity and impair microcirculatory flow and oxygen delivery.

These physiological changes pose significant challenges to perioperative physicians, surgeons, and anaesthetists, as excessive fluid administration may exacerbate or lead to further decompensation of cardiac function. Moreover, the diagnosis or clinical suspicion of fluid imbalance may also be masked by this altered physiology [7,8]. Therefore, the threshold for perioperative echocardiography may be lower in obese patients undergoing major surgery. This investigation may give the clinician a better idea of how well the patient will be able to deal with fluid challenges and how fastidious they must be in their fluid therapy. Cardiopulmonary exercise testing may also provide an estimate of functional capacity and heart failure, and thus the potential tolerance of the obese patient's cardiovascular system to fluid shifts in the perioperative period. For operations on obese patients it may be necessary to use a reverse Trendelenburg position to reduce the effect of the abdomen on the intrathoracic pressure, which will already be significantly elevated due to reduced thoracic wall compliance during intermittent positive pressure ventilation. Increased intrathoracic pressure can have a significant effect on venous return and consequently cardiac preload.

Principles of fluid management

The main aims of fluid administration can be broadly categorized as resuscitation and maintenance therapy. Intravenous fluids are also used for assisting drug delivery but this is often a low-volume and low-rate infusion. The goal of fluid therapy should always be to restore euvolaemia and replace 'like with like'. To that end, one needs to be aware of what 'fluid' has been lost and over what timescale. Plasma loss, as in the case of trauma with intravascular depletion, necessitates rapid resuscitation with fluids which may include blood products. Fluid from the interstitial space is redistributed to the intravascular compartment as an initial compensatory measure. Extracellular fluid loss (which includes interstitial and intravascular loss) can occur with excessive vomiting or gastrointestinal obstruction. Fluid loss in this instance is isotonic; thus, intracellular compensation is not achieved, and instead intravenous crystalloid infusion is required for replacement. Pure water loss which invariably is associated with some electrolyte loss rarely presents as shock unless under severe conditions where intracellular water stores have become depleted.

The choice of which fluid to give and at what rate is the basis of the ongoing fluid debate within the literature. However, overwhelmingly, evidence supports the use of balanced rather than unbalanced

solutions when used for either resuscitative or maintenance intent [9–11]. It is important to consider the integrity of the glycocalyx when selecting the choice of fluid as this plays a crucial role in preserving the intravascular volume and preventing endovascular leak. It is unclear whether the proinflammatory state associated with morbid obesity [8] has any bearing on the functional ability of the glycocalyx.

Surgical specialities common to the obese patient

Intuitively, bariatric surgery is aimed at the obese patient population; however, with the incidence of obesity increasing among the general population, this patient demographic is likely to increase across all surgical specialities. In England, the proportion of adults who were obese had increased from 13.2% in 1993 to 26.0% in 2013 for men, and from 16.4% to 23.8% for women [12]. In 2014, the Sprint National Anaesthesia Project 1 (SNAP-1) took place in the United Kingdom [13]. This project provided a snapshot evaluation of the clinical activity and patent-reported outcomes after anaesthesia. Data from this study demonstrated that obese patients (BMI >30 kg/m^2) present commonly across different surgical subspecialties and varying surgical complexity. This is demonstrated in Table 26.1.

Table 26.1 Distribution of patients with obesity (BMI >30 kg/m^2) in the SNAP-1 study

Specialty	Number of obese patients (over total number of patients in group)	Percentage (%)
Abdomen (endocrine)	1/9	11
Abdomen (bariatric)	34/36	94
Abdomen (gut)	358/1815	20
Abdomen (hepatobiliary)	177/494	36
Orthopaedics	999/4000	25
Head and neck	199/1209	16
Body surface (breast)	145/699	21
Body surface (other)	107/445	24
Thoracics	20/133	15
Endocrine	27/91	30
Vascular	64/346	18
Transplant	2/21	10
Neurosurgery	53/272	19
Urology	342/1799	19
Gynaecology	426/1948	22
Ophthalmology	153/984	16
Cardiac	68/250	27
Interventional radiology	11/45	24
Dental	46/304	15
Endoscopy	26/139	19

Reproduced with permission from Moonesinghe, S.R., Walker, E.M.K., and Bell, M. Design and methodology of SNAP-1: a Sprint National Anaesthesia Project to measure patient reported outcome after anaesthesia. *Perioperative Medicine*, 4(4), 2015 Springer Nature. Distributed under the Creative Commons Attribution 4.0 International (CC BY 4.0). http://creativecommons.org/licenses/by/4.0

From this study we can see that the highest-ranking specialities for having obese patients on their lists include endocrine, cardiac, and orthopaedic surgeries, with an overall prevalence of obesity of 20% in the surgical population in the United Kingdom.

Preoperative evaluation of fluid status

Evaluating the hydration status of an obese patient in the preoperative period is much the same methodology as applied to the normal-weight patient. These can be categorized as using a clinical assessment or objective measurements performed using specialized dynamic monitoring.

Clinically assessing an obese patient for dehydration can be inaccurate. The standard ways of assessing can include:

- Capillary refill
- Mucous membranes
- Pulse
- Blood pressure
- Heart rate
- Skin turgor
- Urine output.

Clinical assessment is notoriously inaccurate and variable between individuals and in most cases patients may, in reality, be more dehydrated than they initially appear. Additionally, some signs and symptoms, such as thirst and dry mouth, may be difficult to interpret in the context of a preoperative surgical patient who has been nil by mouth prior to anaesthesia. Signs such as reduced skin turgor can also be unreliable, whereas hypotension, which is often a late sign of hypovolaemia, may be attributed to antihypertensive medications that many morbidly obese patients may be taking. In assessing for signs of oliguria, determining adequate urine output may also be difficult as the rate can vary considerably depending on which body weight is used, that is, total body weight or ideal body weight.

Obese patients commonly have difficult intravenous access and therefore they may arrive in the operating room under-resuscitated or not resuscitated at all. For patients undergoing bariatric surgery, it is now commonplace for these patients to be prescribed a rapid weight loss diet a few weeks prior to their procedure to facilitate the ease of access for laparoscopic surgery [14,15]. Rapid weight loss diets have been shown to be associated with hypovolaemia in up to 70% of these morbidly obese patients [16]. As such, Pösö and colleagues demonstrated transthoracic echocardiography as an effective tool for assessing preload and thus fluid status in the morbidly obese [17]. They also showed that if the patients were rehydrated with 500 mL of a colloid solution, then a higher mean arterial pressure might be achieved in the intraoperative period. It is very important to be cognisant of the fact that haemodynamic instability may occur particularly during induction and that having a euvolaemic status preoperatively is very important to minimize any cardiac depression that is associated with the pneumoperitoneum as well [18].

Selecting fluids

Looking initially at the type of intravenous fluid that should be used, the age-old debate on whether colloid or crystalloid should be used for fluid management of patients is still ongoing. Two meta-analyses of randomized controlled trials have been performed: in both cases there was no subanalysis of obese patients and only one analysis focused on the surgical patient. The overarching message still seems to be that colloids are associated with a relative risk of 1.24 of developing an acute kidney injury according to Serpa Neto et al. [19] and an odds ratio of 1.24 of developing acute kidney injury or renal failure from Qureshi et al. [20]. Although they did differ in associated morbidity, the congruous outcomes of both meta-analyses are useful in this setting. Added to this, it has been shown that there is an increased incidence of comorbidities such as cardiovascular disease and diabetes mellitus in obese patients [21]. There is also an increased incidence of rhabdomyolysis in prolonged surgical procedures; therefore, it may be pertinent to use crystalloid maintenance fluids to reduce the risk of causing a kidney injury. This may be at odds with the theory that the use of colloids may have the advantage of reducing overall amount of intravenous fluids administered, as they remain intravascular compartment for longer. It has been shown that only 20% of crystalloids remain in the intravascular compartment after 30 minutes and thus the use of colloids may help in preventing morbidity associated with excessive fluid administration [11].

When deciding on the choice of crystalloid, the high prevalence of diabetes mellitus in obese patients must be taken into consideration. As part of many major surgical quality improvement programmes, the maintenance of euglycaemia in the perioperative period, especially in the intraoperative period and the following two postoperative days [22], has been shown to improve surgical outcomes. Lower morbidity and mortality rates have been demonstrated when glucose levels are kept in the range of 140–179 mg/dL (8–10 mmol/L) [23], therefore the selection of which crystalloid is important. Historically it has been advised to avoid Hartmann's solution in diabetic patients undergoing surgery based on a paper by Alberti et al. in 1978 [24] but the findings of this paper have been shown to be biochemically impossible. More recently, the Royal College of Anaesthetists and Joint British Diabetes Societies endorsed guidelines recommending balanced solutions such as Hartmann's as it causes minimal metabolic and electrolyte disturbance provided the blood sugars are stable [25]. If insulin is required, then variable rate intravenous insulin infusions are recommended with 0.45% saline in 5% glucose to prevent hyponatraemia except in the peripartum period and remembering that supplemental potassium may be required [26]. Otherwise, although it is only a weak recommendation, it has been shown that balanced electrolyte solutions, such as Hartmann's, offer a similar electrolyte composition to plasma and so avoid the risk of hyperchloraemic acidosis which is caused by large volumes of normal saline [11].

Which weight to base it on?

Currently there is limited evidence available about dose adjustment of fluids in the obese patient and the selection of appropriate weight parameters on which to base it has been controversial. There are four main dictums that include:

1. Total body weight (TBW)—the actual body weight of the patient
2. Ideal body weight (IBW)—what the patient should weight with a normal ratio of lean mass to fat mass:

$$IBW = height(cm) - x(x = 105 \text{ in females and } 100 \text{ in males})$$

3. Lean body weight (LBW)—the patient's weight excluding fat. It can be simply calculated with the most widely used equation:

$$LBW(kg) = \frac{9270 \times TBW(kg)}{6680 + (216 \times BMI(kg/m^2))} \text{ For Men}$$

$$LBW(kg) = \frac{9270 \times TBW(kg)}{8780 + (244 \times BMI(kg/m^2))} \text{ For women}$$

4. Adjusted body weight (ABW)—this takes into account the fact that obese individuals have increased lean body mass. It is calculated by adding 40% of the excess weight to the IBW:

$$ABW(kg) = IBW(kg) + 0.4(TBW(kg) - IBW(kg))$$

As previously mentioned, there can be a considerable difference in absolute and total body water between the non-obese patient and the obese patient and this has a significant bearing on the choice of the best strategy to adopt in fluid administration.

Choosing a fluid regimen

Debate has surrounded the use of a liberal or restrictive fluid regimen intraoperatively. In open procedures for the non-obese population, McCardle et al. in 2009 reported on restrictive versus standard fluid protocols for abdominal surgery, where the total intraoperative fluid given was 4 mL/kg/h versus 16 mL/kg/h (included an additional preload bolus). The study showed worse outcomes for the standard group with reference to wound, cardiac, respiratory, and cognition complications [27]. They concluded that excessive hydration led to organ dysfunction. This has been followed up by a review of big data in the United States which suggested fluid optimization would lead to improved outcomes [28].

Focusing on the obese patient, it has already been shown by Ettinger et al. that there is an increased risk of rhabdomyolysis following bariatric surgery, especially in prolonged cases, in patients who are hypertensive, diabetic, super-obese, have peripheral vascular disease, or are taking statin medication [29]. Thus, there is a theoretical risk that a more restrictive fluid regimen may have a negative effect on renal function. In addition, multiple studies have shown that monitoring of urine output is a not a good indicator of renal function following both bariatric and non-bariatric laparoscopic operations [18,30,31]. The reasons stem from the increased intra-abdominal pressure affecting the renal blood flow, intraoperative release of certain stress hormones, and the positioning of the bed during laparoscopic procedures.

The few studies on fluid regimens for obese patients have focused on bariatric surgery, as opposed to surgery on obese patients, and thus are limited to laparoscopic procedures. Studies examining this issue have shown heterogeneity in their approach to restrictive versus liberal fluid management. It was originally suggested in 2002 by Ogunnaike et al. that to avoid postoperative acute tubular necrosis, the intravenous maintenance rate of the order of twice that calculated for lean or ideal body weight is required [32]; however, in 2006 an article by McGlinch et al. found that in their clinical experience restricted fluids reduced respiratory dysfunction, hypoxia, and hospital stay [33], while Schuster et al.'s retrospective study of 180 gastric bypass patients showed that patients who had postoperative nausea and vomiting had significantly less fluid compared to those who did not (21.8 ± 6.9 mL/kg vs 24.9 ± 8.8mL/kg) [34].

Following on from this, a randomized controlled study by Matot et al. looked at giving 4 mL/kg/h intraoperatively versus 10 mL/hg/h. Both treatment arms showed low urine output but no change in the serum creatinine in either group [35]. The study did, however, show a non-significant increase in postoperative complications in the high-volume group. Another randomized study by Wool et al. showed that a more restrictive fluid regimen did not change the incidence of rhabdomyolysis, when a regimen of 15 mL/kg/h versus 40 mL/kg/h of TBW intraoperatively was used [31]. More recently, a retrospective study of 224 patients showed in favour of liberal intraoperative fluids, as restricted fluids resulted in a higher incidence of hospital length of stay and a delay in postoperative wound healing [36]. This study was based on less than 5 mL/kg/h versus greater than 7 mL/kg/h. It is clear there is a lack of good, clear evidence into optimal fluid management of the obese patient and that the limited information available is quite dichotomous. The research that is available possibly leans in favour of a somewhat less restrictive level of fluid administration, somewhere between 7 and 15 mL/kg/h.

Monitoring intravascular volume

Deciding on the optimum goal of direct fluid therapy comes with the caveat that there should be a prior assessment of the hydration status of the patient. As described earlier in the chapter, it can sometimes be difficult to assess an obese patient's hydration status clinically and the use of various measuring tools may be necessary. Also, it has been well documented that following urine output is a poor marker of renal function and hydration status [37]. Blood pressure cuffs can also be inaccurate if not fitted correctly; the bladder of the cuff should encircle a minimum of 75% of the upper arm, otherwise it may give a falsely elevated reading.

Depending on the invasiveness and length of time of the surgery and the comorbidities of the patient, it may be pertinent to insert an arterial line. Jain et al. studied pulse contour analysis using a LiDCO® Cardiac Sensor System in laparoscopic cases [38]. The system was initially calibrated with lithium for cardiac output and subsequently the stoke volume variation was obtained from arterial pressure waveform analysis. Using a stroke volume variation of more than 10% as a transfusion trigger, the mean fluid requirements were 2 L for laparoscopic surgery lasting a mean of 206 minutes, which is in keeping with about a 10 mL/kg/h regimen. Monitoring central venous pressure and pulmonary capillary wedge pressure for fluid administration has low sensitivity and specificity [39].

Another common method of monitoring cardiac output is through the use of an oesophageal Doppler probe. Newer models have the advantage that they may be inserted without excessive patient discomfort prior to general anaesthesia and will show clearly the effect of the anaesthetic on volume status and the filling that may be required. The advantage of inserting the oesophageal Doppler probe prior to induction of anaesthesia is that it will give an accurate idea of the patient's hydration status, which is particularly important as perioperative haemodynamic instability can occur for a multitude of reasons, such as cardiac medications, the pneumoperitoneum affecting intra-abdominal pressure, and Trendelenburg positioning. Unfortunately, inserting an oesophageal Doppler probe may not be always possible, given the types of procedures that the obese patient has, and in bariatric surgery this is generally the case. There are also several assumptions that need to be made when using the oesophageal Doppler probe, namely that there is a flat velocity through the aorta, that the probe is correctly aligned perpendicular to the aorta, and that the cross-sectional area is constant. In cases where the patient's position may vary on the operating table, it may be difficult to adjust for this, making an accurate reading difficult to obtain. Pösö et al. in 2013 [16] demonstrated the benefit of peri- and intraoperative use of the newer hand-held cardiac echocardiography machines, which can give good real-time results on cardiac filling and hydration. Unlike the oesophageal Doppler probe, the echocardiogram can give direct views of the heart function itself and the patient's perfusion status, although views may be difficult, given the patient's body habitus and the fact that they are ventilated. Goal-directed fluid therapy has been shown to be of benefit in patients undergoing bariatric surgery [40,41].

Transfusion

Transfusion of obese patients does not need to be adapted, though some studies have reported a reduction in transfusion requirements as the BMI increases [42–46]. These studies, both retrospective and prospective, of large numbers of patients undergoing coronary artery bypass grafting have all shown that obese patients have a reduced requirement for intraoperative transfusion, reduced risk of postoperative bleeding, and lower reoperation rates for bleeding. The theories put forward include that the raised intrathoracic pressure, secondary to mediastinal fat, and pressure from the abdomen compresses minor bleeding sites. Other theories are that there are increased levels of coagulant factors in obese patients, that there is a procoagulant state associated with patients who have syndrome X, and there is better platelet aggregation in patients with hyperlipidaemia. In general, it is important to be aware of the comorbidities of obese patients and that it may be preferable to aim for higher haemoglobin levels as a result.

Postoperative care

Postoperatively, it is beneficial to return patients to enteral fluids and diet as soon as possible. In the case of bariatric patients, there can be issues with intake due to the procedure and also the high risk of nausea and vomiting. Fluid regimens vary between that for IBW and others, basing it on twice the ideal body weight for maintenance [32]. Depending on the type of surgery and the recovery period, it may be helpful to have a central line inserted for access and to keep the patients catheterized to enable assessment of fluid balance.

Rhabdomyolysis

Studies have shown that obese patients undergoing surgery have an increased risk of rhabdomyolysis [29] and that it is more common in men with higher BMIs undergoing prolonged operations [47].

This risk is compounded by the fact that cases tend to be of longer overall duration due to positioning and access, so it is important to be aware of the need to monitor for signs of rhabdomyolysis during and after the procedure. As urine output is not the most reliable yardstick, it may be of benefit to monitor the patient's pH and lactate levels checking for any unexpected rise and then treat accordingly. Creatinine phosphokinase levels tend to peak about the second to fifth postoperative days and take about 2 weeks to resolve [48]. Treatment involves aggressive hydration, alkalization of the urine, and diuresis with mannitol to achieve a urine output of 1.5 mL/kg/h.

The critically ill obese patient

There are increasing numbers of obese patients with critical illness requiring surgery. These patients present unique challenges to the anaesthetist as it has been shown that they have a chronic proinflammatory status in addition to the stress of critical illness. In cases that have massive haemorrhage, polytrauma, or prolonged operating time resulting in large fluid shifts requiring significant volume resuscitation, there is the risk of developing abdominal compartment syndrome [49]. Pressures can be measured via the urinary catheter and signs of developing this syndrome postoperatively include difficulty with ventilation, high peak and plateau pressures, and decreased urine output. Treatment involves decompression of the abdomen by laying it open.

Conclusion

This chapter has explored some physiological principles underlying fluid therapy including fluid compartments and provided a brief overview of the glycocalyx model and its role in fluid homeostasis. Obese patients have a disproportionate reduction in total body water in comparison to the non-obese patient, despite the clear increase in total body mass. The obese population presents significant challenges for fluid management in the perioperative period. This is because of the inaccuracies of clinical assessment and consequent estimation of volume status. This is exacerbated by the cardiovascular and pathological changes that may be present in the obese population. This cohort of patients presents a knowledge gap in the role of perioperative echocardiography with respect to fluid management. Whether the aim is fluid resuscitation or providing a fluid maintenance regimen, the overall goal should be to replace 'like with like' using balanced solutions, with a tendency towards a restrictive regimen and thus prevent any further physiological insults.

CASE REPORT

A 75-year-old woman with a BMI of 38 kg/m² was scheduled for gynaecological surgery. She had a history of asthma, hypertension, previous myocardial infarction 10 years ago, and diabetes mellitus type 2. Routine bloods were done. Her electrocardiogram in preoperative assessment showed that there was left bundle branch block. There was no prior electrocardiogram to compare to and given her cardiac history, an echocardiogram was performed which showed left ventricular hypertrophy, diastolic dysfunction, and ejection fraction of 45%.

Instructions from the pre-assessment team told her to continue with her beta-blocker on the morning of the operation and to omit her angiotensin-converting-enzyme inhibitor. The surgical team had given her oral bowel preparation to be taken the day before surgery as colonic resection was necessary. She was the first on the operating list and was planned for an awake epidural, induction of anaesthesia, and insertion of arterial line asleep. There had been difficulty gaining peripheral access and only a 23-gauge cannula could be inserted in the antecubital fossa. Induction of anaesthesia was done in the semi-recumbent position using a mixture of propofol, fentanyl, and rocuronium. She was intubated successfully but noted to remain hypotensive. Ephedrine was given initially which was followed by metaraminol as she received a fluid bolus. She was placed in the Trendelenburg position not only to assist her blood pressure but it was decided at this point the central venous access was appropriate. The anaesthetist noted the small calibre of the internal jugular vein on ultrasound of her neck; an arterial line was inserted in the left forearm and a swing was identified in her pulse pressure with respiration. When an oesophageal Doppler probe was inserted, the patient was found to be hypovolaemic. Prior to transfer to the operating room, the patient was fluid resuscitated with 1 L of compound sodium lactate.

The operation started as an open procedure on account of her previous surgical history and the extensive nature of her disease. Cardiac output monitoring was done throughout the operation using the oesophageal Doppler monitor. It had been observed 1 hour into the operation that her urine output had remained low for her presumed weight and on that basis the anaesthetist increased her intravenous fluid infusion rate. By the end of the second hour she had received 5 L of crystalloid and was requiring a higher fraction of inspired oxygen. An arterial blood gas was done which showed a relative hypoxaemia with a normal partial pressure of carbon dioxide. On auscultation of the chest there was no wheeze but fine crepitations throughout. She was thought to be overloaded at this point, so was given 20 mg of intravenous furosemide and subsequently had a good diuresis with improvement of oxygenation. The fluid rate was also reduced and it was decided to strictly monitor cardiac output using the oesophageal Doppler probe as opposed to urine output.

Discussion

This case study describes the difficulty in volume assessment of obese patients and that clinical signs of hypovolaemia may not be as obvious compared to non-obese patients. Added to that is the fact that obese patients require a larger total body volume to meet the increased metabolic demands. Because of the associated cardiac dysfunction and therefore medications, their ability to compensate for induction-associated hypotension may be impaired. Best practice would suggest that two intravenous cannulae should be sited while in theatre and that use of ultrasound may be useful in helping to locate peripheral veins. Central venous access should be considered if peripheral is impossible or specifically indicated. Blood pressure monitoring also presents a challenge to the anaesthetist. Surface anatomy can make insertion of intra-arterial blood pressure lines infeasible. Studies have shown that non-invasive measurements are just as accurate and placement of the blood pressure cuff on the forearm is a good surrogate for an ill-fitting upper arm cuff.

The lack of evidence pertaining to the perioperative fluid management of obese patients makes recommendations less evidence based. It would therefore be prudent, given the difficulty in assessment of the volume status of such patients, that some form of cardiac output monitoring would be used to guide fluid administration. Depending on the type and grade of the surgical procedure and the comorbidities of the patient, an oesophageal Doppler probe may be a good choice.

REFERENCES

1. Hankin ME, Munz K Steinbeck AW. Total body water content in normal and grossly obese women. Med J Aus. 1976;**2**(14):533–37.
2. Ingrande J, Brodsky JB. Intraoperative fluid management and bariatric surgery. Int Anesthesiol Clin. 2013;**51**(3):80–89.
3. Lemmens HJ, Bernstein DP Brodsky JB. Estimating blood volume in obese and morbidly obese patients. Obes Surg. 2006;**16**(6):773–76.
4. Woodcock TE, Woodcock TM. Revised Starling equation and the glycocalyx model of transvascular fluid exchange: an improved paradigm for prescribing intravenous fluid therapy. Br J Anaesth. 2012;**108**(3):384–94.
5. Alpert MA. Obesity cardiomyopathy: pathophysiology and evolution of the clinical syndrome. Am J Med Sci. 2001;**321**(4):225–36.
6. Timoh T, Bloom ME, Siegel RR, Wagman G, Lanier GM Vittorio TJ. A perspective on obesity cardiomyopathy. Obes Res Clin Pract. 2012;**6**(3):e175–262.
7. Lotia S, Bellamy MC. Anaesthesia and morbid obesity. Contin Educ Anaesthes Crit Care Pain. 2008;**8**(5):151–56.
8. Ortiz VE, Kwo J. Obesity: physiologic changes and implications for preoperative management. BMC Anesthesiol. 2015;**15**(1):97.
9. Shaw AD, Bagshaw SM, Goldstein SL, Scherer LA, Duan M, Schermer CR, et al. Major complications, mortality, and resource utilization after open abdominal surgery: 0.9% saline compared to Plasma-Lyte. Ann Surg. 2012;**255**(5):821–29.
10. Lobo DN, Stanga Z, Aloysius MM, Wicks C, Nunes QM, Ingram KL, et al. Effect of volume loading with 1 liter intravenous infusions of 0.9% saline, 4% succinylated gelatine (Gelofusine) and 6% hydroxyethyl starch (Voluven) on blood volume and endocrine responses: a randomized, three-way crossover study in healthy volunteers. Crit Care Med. 2010;**38**(2):464–70.
11. Chowdhury AH, Cox EF, Francis ST, Lobo DN. A randomized, controlled, double-blind crossover study on the effects of 2-L infusions of 0.9% saline and plasma-lyte(R) 148 on renal blood flow velocity and renal cortical tissue perfusion in healthy volunteers. Ann Surg. 2012;**256**(1):18–24.
12. Health and Social Care Information Centre. Homepage. http://www.hscic.gov.uk/
13. Moonesinghe SR, Walker EMK, Bell M. Design and methodology of SNAP-1: a Sprint National Anaesthesia Project to measure patient reported outcome after anaesthesia. Perioper Med (Lond). 2015;**4**:4.
14. Liu RC, Sabnis AA, Forsyth C, Chand B. The effects of acute preoperative weight loss on laparoscopic Roux-en-Y gastric bypass. Obes Surg. 2005;**15**(10):1396–402.
15. Fris RJ. Preoperative low energy diet diminishes liver size. Obes Surg. 2004;**14**(9):1165–70.
16. Pösö T, Kesek D, Aroch R, Winsö O. Rapid weight loss is associated with preoperative hypovolemia in morbidly obese patients. Obes Surg. 2013;**23**(3):306–13.

17. Pösö T, Kesek D, Aroch R, Winsö O. Morbid obesity and optimization of preoperative fluid therapy. Obes Surg. 2013;**23**(11):1799–805.

18. Nguyen NT, Wolfe BM. The physiologic effects of pneumoperitoneum in the morbidly obese. Ann Surg. 2005;**241**(2):219–26.

19. Serpa Neto A, Veelo DP, Peireira VGM, de Assunção MSC, Manetta JA, Espósito DC, et al. Fluid resuscitation with hydroxyethyl starches in patients with sepsis is associated with an increased incidence of acute kidney injury and use of renal replacement therapy: a systematic review and meta-analysis of the literature. J Crit Care; 2014;**29**(1):185.e1–7.

20. Qureshi SH, Rizvi SI, Patel NN, Murphy GJ. Meta-analysis of colloids versus crystalloids in critically ill, trauma and surgical patients. Br J Surg. 2016;**103**(1):14–26.

21. Guh DP, Zhang W, Bansback N, Amarsi Z, Birmingham CL, Anis AH. The incidence of co-morbidities related to obesity and overweight: a systematic review and meta-analysis. BMC Public Health. 2009;**9**:88.

22. Rosenberger LH, Politano AD, Sawyer RG. The surgical care improvement project and prevention of post-operative infection, including surgical site infection. Surg Infect (Larchmt). 2011;**12**(3):163–68.

23. Duncan AE, Abd-Elsayed A, Maheshwari A, Xu M, Soltesz E, Koch CG. Role of intraoperative and postoperative blood glucose concentrations in predicting outcomes after cardiac surgery. Anesthesiology. 2010;**112**(4):860–71.

24. Thomas DJB, Alberti KG. Hyperglycaemic effects of Hartmann's solution during surgery in patients with maturity onset diabetes. Br J Anaesth. 1978;**50**(2):185–88.

25. Dhatairiya K, Flanagan D, Hilton L, Kilvery A, Levy N, Rayman G, et al. Management of adults with diabetes undergoing surgery and elective procedures: improving standards. Joint British Diabetes Societies Inpatient Care Group; 2011. http://www.diabetologists-abcd.org.uk/JBDS/JBDS_IP_Surgery_Adults_Full.pdf

26. Rickard L, Cubas V, Ward S, Hanif W. Slipping up on the sliding scale: fluid and electrolyte management in variable rate intravenous insulin infusions. Pract Diabetes. 2016;**33**(5):159–62.

27. McArdle GT, McAuley DF, McKinley A, Blair P, Hoper M, Harkin DW. Preliminary results of a prospective randomized trial of restrictive versus standard fluid regime in elective open abdominal aortic aneurysm repair. Ann Surg. 2009;**250**(1):28–34.

28. Thacker JKM, Mountford WK, Ernst FR, Krukas MR, Mythen MMG. Perioperative fluid utilization variability and association with outcomes: considerations for enhanced recovery efforts in sample us surgical populations. Ann Surg. 2016;**263**(3):502–10.

29. Ettinger JE, Marcílio de Souza CA, Azaro E, Mello CA, Santos-Filho PV, Orrico J, et al. Clinical features of rhabdomyolysis after open and laparoscopic Roux-en-Y gastric bypass. Obes Surg. 2008;**18**(6):635–43.

30. Nishio S, Takeda H, Yokoyama M. Changes in urinary output during laparoscopic adrenalectomny. BJU Int. 1999;**83**(9):944–47.

31. Wool DB, Lemmens HJ, Brodsky JB, Solomon H, Chong KP, Morton JM. Intraoperative fluid replacement and postoperative creatine phosphokinase levels in laparoscopic bariatric patients. Obes Surg. 2010;**20**(6):698–701.

32. Ogunnaike BO, Jones SB, Jones DB, Provost D, Whitten CW. Anesthetic considerations for bariatric surgery. Anesth Analg. 2002;**95**(3):1793–805.

33. McGlinch BP, Que FG, Nelson JL, Wrobleski DM, Grant JE, Collazo-Clavell ML. Perioperative care of patients undergoing bariatric surgery. Mayo Clin Proc. 2006;**81**(10 Suppl):S25–33.

34. Schuster R, Alami RS, Curet MJ, Paulraj N, Morton JM, Brodsky JB, et al. Intra-operative fluid volume influences postoperative nausea and vomiting after laparoscopic gastric bypass surgery. Obes Surg. 2006;**16**(7):848–51.

35. Matot I, Paskaleva R, Eid L, Cohen K, Khalaileh A, Elazary R, et al. Effect of the volume of fluids administered on intraoperative oliguria in laparoscopic bariatric surgery: a randomized controlled trial. Arch Surg. 2012;**147**(3):228–34.

36. Nossaman VE, Richardson WS, Wooldridge JB, Nossaman BD. Role of intraoperative fluids on hospital length of stay in laparoscopic bariatric surgery: a retrospective study in 224 consecutive patients. Surg Endosc Other Interv Tech. 2015;**29**(10):2960–69.

37. Kheterpal S, Tremper KK, Englesbe MJ, O'Reilly M, Shanks AM, Fetterman DM, et al. Predictors of postoperative acute renal failure after noncardiac surgery in patients with previously normal renal function. Anesthesiology. 2007;**107**(6):892–902.

38. Jain AK, Dutta A. Stroke volume variation as a guide to fluid administration in morbidly obese patients undergoing laparoscopic bariatric surgery. Obes Surg. 2010;**20**(6):709–15.

39. Osman D, Ridel C, Ray P, Monnet X, Anguel N, Richard C, et al. Cardiac filling pressures are not appropriate to predict hemodynamic response to volume challenge. Crit Care Med. 2007;**35**(1):64–68.

40. Munoz JL, Gabaldon T, Miranda E, Berrio DL, Ruiz-Tovar J, Ronda JM, et al. Goal-directed fluid therapy on laparoscopic sleeve gastrectomy in morbidly obese patients. Obes Surg. 2016;**26**(11):2648–53.

41. Thorell A, MacCormick AD, Awad S, Reynolds N, Roulin D, Demartines N, et al. Guidelines for perioperative care in bariatric surgery: Enhanced Recovery After Surgery (ERAS) Society recommendations. World J Surg. 2016;**40**(9):2065–83.

42. Nolan H, Davenport D, Ramaiah C. BMI is an independent preoperative predictor of intraoperative transfusion and postoperative chest-tube output. Int J Angiol. 2013;**22**(1):31–36.

43. Birkmeyer NJ, Charlesworth DC, Hernandez F, Leavitt BJ, Marrin CA, Morton JR, et al. Obesity and risk of adverse outcomes associated with coronary artery bypass surgery. Northern New England Cardiovascular Disease Study Group. Circulation. 1998;**97**(17):1689–94.

44. Alam M, Siddiqui S, Lee VV, Elayda MA, Nambi V, Yang EY, et al. Isolated coronary artery bypass grafting in obese individuals: a propensity matched analysis of outcomes. Circ J. 2011;**75**(6):1378–85.

45. Kim J, Hammar N, Jakobsson K, Luepker R V., McGovern PG, Ivert T. Obesity and the risk of early and late mortality after coronary artery bypass graft surgery. Am Heart J. 2003;**146**(3):555–60.

46. Costa VEA, Ferolla SM, Reis TO dos, Rabello RR, Rocha EAV, Couto CMF, et al. Impact of body mass index on outcome in patients undergoing coronary artery bypass grafting and/or valve replacement surgery. Rev Bras Cir Cardiovasc. Brazil; 2015;**30**(3):335–42.

47. Chakravartty S, Sarma DR, Patel AG. Rhabdomyolysis in bariatric surgery: a systematic review. Obes Surg. 2013;**23**(8):1333–40.

48. Bostanjian D, Anthone GJ, Hamoui N, Crookes PF. Rhabdomyolysis of gluteal muscles leading to renal failure: a potentially fatal complication of surgery in the morbidly obese. Obes Surg. 2003;**13**(2):302–305.

49. Sugerman H, Windsor A, Bessos M, Wolfe L. Intra-abdominal pressure, sagittal abdominal diameter and obesity comorbidity. J Intern Med. 1997;**241**(1):71–79.

Venous thromboembolism
Incidence, prophylaxis, and management

Elizabeth A. Valentine

Introduction

Obesity has become a worldwide pandemic. More than one-third of adults in the United States are obese, defined as a body mass index (BMI) greater than or equal to 30 kg/m² [1]. Obesity is associated with significant medical comorbidities including cardiovascular disease, renal disease, metabolic syndrome, obstructive sleep apnoea, cancer, and venous thromboembolism (VTE) [2–8]. Bariatric surgery has been demonstrated to be the most effective treatment for morbidly obese patients (BMI >40 kg/m²) and may result in the reduction or elimination of these comorbidities [9–14]. The majority of non-surgical alternatives (primarily focused on diet modification and exercise) have not been demonstrated to be efficacious over the long-term in this patient population [15–17]. Similarly, bariatric surgery may result in better long-term weight loss in patients with class I obesity (BMI 30–35 kg/m²) than non-surgical therapies [18]. Thus, the number of bariatric surgeries performed worldwide continues to increase, with over 220,000 performed annually in the United States [17,19].

VTE is a spectrum of disease encompassing both deep vein thrombosis (DVT) and pulmonary embolism (PE). Venous thromboembolic disease is one of the leading causes of preventable death in hospitalized patients, and approximately one-third of VTE-related deaths occur in surgical patients [20,21]. Obesity is a known risk factor for VTE in both medical and surgical patients, and VTE continues to be a major source of morbidity and mortality following bariatric surgery [22,23]. VTE is the second leading cause of death following bariatric surgery following anastomotic leak [24–26]. Nearly 40% of postoperative deaths have been attributable to VTE [24], and PE was noted on autopsy in as many as 80% of bariatric surgery patients [26]. The overall incidence of VTE in bariatric surgery varies based on type and invasiveness of procedure. The incidence of VTE in open bariatric surgery has been reported to be anywhere from 0.6% to 3.5% of patients [27–41]. In revisional surgery, the risk is likely greater still and has been reported to be as high as 6.4% [38]. The risk of VTE has decreased with the advent of laparoscopic bariatric surgery, with reported incidences ranging from 0% to 2.9% [30–33,37–40,42–44].

In this chapter, we will review the pathophysiology of venous thromboembolic disease in the bariatric population, the clinical presentation and diagnostic issues encountered, and options for prophylaxis and treatment.

Pathophysiology of venous thromboembolism

Though the coagulation cascade is an essential part of haemostasis, a pathological activation of this mechanism results in the clinical entity known as VTE. Thrombi most commonly originate in the deep veins in the calf and propagate proximally. Thrombi that extend above the popliteal vein are more likely to embolize to the lungs [45]. Approximately 80% of patients who present with PE exhibit evidence of lower extremity DVT; however, only approximately half of patients with proximal DVT progress to PE [46–48].

VTE is associated with three conditions that predispose to thrombus formation, known as Virchow's triad: (1) hypercoagulability, (2) stasis, and (3) endothelial damage (**Fig. 27.1**). It is increasingly recognized that obesity is a proinflammatory, prothrombotic state [7,49]. BMI has been positively correlated with coagulation factor, fibrinogen, and von Willebrand factor levels [50–53]. Increased platelet aggregation, plasma viscosity, and fibrin formation also contribute to the increased risk of VTE in this patient population [49,53]. Elevated BMI is associated with elevated plasminogen activator inhibitor-1 activity, which inhibits normal fibrinolysis and further increases the risk of thrombus formation [52,53]. Finally, visceral adipose tissue produces adipokines such as leptin, which acts peripherally on adenosine diphosphate-induced platelet aggregation and tissue plasminogen activator antigen [49,50,54,55]. Leptin levels are elevated in obesity and may contribute to an imbalance favouring thrombus formation. Obesity-associated hypertriglyceridemia and hyperglycaemia may induce a hypercoagulable, hypofibrinolytic state independent of obesity alone [49,56–58].

Surgery also promotes an inflammatory milieu and is a significant risk factor for VTE [59,60]. The incidence of VTE in surgical patients is approximately 8 per 1000 patients, approximately eight times the incidence in the general population [61,62].

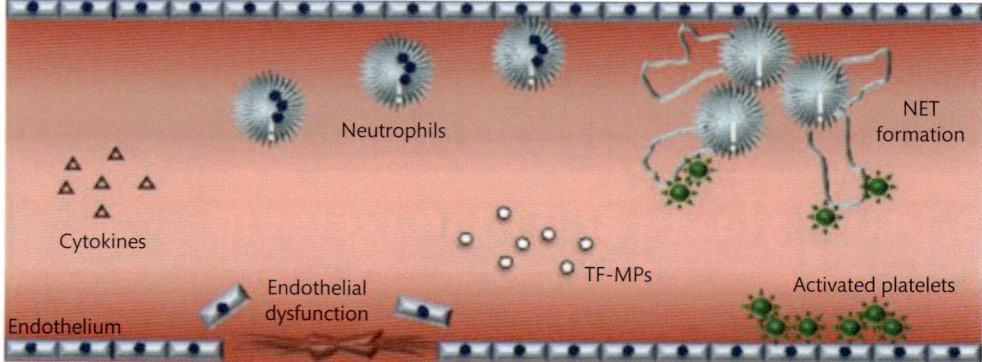

Fig. 27.1 Molecular and cellular mediators of inflammation-induced thrombosis. Schematic representation of inflammatory mediators of venous thrombosis, which include cytokine release, induction of neutrophil extracellular trap (NET) formation, endothelial dysfunction, platelet activation, and tissue factor microparticle (TF-MP) generation.

Reproduced with permission from Albayati, M. A., Grover, S. P., Saha, P., Lwaleed, B. A., Modrai, B., Smith, A., Postsurgical inflammation as a causative mechanism of venous thromboembolism, *Seminars in Thrombosis and Hemostasis*, 41(6): 615–20. Copyright © 2015 Georg Thieme Verlag KG. doi: 10.1055/s-0035-1556726.

Intraoperative tissue manipulation and endothelial damage may release a variety of proinflammatory cytokines such as interleukins 6, 8, and 10; tumour necrosis factor alpha, tissue factor, and C-reactive protein [60]. These cytokines remain upregulated in the postoperative period. Neutrophil extracellular traps, stimulated by proinflammatory cytokines, interact with both platelets and erythrocytes and attract components of the coagulation cascade including von Willebrand factor and fibrinogen [63]. These neutrophil extracellular traps are necessary for thrombus formation and may serve as the nidus for thrombus propagation [60,63]. Surgery also leads to transient platelet activation for the first 24–48 hours postoperatively [64].

Both obesity and surgery contribute to blood stasis which predisposes patients to VTE. Obesity, particularly abdominal obesity, leads to chronic elevations in intra-abdominal pressure and decreased blood velocity in the femoral veins [6,60]. Obesity may contribute to a sedentary lifestyle and impaired gait, also increasing the risk of stasis and VTE [7,45]. Both length of surgery and invasiveness of surgery have been associated with risk of VTE. In the acute postoperative period, pain, residual sedation, or activity restriction may also contribute to inactivity and venous stasis.

When DVT embolizes to the pulmonary circulation, obstruction of the pulmonary arteries by thrombus leads to increased right ventricular (RV) afterload and wall tension. The RV differs both structurally and functionally from the left ventricle (LV) [65]. The concentric-shaped LV, comprised of muscle fibres arranged primarily in parallel, is well suited for withstanding large increases in afterload. The RV, on the other hand, is thinner, crescent-shaped, with muscle fibres arranged in series [66]. This makes the RV much less tolerant of acute increases in afterload such as those that occur with VTE. The pulmonary vasculature is a low-resistance, high-capacitance system and the increase in RV afterload depends on the location and burden of pulmonary thrombus. Approximately one-quarter to one-third of the pulmonary circulation must be occluded in a healthy patient before an increase in pulmonary pressure is noted, and nearly one-half to three-quarters must be obstructed before frank RV failure occurs [48,65,67]. The end result of a significantly increased afterload on the more compliant is RV is dilation, ischaemia, and dysfunction [65]. Both RV volume and pressure increase, and the RV begins to 'fall off' the descending portion of the Frank–Starling curve, resulting in a decrease in stroke volume [65,68]. Increasing RV dilation also leads to progressive dilation of the tricuspid valve annulus, further decreasing forward RV output. Progressive RV overload shifts the interventricular septum towards the LV, which additionally impinges upon RV function [68]. Ultimately, death from PE occurs as a result of progressive 'auto-aggravation' of RV dysfunction, culminating in electromechanical dissociation and RV failure [65,66,68]. While mechanical obstruction is the primary contributor to haemodynamic compromise, the release of vasoactive and bronchoactive substances (including histamine, serotonin, and thromboxane) by platelet and thrombin-rich clots also contribute to the pathophysiological derangements commonly observed with PE [45,65].

Clinical presentation

Venous thromboembolic disease has been called 'the great imitator' because the presentation is frequently non-specific and insidious, requiring a high degree of suspicion. Symptoms depend on where in the circulatory system the disease process is present. The typical site of thrombus origin is in the deep venous system of the leg, which then embolizes to the lungs. Diagnosis may prove difficult in the bariatric patient due to limitations in physical examination and confirmatory diagnostic imaging.

The clinical presentation of DVT may range from the asymptomatic to the atypical but dramatic phlegmasia cerulea dolens (literally: 'painful blue oedema'). The most common signs and symptoms of DVT include leg pain, tenderness, erythema, oedema, cyanosis, and fever. A palpable 'cord' may be felt over the thrombosed vessel. The sensitivity and specificity of history and physical examination for diagnosing DVT is notoriously low, although the diagnostic value is relatively higher in high-risk populations (such as obese and postoperative patients) [69–72]. In the obese patient, the ability to appreciate physical examination findings may be limited due to body habitus. For example, the ability to appreciate cords or swelling in the lower extremities may be hindered by body habitus. Chronic lower extremity oedema and skin changes are very common in obesity. Acute changes in baseline symptoms may alert the clinician to a new diagnose of DVT.

Table 27.1 Common physiological alterations seen in obesity complicating the diagnosis of pulmonary embolism

Suggestive diagnostic criteria for PE	Common physiological alterations in obese and morbidly obese patients
Dyspnoea	Respiratory rates up to 40% higher than normal
Tachycardia	Heart rate increases as BMI increases
Signs of DVT	Leg oedema and chronic skin changes
Hypoxaemia	PaO_2 inversely related to waist circumference
Elevated BNP	Complex BNP alterations with both decreases and elevations seen
Elevated D-dimer	D-dimer is commonly elevated
Pulmonary hypertension	RVSP up to 40 mmHg may be normal

BMI, body mass index; BNP, brain natriuretic protein; DVT, deep vein thrombosis; PaO_2, arterial partial pressure of oxygen; PE, pulmonary embolism; RVSP, right ventricular systolic pressure.

Reproduced with permission from Hawley, P.C., Hawley, M. P. Difficulties in diagnosing pulmonary embolism in the obese patient: a literature review. *Vascular Medicine*, 16(6):444–51. Copyright © SAGE.

When a DVT embolizes to the pulmonary circulation, symptoms depend on both the temporal acuity as well as the extent of pulmonary vasculature obstruction and right heart strain (Table 27.1). A small PE, in which less than 50% of the vasculature is obstructed, is often asymptomatic. It has been demonstrated that close to 40% of patients with DVT who have no symptoms of PE have evidence of the disease on lung imaging [48]. Those with clinical symptomatology most frequently present with dyspnoea, either at rest or on exertion [73]. The clinical picture is often compounded as dyspnoea is also a common complaint in the general obese population [74,75]. Pulmonary infarction may also result in pleuritic chest pain and haemoptysis. Physical signs are frequently non-specific. The patient may present with fever, tachycardia, and/or tachypnoea. Breathing is frequently dyspnoeic or shallow as a result of pleuritic pain; however, both tachycardia [76] and tachypnoea [77] are common in obese patients at baseline. Cyanosis is not present with a small PE because the disturbance in oxygenation will be minor when a minimal amount of pulmonary vasculature is compromised. Signs of pulmonary infarction may include rales, effusion, or a pleural rub. Such physical examination findings may be difficult to appreciate through a large chest wall [78]. Haemodynamics will be maintained, with no evidence of compromised cardiac output or elevated pulmonary arterial pressures.

A massive acute PE, obstructing greater than 50% of the vasculature, may present with syncope, right heart strain, and haemodynamic instability or collapse [48]. This can occur with a large clot that obstructs the pulmonary arteries (known as a 'saddle embolus') or a cumulative result of multiple 'showers' of more distal emboli. Massive PE results in hypoxia for several reasons. Ventilation/perfusion (V/Q) mismatch occurs both as a result of the release of vasoactive mediators as well as by the fact that remaining unobstructed pulmonary vasculature may receive a disproportionate fraction of the cardiac output. This relative overperfusion may overwhelm the ability to fully oxygenate the blood. Shunting occurs as a result of pulmonary collapse and infarction. Finally, a low cardiac output from progressive RV failure leads to a high extraction of blood oxygen content, with an inability to fully adapt as more deoxygenated blood passes through the compromised pulmonary system

[48]. In patients without underlying cardiovascular or pulmonary disease, the degree of arterial hypoxia is proportional to the extent of the embolus. Carbon dioxide elimination may also be affected by the increase in dead-space ventilation, although a compensatory hyperventilation as a result of hypoxia tends to compensate for this problem.

Massive acute PE frequently presents with a more dire clinical presentation. Patients typically appear in acute distress with severe dyspnoea. They may present with syncope related to haemodynamic instability, as the RV has no time to adapt to a sudden increase in vascular resistance. Mental status may range from agitation to confusion to frank obtundation. Patients may be tachypnoeic, dyspnoeic, and cyanotic. A combination of increased myocardial demand and decreased oxygen supply can result in angina chest pain. Physical signs may include those of both left-sided (sinus tachycardia, hypotension, and cool extremities) and right-sided (jugular venous distension, a widely split second heart sound, or a 'gallop' on cardiac auscultation) heart failure. Again, physical signs of left and right heart failure may be more difficult to appreciate in obese patients due to body habitus.

Massive subacute PE occurs over days to weeks, as may occur in the postoperative period. The RV has time to hypertrophy and adapt since the obstruction occurs over a longer period of time. Pulmonary pressures may be higher than those seen in acute massive PE because the RV has time to adjust to the increased pressure without overt failure. As a result of this gradual adaptation, right-sided heart pressures are typically lower than those seen in the acute presentation. Similarly, systemic haemodynamics are reasonably normal because of the well-adapted RV. The main symptoms of a subacute massive PE are dyspnoea (frequently out of proportion to other clinical findings) and fatigue. A third heart sound may be audible at the lower sternal border and the pulmonic component of the second heart sound may be accentuated. Ability to appreciate these findings may be limited in the bariatric population [48].

Diagnostic testing

The ability to accurately diagnose VTE by history and physical examination is notoriously poor [69–72]. Thus, diagnostic testing is generally employed to confirm suspicion of VTE. Hypoxia, diagnosed by pulse oximetry or arterial blood gas, is frequently the first indication of PE; however, resting hypoxia is not uncommon in obese patients due to V/Q mismatch or obesity hypoventilation syndrome [74,79]. Plasma D-dimers are specific cross-linked fibrin derivatives that are formed whenever fibrin is formed and degraded. Plasma D-dimer levels are elevated in a variety of conditions including VTE, surgery, cancer, or infection. Thus, D-dimer levels are sensitive but not specific for VTE. Conversely, D-dimer values are rarely elevated in healthy patients; thus, they have a high negative predictive value as an exclusionary test [80]. The combination of a low pretest probability of VTE and negative D-dimer has been demonstrated as a safe and efficacious way to rule out VTE without further diagnostic imaging [81].

An electrocardiogram (ECG) is generally obtained as part of the diagnostic workup of chest pain or dyspnoea. A variety of ECG changes have been suggested to have diagnostic value in patients with suspected PE, although the role of ECG in diagnosing PE has been called into question [82]. Non-specific ECG findings associated with PE include sinus tachycardia, atrial tachycardia, complete or incomplete right bundle branch block, right axis deviation, T-wave inversion in the anterior precordial and inferior leads, and ST changes [83]. The classic teaching of S1Q3T3 (deep S wave in lead I, Q wave in lead III, and inverted T wave in lead III) is an infrequent finding in acute PE [84]. Obesity in itself results in predictable changes in ECG, including a baseline sinus tachycardia and non-specific repolarization abnormalities, leading to more difficult interpretation in this patient population [85]. Obese patients may also have ECG evidence of right heart compromise from underlying pulmonary hypertension and RV dysfunction, as opposed to VTE.

Echocardiography may be a diagnostic tool employed for patients with suspected PE, particularly for those deemed too unstable to travel to radiology. Transthoracic echocardiography can elucidate indirect signs of PE, based on estimations of pulmonary artery systolic pressure and acute RV pressure overload. Transoesophageal echocardiography may be able to directly demonstrate a saddle thrombus in the main pulmonary arteries but is unable to visualize more distal clot burden [86]. Most patients with a PE have a normal echocardiogram as at least 30% of pulmonary vasculature must be obstructed before evidence of RV dysfunction can be appreciated [87]. The presence of RV dysfunction, dilation, or hypokinesis by echocardiography significantly increases the clinical probability of PE and is a poor prognostic indicator [87]. Elevated pulmonary and RV pressures, however, can be a normal finding in obese patients, especially those with underlying obstructive sleep apnoea or obesity hypoventilation syndrome [88]. It may be difficult to determine, therefore, whether elevated pulmonary artery pressures are due to an acute process without knowing the patient's baseline status. Technical limitations as a result of body habitus may make it difficult or impossible to obtain adequate windows on examination.

Historically, the radiological 'gold standard' for diagnosis of VTE was invasive imaging including contrast venography (for DVT) and pulmonary angiography (for PE). These examinations are invasive, expensive, and fraught with complications such as nephrotoxicity of iodinated contrast agents, risk for allergic reaction, phlebitis, arrhythmia, and haemorrhage. Thus, while these imaging modalities may still be used in rare circumstances, the practice has been largely abandoned in favour of newer, less invasive techniques. If these studies are deemed necessary, weight constraints of the fluoroscopy table may limit the ability to safely perform these procedures.

Venography has been replaced by duplex ultrasonography (US) as the imaging modality of choice for the diagnosis of DVT. It is also often used as part of the decision-making process for patients with suspected PE in whom pulmonary imaging is either non-diagnostic or not obtainable. Diagnostic criteria for DVT include inability to collapse a vein under moderate pressure, increased venous diameter, absence of spontaneous of blood flow, absence of adequate augmentation of blood flow with distal compression, and increased intraluminal echogenicity [89]. Duplex US is both sensitive and specific for the diagnosis of VTE disease. A recent meta-analysis found the overall sensitivity and specificity of duplex US for diagnosis of DVT to be 89.7% and 93.8%, respectively [90]. Both sensitivity and specificity were better in patients at high clinical risk of DVT. Duplex US has the ability to comment on other differential diagnoses (such as aneurysm, tumour, cyst, or musculoskeletal injury) as well as

differentiate between acute or chronic thrombosis [91]. Duplex US also has the additional benefit of being non-invasive and portable.

Obesity may prove a hurdle in the accurate diagnosis of DVT by US. US imaging, compared to other imaging modalities, is compromised by increase tissue depth as a result of obesity [92]. As US waves traverse tissues, they are either transmitted to deeper structures, reflected back to the US probe as echo, or transformed to heat. The amount of echo depends on the acoustic impedance innate to the tissue interface encountered (e.g. air, bone, blood, or muscle). High-frequency (short wavelength) US generates images of high axial resolution; however, low tissue penetration means they are suitable for more superficial structures only [93]. Low-frequency (long wavelength) ultrasound can penetrate deeper structures but offer images of lower resolution. Deep veins, particularly in obese patients, may require the use of lower-frequency US transducers, leading to suboptimal imaging. Increased attenuation of the US beam as it passes through an increased amount of subcutaneous fat further compounds the issue of beam penetration [94]. Calf size has been noted to compromise the technical adequacy of US imaging [95]. Computed tomographic (CT) or magnetic resonance venography may be a more useful imaging tool for morbidly obese patients although body habitus may also preclude the ability to obtain these studies [96–98].

V/Q scintigraphy and CT pulmonary angiography (CTPA) are the diagnostic modalities of choice in the modern era for PE. A V/Q scan is a nuclear medicine procedure that uses radiolabelled tracers to evaluate air flow (ventilation) and blood flow (perfusion) to the lungs. Patients are classified into high, intermediate, and low risk of PE on the basis of size and number of defects noted on the scan [99]. Many early V/Q scans produced an unacceptably high rate of low- or intermediate-probability tests, with truly 'diagnostic' results (either normal study or high probability for PE) in fewer than 30% of cases [47,100,101]. Further study suggested that underlying cardiopulmonary issues (common in bariatric patients) makes interpretation of V/Q scans more difficult [102]. These limitations in diagnostic accuracy led to the increase in popularity of CTPA as the diagnostic imagining of choice for PE [103,104]. More recently, single-photon emission computed topography (V/Q SPECT) has emerged as an option for diagnostic imaging, and a recent meta-analysis suggests no performance difference between V/Q SPECT and CTPA [105]. CTPA has the benefit of 24/7 availability in most institutions (as opposed to more limited availability of nuclear medicine studies), at the cost of increased radiation exposure as well as exposure to iodinated contrast.

No published studies have evaluated the relationship between obesity and quality of imaging for V/Q scans; however, functional limitations may prevent the ability to obtain a diagnostic quality image. Table weight limits may exclude morbidly obese patients. Some patients may not fit between the two heads of the biplanar scanner (typically not adjustable), and while single-plane scanning can be performed, the quality may be compromised. Single-plane scanning also limits the number of images obtainable and results in suboptimal cropping of the images obtained. Though dosing of radioisotope used is weight based, a maximal allowable dose may also result in inadequate images for obtaining a diagnosis [74]. Image quality is degraded by the scatter of photons within adipose and other soft tissue [94].

CTPA has largely replaced V/Q scans in the modern era for diagnosis of PE. CTPA has been demonstrated to be an effective imaging modality in patients weighing up to 125 kg with no significant deterioration of either image quality or diagnostic confidence [106,107]. In general, details of even small structures are discernible in obese patients. Limitations exist, however, including increased noise secondary to beam penetration, limited field of view, and a decrement in image quality due to image cropping [94]. Obesity is frequently cited as a factor when studies are poor or non-diagnostic [108–110]. In addition to poor image quality, weight and girth limitations may prevent the ability to obtain a CT scan. Some patients may meet weight requirements but girth prevents them from fitting through the CT gantry. New 'heavy-weight' scanners for weights up to 300 kg (gantry aperture 80 cm) are improving the ability to obtain CT scans in the bariatric population [74].

Options for venous thromboembolism prophylaxis

As both obesity and surgery are risk factors for VTE, it is reasonable to assume that patients undergoing bariatric surgery are at particularly high risk for perioperative VTE. Risk factors thought to qualify a patient as high risk for VTE in bariatric surgery included male sex, history of DVT, known hypercoagulable status, severe immobility, BMI exceeding 55 kg/m², and arterial partial pressure of oxygen less than 60 mmHg [111]. To date, however, there is no clear consensus on the most appropriate VTE prophylaxis regimen in this population. The efficacy of VTE prophylaxis in bariatric patients, specifically, has been the focus of relatively few prospective studies, all with methodological flaws. Recent surveys of bariatric surgeons suggest that while nearly all surgeons consider this population high risk for thromboembolism, practice variations exist in the type and duration of VTE prophylaxis [112,113]. Perioperative pharmacological prophylaxis was used by the vast majority of respondents (92%), typically in combination with mechanical prophylaxis in the form of sequential compression devices [113]. In clinical practice, however, methods of prophylaxis range from early ambulation to mechanical to pharmacological prophylaxis.

Several societies have released recommendations for prevention of VTE in bariatric surgery (Table 27.2). The American College of Chest Physicians (ACCP) recommended in 2012 that virtually all patients undergoing bariatric surgery are at least moderate risk, if not high risk, for VTE [20]. It was the recommendation of that group that most patients undergoing bariatric surgery should be treated as high risk non-orthopaedic patients, with both pharmacological prophylaxis with low-dose unfractionated heparin (UFH) or low-molecular-weight heparin (LMWH) in combination with mechanical prophylaxis with elastic stockings or intermittent pneumatic compression [20]. The American Society for Metabolic and Bariatric Surgery and a joint position from the American Association of Clinical Endocrinologists, The Obesity Society, and the American Society for Metabolic and Bariatric Surgery released similar statements that a combination of pharmacological and mechanical prophylaxis is appropriate for patients undergoing bariatric surgery [114,115]. The Interdisciplinary European Guidelines on Metabolic and Bariatric Surgery similarly recommend both

mechanical and pharmacological prophylaxis and recommend LMWH in particular [116].

Mechanical strategies that may be employed for VTE prophylaxis include early ambulation and mechanical prophylaxis. Because bariatric patients are generally considered high risk for VTE complications, and mechanical prophylaxis is a reasonably low-risk addition, it is frequently employed in addition to pharmacological prophylaxis as described later in this chapter [113]. Early ambulation, while reported as a preventative strategy for VTE, is primarily used as an adjunctive therapy. Early ambulation helps to prevent VTE formation by reducing venous stasis. Methods of mechanical prophylaxis include graduated compression stockings or intermittent pneumatic compression with sequential compression devices. Literature in the general surgical population suggests a 50–65% reduction in the risk of perioperative DVT when mechanical prophylaxis is used [117,118]. There is no literature directly comparing mechanical to no mechanical prophylaxis in the bariatric surgery population.

Though some studies suggest that mechanical prophylaxis is sufficient for most bariatric patients [119,120], the general consensus is that that pharmacological prophylaxis is appropriate in this patient population [20,121]. Common pharmacological prophylaxis options for VTE prophylaxis include subcutaneous UFH and LMWH. LMWH offers the advantage of higher bioavailability, more predictable anticoagulation effect, lower risk of heparin-induced thrombocytopenia, and a longer half-life allowing for less frequent dosing [122–124]. In the general surgical population, meta-analyses suggest no difference between UFH and low-dose LMWH with respect to VTE incidence or outcomes; high-dose LMWH was associated with a lower risk of PE at the expense of increased risk of major haemorrhage [125,126]. Data comparing UFH to LMWH in the bariatric population are limited. An observational comparison of three perioperative regimens (pre- and postoperative UFH, preoperative UFH and postoperative LMWH, and pre- and postoperative LMWH) found a 57% lower risk of VTE in the UFH/LMWH group and a 66% lower risk of VTE in the LMWH/LMWH group [127]. A non-randomized study of two cohorts who received enoxaparin 40 mg subcutaneously twice daily to UFH 5000 units three times daily found no statistically significant difference in VTE rates but an increased risk of bleeding in the LMWH group [128]. It is notable that the dose of enoxaparin was higher than the recommended prophylactic dose. The paucity of literature does not allow for a recommendation for either UFH or LMWH as superior compared to the other. For preoperative prophylaxis, the majority of practitioners report using UFH (48.0%), with the remainder using enoxaparin (33.4%) or other agents (10.9%) [113]. Postoperatively, enoxaparin was the most commonly utilized agent (49.5%), followed by UFH (33.0%), and other agents (14.5%).

Regardless of the pharmacological agent chosen, recent guidelines agree that standard prophylactic doses of parenteral anticoagulants may not be sufficient to adequately prevent VTE in obese patients [20,121,123]. Both the ACCP 2012 Guidelines [20] and American Society for Metabolic and Bariatric Surgery Position Statement [114] on anticoagulation offer vague guidance that both choice and dose of agent is controversial. ACCP recommendations include consideration of consultation with a pharmacist regarding dosing in obese patients [20]. A number of clinical trials have demonstrated that standard dosing of prophylactic anticoagulants results in a

Table 27.2 Summary of published guidelines for prevention of venous thromboembolism in bariatric surgery

Guidelines (year)	Early ambulation	Lower extremity compression	Pharmacologic prophylaxis	Adjusted-dose heparin	Post-discharge pharmacologic prophylaxis	Prophylactic vena cava filter	Other recommendations
American Association of Clinical Endocrinologists/The Obesity Society/American Society for Metabolic and Bariatric Surgery (2013)	Recommended	Recommended SCD	SC UFH or LMWH given within 24 hours of surgery. Dose not specified	Not mentioned	Consider for high-risk patients (history of DVT)	Risk may exceed benefit	Discontinue oestrogen therapy preoperatively. Patients with history of DVT or cor pulmonale should undergo evaluation for DVT
American Society for Metabolic and Bariatric Surgery (2013)	Recommended	Recommended for all (unless not practical)	Combination of mechanical and chemical, should be considered based on clinical judgement and risk of bleeding. Conflicting data but data suggest LMWH over UFH	Not mentioned	Consider but insufficient data to recommend specific dose or duration	VCF as only method not recommended. Consider addition of VCF in high-risk patients where VTE risk > risk of filter-related complications	None
American College of Chest Physicians (2012)	Recommended	Rogers or Caprini score recommended: Low VTE risk: IPC. Moderate VTE risk: • Not high bleeding risk: SC UFH or LMH or IPC • High bleeding risk: IPC. High VTE risk: • Not high bleeding risk: SC UFH or LMWH and ES/IPC • High bleeding risk: IPC		Not mentioned	Not mentioned	Not recommended	If heparin contraindicated and not high risk of bleeding, consider low-dose aspirin, fondaparinux or IPC
Interdisciplinary European Guidelines on Metabolic and Bariatric Surgery (2013)	Recommended	Recommended ES and IPC	SC LMWH Dose not specified	Not mentioned	Not mentioned	Not mentioned	None

DVT, deep vein thrombosis; ES, elastic stockings; IPC, intermittent pneumatic compression; LMWH, low molecular weight heparin; SC, subcutaneous; SCD, sequential compression devices; UFH, unfractionated heparin; VCF, vena cava filters; VTE, venous thromboembolism.

subtherapeutic level of anticoagulation in more than 75% of patients [129,130]. A recent retrospective cohort study studied more than 9000 obese patients who received either standard-dose (enoxaparin 40 mg daily or UFH 5000 units two or three times daily) or high-dose (enoxaparin 40 mg twice daily or UFH 7500 units two or three times daily) VTE prophylaxis [131]. Patients were further stratified by BMI less than 40 kg/m² or BMI greater than or equal to 40 kg/m². While no difference in VTE rates was noted in the BMI less than 40 kg/m² group, a statistically significantly reduced incidence of VTE was noted in the high-dose prophylaxis group for those patients with BMI of at least 40 kg/m². It seems prudent, then, that an increased prophylactic dose of UFH 7500 units three times daily should be considered for patients with a BMI greater than 40 kg/m². Other studies have replicated a decreased risk of VTE in bariatric patients on higher-dose enoxaparin prophylaxis [132] and that higher-dose regimens are well tolerated [133]. Other LMWHs have not been as extensively studied as enoxaparin, but best expert consensus suggests that clinicians may consider increasing the total daily dose by 25–30% [134–136].

VTE events may occur in the immediate postoperative period or may be delayed after hospital discharge. Current guidelines suggest consideration of post discharge prophylaxis for high-risk patient populations, although the appropriate length of VTE prophylaxis following bariatric surgery is unclear [20]. Evidence from the Bariatric Outcomes Longitudinal Database suggests the overall risk of VTE within 90 days of surgery was 0.42%, and nearly 75% of these events occurred after hospital discharge [37]. Outcomes from the Mayo Bariatric Surgery Registry demonstrated the cumulative incidence of VTE at 7, 30, 90, and 180 days was 0.3, 1.9, 2.1, and 2.1%, respectively [29]. The majority of events occurred after hospital discharge but within 1 month of surgery. Recent evaluation of in-hospital only versus extended 10-day post-discharge pharmacological VTE prophylaxis demonstrated that two-thirds of thrombotic events occurred after cessation of prophylaxis, and rates were significantly higher in the in-hospital only group [137]. There was no significant difference in bleeding or reoperation rates in the group receiving extended VTE prophylaxis. While the appropriate duration of postoperative VTE prophylaxis remains uncertain, current literature suggests that continuation beyond hospital discharge, particularly for high-risk patients, is reasonable.

There are limited data on either traditional (i.e. warfarin) or novel oral anticoagulants in the bariatric surgery population. One study evaluating the use of postoperative warfarin for 30 days postoperatively (targeting and international normalized ratio <1.8) reports a decreased incidence of VTE events in the warfarin group; however, methodological flaws in the study limit the conclusions that can be drawn [138]. Dabigatran, a direct thrombin inhibitor, and rivaroxaban, a factor Xa inhibitor, are absorbed in the proximal gastrointestinal tract which is manipulated by bariatric procedures. Thus, the absorption of these drugs is likely to be altered following bariatric surgery [139]. Apixaban, another direct factor Xa inhibitor, is absorbed more distally in the gastrointestinal tract and may be less likely to be affected [139]. Neither the efficacy nor the safety of these agents has been adequately studied for postoperative VTE prophylaxis in the bariatric population [122]. Given the lack of data, oral anticoagulants cannot be recommended for VTE prophylaxis in this population.

The recognition of bariatric patients as high risk for VTE has resulted in an increased interest of prophylactic inferior vena cava (IVC) filters to prevent the downstream effects of PE. IVC filters represent the most aggressive and invasive method of VTE prophylaxis [24]. Reported complications related to IVC filter placement include IVC thrombosis, IVC perforation, filter migration requiring emergent cardiac surgery for retrieval/repair, hemopericardium, pneumothorax, contrast nephropathy, and infection [140,141]. Several studies have looked at the efficacy of IVC filters for VTE prophylaxis in the bariatric population [24,33,127,142,143]. Two meta-analysis have addressed the use of IVC filters in the bariatric surgery population [144,145]. Kaw and colleagues found that the use of IVC filters was associated with no difference in the incidence of PE, but an approximately threefold higher risk of DVT and death [144]. Brotman and colleagues also found an increased incidence of DVT and death in the IVC filter group with no difference in rate of PE [145]. It is difficult to make recommendations based on current literature, however, as it is all observational in nature. Selection bias exists as those patients who undergo prophylactic IVC filters are frequently those at highest risk for postoperative VTE. For example, patients in one study were more likely to be male and had a higher BMI (both associated with an increased risk of VTE) in the IVC filter group as compared to the no IVC filter group [33]. Patients who received filters may be more likely to also receive pharmacological prophylaxis [127], which may be a surrogate for patients considered high risk for VTE event. It is impossible to know what the postoperative rate of PE may have been for these high-risk patients had they not received a prophylactic IVC filter. Furthermore, the heterogeneity in pharmacological and mechanical prophylaxis employed in addition to IVC filters makes it difficult to generalize results. Randomized controlled trials are needed to make more definitive recommendations, but the available literature does not seem to support the placement of IVC filters as a routine method of VTE prophylaxis in the bariatric population. Current guidelines generally recommend against routine use of IVC filters for prophylaxis [20,114,116]. Nevertheless, in practice, 28.1% of recent survey respondents report routinely using retrievable IVC filters as VTE prophylaxis in this population [113]. If a retrievable filter was placed, it was most typically removed 30–90 days postoperatively [113].

Treatment of venous thromboembolism

Treatment of uncomplicated DVT is important to prevent post-thrombotic syndrome as well as propagation to acute PE. Up to 50% with proximal (above knee) lower extremity DVT will progress to PE without treatment [111,146]. Current treatment guidelines recommend patients with uncomplicated DVT be treated using LMWH, UFH, fondaparinux, or a hirudin derivative [146]. LMWH or fondaparinux is recommended rather than intravenous or subcutaneous UFH as LMWH is associated with decreased mortality, lower recurrence of VTE, and decreased incidence of major bleeding compared with UFH. An oral vitamin K antagonist such as warfarin is warranted for at least 3 months (and potentially longer if patient is at high risk of recurrence). Isolated deep distal (below knee) DVT without severe symptoms or risk for extension can be managed expectantly with serial imaging of the deep veins rather than initiating anticoagulation [146]. If at any point the thrombus extends (occurs in 10–20%), then anticoagulation management as previously mentioned is warranted. IVC filters are not recommended for routine management of lower extremity DVT but are recommended for patients with contraindications to anticoagulation and in those who failed therapy (i.e. PE despite adequate anticoagulation) [146].

In the case of a known diagnosis or high clinical suspicion of PE, treatment with parenteral anticoagulation (LMWH, fondaparinux, or UFH) should begin without delay and be continued for at least 5 days [146]. Current guidelines recommend LMWH or fondaparinux over UFH (either intravenous or subcutaneous). Enoxaparin should be dosed at 1 mg/kg twice daily, although caution must be utilized in obese patients (particularly those weighing >130 kg) as this population was not well represented in clinical trials for treatment of VTE [139]. Fondaparinux should be dosed 10 mg subcutaneously once daily for patients over 100 kg [139]. UFH should be dosed according to institutional protocol to maintain a goal-activated partial thromboplastin time of 1.5–2 times the normal value [139]. Early (same day) initiation of oral vitamin K antagonists is recommended, with documented international normalized ratio greater than 2 for at least 24 hours prior to discontinuing parenteral anticoagulation. Oral vitamin K antagonists should be continued for at least 3 months or longer if high risk. Thrombolytic therapy should be considered in patients with systemic hypotension (systolic blood pressure <90 mmHg) if no contraindication or bleeding risk.

Conclusion

Venous thromboembolic disease is a common postoperative complication and is more common in obese medical and surgical patients. It continues to be a significant source of both morbidity and mortality following bariatric surgery. Randomized controlled trials are lacking in the literature to recommend a best practice for prophylactic management. If pharmacological prophylaxis is to be employed, the literature lacks consensus on the best agent or dosing strategy. It is reasonable and recommended to consider bariatric patients a high-risk population and employ both pharmacological and mechanical prophylactic strategies. IVC filters cannot be routinely recommended for prophylaxis at this time. It is also reasonable to consider VTE prophylaxis in the post-hospital discharge due to the continued risk of VTE in the early postoperative period.

REFERENCES

1. Ogden CL, Carroll MD, Kit BK, Flegal KM. Prevalence of childhood and adult obesity in the United States, 2011–2012. JAMA 2014;311:806–14.
2. Ashrafian H, le Roux CW, Darzi A, Athanasiou T. Effects of bariatric surgery on cardiovascular function. Circulation 2008;118:2091–102.
3. Fenske W, Athanasiou T, Harling L, Drechsler C, Darzi A, Ashrafian H. Obesity-related cardiorenal disease: the benefits of bariatric surgery. Nature Reviews Nephrology 2013;9:539–51.
4. Ashrafian H, le Roux CW, Rowland SP, et al. Metabolic surgery and obstructive sleep apnoea: the protective effects of bariatric procedures. Thorax 2012;67:442–49.
5. Ashrafian H, Ahmed K, Rowland SP, et al. Metabolic surgery and cancer: protective effects of bariatric procedures. Cancer 2011;117:1788–99.
6. Braekkan SK, Hald EM, Mathiesen EB, et al. Competing risk of atherosclerotic risk factors for arterial and venous thrombosis in a general population: the Tromso study. Arteriosclerosis, Thrombosis, and Vascular Biology 2012;32:487–91.
7. Darvall KA, Sam RC, Silverman SH, Bradbury AW, Adam DJ. Obesity and thrombosis. European Journal of Vascular and Endovascular Surgery 2007;33:223–33.
8. Cello JP, Rogers SJ. Morbid obesity—the new pandemic: medical and surgical management, and implications for the practicing gastroenterologist. Clinical and Translational Gastroenterology 2013;4:e35.
9. Buchwald H. Consensus conference statement bariatric surgery for morbid obesity: health implications for patients, health professionals, and third-party payers. Surgery for Obesity and Related Diseases 2005;1:371–81.
10. Fried M, Hainer V, Basdevant A, et al. Interdisciplinary European guidelines on surgery of severe obesity. Obesity Facts 2008;1:52–59.
11. Sjostrom L, Peltonen M, Jacobson P, et al. Association of bariatric surgery with long-term remission of type 2 diabetes and with microvascular and macrovascular complications. JAMA 2014;311:2297–304.
12. Sjostrom L. Review of the key results from the Swedish Obese Subjects (SOS) trial—a prospective controlled intervention study of bariatric surgery. Journal of Internal Medicine 2013;273:219–34.
13. Sjostrom L, Peltonen M, Jacobson P, et al. Bariatric surgery and long-term cardiovascular events. JAMA 2012;307:56–65.
14. Sjostrom L, Narbro K, Sjostrom CD, et al. Effects of bariatric surgery on mortality in Swedish obese subjects. New England Journal of Medicine 2007;357:741–52.
15. Ashrafian H, Darzi A, Athanasiou T. Bariatric surgery—can we afford to do it or deny doing it? Frontline Gastroenterology 2011;2:82–89.
16. Safer DJ. Diet, behavior modification, and exercise: a review of obesity treatments from a long-term perspective. Southern Medical Journal 1991;84:1470–74.
17. Maggard MA, Shugarman LR, Suttorp M, et al. Meta-analysis: surgical treatment of obesity. Annals of Internal Medicine 2005;142:547–59.
18. Busetto L, Dixon J, De Luca M, Shikora S, Pories W, Angrisani L. Bariatric surgery in class I obesity: a Position Statement from the International Federation for the Surgery of Obesity and Metabolic Disorders (IFSO). Obesity Surgery 2014;24:487–519.
19. Buchwald H, Oien DM. Metabolic/bariatric surgery worldwide 2008. Obesity Surgery 2009;19:1605–11.
20. Gould MK, Garcia DA, Wren SM, et al. Prevention of VTE in nonorthopedic surgical patients: Antithrombotic Therapy and Prevention of Thrombosis, 9th ed: American College of Chest Physicians Evidence-Based Clinical Practice Guidelines. Chest 2012;141:e227S–77S.
21. Horlander KT, Mannino DM, Leeper KV. Pulmonary embolism mortality in the United States, 1979–1998: an analysis using multiple-cause mortality data. Archives of Internal Medicine 2003;163:1711–17.
22. Rocha AT, de Vasconcellos AG, da Luz Neto ER, Araujo DM, Alves ES, Lopes AA. Risk of venous thromboembolism and efficacy of thromboprophylaxis in hospitalized obese medical

patients and in obese patients undergoing bariatric surgery. Obesity Surgery 2006;**16**:1645–55.

23. Sapala JA, Wood MH, Schuhknecht MP, Sapala MA. Fatal pulmonary embolism after bariatric operations for morbid obesity: a 24-year retrospective analysis. Obesity Surgery 2003;**13**:819–25.

24. Li W, Gorecki P, Semaan E, Briggs W, Tortolani AJ, D'Ayala M. Concurrent prophylactic placement of inferior vena cava filter in gastric bypass and adjustable banding operations in the Bariatric Outcomes Longitudinal Database. Journal of Vascular Surgery 2012;**55**:1690–95.

25. Podnos YD, Jimenez JC, Wilson SE, Stevens CM, Nguyen NT. Complications after laparoscopic gastric bypass: a review of 3464 cases. Archives of Surgery (Chicago, Ill: 1960) 2003;**138**:957–61.

26. Melinek J, Livingston E, Cortina G, Fishbein MC. Autopsy findings following gastric bypass surgery for morbid obesity. Archives of Pathology & Laboratory Medicine 2002;**126**:1091–95.

27. Rowland SP, Dharmarajah B, Moore HM, et al. Inferior vena cava filters for prevention of venous thromboembolism in obese patients undergoing bariatric surgery: a systematic review. Annals of Surgery 2015;**261**:35–45.

28. Mason EE, Ito C. Gastric bypass. Annals of Surgery 1969;**170**:329–39.

29. Froehling DA, Daniels PR, Mauck KF, et al. Incidence of venous thromboembolism after bariatric surgery: a population-based cohort study. Obesity Surgery 2013;**23**:1874–79.

30. Smith SC, Edwards CB, Goodman GN, Halversen RC, Simper SC. Open vs laparoscopic Roux-en-Y gastric bypass: comparison of operative morbidity and mortality. Obesity Surgery 2004;**14**:73–76.

31. Carmody BJ, Sugerman HJ, Kellum JM, et al. Pulmonary embolism complicating bariatric surgery: detailed analysis of a single institution's 24-year experience. Journal of the American College of Surgeons 2006;**203**:831–37.

32. Gonzalez R, Haines K, Nelson LG, Gallagher SF, Murr MM. Predictive factors of thromboembolic events in patients undergoing Roux-en-Y gastric bypass. Surgery for Obesity and Related Diseases 2006;**2**:30–35.

33. Obeid FN, Bowling WM, Fike JS, Durant JA. Efficacy of prophylactic inferior vena cava filter placement in bariatric surgery. Surgery for Obesity and Related Diseases 2007;**3**:606–608.

34. Caruana JA, McCabe MN, Smith AD, Stawiasz KA, Kabakov E, Kabakov JM. Roux en Y gastric bypass by single-incision mini-laparotomy: outcomes in 3,300 consecutive patients. Obesity Surgery 2011;**21**:820–24.

35. Smith MD, Patterson E, Wahed AS, et al. Thirty-day mortality after bariatric surgery: independently adjudicated causes of death in the longitudinal assessment of bariatric surgery. Obesity Surgery 2011;**21**:1687–92.

36. Biertho L, Lebel S, Marceau S, et al. Perioperative complications in a consecutive series of 1000 duodenal switches. Surgery for Obesity and Related Diseases 2013;**9**:63–68.

37. Winegar DA, Sherif B, Pate V, DeMaria EJ. Venous thromboembolism after bariatric surgery performed by Bariatric Surgery Center of Excellence Participants: analysis of the Bariatric Outcomes Longitudinal Database. Surgery for Obesity and Related Diseases 2011;**7**:181–88.

38. Jamal MH, Corcelles R, Shimizu H, et al. Thromboembolic events in bariatric surgery: a large multi-institutional referral center experience. Surgical Endoscopy 2015;**29**:376–80.

39. Stein PD, Matta F. Pulmonary embolism and deep venous thrombosis following bariatric surgery. Obesity Surgery 2013;**23**:663–68.

40. Nguyen NT, Hinojosa M, Fayad C, Varela E, Wilson SE. Use and outcomes of laparoscopic versus open gastric bypass at academic medical centers. Journal of the American College of Surgeons 2007;**205**:248–55.

41. Escalante-Tattersfield T, Tucker O, Fajnwaks P, Szomstein S, Rosenthal RJ. Incidence of deep vein thrombosis in morbidly obese patients undergoing laparoscopic Roux-en-Y gastric bypass. Surgery for Obesity and Related Diseases 2008;**4**:126–30.

42. Higa KD, Ho T, Boone KB. Laparoscopic Roux-en-Y gastric bypass: technique and 3-year follow-up. Journal of Laparoendoscopic & Advanced Surgical Techniques Part A 2001;**11**:377–82.

43. Shepherd MF, Rosborough TK, Schwartz ML. Heparin thromboprophylaxis in gastric bypass surgery. Obesity Surgery 2003;**13**:249–53.

44. McCarty TM, Arnold DT, Lamont JP, Fisher TL, Kuhn JA. Optimizing outcomes in bariatric surgery: outpatient laparoscopic gastric bypass. Annals of Surgery 2005;**242**:494–98.

45. Tapson VF. Acute pulmonary embolism. New England Journal of Medicine 2008;**358**:1037–52.

46. Sandler DA, Martin JF. Autopsy proven pulmonary embolism in hospital patients: are we detecting enough deep vein thrombosis? Journal of the Royal Society of Medicine 1989;**82**:203–205.

47. Goldhaber SZ, Visani L, De Rosa M. Acute pulmonary embolism: clinical outcomes in the International Cooperative Pulmonary Embolism Registry (ICOPER). Lancet 1999;**353**:1386–89.

48. Riedel M. Acute pulmonary embolism 1: pathophysiology, clinical presentation, and diagnosis. Heart (British Cardiac Society) 2001;**85**:229–40.

49. Allman-Farinelli MA. Obesity and venous thrombosis: a review. Seminars in Thrombosis and Hemostasis 2011;**37**:903–907.

50. Chu NF, Spiegelman D, Hotamisligil GS, Rifai N, Stampfer M, Rimm EB. Plasma insulin, leptin, and soluble TNF receptors levels in relation to obesity-related atherogenic and thrombogenic cardiovascular disease risk factors among men. Atherosclerosis 2001;**157**:495–503.

51. Steffen LM, Cushman M, Peacock JM, et al. Metabolic syndrome and risk of venous thromboembolism: Longitudinal Investigation of Thromboembolism Etiology. Journal of Thrombosis and Haemostasis: JTH 2009;**7**:746–51.

52. Rosito GA, D'Agostino RB, Massaro J, et al. Association between obesity and a prothrombotic state: the Framingham Offspring Study. Thrombosis and Haemostasis 2004;**91**:683–89.

53. Mertens I, Van Gaal LF. Obesity, haemostasis and the fibrinolytic system. Obesity Reviews 2002;**3**:85–101.

54. Dellas C, Schafer K, Rohm I, et al. Absence of leptin resistance in platelets from morbidly obese individuals may contribute to the increased thrombosis risk in obesity. Thrombosis and Haemostasis 2008;**100**:1123–29.

55. Nakata M, Yada T, Soejima N, Maruyama I. Leptin promotes aggregation of human platelets via the long form of its receptor. Diabetes 1999;**48**:426–29.

56. Tsai AW, Cushman M, Rosamond WD, Heckbert SR, Polak JF, Folsom AR. Cardiovascular risk factors and venous thromboembolism incidence: the longitudinal investigation of thromboembolism etiology. Archives of Internal Medicine 2002;**162**:1182–89.

57. Ay C, Tengler T, Vormittag R, et al. Venous thromboembolism—a manifestation of the metabolic syndrome. Haematologica 2007;**92**:374–80.

58. Lemkes BA, Hermanides J, Devries JH, Holleman F, Meijers JC, Hoekstra JB. Hyperglycemia: a prothrombotic factor? Journal of Thrombosis and Haemostasis: JTH 2010;**8**:1663–69.

59. Anderson FA, Jr, Spencer FA. Risk factors for venous thromboembolism. Circulation 2003;**107**:I9–16.

60. Albayati MA, Grover SP, Saha P, Lwaleed BA, Modarai B, Smith A. Postsurgical inflammation as a causative mechanism of venous thromboembolism. Seminars in Thrombosis and Hemostasis 2015;**41**:615–20.

61. White RH, Zhou H, Romano PS. Incidence of symptomatic venous thromboembolism after different elective or urgent surgical procedures. Thrombosis and Haemostasis 2003;**90**:446–55.

62. Heit JA. The epidemiology of venous thromboembolism in the community. Arteriosclerosis, Thrombosis, and Vascular Biology 2008;**28**:370–72.

63. Fuchs TA, Brill A, Duerschmied D, et al. Extracellular DNA traps promote thrombosis. Proceedings of the National Academy of Sciences of the United States of America 2010;**107**:15880–85.

64. Samama CM, Thiry D, Elalamy I, et al. Perioperative activation of hemostasis in vascular surgery patients. Anesthesiology 2001;**94**:74–78.

65. Matthews JC, McLaughlin V. Acute right ventricular failure in the setting of acute pulmonary embolism or chronic pulmonary hypertension: a detailed review of the pathophysiology, diagnosis, and management. Current Cardiology Reviews 2008;**4**:49–59.

66. Bristow MR, Zisman LS, Lowes BD, et al. The pressure-overloaded right ventricle in pulmonary hypertension. Chest 1998;**114**:S101–106.

67. McIntyre KM, Sasahara AA. The hemodynamic response to pulmonary embolism in patients without prior cardiopulmonary disease. American Journal of Cardiology 1971;**28**:288–94.

68. Mebazaa A, Karpati P, Renaud E, Algotsson L. Acute right ventricular failure--from pathophysiology to new treatments. Intensive Care Medicine 2004;**30**:185–96.

69. Oudega R, Moons KG, Hoes AW. Limited value of patient history and physical examination in diagnosing deep vein thrombosis in primary care. Family Practice 2005;**22**:86–91.

70. Oudega R, Hoes AW, Toll DB, Moons KG. The value of clinical findings and D-dimer tests in diagnosing deep vein thrombosis in primary care. Seminars in Thrombosis and Hemostasis 2006;**32**:673–77.

71. Toll DB, Oudega R, Vergouwe Y, Moons KG, Hoes AW. A new diagnostic rule for deep vein thrombosis: safety and efficiency in clinically relevant subgroups. Family Practice 2008;**25**:3–8.

72. Criado E, Burnham CB. Predictive value of clinical criteria for the diagnosis of deep vein thrombosis. Surgery 1997;**122**:578–83.

73. Stein PD, Terrin ML, Hales CA, et al. Clinical, laboratory, roentgenographic, and electrocardiographic findings in patients with acute pulmonary embolism and no pre-existing cardiac or pulmonary disease. Chest 1991;**100**:598–603.

74. Hawley PC, Hawley MP. Difficulties in diagnosing pulmonary embolism in the obese patient: a literature review. Vascular Medicine (London, England) 2011;**16**:444–51.

75. Sahebjami H. Dyspnea in obese healthy men. Chest 1998;**114**:1373–77.

76. Frank S, Colliver JA, Frank A. The electrocardiogram in obesity: statistical analysis of 1,029 patients. Journal of the American College of Cardiology 1986;**7**:295–99.

77. Burki NK, Baker RW. Ventilatory regulation in eucapnic morbid obesity. American Review of Respiratory Disease 1984;**129**:538–43.

78. Silk AW, McTigue KM. Reexamining the physical examination for obese patients. JAMA 2011;**305**:193–94.

79. Holley HS, Milic-Emili J, Becklake MR, Bates DV. Regional distribution of pulmonary ventilation and perfusion in obesity. Journal of Clinical Investigation 1967;**46**:475–81.

80. Kelly J, Rudd A, Lewis RR, Hunt BJ. Plasma D-dimers in the diagnosis of venous thromboembolism. Archives of Internal Medicine 2002;**162**:747–56.

81. Wells PS, Anderson DR, Rodger M, et al. Excluding pulmonary embolism at the bedside without diagnostic imaging: management of patients with suspected pulmonary embolism presenting to the emergency department by using a simple clinical model and D-dimer. Annals of Internal Medicine 2001;**135**:98–107.

82. Van Mieghem C, Sabbe M, Knockaert D. The clinical value of the ECG in noncardiac conditions. Chest 2004;**125**:1561–76.

83. Digby GC, Kukla P, Zhan ZQ, et al. The value of electrocardiographic abnormalities in the prognosis of pulmonary embolism: a consensus paper. Annals of Noninvasive Electrocardiology 2015;**20**:207–23.

84. Richman PB, Loutfi H, Lester SJ, et al. Electrocardiographic findings in Emergency Department patients with pulmonary embolism. Journal of Emergency Medicine 2004;**27**:121–26.

85. Eisenstein I, Edelstein J, Sarma R, Sanmarco M, Selvester RH. The electrocardiogram in obesity. Journal of Electrocardiology 1982;**15**:115–18.

86. Pavan D, Nicolosi GL, Antonini-Canterin F, Zanuttini D. Echocardiography in pulmonary embolism disease. International Journal of Cardiology 1998;**65**(Suppl 1):S87–90.

87. Torbicki A, Pruszczyk P. The role of echocardiography in suspected and established PE. Seminars in Vascular Medicine 2001;**1**:165–74.

88. McQuillan BM, Picard MH, Leavitt M, Weyman AE. Clinical correlates and reference intervals for pulmonary artery systolic pressure among echocardiographically normal subjects. Circulation 2001;**104**:2797–802.

89. Lensing AW, Prandoni P, Brandjes D, et al. Detection of deep-vein thrombosis by real-time B-mode ultrasonography. New England Journal of Medicine 1989;**320**:342–45.

90. Goodacre S, Sampson F, Stevenson M, et al. Measurement of the clinical and cost-effectiveness of non-invasive diagnostic testing strategies for deep vein thrombosis. Health Technology Assessment (Winchester, England) 2006;**10**:1–168, iii–iv.

91. Labropoulos N, Leon M, Kalodiki E, al Kutoubi A, Chan P, Nicolaides AN. Colour flow duplex scanning in suspected acute deep vein thrombosis; experience with routine use. European Journal of Vascular and Endovascular Surgery 1995;**9**:49–52.

92. Uppot RN. Impact of obesity on radiology. Radiologic Clinics of North America 2007;**45**:231–46.

93. Lawrence JP. Physics and instrumentation of ultrasound. Critical Care Medicine 2007;**35**:S314–22.

94. Uppot RN, Sahani DV, Hahn PF, Gervais D, Mueller PR. Impact of obesity on medical imaging and image-guided intervention. AJR American Journal of Roentgenology 2007;**188**:433–40.

95. Rose SC, Zwiebel WJ, Murdock LE, et al. Insensitivity of color Doppler flow imaging for detection of acute calf deep venous thrombosis in asymptomatic postoperative patients. Journal of Vascular and Interventional Radiology 1993;**4**:111–17.

96. Hofmann LV, Bluemke DA, Fishman EK. Thrombosis of the deep femoral vein: a potential pitfall of color flow duplex Doppler ultrasonography. Southern Medical Journal 1997;**90**:1244–47.

97. Abdalla G, Fawzi Matuk R, Venugopal V, et al. The diagnostic accuracy of magnetic resonance venography in the detection of deep venous thrombosis: a systematic review and meta-analysis. Clinical Radiology 2015;**70**:858–71.

98. Garg K, Kemp JL, Wojcik D, et al. Thromboembolic disease: comparison of combined CT pulmonary angiography and venography with bilateral leg sonography in 70 patients. AJR American Journal of Roentgenology 2000;**175**:997–1001.

99. Biello DR, Mattar AG, McKnight RC, Siegel BA. Ventilation-perfusion studies in suspected pulmonary embolism. AJR American Journal of Roentgenology 1979;**133**:1033–37.

100. PIOPED Investigators. Value of the ventilation/perfusion scan in acute pulmonary embolism. Results of the prospective investigation of pulmonary embolism diagnosis (PIOPED). JAMA 1990;**263**:2753–59.

101. Goldhaber SZ, Visani L, De Rosa M. Acute pulmonary embolism: clinical outcomes in the International Cooperative Pulmonary Embolism Registry (ICOPER). Lancet 1999;**353**:1386–89.

102. Onyedika C, Glaser JE, Freeman LM. Pulmonary embolism: role of ventilation-perfusion scintigraphy. Seminars in Nuclear Medicine 2013;**43**:82–87.

103. Perrier A, Howarth N, Didier D, et al. Performance of helical computed tomography in unselected outpatients with suspected pulmonary embolism. Annals of Internal Medicine 2001;**135**:88–97.

104. Fedullo PF, Tapson VF. Clinical practice. The evaluation of suspected pulmonary embolism. New England Journal of Medicine 2003;**349**:1247–56.

105. Phillips JJ, Straiton J, Staff RT. Planar and SPECT ventilation/perfusion imaging and computed tomography for the diagnosis of pulmonary embolism: a systematic review and meta-analysis of the literature, and cost and dose comparison. European Journal of Radiology 2015;**84**:1392–400.

106. Szucs-Farkas Z, Megyeri B, Christe A, Vock P, Heverhagen JT, Schindera ST. Prospective randomised comparison of diagnostic confidence and image quality with normal-dose and low-dose CT pulmonary angiography at various body weights. European Radiology 2014;**24**:1868–77.

107. Megyeri B, Christe A, Schindera ST, et al. Diagnostic confidence and image quality of CT pulmonary angiography at 100 kVp in overweight and obese patients. Clinical Radiology 2015;**70**:54–61.

108. Jones SE, Wittram C. The indeterminate CT pulmonary angiogram: imaging characteristics and patient clinical outcome. Radiology 2005;**237**:329–37.

109. Stein PD, Fowler SE, Goodman LR, et al. Multidetector computed tomography for acute pulmonary embolism. New England Journal of Medicine 2006;**354**:2317–27.

110. Roggenland D, Peters SA, Lemburg SP, Holland-Letz T, Nicolas V, Heyer CM. CT angiography in suspected pulmonary embolism: impact of patient characteristics and different venous lines on vessel enhancement and image quality. AJR American Journal of Roentgenology 2008;**190**:W351–59.

111. Buesing KL, Mullapudi B, Flowers KA. Deep venous thrombosis and venous thromboembolism prophylaxis. Surgical Clinics of North America 2015;**95**:285–300.

112. Barba CA, Harrington C, Loewen M. Status of venous thromboembolism prophylaxis among bariatric surgeons: have we changed our practice during the past decade? Surgery for Obesity and Related Diseases 2009;**5**:352–56.

113. Pryor HI, 2nd, Singleton A, Lin E, Lin P, Vaziri K. Practice patterns in high-risk bariatric venous thromboembolism prophylaxis. Surgical Endoscopy 2013;**27**:843–48.

114. American Society for Metabolic and Bariatric Surgery Clinical Issues Committee. ASMBS updated position statement on prophylactic measures to reduce the risk of venous thromboembolism in bariatric surgery patients. Surgery for Obesity and Related Diseases 2013;**9**:493–97.

115. Mechanick JI, Youdim A, Jones DB, et al. Clinical practice guidelines for the perioperative nutritional, metabolic, and nonsurgical support of the bariatric surgery patient—2013 update: cosponsored by American Association of Clinical Endocrinologists, The Obesity Society, and American Society for Metabolic & Bariatric Surgery. Obesity (Silver Spring, Md) 2013;**21**(Suppl 1):S1–27.

116. Fried M, Yumuk V, Oppert JM, et al. Interdisciplinary European Guidelines on metabolic and bariatric surgery. Obesity Facts 2013;**6**:449–68.

117. Urbankova J, Quiroz R, Kucher N, Goldhaber SZ. Intermittent pneumatic compression and deep vein thrombosis prevention. A meta-analysis in postoperative patients. Thrombosis and Haemostasis 2005;**94**:1181–85.

118. Sachdeva A, Dalton M, Amaragiri SV, Lees T. Elastic compression stockings for prevention of deep vein thrombosis. Cochrane Database of Systematic Reviews 2010;**12**:CD001484.

119. Frantzides CT, Welle SN, Ruff TM, Frantzides AT. Routine anticoagulation for venous thromboembolism prevention following laparoscopic gastric bypass. JSLS: Journal of the Society of Laparoendoscopic Surgeons 2012;**16**:33–37.

120. Gagner M, Selzer F, Belle SH, et al. Adding chemoprophylaxis to sequential compression might not reduce risk of venous thromboembolism in bariatric surgery patients. Surgery for Obesity and Related Diseases 2012;**8**:663–70.

121. Prophylactic measures to reduce the risk of venous thromboembolism in bariatric surgery patients. Surgery for Obesity and Related Diseases 2007;**3**:494–95.

122. Bartlett MA, Mauck KF, Daniels PR. Prevention of venous thromboembolism in patients undergoing bariatric surgery. Vascular Health and Risk Management 2015;**11**:461–77.

123. Garcia DA, Baglin TP, Weitz JI, Samama MM. Parenteral anticoagulants: Antithrombotic Therapy and Prevention of Thrombosis, 9th ed: American College of Chest Physicians Evidence-Based Clinical Practice Guidelines. Chest 2012;**141**:e24S43S.

124. Weitz JI. Low-molecular-weight heparins. New England Journal of Medicine 1997;**337**:688–98.

125. Mismetti P, Laporte S, Darmon JY, Buchmuller A, Decousus H. Meta-analysis of low molecular weight heparin in the prevention of venous thromboembolism in general surgery. British Journal of Surgery 2001;**88**:913–30.

126. Koch A, Ziegler S, Breitschwerdt H, Victor N. Low molecular weight heparin and unfractionated heparin in thrombosis prophylaxis: meta-analysis based on original patient data. Thrombosis Research 2001;**102**:295–309.

127. Birkmeyer NJ, Finks JF, Carlin AM, et al. Comparative effectiveness of unfractionated and low-molecular-weight heparin for prevention of venous thromboembolism following bariatric surgery. Archives of Surgery (Chicago, Ill: 1960) 2012;**147**:994–98.

128. Kothari SN, Lambert PJ, Mathiason MA. Best Poster Award. A comparison of thromboembolic and bleeding events following laparoscopic gastric bypass in patients treated with prophylactic regimens of unfractionated heparin or enoxaparin. American Journal of Surgery 2007;**194**:709–11.

129. Freeman A, Horner T, Pendleton RC, Rondina MT. Prospective comparison of three enoxaparin dosing regimens to achieve target anti-factor Xa levels in hospitalized, medically ill patients with extreme obesity. American Journal of Hematology 2012;**87**:740–43.

130. Rowan BO, Kuhl DA, Lee MD, Tichansky DS, Madan AK. Anti-Xa levels in bariatric surgery patients receiving prophylactic enoxaparin. Obesity Surgery 2008;**18**:162–66.

131. Wang TF, Milligan PE, Wong CA, Deal EN, Thoelke MS, Gage BF. Efficacy and safety of high-dose thromboprophylaxis in morbidly obese inpatients. Thrombosis and Haemostasis 2014;**111**:88–93.

132. Scholten DJ, Hoedema RM, Scholten SE. A comparison of two different prophylactic dose regimens of low molecular weight heparin in bariatric surgery. Obesity Surgery 2002;**12**:19–24.

133. Borkgren-Okonek MJ, Hart RW, Pantano JE, et al. Enoxaparin thromboprophylaxis in gastric bypass patients: extended duration, dose stratification, and antifactor Xa activity. Surgery for Obesity and Related Diseases 2008;**4**:625–31.

134. Vandiver JW, Ritz LI, Lalama JT. Chemical prophylaxis to prevent venous thromboembolism in morbid obesity: literature review and dosing recommendations. Journal of Thrombosis and Thrombolysis 2016;**41**:475–81.

135. Nutescu EA, Spinler SA, Wittkowsky A, Dager WE. Low-molecular-weight heparins in renal impairment and obesity: available evidence and clinical practice recommendations across medical and surgical settings. Annals of Pharmacotherapy 2009;**43**:1064–83.

136. Hirsh J, Raschke R. Heparin and low-molecular-weight heparin: the Seventh ACCP Conference on Antithrombotic and Thrombolytic Therapy. Chest 2004;**126**:188s–203s.

137. Raftopoulos I, Martindale C, Cronin A, Steinberg J. The effect of extended post-discharge chemical thromboprophylaxis on venous thromboembolism rates after bariatric surgery: a prospective comparison trial. Surgical Endoscopy 2008;**22**:2384–91.

138. Heffline MS. Preventing vascular complications after gastric bypass. Journal of Vascular Nursing 2006;**24**:50–54.

139. Quidley AM, Bland CM, Bookstaver PB, Kuper K. Perioperative management of bariatric surgery patients. American Journal of Health-System Pharmacy 2014;**71**:1253–64.

140. Van Ha TG. Complications of inferior vena caval filters. Seminars in Interventional Radiology 2006;**23**:150–55.

141. Birkmeyer NJ, Finks JF, English WJ, et al. Risks and benefits of prophylactic inferior vena cava filters in patients undergoing bariatric surgery. Journal of Hospital Medicine 2013;**8**:173–77.

142. Halmi D, Kolesnikov E. Preoperative placement of retrievable inferior vena cava filters in bariatric surgery. Surgery for Obesity and Related Diseases 2007;**3**:602–605.

143. Gargiulo NJ, 3rd, Veith FJ, Lipsitz EC, Suggs WD, Ohki T, Goodman E. Experience with inferior vena cava filter placement in patients undergoing open gastric bypass procedures. Journal of Vascular Surgery 2006;**44**:1301–305.

144. Kaw R, Pasupuleti V, Wayne Overby D, et al. Inferior vena cava filters and postoperative outcomes in patients undergoing bariatric surgery: a meta-analysis. Surgery for Obesity and Related Diseases 2014;**10**:725–33.

145. Brotman DJ, Shihab HM, Prakasa KR, et al. Pharmacologic and mechanical strategies for preventing venous thromboembolism after bariatric surgery: a systematic review and meta-analysis. JAMA Surgery 2013;**148**:675–86.

146. Kearon C, Akl EA, Comerota AJ, et al. Antithrombotic therapy for VTE disease: Antithrombotic Therapy and Prevention of Thrombosis, 9th ed: American College of Chest Physicians Evidence-Based Clinical Practice Guidelines. Chest 2012;**141**:e419S–94S.

Tissue oxygenation in the obese patient

Shubhangi Singh, Prashant Singh, and Preet M. Singh

Introduction

Obesity is defined as a body mass index (BMI) greater than 30 kg/m². Morbid obesity is defined as a BMI greater than 40 kg/m² or greater than 35 kg/m² with the presence of comorbidities such as diabetes and hypertension. Obesity is a rampantly increasing medical condition all over the world. It affects over one-third of American adults [1] and its incidence continues to rise yearly. This proportionate increase in obesity is probably related to increased incidence and survival with chronic medical conditions such as type 2 diabetes, hypertension, and atherosclerotic disease including stroke and coronary artery disease. It poses unique challenges for the anaesthesiologist. This chapter focuses on pathophysiological changes occurring at micro-circulation level in the obese patient that may actually be an indirect consequence of the above-mentioned comorbidities.

Obesity is associated with many physiological changes. With the increase in body mass, there is also an increase in the blood volume. However, the increase in blood volume is disproportionately less as compared to the body mass and the adipose tissue. Thus, it follows that the blood supply (per gram) to various tissues, including the adipose tissues, is relatively less as compared to lean individuals. Pasarica et al. also found that obese patients have 44% less capillary density in the subcutaneous fat as compared to their lean counterparts [2]. In addition, it is known that during the adipose tissue expansion, areas of relative oxygen deficit develop due to insufficient angiogenesis in comparison to expansion of the adipose tissue. Thus, a situation of relatively lower oxygen/blood supply persists at the basal level.

Further, due to an increase in the soft tissue in the upper airway, the obese are also more prone to obstructive sleep apnoea as compared to their leaner counterparts. Thus, these individuals may undergo periods of extremely low oxygen tension during sleep. The basal partial pressures of oxygen are lower in morbidly obese patients and are further compromised in obese patients with obesity hypoventilation syndrome, therefore oxygen delivery to the tissue suffers.

Other changes involved with obesity include a decreased functional residual capacity. This occurs mostly due to a decrease in the expiratory reserve volume. The anatomical changes associated with obesity contribute to the mechanical disadvantage towards diaphragmatic excursion during basal breathing efforts. The interstitial pressure increases significantly, contributing to the collapse of conducting airways, at much higher lung residual volumes. Even at normal tidal volumes lung collapse starts to occur (higher closing capacity) and eventually the ventilation/perfusion mismatch worsens. This, in addition to lower functional residual capacity, is of importance as it decreases the time for tolerance of hypoxia in the obese population, leads to a faster apnoea time, and makes them more prone to tissue hypoxia. Also, the increased metabolic activity that the increase in the body weight affords makes the obese patients more prone to hypoxia.

Understanding why the morbidly obese patient has low baseline tissue oxygen saturation levels, and how they are more prone to further dips in oxygen levels as compared to their healthier counterparts, requires an understanding of the microcirculation and tissue oxygenation. The next section covers the details of how these variables are affected by obesity.

Microcirculation and cellular homeostasis

Human physiology is geared towards maintaining a steady state. Maintaining an organism as a whole in a steady state is dependent on maintaining homeostasis at the cellular level. It is well understood at this time that most of the traditional clinical parameters that are often used to represent homeostatic status of the body (blood pressure, arterial oxygen saturation) do not represent accurately the blood or oxygen delivered at the cellular level. Intuitively, mixed venous saturation (SvO_2) and the central venous oxygen saturation ($ScvO_2$) are often used to interpret the status of availability/extraction of oxygen and nutrients to the tissues. Lower values represent higher oxygen extraction and hence decreased oxygen or blood supply or increased tissue oxygen demand. However, since these entities essentially provide pooled data from all of the tissues of the body, they are prone to missing hypoxia or hypoperfusion in certain tissues of the body since lower oxygen levels in the blood coming from high-oxygen-extraction tissues can be counterbalanced by the highly saturated blood coming from less metabolically active tissues.

These concepts get more complicated in the obese patient. Obesity is associated with an overall increase in blood volume. However, the increase in the blood volume is not proportional to the increase in body weight or body fat. Hodson et al. found that the blood flow per 100 g of adipose tissue was about 3.2 mL/min in obese individuals as compared to 4.7 mL/min in their leaner counterparts [3]. Although this difference was not statistically significant, it can be extrapolated that the adipose tissue actually gets less blood supply per unit mass of tissue in an obese person as compared to a lean person. This has implications both for the chronic health and acute critical conditions in the obese. Although this concept leads to the idea of adipose tissue hypoxia, it needs further research for substantial evidence [4].

Microcirculation

Microcirculation refers to the vessels that are too small to be seen by the naked eye. These are the vessels that are directly responsible for carrying oxygen and other nutrients to the tissues. The adequacy of this blood flow can be assessed by either directly measuring the microvascular perfusion or indirectly by assessing the tissue oxygenation, which, gives an idea of the balance between supply to and demand of the tissue [5].

Tissue oxygenation

Tissue oxygenation refers to the amount of oxygen available at the tissue level. It can be estimated by two entities that are inter-related:

1. Tissue oxygen tension (tPO_2): tPO_2 refers to the tension or the partial pressure of the oxygen in the interstitial or the extra-vascular space. It represents a balance between the oxygen delivered by the capillaries to the cells and the consumption by the cells [6].
2. Tissue oxygen saturation (StO_2): StO_2 refers to the percentage of saturated haemoglobin in the tissue capillaries. Again, representing the balance between oxygen supply and demand, it is related to the tPO_2 by a complex sigmoid oxygen dissociation curve [7].

It is very important to emphasize that the microvasculature anatomy as well as the physiological parameters such as tPO_2, StO_2, and oxygen extraction vary widely from tissue to tissue. Additionally, a value that may be physiologically normal in one tissue, may actually represent severe hypoxia in the other. An example of this is that the normal oxygen extraction is about 60% in the cardiac muscle and only 15% in the kidneys under normal conditions. Thus, even in completely healthy states the tissue oxygenation in the cardiac tissue is likely to be much lower than that in the renal tissue. Therefore, equating cardiac and renal values may actually miss tissue level hypoxia occurring at the renal level manifesting only as a small drop in venous saturations.

Critical oxygen delivery point

The normal response of the tissue capillaries to an imbalance in the demand and supply is to dilate and increase the tissue perfusion to increase the oxygen supply, so that the metabolic demands are met. Under these conditions the cellular metabolism is aerobic. This also happens in cases where there is a fall in the oxygen saturation or blood pressure. This response is further enhanced by increases in metabolites such as bicarbonate, hydrogen ions, adenosine, hypoxia-related factors, and so on. In the vascular beds that are already maximally dilated, in the case of a fall in tissue perfusion, the oxygen

extraction increases without any change in oxygen consumption [8]. However, at a point referred to as the critical point, there cannot be any further increase in the oxygen extraction ratio and a switch from aerobic to anaerobic metabolism takes place. In addition to tissue metabolic rate, biochemical factors such as carbon dioxide (CO_2), 2,3-diphosphoglycerate, and products of metabolism determine this point. As a result, the absolute value of this physiological shift shows marked inter-tissue variability. Thus, recognizing when a particular tissue reaches this point can help in recognizing the temporal proximity to tissue damage. By the time the traditionally measurable parameters, such as arterial oxygen saturation, arterial oxygen tension, and blood pressure, get deranged, the tissues, especially, the ones with high metabolic requirements that are more prone to hypoxic damage, may have already sustained some degree of irreversible damage. Thus, the importance of measuring StO_2 and tension at individual tissue (metabolic units) cannot be overemphasized.

Measurement of tissue oxygen content

Clark et al. were the first to suggest measurement of tissue oxygen content in 1956. They used an electrode that used polarography to measure tPO_2 [9]. The more recent technologies are described in the following sections.

Reflectance spectroscopy

Reflectance spectroscopy-based technology has been used to measure tissue haemoglobin and relative oxyhaemoglobin concentration. This is then used to estimate tissue oxygenation. More recently, it has been used in the detection of dysplastic tissue [10].

Near-infrared spectroscopy

Near-infrared spectroscopy (NIRS) has been used to measure the ratio of haemoglobin to oxygenated haemoglobin and cytochrome CC3 (a high-molecular-weight cytochrome c) in tissues. This then estimates tissue oxygen availability [7,11]. It is extensively used to monitor cerebral oxygenation, often termed as $rScO_2$, in cardiac as well as non-cardiac surgeries [12]. It is important to note some limitations of NIRS in obese patients. First of all, penetration of infrared rays is limited in this patient population, due to increased tissue thickness. Also, in the obese, at baseline, the level of tissue oxygenation is lower than in the leaner counterparts to begin with. This number is expected to further decrease with development of a pathological state such as shock.

Microvascular perfusion

This can be directly measured as blood flow at tissue level assisted by laser Doppler flowmetry, nail fold microscopy, orthogonal polarization spectral imaging, or by sidestream dark field imaging, or indirectly by regional capnometry or by optode sensors.

Microvascular function

This can be assessed by venous occlusion plethysmography. This technology measures the microvascular permeability, which is expected to be deranged in the presence of microvascular dysfunction. The disadvantages of this technology include long measurement time and decreased utility in patients with low blood pressure. Also, with the currently available equipment, this can only be used in the extremities.

Tissue oxygenation and the morbidly obese

Obese patients are usually, chronically, in a state of mildly lower adipose tissue perfusion as compared to their leaner counterparts. This state of relative hypoperfusion promotes the generation of inflammatory cytokines via a pathway that involves the hypoxia-inducible factor [13]. It also leads to downregulation of the anti-inflammatory cytokine adiponectin [14], perpetuating towards a proinflammatory state. It is not clear, currently, if this leads to a generalized, global inflammation or to a relatively localized area of inflammation in the adipose tissue [13]. As mentioned earlier, obese individuals are more prone to obstructive sleep apnoea. During these episodes of apnoea, it is very likely that the above-mentioned expression of the pro-inflammatory cytokines such as hypoxia-inducible factor is exaggerated. It also follows that this further enhances the downregulation of the anti-inflammatory entities such as adiponectin. This inflammatory state is often not confined to the unhealthy tissue and is likely to cause dysfunction of the non-adipose adequately perfused tissue as well. Also, the downregulation of adiponectin is known to alter glucose/fatty acid metabolism and promote localized inflammation [15]. Furthermore, due to the inflammatory state, the levels of interleukin-6 are also elevated and this further contributes to the pathological inflammatory cascade process. All of these alterations lead to an adverse metabolic milieu that has a significant effect on the chronic health of the obese patient [16].

The obese patient in the perioperative period

The anaesthesia literature is well versed with the many anaesthetic challenges that the obese patient poses. These include increased incidence of difficult airway, reduced allowable apnoea time due to factors such as decreased functional residual capacity, increased incidence of difficult intravenous line placement, difficulty in regional and neuraxial blocks, difficulty in positioning, and so on. Often missed are pathological processes that are not clinically documented. Lower basal oxygen tension at tissue level is one of the frequently understated problems.

It is well known in the surgical world that subcutaneous tPO$_2$ determines the pace and quality of wound healing. Decreased tissue oxygenation, therefore, slows down wound healing in the obese and they need a higher inspired oxygen tension to heal surgical wounds as compared to lean patients [17]. Also, neutrophils need oxygen for their oxidative killing process. Lower oxygen tension in the tissues hampers this mechanism, thus rendering the obese patient more prone to wound infections [18]. As such, due to ample subcutaneous tissue, wound closure is mechanically more challenging in the obese.

Effect of neuraxial analgesia on tissue oxygenation in the obese

Pain that is inevitably associated with most surgical procedures also augments the sympathetic tone of the body. This increases metabolism and oxygen consumption, thus further lowering the tPO$_2$. Pain control itself is challenging in the obese population. Traditional intravenous medications such as opioids make the obese patient more prone to respiratory depression and increase the incidence of obstructive sleep apnoea. Thus, the medications that are used to alleviate pain can also precipitate a decrease in tissue oxygenation by associated respiratory depression. Regional anaesthesia techniques such as epidurals and nerve blocks are thus invaluable in the obese. They not only decrease the oxygen demand by decreasing the pain, but also lead to improved oxygen supply by causing vasodilation and hence increasing the blood flow to the tissue. Kabon et al. [19] compared general anaesthesia to a combination of general and thoracic epidural anaesthesia for major abdominal surgery in terms of tPO$_2$ in the obese patient. They found that although the haemodynamic responses and global or macroscopic oxygen variables, such as oxygen saturation of the arterial blood, were similar in both groups, tPO$_2$ was higher in the combined group as compared to the general anaesthesia group. Thus, they concluded that thoracic epidural anaesthesia improved the tPO$_2$ outside the pain control area covered by the epidural. Decrease in sympathetic tone due to pain relief plays an important role in this. However, as mentioned previously, these procedures are also more challenging technically in these patients due to excessive body fat and subcutaneous tissue obscuring the landmarks.

Effect of mild hypercapnia on tissue oxygenation in the obese

Hager et al. studied the effects of mild hypercapnia in obese patients undergoing gastric bypass on tissue oxygenation. They divided these patients into a normocapnia group (end-tidal CO$_2$ of 35 mmHg) and a mild hypercapnia group (end-tidal CO$_2$ of 50 mmHg). They measured the subcutaneous tissue oxygenation in both groups and found that the patients in the mild hypercapnia group had higher subcutaneous tPO$_2$. Thus, they concluded that mild hypercapnia could reduce the risk of surgical infections in obese patients [20].

Effect of postoperative oxygen supplementation on tissue oxygenation in the obese

Kabon et al. studied the effect of postoperative oxygen supplementation on tissue oxygenation in the morbidly obese patient. They compared the tissue and wound oxygen tension in a group of postoperative obese patients treated with 80% oxygen supplementation to another group who were supplemented with a fraction of inspired oxygen (FiO$_2$) of 30%. They found that tPO$_2$ was significantly higher in the obese patients who received oxygen supplementation at FiO$_2$ of 80% for 10–12 hours postoperatively as compared to those who received a FiO$_2$ of 30%. This was also true for wound oxygen tension [21]. Long-term improvement in outcome is still a matter of further research.

Thus, the obese patient in the perioperative period is a unique challenge in terms of tissue oxygenation. Use of regional techniques for pain control should be encouraged as far as possible. Although mild hypercapnia and increasing the FiO$_2$ of supplemental oxygen do improve the tPO$_2$, this has not been adopted as a clinical practice. More research needs to be done for risk:benefit assessment, before these practices can be accepted clinically.

Pathological states and tissue oxygen tension

Tissue oxygenation in states of decreased systemic perfusion

In pathological states of hypotension, due to compensatory vasoconstriction, it is easily understandable that the peripheral organs (e.g. skin and subcutaneous adipose tissue) will show a fall in the tissue oxygenation or StO_2 much earlier as compared to the central organs (e.g. brain, kidneys, and heart). This earlier fall in tissue oxygenation in the peripheral organs can thus be used to detect a pathological insult before the tissue oxygenation falls in the central organs leading to organ dysfunction. Alteration in the haemodynamic parameters (heart rate and blood pressure) and arterial oxygen saturation also occurs only after these compensatory mechanisms have failed. This fall in peripheral tissue oxygenation is expected to be more exaggerated in the obese patient due to their increased subcutaneous fat distribution and relatively lower adipose tissue perfusion. As mentioned previously, this leads to propagation of inflammatory pathways. It can thus be conjectured that the obese patients release far more inflammatory substances as compared to their leaner counterparts during these pathological states. It can be extrapolated from this that they can have a relatively faster clinical decline. The positive aspect of this is that a large-sized sampling tissue is available for monitoring and detection of such pathological states in the obese patients and can lead to the detection of a pathology early on. The next sections deal with some specific pathological conditions.

Haemorrhage and trauma

Drucker et al. studied the effects of haemorrhage in trauma patients on StO_2 and the mean arterial pressure (MAP). They used an optical method using fluorescent technology to study the subcutaneous tissue oxygen tension $(P(sg)O_2)$. They found that with 20% loss of blood volume the subcutaneous tissue oxygen tension declined rapidly and paralleled the change in the MAP. However, after the resuscitation, the MAP returned to normal rapidly, but the $P(sg)O_2$ did not return to normal until after 2 hours [22]. In a similar trial, Lima et al. studied the relationship between peripheral StO_2 measured by NIRS and haemodynamic parameters such as MAP, heart rate, and $ScvO_2$. They found that StO_2 did not show any correlation to the global haemodynamic parameters (MAP, $ScvO_2$, and heart rate). However, a lower StO_2 was found to be associated with a worse outcome [23]. Thus, traditional parameters such as blood pressure do not give an adequate idea of microcirculation and peripheral vasoconstriction may not have resolved by the time blood pressure has come back to normal. This microcirculatory deficiency continues to trigger inflammatory processes that lead to continued deterioration of the clinical status. It can thus be used to predict the possibility of an impending fall in blood pressure.

Biochemical markers have been used to indirectly assess the tissue perfusion. Lactate is one metabolite that is generated in the setting of anaerobic respiration at the cellular level. It is therefore logical that a decrease in tissue perfusion would lead to an increase in lactate levels. However, lactate is aerobically metabolized in the liver. This metabolism of lactate by the liver increases with increases in the FiO_2, by supplemental oxygen [7]. Thus, in the presence of supplemental oxygen, lactate levels may be normal, in spite of tissue hypoperfusion. Another biochemical parameter that has been used is the base deficit. Cohn et al. found that StO_2 measured using NIRS performed as well as base deficit in identifying multiorgan dysfunction syndrome among 383 trauma patients. The two were also equally good predictors of mortality [24].

Hypotension often prompts initiation of vasopressor support. Use of vasopressors can further decrease the peripheral tissue perfusion by increasing peripheral vasoconstriction. In a search for agents that can prevent tissue hypoperfusion, Nordin et al. conducted an interesting study on the effects of pentoxifylline on hepatic, gut, and peripheral tissue oxygenation in piglets in which haemorrhagic shock was induced. They found that although pentoxifylline improved the hepatic oxygen content, it did not have any effect on peripheral tissue oxygen content, until the blood volume was restored [25]. Thus, in order to counter a decrease in blood pressure, vasopressors may show improvement in global perfusion indices such as blood pressure and central venous pressure, although at tissue level the blood flow per unit mass actually falls and this compounds as tissue level hypoxia. Understanding the concept behind tissue level hypoxia may actually prompt the use of flow enhancers such as pentoxifylline in combination with vasoconstrictors in the near future.

Haemorrhage and trauma in the obese

Due to the increase in blood volume, it is understandable that obese trauma patients will require larger amounts of fluid for resuscitation as compared to those with normal BMI. Nelson et al. retrospectively studied the adequacy of resuscitation and its resulting outcome in over 1000 trauma patients. They found that, when corrected for BMI, the obese patients were under-resuscitated. Also, the day 0 mortality was about three times higher in the obese patients when compared to the leaner patients [26]. Therefore, the obese trauma patient is not only at a higher risk of mortality, but also is typically difficult to assess in terms of fluid resuscitation. The need for a parameter that can serve as a guide for fluid resuscitation with improved clinical outcome is thus obvious. Additionally, this also highlights the inadequacy of current conventional perfusion parameters in predicting patient survival outcomes.

Belzberg et al. studied 625 trauma patients in hypovolaemic shock. They studied the transcutaneous oxygen tension and oxygen delivery to the tissues (DO_2) along with traditional haemodynamic parameters. They found that obese patients in general had a higher risk of complications such as sepsis, renal failure, and acute respiratory distress syndrome as compared to their leaner counterparts. They also found that obese non-survivors had a lower tissue oxygenation (almost 50% lower) as well as lower tissue DO_2 as compared to the survivors [27]. The obese trauma patients are thus more likely to be under-resuscitated as assessment of volume status is difficult. Tissue oxygenation not only serves as a clinical target to guide resuscitation, but also helps in prognostication of such patients and should be used whenever possible.

Tissue oxygenation in sepsis

Sepsis is a complex pathological state where the alteration in the physiological variables varies with the stage of sepsis. The initial stage is comprised of systemic vasodilatation that is associated with augmentation of cardiac output. During this phase, an increase in tissue oxygen delivery occurs. As the cardiac compensation fails, the tissue oxygen delivery decreases and the StO_2 and tPO_2 also decrease.

In addition, microcirculatory dysfunction plays an important role in sepsis [28]. It contributes to systemic inflammation and multiorgan dysfunction. The pathological mechanisms are related to endothelial cell injury, mitochondrial dysfunction, activation of coagulation cascade, and tissue hypoxia.

As with haemorrhagic shock, there seems to be a discrepancy between the macro- and the microcirculation in states of sepsis. Normalization of the haemodynamic and oxygenation parameters at the level of macrocirculation may not reflect a normal microcirculation. There also exists a discrepancy between arterial and tissue oxygen levels in sepsis that can partially be explained by arteriovenous shunting and partially by improper substrate handling at the cellular level. Creteur et al. found that recovery of tissue oxygen levels, from ischaemic challenge, was much slower in patients with sepsis. When followed over 48 hours the recovery was faster and improved over time in survivors as compared to non-survivors [29].

Anning et al. induced endotoxaemia in rats and studied the effects of volume resuscitation and nitric oxide synthase inhibition on the tPO_2 measured in the skeletal muscle tissues. They found that the tPO_2 was lower in the endotoxaemic rats and had a significantly attenuated response to an increase in FiO_2 as compared to normal rats. Nitric oxide synthase inhibition also significantly attenuated the response of tPO_2 to hyperoxia. However, volume resuscitation helped to reverse the changes induced from the endotoxaemia [30].

Sepsis and toxaemia, therefore, lead to microcirculatory dysfunction that further exacerbates the tissue hypoperfusion caused by hypotension associated with sepsis. This tissue hypoperfusion is reversible with fluid resuscitation. Therefore, fluid resuscitation forms the mainstay of initial therapy in sepsis along with antibiotics. Unfortunately, there have been no targeted studies on sepsis in obese patients. It is very likely that the above-described pathophysiological mechanisms hold true in the obese patients as well. Their baseline low tissue oxygenation is likely to make the prognosis worse. Also, fluid requirements may be higher in settings of higher baseline blood volume. Further studies are, however, needed to evaluate the behaviour of this patient population in sepsis, especially in relation to tissue oxygenation. Research on this subject will have huge implications for the care of this patient population.

Conclusion

Obesity is a continuously worsening pathophysiological state. Its unique effects on tissue oxygenation present special challenges in optimally measuring the homeostatic state of a patient. From the discussion in this chapter, it is clear that global haemodynamic parameters do not provide adequate information on haemodynamics at the microcirculatory level. This discrepancy is further exaggerated in obese patients and more so in pathological states associated with hypoperfusion. The under-resuscitation of obese patients that is often associated with using global haemodynamic parameters to determine adequacy of resuscitation, can lead to tissue hypoxia and propagation of inflammatory pathways, which can have a serious impact on morbidity and mortality. Tissue oxygenation is also adversely affected in sepsis through various mechanisms at the cellular and microcirculatory levels. Volume resuscitation guided by tissue-level parameters can partially help attenuate this problem.

There are still many avenues that need to be studied to promote better understanding of how the obese patient population behaves, especially in pathological conditions, and ultimately promote appropriate medical care.

REFERENCES

1. Ogden CL, Carroll MD, Flegal KM. Prevalence of obesity in the United States. JAMA. 2014;**312**(2):189–90.
2. Pasarica M, Sereda OR, Redman LM, Albarado DC, Hymel DT, Roan LE, et al. Reduced adipose tissue oxygenation in human obesity: evidence for rarefaction, macrophage chemotaxis, and inflammation without an angiogenic response. Diabetes. 2009;**58**(3):718–25.
3. Hodson L, Humphreys SM, Karpe F, Frayn KN. Metabolic signatures of human adipose tissue hypoxia in obesity. Diabetes. 2013;**62**(5):1417–25.
4. Landini L, Honka MJ, Ferrannini E, Nuutila P. Adipose tissue oxygenation in obesity: a matter of cardiovascular risk? Current Pharmaceutical Design. 2016;**22**(1):68–76.
5. Sakr Y. Techniques to assess tissue oxygenation in the clinical setting. Transfusion and Apheresis Science. 2010;**43**(1):79–94.
6. Duling BR, Berne RM. Longitudinal gradients in periarteriolar oxygen tension. A possible mechanism for the participation of oxygen in local regulation of blood flow. Circulation Research. 1970;**27**(5):669–78.
7. Alvarez A, Singh PM, Sinha AC. Tissue oxygenation in morbid obesity—the physiological and clinical perspective. Trends in Anaesthesia and Critical Care. 2013;**3**:310–15.
8. Soni N, Fawcett WJ, Halliday FC. Beyond the lung: oxygen delivery and tissue oxygenation. Anaesthesia. 1993;**48**(8):704–11.
9. Severinghaus JW. First electrodes for blood PO2 and PCO2 determination. Journal of Applied Physiology (Bethesda, Md: 1985). 2004;**97**(5):1599–600.
10. Wallace MB, Wax A, Roberts DN, Graf RN. Reflectance spectroscopy. Gastrointestinal Endoscopy Clinics of North America. 2009;**19**(2):233–42.
11. Lipcsey M, Woinarski NC, Bellomo R. Near infrared spectroscopy (NIRS) of the thenar eminence in anesthesia and intensive care. Annals of Intensive Care. 2012;**2**(1):11.
12. Nielsen HB. Systematic review of near-infrared spectroscopy determined cerebral oxygenation during non-cardiac surgery. Frontiers in Physiology. 2014;**5**:93.
13. Trayhurn P, Wood IS. Adipokines: inflammation and the pleiotropic role of white adipose tissue. British Journal of Nutrition. 2004;**92**(3):347–55.
14. Wree A, Mayer A, Westphal S, Beilfuss A, Canbay A, Schick RR, et al. Adipokine expression in brown and white adipocytes in response to hypoxia. Journal of Endocrinological Investigation. 2012;**35**(5):522–27.
15. Kim DH, Kim C, Ding EL, Townsend MK, Lipsitz LA. Adiponectin levels and the risk of hypertension: a systematic review and meta-analysis. Hypertension. 2013;**62**(1):27–32.
16. Wood IS, de Heredia FP, Wang B, Trayhurn P. Cellular hypoxia and adipose tissue dysfunction in obesity. Proceedings of the Nutrition Society. 2009;**68**(4):370–77.
17. Greif R, Akca O, Horn EP, Kurz A, Sessler DI. Supplemental perioperative oxygen to reduce the incidence of surgical-wound infection. New England Journal of Medicine. 2000;**342**(3):161–67.
18. Hopf HW, Hunt TK, West JM, Blomquist P, Goodson WH 3rd, Jensen JA, et al. Wound tissue oxygen tension predicts the risk of wound infection in surgical patients. Archives of Surgery (Chicago, Ill: 1960). 1997;**132**(9):997–1004.
19. Kabon B, Fleischmann E, Treschan T, Taguchi A, Kapral S, Kurz A. Thoracic epidural anesthesia increases tissue oxygenation

during major abdominal surgery. Anesthesia and Analgesia. 2003;**97**(6):1812–17.

20. Hager H, Reddy D, Mandadi G, Pulley D, Eagon JC, Sessler DI, et al. Hypercapnia improves tissue oxygenation in morbidly obese surgical patients. Anesthesia and Analgesia. 2006;**103**(3):677–81.

21. Kabon B, Rozum R, Marschalek C, Prager G, Fleischmann E, Chiari A, et al. Supplemental postoperative oxygen and tissue oxygen tension in morbidly obese patients. Obesity Surgery. 2010;**20**(7):885–94.

22. Drucker W, Pearce F, Glass-Heidenreich L, Hopf H, Powell C, Ochsner MG, et al. Subcutaneous tissue oxygen pressure: a reliable index of peripheral perfusion in humans after injury. Journal of Trauma. 1996;**40**(3 Suppl):S116–22.

23. Lima A, van Bommel J, Jansen TC, Ince C, Bakker J. Low tissue oxygen saturation at the end of early goal-directed therapy is associated with worse outcome in critically ill patients. Critical Care (London, England). 2009;**13**(Suppl 5):S13.

24. Cohn SM, Nathens AB, Moore FA, Rhee P, Puyana JC, Moore EE, et al. Tissue oxygen saturation predicts the development of organ dysfunction during traumatic shock resuscitation. Journal of Trauma. 2007;**62**(1):44–54.

25. Nordin A, Mildh L, Makisalo H, Harkonen M, Hockerstedt K. Hepatosplanchnic and peripheral tissue oxygenation during treatment of hemorrhagic shock: the effects of pentoxifylline administration. Annals of Surgery. 1998;**228**(6):741–47.

26. Nelson J, Billeter AT, Seifert B, Neuhaus V, Trentz O, Hofer CK, et al. Obese trauma patients are at increased risk of early hypovolemic shock: a retrospective cohort analysis of 1,084 severely injured patients. Critical Care (London, England). 2012;**16**(3):R77.

27. Belzberg H, Wo CC, Demetriades D, Shoemaker WC. Effects of age and obesity on hemodynamics, tissue oxygenation, and outcome after trauma. Journal of Trauma. 2007;**62**(5):1192–200.

28. Trzeciak S, Rivers EP. Clinical manifestations of disordered microcirculatory perfusion in severe sepsis. Critical Care (London, England). 2005;**9**(Suppl 4):S20–26.

29. Creteur J, Carollo T, Soldati G, Buchele G, De Backer D, Vincent JL. The prognostic value of muscle StO2 in septic patients. Intensive Care Medicine. 2007;**33**(9):1549–56.

30. Anning PB, Sair M, Winlove CP, Evans TW. Abnormal tissue oxygenation and cardiovascular changes in endotoxemia. American Journal of Respiratory and Critical Care Medicine. 1999;**159**(6):1710–15.

SECTION 6
Other important aspects

Perioperative paediatric obesity

Alissa Doll and Aditee P. Ambardekar

Introduction: epidemiology and definitions

Paediatric obesity is a worldwide epidemic with estimations of the prevalence of overweight and obese as high as 23.8% and 22.6% in paediatric and adolescent males and females, respectively [1]. In the United States, significant increases in the prevalence of obesity in children were noted in the 1980s and 1990s but have since levelled off in 2010 at 16.9% overall [2]. Moreover, about 12% of infants 6–23 months of age in the United States are considered overweight [3]. The World Health Organization and the United States Centers for Disease Control and Prevention have slightly different definitions of paediatric obesity based on body mass index (BMI), which leads to somewhat varied estimations of prevalence. Despite this, recent trends suggest the number of overweight and obese children presenting for elective and emergent procedures is increasing [3].

A serious public health concern, paediatric obesity can accompany congenital or genetic comorbidities or be the cause of accelerated comorbidities such as cardiovascular disease, diabetes, and cancers that are typically associated with adult morbidity and mortality (**Fig. 29.1**). This chapter will describe the comorbidities that

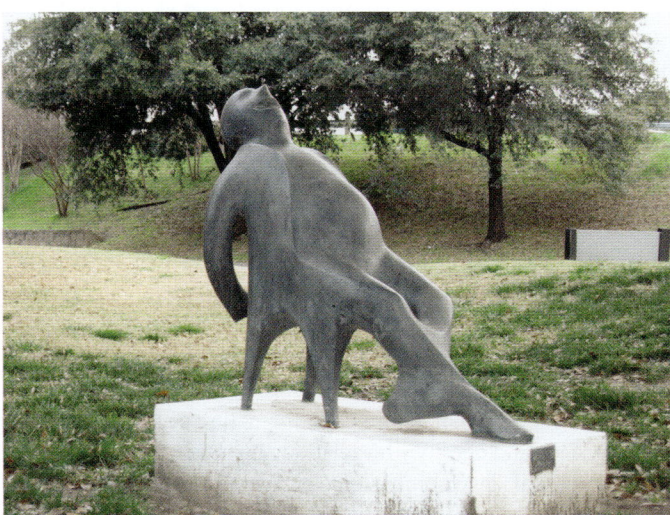

Fig. 29.1 *Laughing Man* by Harry Marinsky.
Reproduced courtesy of Edward Prejean, MD.

are typically associated with paediatric obesity as they become relevant in the perioperative period, summarize surgical procedures in which paediatric obesity is common, and discuss peri-anaesthetic implications of the obese child or adolescent.

Aetiology and risk factors

The aetiology of paediatric obesity is multifactorial in nature. The summative downstream effects of excessive consumption and sedentary lifestyle create an imbalance of caloric supply and demand. Many of the environmental factors, as summarized in **Fig. 29.2**, are not directly relevant in the considerations for planning the anaesthetic but must be considered in the broader picture of a child's perioperative experience [4]. Those environmental, genetic, pathological, and iatrogenic contributions to obesity that are more relevant to anaesthesiologists in the perioperative period will be discussed in the following sections.

Neurodevelopmental or physical disability

Children with intellectual or developmental disabilities tend to experience overweight and obesity at higher rates than their typically developing peers [5]. In addition to the many environmental risk factors, many children with disability require psychotropic medications that distort eating habits, manipulate hormone production or metabolism, or cause fluid retention [6]. Physical disability adds the challenge of limited mobility. Obesity therefore adds to the complexity of patients that often are anxious, are fearful of medical professionals, and require specialized distraction techniques simply to initiate an encounter in the perioperative suite.

Genetic causes

Syndromic causes of obesity, although rare, are worth mentioning as these patients may present to anaesthetizing locations for a variety of procedures [3,7]. There are approximately 30 such syndromes with obesity reported as an omnipresent or variable clinical feature. These patients are obese and are also characterized by developmental delay, organ abnormalities, and dysmorphic features [8]. Of the many syndromic causes of obesity (**Table 29.1**), Prader–Willi syndrome is the most common [8].

There are severe forms of obesity caused by a single-gene variant characterized by early-onset obesity and associated with

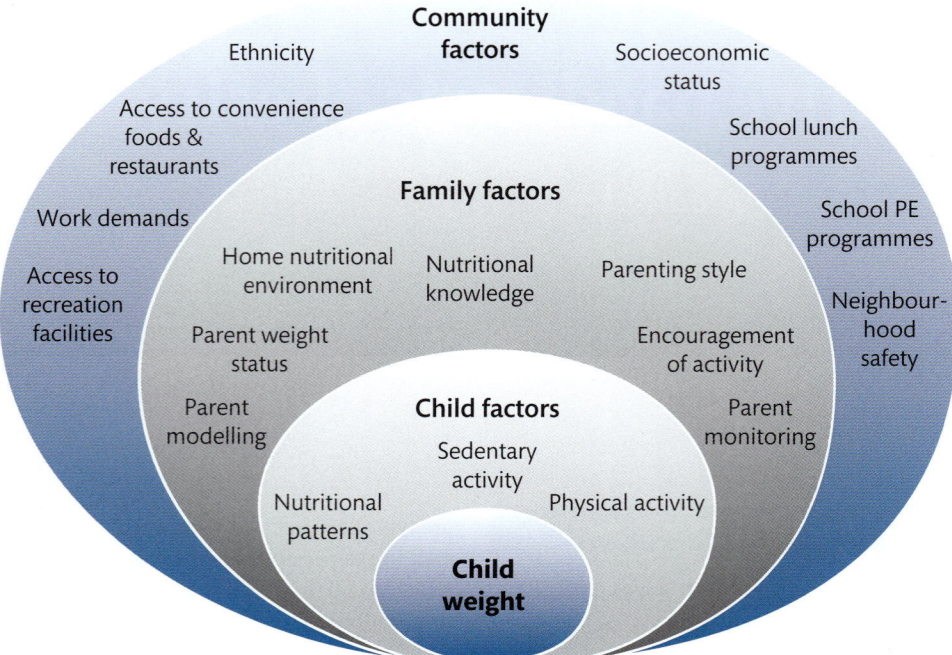

Fig. 29.2 Environmental risk factors as they impact child weight.

Reproduced with permission from Brown, C. L., Halvorson, E. E., Cohen, G. M. et al. Addressing Childhood Obesity Opportunities for Prevention, *Pediatric Clinics*, 62(5): 1241–1261. Copyright (c) 2015 with permission from Elsevier. https://doi.org/10.1016/j.pcl.2015.05.013

hypogonadism and hyperphagia [8]. These genetic variants typically affect the leptin–melanocortin pathway, in which congenital leptin deficiency is implicated [9]. Leptin is a protein secreted mostly by adipocytes whose main function is to control the body fat mass by inhibiting food intake via the central nervous system [9]. Deficiency causes impaired satiety resulting in hyperphagia and early-onset obesity. These patients can be treated with recombinant human leptin [9,10]. Other abnormalities of this pathway associated with obesity include leptin receptor deficiency, pro-opiomelanocortin mutations, and melanocortin-4 receptor mutations.

Endocrinopathies

Endocrinopathies are rare but when present can be significant contributors to obesity in children and adolescents. Hypothyroidism is the most common cause of endocrine-related weight gain [7]. Other hormone abnormalities such as hypercortisolaemia (Cushing syndrome), growth hormone deficiency, and pseudohypoparathyroidism can cause accelerated weight gain and slowed vertical growth [7]. These can occur in the presence of central nervous system tumours of the hypothalamus or pituitary gland that require surgical resection. It is important to remember that even surgical debulking and removal of secreting tumours can cause autonomic dysregulation and subsequent weight gain [11].

Medications

Certain classes of prescription drugs can contribute to obesity. In addition to the antipsychotics, antidepressants, and anticonvulsants that are often used in children with neurodevelopmental or psychiatric diagnoses, long-standing glucocorticoid use has been implicated in lipogenesis and increased adiposity [12]. Hollman

et al. report the case of an asthmatic child with overt glucocorticoid excess in the setting of inhaled triamcinolone therapy alone. Her hypothalamic–pituitary–adrenal axis suppression manifested as obesity, hirsutism, and growth restriction [13]. Glucocorticoids are commonly used in treatment for asthma and reactive airway disease, autoimmune diseases, and certain cancers, comorbidities that are frequently seen in patients requiring anaesthesia for surgical or procedural intervention.

Environmental factors

Environmental factors such as parental BMI, maternal health during pregnancy, nutrition, sociodemographics, stress, and quantity of physical activity all require consideration in the global health and medical care of an obese patient [4]. Rarely, these factors impact peri-anaesthetic care. Of relevance to the anaesthesiologist, however, is the body of literature that discusses quantity of sleep and its relationship to the development of obesity in childhood and adolescence.

Studies show that even as early as infancy, less sleep time during the night and day may increase the likelihood of obesity later in childhood [14,15]. Furthermore, a meta-analysis of longitudinal studies examining the impact of sleep duration on the rates of overweight and obesity showed that children and adolescents sleeping for short duration had twice the risk of being overweight or obese compared with subjects sleeping for long duration [16].

There are several hypotheses as to the nature of this relationship between sleep and obesity. This relationship is certainly exacerbated by the eventual development of obstructive sleep apnoea (OSA) as the obesity worsens. As the sleep apnoea worsens, so do quality and quantity of sleep; the vicious cycle of poor sleep and apnoea continues.

Table 29.1 Summary of syndromes associated with severe obesity

	Syndrome	Mode of inheritance	Clinical features	Locus	Gene/locus
1	Prader–Willi syndrome	Autosomal dominant	Diminished fetal activity, muscular hypotonia, mental retardation, short stature, hypogonadotropic hypogonadism, and small hands and feet	15q11.2–q12	NDN and SNRPN
2	Bardet–Biedl syndrome	Autosomal recessive	Mental retardation, dysphormic extremities, retinal dystrophy or pigmentary retinopathy, hypogonadism, and structural abnormalities of the kidney or functional renal impairment	2q311, 4q27, 11q13.2, 12q21.2, 15q24,1, 16q12,2, and others	BBS5, BBS7, BBS12, BBS1, BBS10, BBS4, BBS2, and others
3	Alström syndrome	Autosomal recessive	Retinal dystrophy, neurosensory deafness, diabetes, and dilated cardiomyopathy	2p13.1	ALMS1
4	Albright hereditary osteodystrophy	Autosomal dominant	Short stature, skeletal defects, and impaired olfaction (pseudohypoparathyroidism)	20q13.32	GNAS
5	Fragile X syndrome	Autosomal dominant	Mental retardation, macro-orchidism, and high-pitched jocular speech	Xq27.3	FMR1
6	Cohen syndrome	Autosomal recessive	Prominent central incisors, ophthalmopathy, and microcephaly	8q22.2	VPS13B
7	Borjeson–Forssman–Lehmann syndrome	X-linked	Mental retardation, hypogonadism, and large ears	Xq26.2	PHF6
8	Mehmo syndrome	X-linked	Mental retardation, epilepsy, hypogonadism, and microcephaly	Xp22.13–p21.1	Mitochondrial DNA
9	Simpson–Golabi–Behmel syndrome	X-linked	Craniofacial defects and skeletal and visceral abnormalities	Xp22.2	OFD1
10	Wilson–Turner syndrome	X-linked	Mental retardation, tapering fingers, and gynaecomastia	Xq13.1	HDAC8
11	Achondroplasia	75% sporadic and 25% Autosomal dominant	Dwarfism (short stature)	4p16.3	FGFR3
12	Bannayan–Riley–Ruvalcaba syndrome	Autosomal dominant	Multiple subcutaneous lipomas, macrocephaly, and haemangiomas	10q23.31	PTEN
13	Beckwith–Wiedemann syndrome	Sporadic	Macroglossia, macrosomia, midline abdominal wall defects (omphalocele/exomphalos, umbilical hernia, and diastasis recti), and neonatal hypoglycaemia	5q35.2–q35.3 and 11p15.4	NSD1, KCNQ1OT1, H19, and CDKN 1C
14	Carpenter syndrome	Autosomal recessive	Craniofacial malformations, syndactyly, and variable mental retardation	6p11.2	RAB23
15	CDG 1a	Autosomal recessive	Psychomotor retardation, ataxia, strabismus, coagulopathy, and peripheral neuropathy	16p13.3–p13.2	PMM2
16	Smith–Magenis syndrome	Sporadic	Mild to moderate mental retardation, distinctive facial features, sleep disturbances, and behavioural problems	17p11.2	RA11
17	Sotos syndrome	Sporadic	Autism, mild mental retardation, delayed motor, cognitive and social development, hypotonia, macrocephaly, hypertelorism, and aggressiveness and irritability	5q35.2–q35.3	NSD1
18	Ulnar–mammary Schinzel syndrome	Autosomal dominant	Posterior limb deficiencies or duplications, apocrine/mammary gland hypoplasia and/or dysfunction, abnormal dentition, delayed puberty in males, and genital anomalies	12q24.21	TBX3

Reproduced with permission from Alqahtani, A. R., Elahmedi, M., Alqahtani, Y., A. Bariatric surgery in monogenic and syndromic forms of obesity, *Seminars in Pediatric Surgery*, 23(1): 37–42. Copyright (c) 2014, with permission from Elsevier. https://doi.org/10.1053/j.sempedsurg.2013.10.013

Treatment

With 43 million children considered overweight or obese globally and 92 million at risk, the most cost-effective intervention is prevention [17]. Ultimately, the goal is a balance of caloric intake and expenditure through physical activity. A public health effort to ensure school-aged children have access to balanced meals and healthy beverages is one example of policy initiatives to curb childhood obesity. Lifestyle modification, dietary restrictions, and prescription therapy are conservative strategies once a child is overweight or obese; however, weight-loss programmes for adolescents and children have had limited success, leading to an increase in surgical management for severely obese adolescents [18]. The following sections will summarize surgical management for severe obesity.

Selection for surgical management

Bariatric surgery can lead to clinically significant and sustained weight loss in the correctly chosen patient. Only severely obese patients who have already attempted to achieve weight loss via conservative measures should be evaluated. A multidisciplinary approach to evaluation is recommended and should include at minimum an ethicist, bariatric surgeon, nutritionist, gastroenterologist, pulmonologist, endocrinologist, and an adolescent medicine physician [19]. Of course, other specialists should be included on a case-by-case basis; an anaesthesia consultation prior to the day of surgery may add value to the perioperative preparation of these patients.

Patient requirements for adolescent bariatric surgery can safely follow adult recommendations, based on a detailed review of the literature by the American Society for Metabolic and Bariatric Surgery Pediatric Committee [20]. These recommendations suggest a fixed BMI cut-off with the presence of comorbidities is reasonable and safe. Thus, adolescents are candidates for bariatric surgery if they have (1) a BMI greater than 35 kg/m² with major comorbidities (e.g., diabetes mellitus type 2, moderate to severe OSA, or severe non-alcoholic steatohepatitis) or (2) a BMI greater than 40 kg/m² in the presence of other comorbidities (e.g., glucose intolerance, impairment of activities of daily life, or any degree of sleep apnoea) [20].

There is some concern that specific bariatric techniques could impair skeletal maturation due to the resulting metabolic milieu. Thus, some adolescent bariatric surgery programmes have age-based criteria to lessen these adverse effects. Females older than 13 years and males older than 15 years have attained the majority of their skeletal maturity, particularly in the setting of early puberty. While there is less concern for growth impairment when adolescents reach the 50th percentile of height for age, the general recommendation is that physicians should defer surgical intervention until patients reach 95% of their adult stature [19,21]. This can be guided by radiological studies of long bones to measure the degree of epiphyseal closure [22].

Surgical techniques

Bariatric surgery in the adolescent population has been reported to be not only highly effective with a reduction of excess weight in the range of 58–73%, but also has the potential to prevent and even reverse comorbid states such as diabetes, hypertension, and OSA [23–25]. Three techniques are commonly used. The laparoscopic sleeve gastrectomy reduces the stomach into a smaller, tubular viscus without diversion. It has been reported to be particularly effective in children with certain genetic and syndromic causes of severe obesity [8]. Adjustable gastric banding is another laparoscopic technique that has been advocated for specifically in adolescents as it theoretically has less postoperative nutritional deficiencies, has less potential for surgical complication, and is reversible [24]. The Roux-en-Y gastric bypass can be done using a laparoscopic or open technique. Bariatric surgeons may prefer to perform the more technically challenging laparoscopic method due to decreased morbidity in the perioperative period compared to the open approach [26]. Regardless of approach, the Roux-en-Y gastric bypass causes nutritional deficiencies

due to diversion and resultant non-absorption of ingested food and thus may be a less desirable technique in adolescence.

Preoperative evaluation

A thorough history and physical identifies the many, often severe comorbidities that can exist in the obese adolescent. The presence of the multidisciplinary team supports proper identification, treatment, and optimization of comorbidities prior to presentation for surgery, although this may not be available in the setting of non-bariatric surgery or procedures. Review of this information pre-emptively and deliberately ensures careful planning for the care of the adolescent in the perioperative period. A systems-based discussion of the possible comorbidities and their peri-anaesthetic implications follows. **Box 29.1** provides a summary of those comorbidities that have important anaesthetic implications [27].

Box 29.1 Summary of comorbidities that impact the perioperative period

Respiratory

Decrease in:
- Lung volume:
  − Functional residual capacity, vital capacity, inspiratory capacity.
- Diffusion capacity.
- Compliance of the lung.

Increase in:
- Work of breathing.
- Obstruction of the lower airway.
- Exercise-induced asthma bronchiale in 30% of overweight and obese paediatric patients.
- Sleep apnoea disease in about 17% of obese children greater than 150th percentile, chronic nocturnal hypoxaemia leads progressively to pulmonary hypertension.

Cardiovascular

Increase in:
- Stiffness and wall thickness of the carotid artery as early signs of arteriosclerotic process in school children:
  − Early development of arterial hypertension, approximately a three-fold higher risk than non-obese children.
- Activity of sympathetic nervous system:
  − Higher heart rate and blood pressure at rest.
- Left ventricular mass and hypertrophy.
- Left ventricular dysfunction.
- Vascularization of the adipose tissue:
  − Increase in cardiac output and blood volume.

Gastrointestinal/endocrine
- Ambiguous data about reflux: higher incidence of reflux in obese children, and no difference between normal-weight obese children.
- Residual gastric volume after 6 hours of fasting and 2 hours without liquid is not different between obese and normal-weight children.
- Metabolic syndrome and resistance to insulin in 50% of severely obese adolescents.
- Non-alcoholic fatty liver disease; progress from hepatic steatosis to fibrosis (histologically).

Reproduced with permission from Philippi-Höhne, C., Anaesthesia in the obese child, *Best Practice & Research Clinical Anaesthesiology*, 25(1): 53–60. Copyright 2011, with permission from Elsevier.

Psychiatric and neurological considerations

There is a convincing body of literature to suggest the increased prevalence of neuropsychiatric diagnoses in the overweight and obese adolescent compared to non-obese adolescents [28–30]. Depression and anxiety are complicated by impaired social relationships and overt bullying, low self-esteem, and stigma of obesity. This, in the setting of an already high-stress environment, i.e., the perioperative period, requires care in the most compassionate of ways. Judicious administration of anxiolysis should be considered to allay fears of transport to the operating room, particularly in the setting of stress of separation from caregivers.

Idiopathic intracranial hypertension (IIH), or primary pseudotumor cerebri syndrome, is a constellation of symptoms caused by idiopathic increases in intracranial pressure (ICP) causing visual disturbances and headache. Its association with obese adults and adolescents, particularly in women of reproductive age, is well documented in the literature and summarized by Andrews et al. [31]. Weight loss causes reversal of IIH symptomatology and thus obese patients with IIH are ideal candidates for bariatric surgery [32]. The obese parturient with IIH presents a clinical dilemma about the safety of neuraxial technique for labour analgesia; Karmaniolou et al. discuss the safety of such techniques despite the presence of elevated ICP [33].

Pulmonary and airway considerations

Respiratory mechanics, airway compliance, and alveolar function are impaired in the obese child just as in adults. There is an inverse relationship between maximal voluntary ventilation and BMI, resulting in reduced expiratory flows and volumes attributed to restriction caused by an increase in chest wall adiposity [34]. Obese patients tend to also have more atelectasis at rest [35]. In children, this extrinsic compression causes reduced expiratory volumes and flows and diminished maximal voluntary ventilation, contributing to decreased diffusion capacity of the alveoli and fatigued extrinsic muscles [36]. The restrictive pathophysiology is accompanied by an increased incidence and severity of obstructive disease as well. A report from the American Thoracic Society Workshop on Obesity and Asthma summarizes an extensive literature review [37]. There is evidence to suggest that there is an increased incidence of asthma in the obese child compared to the non-obese child; however, a causal or contributory relationship is harder to prove [38]. Nevertheless, the severity of disease, relative resistance to conventional therapies, and potential synergy of mechanical and metabolic factors make obstructive disease in this population more challenging [37].

It is imperative that the anaesthesiologist understands the interplay between the restrictive and obstructive pathophysiology for each patient. Severe disease may necessitate pulmonary function testing and optimization, including consultation with a pulmonologist. Medications for treatment of acute bronchospasm should be readily available in the perioperative period.

The association between obesity and OSA in children has been known for nearly three decades [39]. Numerous studies have since demonstrated that obesity is a major risk factor for OSA [40]. Polysomnography results and detailed questions regarding daytime sleepiness, respiratory pauses during sleep, snoring, and attention disorders are useful to estimate severity of disease. Long-standing, abnormal sleep patterns associated with OSA can lead to systemic oxygen desaturation, polycythemia, chronic hypercapnia, and respiratory acidosis; hypercapnia, pulmonary hypertension, and heart failure are known as Pickwickian syndrome. This poses several challenges for the anaesthesiologist in the setting of both bariatric and non-bariatric surgery. Narcotic sensitivity in this population is well documented, likely related to chronic hypoxaemia changing the sensitivity of mu receptors, and suggests that obese children with OSA require lower doses of opiate to achieve analgesia compared to non-obese patients without sleep apnoea [40]. Furthermore, the need for non-invasive ventilation techniques in the postoperative period and the benefit of post-procedure admission for adequate yet safe analgesia should be considered when planning the perioperative period.

As always, a thorough airway examination allows for proper planning of the necessary equipment for airway manipulation. While obese children are more likely to receive a Mallampati classification greater than two compared to non-obese, age-matched individuals, rigorous prospective studies are missing which link obesity to difficulty with management of the airway [3,41]. In contrast, we do know that the incidence of perioperative respiratory complications is higher in obese compared to age-matched non-obese children [41]. This emphasizes the need for careful review of, and deliberate planning for, these children, particularly with respect to their pulmonary comorbidities.

Cardiovascular considerations

Obesity during childhood is associated with early non-congenital changes in cardiovascular structure and function. Well-vascularized adipose tissue not only leads to increased blood volume but also increased metabolic demand. This increase in preload with concomitant increase in afterload due to worsening arterial stiffness accelerates cardiovascular disease that is often seen in the fourth or fifth decade of life [42]. This is exacerbated by the presence of glucose and insulin intolerance, elevated C-reactive protein levels, dyslipidaemia, hypertension, and overall cardiac deconditioning: all well-known cardiovascular risk factors [43]. Cote et al. present a simple yet informative schematic of the various metabolic, genetic, and environmental factors that influence the development of cardiac dysfunction (**Fig. 29.3**) [42].

Clinically, obesity-related changes in cardiovascular structure and function manifest most commonly as hypertension. There are convincing data in the literature, based on several large studies, that the risk of hypertension can be as high as threefold in obese children compared to their lean peers [44]. Left ventricular dysfunction and overload are late findings in the extremely obese and fortunately are rarely seen in children with severe OSA, but can be if left untreated.

If any of the above-mentioned factors is present, consultation with a cardiologist may be beneficial to obtain additional information about advanced disease and for pharmacological treatment for the optimal perioperative state. Baseline information obtained from electrocardiography, echocardiography, heart rate, and blood pressure may all prove useful in the management of intraoperative events. Rarely, if pulmonary hypertension is critical in nature, cardiac-trained paediatric anaesthesiologists may be consulted for specialized intraoperative management.

Gastrointestinal and hepatic considerations

Gastrointestinal diagnoses are common comorbidities in the obese adolescent. Functional abdominal pain syndrome, constipation, and irritable bowel syndrome have been found to be more prevalent in overweight and obese patients and can be associated with depression,

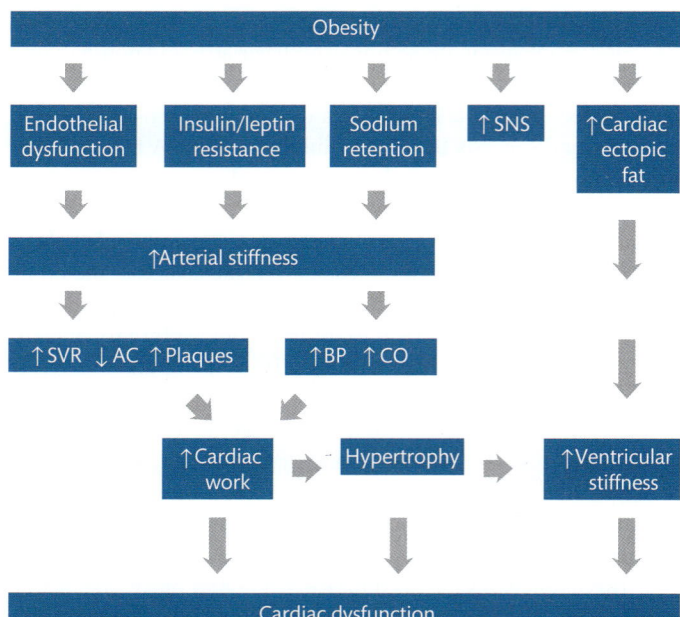

Fig. 29.3 Impact of changes during obesity as they affect cardiac dysfunction. AC, arterial compliance; BP, blood pressure; CO, cardiac output; SNS, sympathetic nervous system; SVR, systemic vascular resistance.

anxiety, and social phobias [45]. Non-alcoholic fatty liver disease (NAFLD) describes a spectrum of pathophysiology that encompasses simple steatosis, non-alcoholic steatohepatitis (NASH), and cirrhosis that is commonly found in obese children. While NAFLD has notable immune and metabolic consequences, the prevalence of severe or cirrhotic NASH is actually quite low even in the majority of the adolescents receiving bariatric surgery who show evidence of NAFLD [46]. More clinically relevant to the anaesthesiologist is the increased prevalence of gastro-oesophageal reflux in obese children irrespective of age, race, and sex. This risk of gastro-oesophageal reflux increases as BMI increases [47]. The presence of gastro-oesophageal reflux is concerning due to an increased risk of aspiration in the perioperative period, and thus symptomatology should be elicited in the perioperative period. Notably, obesity alone does not increase gastric fluid volumes or risk of aspiration in children having day surgical procedures. That is, gastric fluid volume, measured in millilitres per kilogram, in children who ingested clear liquids 2–4 hours prior to surgery remained constant in lean, overweight, and obese children alike [48]. Furthermore, Cook-Sather et al. noted there was no difference in gastric fluid volumes for the patients who fasted 2–4 hours when compared to those who fasted up to 24 hours. This study demonstrates that the American Society of Anesthesiologists fasting guidelines (clear liquids 2 hours prior to surgery) can be safely extended to include overweight and obese children.

Renal considerations

Rather than a simple comorbidity, obesity is proving to be an independent risk factor for chronic kidney disease and end-stage renal disease. Increased prevalence in chronic kidney disease and

end-stage renal disease in the paediatric population has been observed over the last three decades, paralleling the increased prevalence of paediatric obesity [49]. Obesity-related glomerulopathy is described as a secondary form of focal segmental glomerulosclerosis that may be due to glomerular hyperperfusion and hyperfiltration. Furthermore, with coexistence of hypertension and glucose intolerance in this fragile population, renal function may be at risk for further decline. As such, monitoring of renal function and electrolytes in the preoperative period may be beneficial for safe drug delivery as well as electrolyte management, particularly in situations where large volume shifts could occur.

Endocrine considerations

Glucose intolerance and insulin resistance are both endocrine derangements that are widely noted as comorbidities in the obesity literature. Analysis of two large cohorts of children and adolescents presenting for elective surgery demonstrates higher statistically significant prevalence of diabetes in the obese compared to the non-obese [41,50]. Careful monitoring of perioperative glucose with attention to insulin requirements, if any, should be considered. Endocrinology consultation may be warranted in those patients with difficult-to-manage glucose intolerance.

Intraoperative considerations

Monitoring

Standard monitors should include an electrocardiogram, blood pressure cuff, and pulse oximetry. More invasive monitors should be placed in accordance with comorbidities or the procedure being performed. Non-invasive blood pressure monitoring may be challenging in this population, as the upper arms may be large or have a conical shape, making placement of a standard paediatric blood pressure cuff difficult. There is a brief report in the literature about reasonable blood pressure readings measured by a small cuff placed directly on the wrist [51]. This may be a safe option in short cases. Theoretically, pulse oximetry could also be unreliable due to the increased soft tissue thickness between the illuminated sensors.

Peripheral intravenous catheterization can be more challenging in obese children and may require more than one attempt [52]. The excess adipose tissue may also make intravenous cannulation difficult [52]. If available, ultrasound guidance or transcutaneous vein illuminating devices may be helpful for obtaining venous access, particularly in locations where subcutaneous fat make veins difficult to visualize.

Oxygenation, ventilation, and airway management

As discussed earlier, obesity causes restrictive, obstructive, and intrinsic alveolar impairments that make oxygenation and ventilation more challenging. The increased metabolic demands of children, and in particular obese children, make this oxygen desaturation even more rapid. It is not unexpected, then, that respiratory complications in the intraoperative period are among the most common complications [41,50]. A study by Gleich and colleagues showed that severely obese children had an increased occurrence of intraoperative severe hypoxaemia (SpO_2 <70%) as compared to their normal weight counterparts [53]. This requires skilful airway management,

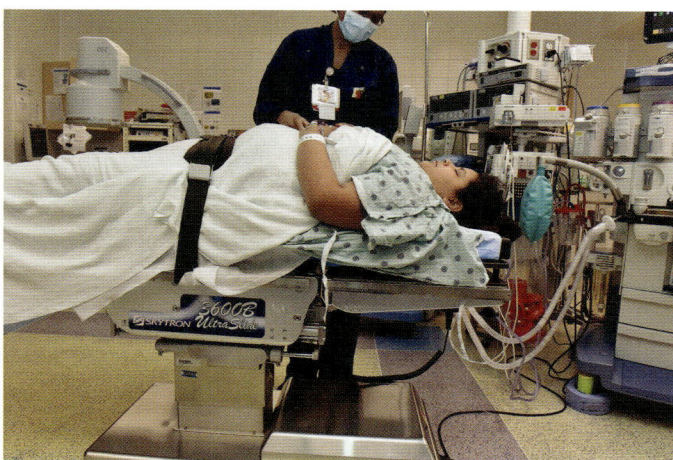

Fig. 29.4 Patient lying supine on operating room table prior to proper positioning. Note that patient's chest wall would likely lead to challenging intubating conditions when positioning is not optimized.

prudent ventilator management, and careful attention to pulmonary mechanics in the intraoperative and postoperative period.

Increased incidence of upper airway obstruction, sleep-disordered breathing or OSA, slightly higher Mallampati classification, and obtrusive chest wall and upper torso fat can make induction of anaesthesia and mask ventilation challenging. Proper positioning with a shoulder roll while in the supine position (**Fig. 29.4** and **Fig. 29.5**), thorough preoxygenation and denitrogenation, and availability of properly sized oro- and nasopharyngeal airways may improve the quality of mask ventilation and mitigate the degree of desaturation that can occur. Holding a proper mask seal and providing continuous positive airway pressure may also lessen upper and lower airway collapse, particularly at a time during which hypoventilation and desaturation is common.

Decreased lung volumes and poor chest wall compliance in the supine but anaesthetized state can accentuate the ventilation/perfusion mismatch that occurs even in healthy individuals. Higher airway pressures may be necessary to achieve adequate minute ventilation. Thus, endotracheal intubation and positive pressure ventilation should be considered for all but the shortest procedures [3].

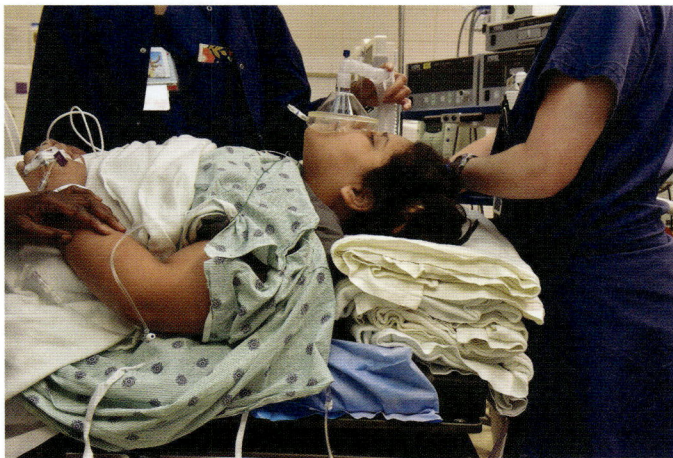

Fig. 29.5 Patient positioned on shoulder roll with blankets used to obtain proper sniffing position for intubation.

Optimizing alveolar recruitment with positive end-expiratory pressure should also be considered.

The current body of literature does not support the notion that laryngoscopy and intubation in obese adolescents is any more challenging than in those who are non-obese, and thus prospective studies are needed to better elucidate this [3]. The anaesthetic plan should include, as always, contingency plans should difficulty arise.

Induction and aspiration

There is concern that obesity may be associated with an increased risk of pulmonary aspiration. However, studies do not reveal a significant difference of aspiration events occurring in obese children compared with non-obese children [41,48]. In one study of 1000 paediatric day surgery patients, 27% of whom were overweight or obese, there were no aspiration events [48]. This study revealed that the average gastric fluid volume in mL/kg of ideal body weight (IBW) was no different between obese, overweight, or lean/normal BMI categories. Thus, indications for a rapid sequence induction should be thoroughly questioned in fasting obese children as the risk of hypoxia during rapid sequence induction is higher than the potential risk of pulmonary aspiration [27].

Pharmacology in obesity

A retrospective study of over 10,000 anaesthetics in children aged 2–17 suggests that obese and overweight children and adolescents were more likely to receive drug doses outside the recommended dosing guidelines [54]. This, in the setting of comorbid states and increased peri-anaesthetic risk, puts an already vulnerable population at greater risk. It is therefore imperative we understand how best to dose our anaesthetics in the setting of obesity and the comorbidities that are often present.

The relationship between total body weight (TBW), IBW, and lean body mass (LBM) is important to consider when calculating drug dosages. IBW is considered the weight measured at the 50th percentile for any given age. Thus, IBW can be calculated using the following formula: IBW (kg) = (BMI at the 50th percentile for the child's age) × (height (m)) ^{2} [55]. LBM is calculated as LBM (kg) = 3.8 × (0.0215 × $W^{0.65}$ × $H^{0.72}$ [56]. LBM increases in obesity also; thus, many of the calculations for drug dosages either use TBW or IBW.

As a general rule, hydrophilic drugs are dosed using IBW while lipophilic drugs are dosed using TBW. This assumes that lipophilic drugs have larger volumes of distribution in the adipose tissue and thus are needed at higher doses to achieve appropriate plasma concentrations. Barbiturates and benzodiazepines are examples of such drugs [18]. Hydrophilic drugs, such as non-depolarizing muscle relaxants, distribute to the lean tissues and thus should be dosed by IBW and, in fact, dosing with TBW may prolong neuromuscular blockade and weakness [18]. Cisatracurium, which relies on plasma esterases for offset of action, should be more independent of body weight, but still shows prolonged duration when dosed based on TBW. Thus, it is reasonable to start with a dose based on IBW and titrate to effect as necessary [3,18,57]. Rose and colleagues found that the potency of succinylcholine in obese adolescents is similar to that observed in non-obese adolescents [58]. It follows that succinylcholine dosing should be based on TBW to obtain adequate neuromuscular blockade. Acetylcholinesterase inhibitors used for reversal of neuromuscular blocking agents, such as neostigmine, should be dosed according to TBW [54]. A retrospective study by Burke and colleagues revealed that both succinylcholine and neostigmine were more likely to be underdosed in overweight and obese children as compared to normal-weight children, with odds ratios of 2 and 1.7, respectively, for being underdosed [54]. Inadequate dosing of succinylcholine can lead to suboptimal intubating conditions, while that of neostigmine could lead to insufficient postoperative ventilation due to residual neuromuscular blockade, and either of these situations can lead to adverse events.

Inadequate dosing of opioids can lead to poor postoperative pain control, while overdosing opioids can lead to respiratory depression and airway obstruction. A study showed that overweight children receiving morphine were 3.5 times more likely to receive an overdose and 70% less likely to receive an underdose [54]. Long-acting opioids should be dosed based on IBW. There may be some advantage in using ultra-short acting agents, such as remifentanil, where relative overdosing can be overcome quickly, but a longer-acting agent will still be needed for postoperative analgesia [3]. Opioids should be used with caution in children with OSA, as the chronic hypoxaemia experienced by these patients leads to upregulation of opioid receptors and, thus, increased sensitivity to opioids [59–61].

Volatile agents accumulate in adipose tissue over time and may lead to prolonged recovery. The less soluble agents, such as sevoflurane and desflurane, have shorter recovery times compared with isoflurane and halothane [3]. Exceptions to this rule do exist and therefore the pharmacokinetics and dynamics should be considered on an individual drug basis to avoid overdose and adverse events.

Propofol is one of these exceptions in which lower than expected doses are required for amnesia in the obese population. Olutoye and colleagues measured the induction dose of propofol necessary for loss of lash reflex and consciousness in 95% of the paediatric population and compared this dosage in obese and non-obese (BMI <85th percentile) children who received general anaesthesia for day surgical cases. Obese patients required 2 mg/kg propofol for loss of lash reflex while non-obese, age-matched children required 3.2 mg/kg using TBW in the calculation [62]. Furthermore, total body clearance and steady-state volume of distribution for propofol have been correlated to TBW, thus it is recommended that the steady-state continuous infusion should be based on TBW [63].

Anaesthetic type

Procedural sedation by providers other than anaesthesiologists is often done outside of the operating room in locations such as endoscopy suites, emergency rooms, oncology units, dentists' offices, and interventional suites. There is convincing literature that obesity is an independent risk factor for adverse events during the sorts of procedures in which children receive procedural sedation [64–67]. Respiratory adverse events are among the highest adverse events reported in these large studies and although not classified as 'major adverse events' did require the need for unexpected interventions such as jaw thrust, oral/nasopharyngeal airway placement, and bag-valve-mask ventilation [65]. Additionally, inability to complete the scheduled procedure and prolonged recovery occurred with increasing frequency in children with OSA and obesity [66].

Scherrer et al. note that this association between obesity and adverse events during procedural sedation is concurrent with the data linking adverse events and obesity while children are under general anaesthesia. Often the same medications are used; specifically, the use of propofol, pentobarbital, ketamine, and midazolam was associated with increased risk of adverse events [65]. This association between respiratory adverse effects and general anaesthesia has been discussed earlier in this chapter. It therefore seems prudent that these procedural sedations, particularly those for patients with obesity and comorbid states, should be performed by those skilled in airway management.

Given the increased sensitivity to opioids and other centrally acting medications in the obese population, regional anaesthesia and local anaesthesia techniques are useful to minimize some of the adverse effects of opioids.

Postoperative considerations

Paediatric obesity is associated with increased perioperative adverse events. One might suspect that, due to the risk of potential overdosing of anaesthetic medications in obese children, anaesthesia duration may be prolonged in this population. Some studies do indeed show a slightly prolonged duration of anaesthesia [53], while others do not. Lee and colleagues found that anaesthesia duration in a cohort of children undergoing tonsillectomy and/or adenoidectomy was not significantly different in obese children compared to that of normal weight children [68].

Postoperative adverse respiratory events appear to occur more commonly in obese children as compared to normal weight children and include airway obstruction [53]. Placing the patient in a semi-recumbent position will decrease atelectasis and improve oxygenation.

Severe obesity is associated with an increased incidence of unplanned hospital admissions [53]. Obesity is also correlated with longer length of stay in hospitals [50]. Depending on the invasiveness of the procedure performed and the intraoperative course, patients with severe sleep apnoea or cardiac pathology may require admission to the intensive care unit (ICU) postoperatively for close monitoring or cardiopulmonary support [8]. Children with severe OSA may need to be managed with continuous positive airway pressure or bi-level positive airway pressure [55]. As mentioned previously, a head-up position will decrease atelectasis and improve respiratory mechanics.

Postoperative pain control is an important issue. Opioid dosage should be based on IBW and respiration should be carefully monitored [55]. Regional anaesthetic techniques should be considered to minimize opioid consumption. Non-opioid adjunctive medications will also be helpful in this population.

In adults, obesity is a risk factor for venous thromboembolism [69]. This is also true for obese children. There has been a recent increase in incidence of in-hospital venous thromboembolism in children across the United States [70]. In a systematic literature review by Halvorson et al., several studies suggested that paediatric obesity may be associated with an increased incidence of thrombosis. Patients in most of these studies had additional risk factors such as limited mobility, malignancy, or presence of a central venous catheter [71]. This is of particular interest in the postoperative period, when patients may have limited mobility. A small pilot study of thromboprophylaxis in obese adolescents undergoing bariatric surgery showed that using a BMI-stratified fixed enoxaparin dose (40 mg subcutaneous twice daily in patients with a BMI ≤50 kg/m² and 60 mg subcutaneous twice daily in patients with a BMI ≥50 kg/m²) achieved therapeutic anti-factor Xa activity [70]. No venous thromboembolism occurred in the study population. These findings reveal the potential need for and the therapeutic value of venous thromboembolism prophylaxis in obese children.

Patients who undergo bariatric surgery need to have frequent medical follow-ups focusing on dietary assessment and instruction, especially during the first year after surgery [8,26,72]. Additionally, there are many surgical complications after bariatric surgery, including anastomotic breakdown, stomal line stenosis, hernias, and bowel obstructions [73]. Patients may present to the emergency department with these postoperative problems, among others. Physical examination findings may be unreliable in these patients, so early surgical consultation may be helpful in the evaluation and management of this population.

Trauma and resuscitation

Obesity may have an effect on trauma and resuscitation outcomes. In a retrospective review study by Brown and colleagues, obese children were found to experience more complications and to require longer ICU stays after severe trauma compared to their lean counterparts [74]. In contrast, a retrospective review of paediatric trauma data by Alselaim et al. showed no significant differences in hospital length of stay, ventilator days, or ICU days between obese and lean patients [75]. Significantly, neither of the aforementioned studies demonstrated any substantial difference in mortality rates between the lean and obese groups.

Obese children may have poor outcomes after paediatric cardiopulmonary resuscitation (CPR). In obese children experiencing cardiac arrest, CPR may be complicated by difficulty with the quality of CPR and problems with dosing of medications. A review by Srinivasan et al. demonstrated that, in obese children undergoing in-hospital CPR, deviations from paediatric advanced life support protocols, invasive airway problems, longer durations of CPR, and vascular access problems were more common than in normal-weight or underweight patients [76]. The same authors found that obesity was associated with lower rates of CPR survival and rates of survival to discharge. These results may indicate a need to address potential differences in resuscitation standards for obese children.

CASE REPORT

A 10-year-old male with a past medical history of obesity, attention-deficit/hyperactivity disorder, allergic rhinitis, snoring, and tonsillar hypertrophy was scheduled for a tonsillectomy and adenoidectomy. Preoperative polysomnography revealed an apnoea–hypopnea index (AHI) of 19 with desaturation to the mid-80s and hypercapnia to 52. His longest apnoea period was 16 seconds. This is suggestive of severe OSA.

On physical examination, the patient was noted to be obese, weighing 85.5 kg at a height of 157 cm, resulting in a BMI of 34.7 kg/m² (99.5th percentile). He had acanthosis nigricans on his neck. An airway exam revealed tonsillar hypertrophy, a Mallampati score of 1, and a thyromental distance greater than three fingerbreadths.

On the day of surgery, the patient was premedicated with 15 mg midazolam orally (0.35 mg/kg of IBW) to provide anxiolysis. The patient underwent an inhalational induction with sevoflurane in 70% nitrous oxide/30% oxygen mixture. Continuous positive airway pressure of approximately 5 cmH$_2$O was held on the bag while the patient was spontaneously ventilating in an attempt to stent the airways open during the inhalational induction. A peripheral intravenous catheter was placed after three attempts and the patient was given ketamine 1 mg/kg intravenously (based on TBW) prior to intubation. The airway table in the operating room was prepared with two laryngoscope blades (one straight blade and one curved blade), two oral airways of different sizes, and nasal trumpets available in case of severe upper airway obstruction. Laryngoscopy revealed a grade 1 view, based on the modified Cormack–Lehane classification system, with a Miller 2 laryngoscope blade. Intubation was atraumatic. Dexmedetomidine 0.5 mcg/kg (based on TBW) was titrated in slow boluses during the case. Our goal for surgery was to minimize opioids; the patient received acetaminophen 750 mg intravenously given over 15 minutes in addition to ketamine and dexmedetomidine as discussed previously. He was not given any opioids during his surgery.

The intraoperative course was uncomplicated. Prior to extubation, a 26-French nasal trumpet was easily inserted prophylactically to prevent postoperative airway obstruction. Extubation occurred after full emergence uneventfully and the patient received blowby oxygen for transport to the post-anaesthesia care unit (PACU).

The patient's PACU course was relatively uneventful. He was positioned in PACU on a shoulder roll to mitigate upper airway obstruction. The nasal trumpet remained in place until the patient was fully awake. The patient's pain scores upon awakening were 0/5. In our institution patients with severe OSA are routinely admitted overnight for observation. His postoperative pain scores on the floor ranged from 0/5 to 2/5, and the patient was treated with oral ibuprofen and acetaminophen as needed. Our multimodal analgesic technique resulted in significant opioid sparing for this patient. He had no postoperative issues and was discharged home the following morning.

REFERENCES

1. Ng M, Fleming T, Robinson M, Thomson B, Graetz N, Margono C, et al. Global, regional, and national prevalence of overweight and obesity in children and adults during 1980–2013: a systematic analysis for the Global Burden of Disease Study 2013. Lancet. 2014;**384**(9945):766–81.
2. Ogden CL, Carroll MD, Kit BK, Flegal KM. Prevalence of obesity and trends in body mass index among US children and adolescents, 1999–2010. JAMA. 2012;**307**(5):483–90.
3. Baines D. Anaesthetic considerations for the obese child. Paediatr Respir Rev. 2011;**12**(2):144–47.
4. Brown CL, Halvorson EE, Cohen GM, Lazorick S, Skelton JA. Addressing childhood obesity: opportunities for prevention. Pediatr Clin North Am. 2015;**62**(5):1241–61.
5. Grondhuis SN, Aman MG. Overweight and obesity in youth with developmental disabilities: a call to action. J Intellect Disabil Res. 2014;**58**(9):787–99.

6. Correll CU. Weight gain and metabolic effects of mood stabilizers and antipsychotics in pediatric bipolar disorder: a systematic review and pooled analysis of short-term trials. J Am Acad Child Adolesc Psychiatry. 2007;**46**(6):687–700.

7. Gurnani M, Birken C, Hamilton J. Childhood obesity: causes, consequences, and management. Pediatr Clin North Am. 2015;**62**(4):821–40.

8. Alqahtani AR, Elahmedi M, Alqahtani YA. Bariatric surgery in monogenic and syndromic forms of obesity. Semin Pediatr Surg. 2014;**23**(1):37–42.

9. Funcke JB, von Schnurbein J, Lennerz B, Lahr G, Debatin KM, Fischer-Posovszky P, et al. Monogenic forms of childhood obesity due to mutations in the leptin gene. Mol Cell Pediatr. 2014;**1**(1):3.

10. O'Rahilly S, Farooqi IS, Yeo GS, Challis BG. Minireview: human obesity-lessons from monogenic disorders. Endocrinology. 2003;**144**(9):3757–64.

11. Hamilton JK, Conwell LS, Syme C, Ahmet A, Jeffery A, Daneman D. Hypothalamic obesity following craniopharyngioma surgery: results of a pilot trial of combined diazoxide and metformin Therapy. Int J Pediatr Endocrinol. 2011;**2011**:417949.

12. John K, Marino JS, Sanchez ER, Hinds TD. The glucocorticoid receptor: cause of or cure for obesity? Am J Physiol Endocrinol Metab. 2016;**310**(4):E249–57.

13. Hollman GA, Allen DB. Overt glucocorticoid excess due to inhaled corticosteroid therapy. Pediatrics. 1988;**81**(3):452–55.

14. Reilly JJ, Armstrong J, Dorosty AR, Emmett PM, Ness A, Rogers I, et al. Early life risk factors for obesity in childhood: cohort study. BMJ. 2005;**330**(7504):1357.

15. Agras WS, Hammer LD, McNicholas F, Kraemer HC. Risk factors for childhood overweight: a prospective study from birth to 9.5 years. J Pediatr. 2004;**145**(1):20–5.

16. Fatima Y, Doi SA, Mamun AA. Longitudinal impact of sleep on overweight and obesity in children and adolescents: a systematic review and bias-adjusted meta-analysis. Obes Rev. 2015;**16**(2):137–49.

17. Ickes MJ, McMullen J, Haider T, Sharma M. Global school-based childhood obesity interventions: a review. Int J Environ Res Public Health. 2014;**11**(9):8940–61.

18. Brenn BR. Anesthesia for pediatric obesity. Anesthesiol Clin North America. 2005;**23**(4):745–64.

19. Inge TH, Garcia V, Daniels S, Langford L, Kirk S, Roehrig H, et al. A multidisciplinary approach to the adolescent bariatric surgical patient. J Pediatr Surg. 2004;**39**(3):442–47.

20. Michalsky M, Reichard K, Inge T, Pratt J, Lenders C, American Society for Metabolic and Bariatric Surgery. ASMBS Pediatric Committee best practice guidelines. Surg Obes Relat Dis. 2012;**8**(1):1–7.

21. Inge TH, Krebs NF, Garcia VF, Skelton JA, Guice KS, Strauss RS, et al. Bariatric surgery for severely overweight adolescents: concerns and recommendations. Pediatrics. 2004;**114**(1):217–23.

22. Inge TH, Donnelly LF, Vierra M, Cohen AP, Daniels SR, Garcia VF. Managing bariatric patients in a children's hospital: radiologic considerations and limitations. J Pediatr Surg. 2005;**40**(4):609–17.

23. Stefater MA, Jenkins T, Inge TH. Bariatric surgery for adolescents. Pediatr Diabetes. 2013;**14**(1):1–12.

24. Sachdev P, Makaya T, Marven SS, Ackroyd R, Wales JK, Wright NP. Bariatric surgery in severely obese adolescents: a single-centre experience. Arch Dis Child. 2014;**99**(10):894–98.

25. Willcox K, Brennan L. Biopsychosocial outcomes of laparoscopic adjustable gastric banding in adolescents: a systematic review of the literature. Obes Surg. 2014;**24**(9):1510–19.

26. Miyano G, Jenkins TM, Xanthakos SA, Garcia VF, Inge TH. Perioperative outcome of laparoscopic Roux-en-Y gastric bypass: a children's hospital experience. J Pediatr Surg. 2013;**48**(10):2092–98.

27. Philippi-Höhne C. Anaesthesia in the obese child. Best Pract Res Clin Anaesthesiol. 2011;**25**(1):53–60.

28. Esposito M, Gallai B, Roccella M, Marotta R, Lavano F, Lavano SM, et al. Anxiety and depression levels in prepubertal obese children: a case-control study. Neuropsychiatr Dis Treat. 2014;**10**:1897–902.

29. Hebebrand J, Herpertz-Dahlmann B. Psychological and psychiatric aspects of pediatric obesity. Child Adolesc Psychiatr Clin N Am. 2009;**18**(1):49–65.

30. Vander Wal JS, Mitchell ER. Psychological complications of pediatric obesity. Pediatr Clin North Am. 2011;**58**(6):1393–401.

31. Andrews LE, Liu GT, Ko MW. Idiopathic intracranial hypertension and obesity. Horm Res Paediatr. 2014;**81**(4):217–25.

32. Sugerman HJ, Felton WL, Salvant JB, Sismanis A, Kellum JM. Effects of surgically induced weight loss on idiopathic intracranial hypertension in morbid obesity. Neurology. 1995;**45**(9):1655–59.

33. Karmaniolou I, Petropoulos G, Theodoraki K. Management of idiopathic intracranial hypertension in parturients: anesthetic considerations. Can J Anesth. 2011;**58**(7):650.

34. Ladosky W, Botelho MA, Albuquerque JP, Jr. Chest mechanics in morbidly obese non-hypoventilated patients. Respir Med. 2001;**95**(4):281–86.

35. Eichenberger A, Proietti S, Wicky S, Frascarolo P, Suter M, Spahn DR, et al. Morbid obesity and postoperative pulmonary atelectasis: an underestimated problem. Anesth Analg. 2002;**95**(6):1788–92.

36. Inselma LS, Milanese A, Deurloo A. Effect of obesity on pulmonary function in children. Pediatr Pulmonol. 1993;**16**(2):130–37.

37. Dixon AE, Holguin F, Sood A, Salome CM, Pratley RE, Beuther DA, et al. An official American Thoracic Society Workshop report: obesity and asthma. Proc Am Thorac Soc. 2010;**7**(5):325–35.

38. Ford ES. The epidemiology of obesity and asthma. J Allergy Clin Immunol. 2005;**115**(5):897–909.

39. Silvestri JM, Weese-Mayer DE, Bass MT, Kenny AS, Hauptman SA, Pearsall SM. Polysomnography in obese children with a history of sleep-associated breathing disorders. Pediatr Pulmonol. 1993;**16**(2):124–29.

40. Coté CJ. Anesthesiological considerations for children with obstructive sleep apnea. Curr Opin Anaesthesiol. 2015;**28**(3):327–32.

41. El-Metainy S, Ghoneim T, Aridae E, Abdel Wahab M. Incidence of perioperative adverse events in obese children undergoing elective general surgery. Br J Anaesth. 2011;**106**(3):359–63.

42. Cote AT, Harris KC, Panagiotopoulos C, Sandor GG, Devlin AM. Childhood obesity and cardiovascular dysfunction. J Am Coll Cardiol. 2013;**62**(15):1309–19.

43. Michalsky MP, Inge TH, Simmons M, Jenkins TM, Buncher R, Helmrath M, et al. Cardiovascular risk factors in severely obese adolescents: the teen longitudinal assessment of bariatric surgery (teen-LABS) study. JAMA Pediatr. 2015;**169**(5):438–44.

44. Sorof J, Daniels S. Obesity hypertension in children: a problem of epidemic proportions. Hypertension. 2002;**40**(4):441–47.

45. Phatak UP, Pashankar DS. Prevalence of functional gastrointestinal disorders in obese and overweight children. Int J Obes (Lond). 2014;**38**(10):1324–27.

46. Xanthakos SA, Jenkins TM, Kleiner DE, Boyce TW, Mourya R, Karns R, et al. High prevalence of nonalcoholic fatty liver disease in adolescents undergoing bariatric surgery. Gastroenterology. 2015;149(3):623–34.

47. Pashankar DS, Corbin Z, Shah SK, Caprio S. Increased prevalence of gastroesophageal reflux symptoms in obese children evaluated in an academic medical center. J Clin Gastroenterol. 2009;43(5):410–13.

48. Cook-Sather SD, Gallagher PR, Kruge LE, Beus JM, Ciampa BP, Welch KC, et al. Overweight/obesity and gastric fluid characteristics in pediatric day surgery: implications for fasting guidelines and pulmonary aspiration risk. Anesth Analg. 2009;109(3):727–36.

49. Gunta SS, Mak RH. Is obesity a risk factor for chronic kidney disease in children? Pediatr Nephrol. 2013;28(10):1949–56.

50. Nafiu OO, Green GE, Walton S, Morris M, Reddy S, Tremper KK. Obesity and risk of peri-operative complications in children presenting for adenotonsillectomy. Int J Pediatr Otorhinolaryngol. 2009;73(1):89–95.

51. Weeratunga GU. Measuring non-invasive blood pressure in obese patients. Anaesthesia. 2003;58(6):616.

52. Nafiu OO, Burke C, Cowan A, Tutuo N, Maclean S, Tremper KK. Comparing peripheral venous access between obese and normal weight children. Pediatr Anesth. 2010;20(2):172–76.

53. Gleich SJ, Olson MD, Sprung J, Weingarten TN, Schroeder DR, Warner DO, et al. Perioperative outcomes of severely obese children undergoing tonsillectomy. Pediatr Anesth. 2012;22(12):1171–78.

54. Burke CN, Voepel-Lewis T, Wagner D, Lau I, Baldock A, Malviya S, et al. A retrospective description of anesthetic medication dosing in overweight and obese children. Pediatr Anesth. 2014;24(8):857–62.

55. Mortensen A, Lenz K, Abildstrøm H, Lauritsen TL. Anesthetizing the obese child. Pediatr Anesth. 2011;21(6):623–29.

56. Peters AM, Snelling HLR, Glass DM, Bird NJ. Estimation of lean body mass in children. Br J Anaesth. 2011;106(5):719–23.

57. Maxwell BG, Ingrande J, Rosenthal DN, Ramamoorthy C. Perioperative management of the morbidly obese adolescent with heart failure undergoing bariatric surgery. Pediatr Anesth. 2012;22(5):476–82.

58. Rose JB, Theroux MC, Katz MS. The potency of succinylcholine in obese adolescents. Anesth Analg. 2000;90(3):576–78.

59. Stepanova NA, Krasovskiĭ VA, Oleĭnikov Ia V, Tabakina TE, Pogrebova TK, Tkachenko BA, et al. [Characteristics of anesthesia in trauma surgery in children with severe burn injuries]. Anesteziol Reanimatol. 1999;4(4):23–6.

60. Kirkwood A, Fernandez E. Associated medical conditions in children. Anaesth Intensive Care Med. 2015;16(8):401–12.

61. Hannallah RS. Ambulatory anesthesia in children. Semin Anesth. 1992;11(4):303–8.

62. Olutoye OA, Yu X, Govindan K, Tjia IM, East DL, Spearman R, et al. The effect of obesity on the ED(95) of propofol for loss of consciousness in children and adolescents. Anesth Analg. 2012;115(1):147–53.

63. Chidambaran V, Venkatasubramanian R, Sadhasivam S, Esslinger H, Cox S, Diepstraten J, et al. Population pharmacokinetic-pharmacodynamic modeling and dosing simulation of propofol maintenance anesthesia in severely obese adolescents. Pediatr Anesth. 2015;25(9):911–23.

64. Biber JL, Allareddy V, Allareddy V, Gallagher SM, Couloures KG, Speicher DG, et al. Prevalence and predictors of adverse events during procedural sedation anesthesia-outside the operating room for esophagogastroduodenoscopy and colonoscopy in children: age is an independent predictor of outcomes. Pediatr Crit Care Med. 2015;16(8):e251–59.

65. Scherrer PD, Mallory MD, Cravero JP, Lowrie L, Hertzog JH, Berkenbosch JW, et al. The impact of obesity on pediatric procedural sedation-related outcomes: results from the Pediatric Sedation Research Consortium. Pediatr Anesth. 2015;25(7):689–97.

66. Grunwell JR, McCracken C, Fortenberry J, Stockwell J, Kamat P. Risk factors leading to failed procedural sedation in children outside the operating room. Pediatr Emerg Care. 2014;30(6):381–87.

67. Baker S, Yagiela JA. Obesity: a complicating factor for sedation in children. Pediatr Dent. 2006;28(6):487–93.

68. Lee JJ, Sun LS, Gu B, Kim M, Wang S, Han S. Does obesity prolong anesthesia in children undergoing common ENT surgery? Pediatr Anesth. 2014;24(10):1037–43.

69. Stein PD, Beemath A, Olson RE. Obesity as a risk factor in venous thromboembolism. Am J Med. 2005;118(9):978–80.

70. Mushtaq A, Vaughns JD, Ziesenitz VC, Nadler EP, van den Anker JN. Use of enoxaparin in obese adolescents during bariatric surgery—a Pilot study. Obes Surg. 2015;25(10):1869–74.

71. Halvorson EE, Irby MB, Skelton JA. Pediatric obesity and safety in inpatient settings: a systematic literature review. Clin Pediatr (Phila). 2014;53(10):975–87.

72. Inge TH, Garcia V, Daniels S, Langford L, Kirk S, Roehrig H, et al. A multidisciplinary approach to the adolescent bariatric surgical patient. J Pediatr Surg. 2004;39(3):442–7.

73. Luber SD, Fischer DR, Venkat A. Care of the bariatric surgery patient in the emergency department. J Emerg Med. 2008;34(1):13–20.

74. Brown CV, Neville AL, Salim A, Rhee P, Cologne K, Demetriades D. The impact of obesity on severely injured children and adolescents. J Pediatr Surg. 2006;41(1):88–91.

75. Alselaim N, Malaekah H, Saade M, Hussein M, Altokhais T, Albedah K, et al. Does obesity impact the pattern and outcome of trauma in children? J Pediatr Surg. 2012;47(7):1404–409.

76. Srinivasan V, Nadkarni VM, Helfaer MA, Carey SM, Berg RA, American Heart Association National Registry of Cardiopulmonary Resuscitation Investigators. Childhood obesity and survival after in-hospital pediatric cardiopulmonary resuscitation. Pediatrics. 2010;125(3):e481–88.

Obesity in pregnancy

Onyi C. Onuoha

Introduction

In both affluent and developing countries, obesity continues to approach epidemic proportions [1,2] and has become a major contributor to the global burden of chronic disease and disability [3]. Although recent data may indicate the exponential increase in obesity in the United States may be levelling off, the prevalence of obesity remains high with 34.9% [4,5] of adults being obese according to recent estimates in 2011–2012. In the United States, women are more affected than men [3,6]. In 2000, the percentage of women with a body mass index (BMI) of 50 kg/m² or more had increased by fivefold in the past 20 years [7]. The National Health and Nutrition Examination Survey in 2010 estimated the incidence of obesity in adult women as 35.8% [2,4].

Unfortunately, women of reproductive age are not spared by this epidemic [8]. Particularly in pregnancy, obesity is a public health issue of concern. Maternal obesity is defined as a BMI of greater than 30 kg/m² at the first antenatal consultation [9]. According to Pan et al. [10], 50% of pregnant women are overweight or obese and as many as 8% of women in their reproductive childbearing age are morbidly obese with a BMI of over 40 kg/m². The confusion among women as to what normal physiological weight gain in pregnancy is, drove the Institute of Medicine in 2009 to revise their prior recommendations for allowable gestational weight gain using pre-pregnancy BMI and to provide a restricted weight range for the obese parturient (**Table 30.1**) [11].

Indisputably, obesity has been associated with significant obstetric and anaesthetic risk [9,12] including being identified as an independent risk factor for maternal mortality by the CEMACH Maternal Death Enquiry [5]. A basic understanding of the general impact of obesity on pregnancy is therefore critical. The goal of this chapter is to (1) discuss the physiological changes that occur in the obese parturient, (2) highlight the resulting implications or challenges encountered, and finally (3) review the potential strategies to ensure the delivery of safe anaesthetic care in this patient population.

Physiological changes in the obese parturient

Normal pregnancy is associated with a myriad of physiological changes in several organ systems of importance in the body [13,14]. Pregnancy as a sole entity can be considered a stressful state that is able to challenge the physiological reserve of a woman of childbearing age [13]. With obesity or morbid obesity superimposed on the pregnancy state, a 'double-hit phenomenon' occurs and a significant burden is added to an already existing compromised state and reserve. Hence, obesity compounds most of the physiological changes that occur in pregnancy [15].

Airway changes

1. *With normal pregnancy*: the increase in blood volume during pregnancy increases the generalized vascularity of vital organs resulting in an increased incidence of interstitial oedema of the airway, engorged oral and pharyngeal mucous membranes, bleeding, and narrowing of the air passages [13,15]. Breast enlargement in pregnancy also increases the difficulty of securing the airway [15].

2. *With obesity*: excessive adipose tissue deposition leads to a distorted anatomy and a generalized increase in soft tissue volume, especially around the neck circumference and pharynx, resulting in additional compression and narrowing of the airway [8,15,16]. Limited mouth opening and neck movement and an enlarged tongue are common in obesity and increase the difficulty of mask ventilation [8,15]. In addition, these patients may present with associated pre-existing comorbidities such as obstructive sleep apnoea (OSA) and obesity hypoventilation syndrome (OHS) [14,15,17].

3. *Double-hit phenomenon*: the synergistic combination of airway oedema, friable mucous membranes from pregnancy, and increased soft tissue deposition from obesity can lead to significant airway challenges with both ventilation and intubation. Obesity

Table 30.1 Recommended weight gain during pregnancy

Prepregnancy BMI (kg/m²)	Recommended weight gain (kg)
<18.5	12.5–18
18.5–24.9	11.5–16
25–29.9	7–11.5
> 30	5–9

Source: Data from *Weight Gain During Pregnancy: Reexamining the Guidelines*, 2009.

and pregnancy each increase the risk of difficult intubation [6]. The incidence can be up to 15.5% [19] in patients with a BMI of greater than 35 kg/m² and as high as 33% [18] in morbidly obese pregnant patients as noted in other sources.

Pulmonary system changes

1. *With normal pregnancy*: early in pregnancy, women develop a sensation of dyspnoea secondary to increased alveolar ventilation from the effects of progesterone on the respiratory centre in the brainstem [3,15]. With elevated progesterone levels, both respiratory rate and tidal volume is increased in pregnancy leading to an increase in minute ventilation [13,14]. There is also a reduction in the expiratory reserve volume (ERV), residual volume, and functional residual capacity (FRC) due to the enlargement of the gravid uterus [6,14]. The oxygen requirement increases from 2 mL/min to 5–6 mL/min during pregnancy due to an increase in metabolic demand and oxygen consumption by the fetus [13]. These physiological changes make the parturient particularly prone to rapid desaturation.

2. *With obesity*: obesity in non-pregnant patients is also associated with a decrease in ERV, residual volume, and FRC, most likely due to the added weight of excess fat on the chest and abdomen and decreased chest compliance [15,20]. Obesity increases oxygen consumption and carbon dioxide (CO_2) production, thus increasing the work of breathing, which in morbidly obese patients can be increased even during quiet breathing at rest [21]. This can lead to chronic hypoventilation and CO_2 retention promoting the development of ventilation/perfusion mismatch, hypoxaemia, and a subsequent gradual onset of pulmonary hypertension [13]. The supine, lithotomy, or particularly the Trendelenburg position, or the induction of general anaesthesia can further reduce the FRC causing the closing capacity to exceed the FRC and resulting in the collapse of the small distal airways, ventilation/perfusion mismatch, shunting, and hypoxaemia [22]. These physiological changes make the obese patient particularly prone to rapid desaturation [14,17]. Obesity also increases the risk of OSA in the parturient. OHS is seen in 8% of obese parturient and is characterized by morbid obesity, alveolar hypoventilation, and daytime somnolence [15].

3. *Double-hit phenomenon*: the combination of an increase in oxygen demand resulting from a decrease in FRC in pregnancy and obesity, increase in oxygen consumption by the fetus, increase in CO_2 production and work of breathing in obesity, an increase in the closing capacity, and the collapse of the distal airways in obesity all significantly reduce the maternal oxygen reserve in the obese parturient, particularly increasing the tendency to rapid desaturation [13,14,17,23].

Cardiovascular system changes

1. *With normal pregnancy*: during the first trimester, the blood volume (BV) and cardiac output (CO) increase by 30–35%. A substantial increase of about 50–70% is seen in both the BV and CO during the third trimester and especially in the immediate postpartum period [13,14,17]. In labour, uterine contractions further increase CO by 10–15% [13–15]. With smooth muscle dilation from elevated levels of progesterone, the peripheral vascular resistance is significantly decreased with a subsequent decrease in maternal blood pressure [6,14]. Maternal heart rate increases by 25–35% [13]. With the progression of pregnancy and the enlargement of the gravid uterus, the presence of aortocaval compression in the supine position decreases the venous return to the heart with a subsequent decrease in CO and organ perfusion. By the second trimester, left uterine displacement of the uterus is often necessary in preventing significant compression and a subsequent reduction in uterine perfusion [13].

2. *With obesity*: with every 100 g of fat, the CO increases by about 30–50 mL/min [24]. In other words, obesity independently increases BV by about 20–25% and CO is subsequently increased to meet the demands from additional adiposity [6,13]. An increase in BV may lead to an increased risk of pulmonary hypertension due to increased pulmonary blood flow and in extreme cases, right heart failure may develop [6,15]. Morbid obesity is also associated with a constellation of other comorbidities including hypertension with left ventricular hypertrophy and diastolic dysfunction, coronary artery disease, early-onset myocardial ischaemia, and peripartum cardiomyopathy [8,24,25].

3. *Double-hit phenomenon*: unlike the non-obese parturient who is able to maintain their contractile performance throughout pregnancy by adjusting their heart rate, stroke volume, and CO appropriately, the obese parturient depicts a maladaptive physiology [26]. In obese parturients, afterload reduction may be impaired due to increased peripheral resistance and greater arterial stiffness [26]. With a hyperdynamic circulation, left ventricular hypertrophy with diastolic dysfunction and late-onset systolic dysfunction could eventually result [15]. Supine hypotension syndrome is often exaggerated in the obese parturient due to the additional aortocaval compression and a significant decrease in the venous return from the panniculus [13,15]. Tseuda et al. reported two cases of sudden death in morbidly obese patients in the supine position [27]. Additionally, with obesity and the increasing maternal age in pregnancy, the risk of myocardial ischaemia is increased due to an increased metabolic demand and hyperdynamic state [28].

Gastrointestinal system changes

1. *With normal pregnancy*: both the presence of elevated levels of progesterone and an increasing gravid uterus during pregnancy can alter the reliability of the lower oesophageal sphincter tone, thus increasing the risk of aspiration of gastric contents and Mendelson's syndrome [13,15,29]. In addition, the placenta secretes gastrin, thus increasing the production of gastric acid and subsequent acid reflux throughout pregnancy [13].

2. *With obesity*: obese patients often have additional risk factors which increase the risk for acid reflux and subsequent aspiration. Abdominal obesity increases intragastric pressure, hence increasing the frequency of transient lower oesophageal sphincter relaxation and/or hiatal hernia formation [30]. Other factors include diabetes mellitus and gestational diabetes which delay gastric emptying due to gastroparesis, and a decreased lower oesophageal sphincter tone [3,13,15].

3. *Double-hit phenomenon*: the presence of an increased risk of aspiration due to additional decrease in gastric motility and emptying in the setting of pregnancy and obesity remains controversial, as conflicting studies exist on this issue. Wong et al. [31] showed no difference in the gastric emptying of water in obese and non-obese pregnant women. Both Juvin et al. [32] and Maltby et al. [33] found no difference in gastric content or pH in obese patients compared to normal-weight patients. Other older studies, however, have shown the contrary, that gastric volume in obese parturients could be up to five times greater than controls [34–36]. Roberts and Shirley [34] demonstrated weight to be a significant factor in gastric content volume during labour but not in patients scheduled for elective caesarean delivery. Vaughan et al. showed that obese non-pregnant patients scheduled for elective surgery had a larger gastric volume and a lower gastric pH than their non-obese non-pregnant counterparts [37].

Haematological function changes

1. *With normal pregnancy*: the increase in procoagulant factors, most notably fibrinogen, and the decrease in endogenous anti-coagulant factors (protein S and activated protein C resistance) characterize pregnancy as a hypercoagulable state [14,38]. Consequently, fibrinolytic activity is impaired [14] and the risk of venous thromboembolism including the occurrence of deep venous thrombosis or pulmonary embolism is four to five times increased in pregnancy and the postpartum period [39]. In the developed world, thromboembolic events remain one of the leading causes of maternal death compared to haemorrhage in the rest of the world [40].

2. *With obesity*: obesity is associated with higher levels of fi-brinogen, factor VII, and factor VIII, which predispose to hypercoagulability [30]. Elevated levels of von Willebrand factor and factor VIII lead to fibrin formation and increased plasminogen activator inhibitor-1 inhibits the fibrinolytic system, further increasing hypercoagulability in the obese state [30]. Obesity also promotes a chronic systemic inflammatory response with an elevation of mediators such as C-reactive protein and interleukin levels [41]. Hence, obesity remains one of the most significant risk factors for venous thromboembolism [13].

3. *Double-hit phenomenon*: given the presence of both pregnancy and obesity as independent risk factors, the risk of thromboembolism in the obese parturient is more significant than in the non-obese patient. Endothelial-dependent vasodilation, which is increased in pregnancy, is often blunted in the obese parturient [42].

Implications of obesity in pregnancy

Maternal implications

1. *Antepartum*: obesity can independently increase the risk of miscarriage after both spontaneous conception and assisted reproductive therapy [13]. Gestational diabetes mellitus and preeclampsia significantly contribute to the substantial medical burden and morbidity seen in obstetric care. The incidence of chronic hypertension and pregnancy-induced hypertension including the more severe form of HELLP syndrome (haemolysis, elevated liver enzymes, and low platelets) are more common in the obese parturient [8,13,15]. The risk of developing gestational diabetes and subsequent type 2 diabetes mellitus also increases with increasing weight in pregnancy [13]. OSA and venous thromboembolism, specifically deep venous thrombosis or pulmonary embolism, are not uncommon in the obese parturient [13,15].

2. *Intrapartum—intraoperative*: the obese parturient is at an increased risk of slower cervical dilatation rates, ineffective uterine contractions, augmentation with oxytocin during labour, induction of labour, a failed induction of labour, fetal intolerance of labour, instrumental delivery, and emergency caesarean delivery compared to their non-obese counterparts [8,13,15]. In addition, they have a higher incidence of prolonged operative times and acute blood loss greater than 1000 mL [15]. Ultimately, obesity is a risk factor for maternal death during pregnancy [2].

   Technical and anaesthetic-related challenges include difficulty acquiring an appropriately sized operating table; difficulty with transfers and intravenous catheter placement; the occasional need for arterial catheter placement for BP monitoring given the unavailability of appropriate cuff sizes; the need for a central venous catheter for access; the need for different sizes of epidural and spinal needles for neuraxial anaesthesia; and difficulty with the placement of an epidural or spinal block [8,13,43]. Mask ventilation and endotracheal intubation have also been shown to be a challenge in this patient population [13].

3. *Postpartum—postoperative*: the risk of major postpartum haemorrhage increases with increasing BMI [13,15]. In addition, the obese parturient has been shown to have a higher risk of postoperative wound infections or dehiscence, endometritis, genital tract infection, urinary tract infection, and respiratory sensitivity to opiates if needed [15,43]. Obesity and pregnancy are each independent risk factors for deep venous thrombosis and on average, the obese women can spend up to five more days in the hospital than their non-obese equivalents resulting in a five-fold increase in the cost of care [3,13,15].

Fetal implications

The obese parturient is at an increased risk of having a large-for-gestational age macrosomic fetus, independent of maternal diabetes [13,15]. There is a threefold increased risk of shoulder dystocia in the morbidly obese parturient. The risks of stillbirth (fetal demise) and infant birth defects are also increased—including neural tube defects such as anencephaly, anomalies of the heart and intestinal tract, omphaloceles, orofacial clefts, and multiple congenital anomalies of the central nervous system [13,15]. With a stable mother, the anaesthesiologist may occasionally be needed to assist in neonatal resuscitation.

Technical challenges include difficulties with fetal heart rate monitoring using external transducers due to the increased depth of maternal adipose tissue [15]. Difficulty with accurate fetal heart rate monitoring can further increase the risk of an operative delivery in this patient population due to perceived fetal indications. The use of fetal scalp electrodes and intrauterine pressure catheters may be needed for accurate monitoring [15] but involve the rupture of membranes, which may increase the risk of infection in a slow and prolonged labour process.

Peripartum anaesthetic management of the obese parturient

The anaesthetic management of the obese parturient presents special challenges due to multiple factors including synergistic physiological processes, numerous coexisting disease conditions, and a variety of logistic or technical issues that make management difficult. Special antepartum counselling is recommended by the American Congress of Obstetricians and Gynecologists to address issues about the risk of obesity to the fetus and mother; encourage a preconception weight-reduction programme; discuss the allowable weight gain during pregnancy; and recommend nutrition counselling and an exercise plan during pregnancy [13,44]. The morbidly obese parturient is therefore often considered a *high-risk* patient and in some cases, is closely followed by maternal fetal medicine specialists in the antenatal period and subsequently recommended for a 'presurgical anaesthesia consultation' [9,13], especially when associated with a diagnosis of OSA, OHS, or known difficult intubation [13]. The goals of an anaesthesia consultation include to establish a rapport with the patient; optimize pre-existing conditions; generate an anaesthetic plan based on risk; and create a general increased awareness of the soon-arrival of this patient to the labour floor. A clear care plan should be formulated, documented, and easily accessible for the staff that may be involved in the delivery process during on-call hours. The criteria or exact BMI cut-off warranting consultation varies with institutions.

Antenatal/antepartum evaluation

Detailed medical history

The evaluation process always begins with obtaining a general history of the patient's health status to assess peripartum risk and optimize management [13]. The general medical history contains data about the patient's general health condition briefly addressing all pertinent systems (cardiopulmonary—functional status, neurological, gastrointestinal, haematological), prior surgical history including abdominal surgery, pertinent family history, any personal history of drug or alcohol use, allergies to any substances, and a medication list including herbal medications. For these patients, establishing the presence of associated findings such as OSA or OHS with or without the use of continuous positive airway pressure, the use of bronchodilators, a pre-existing history of chronic or pulmonary hypertension, gastric reflux, ischaemic heart disease, pre-existing diabetes, or gestational diabetes, is important. The history should include a complete review of systems to identify undiagnosed disease or inadequately controlled chronic disease. In addition, a focused obstetric history including parity, position of placenta, current plan for induction of labour, or a planned elective caesarean section should be obtained [13].

Physical examination

A focused physical examination with specific attention to the cardiopulmonary system and airway is warranted in this patient population. It is important to note that there is often a worsening of the airway during pregnancy and the course of labour [45]. Other pertinent areas of focus include the evaluation of the upper extremities for potential vascular access or monitoring of accurate blood pressures, examination of the back to anticipate technical challenges with establishing neuraxial analgesia, and examination of the exact size of the pannus to assess the availability of the necessary equipment needed for optimal patient care [8,9,13,46].

Preoperative testing

Based on the elicited history and physical examination, preoperative tests and consults are obtained as needed. Although most of the literature still recommends routine screening (12-lead electrocardiogram, echocardiogram, cardiology consult, chest radiograph, complete blood count, electrolyte panel with liver function tests, and coagulation studies) [8,46] based on obesity alone, the need for these additional tests should be driven by clear indications in the history, or physical examination. Tests should be ordered when the history or physical examination would have indicated the need for testing even if delivery or surgery had not been planned.

Education/informed consent

A thorough and well-documented consent form delineating details and risk of anaesthesia should be completed to ensure that the patient's expectations of labour, labour analgesia, conversion of labour analgesia for caesarean section, alternative plan in case of regional failure, the need for emergency caesarean delivery, the need for general anaesthesia, and postoperative pain control are realistic and appropriate [13]. The patient should be aware of the existing challenges that can occur during her intrapartum course. These may include difficult venous access, technical challenges with successful placement of the regional anaesthesia, the risks of general anaesthesia, and the need for the placement of invasive monitors like a continuous arterial catheter or central venous catheter due to suboptimal measurements via non-invasive modalities [8,9,13]. Patient education is especially important in the obese parturient with a rigid birth plan, doula, or adamantly requesting a natural delivery. The clinician should be careful to relate the pertinent information without making the patient feel humiliated about her weight [47].

Intrapartum care

Anaesthetic options

Vaginal delivery (labour analgesia)

The higher incidence of slower cervical dilatation rates, ineffective uterine contractions, a failed induction of labour, fetal intolerance of labour, and emergency caesarean delivery in the obese parturient makes the need for a *functional* neuraxial catheter for labour analgesia in this patient population critical [13,15]. **Table 30.2** illustrates the several options for labour analgesia in the obese parturient. **Table 30.3** provides recommendations for the use of neuraxial analgesia in the obese parturient [8,13,15,43,46,48–52]. The anaesthesiologist should have a high level of suspicion for a possible intrapartum conversion from labour to operative delivery when caring for this patient population. Continuous communication among *all* teams (obstetrician, anaesthesiologist, nursing) caring for the patient should be maintained during the labour course and should address any concerns about fetal heart rate tracing, inadequate analgesia, or new laboratory or radiographic findings early in the process [13].

Caesarean/operative delivery (surgical anaesthesia)

The existing literature does not clearly validate the superiority of one technique over the other (general versus neuraxial anaesthesia)

Table 30.2 Analgesic and anaesthetic options for delivery in the obese parturient

	Advantages	Disadvantages
Labour analgesia		
Epidural	• Reliable • Able to extend the duration of the anaesthetic for an unanticipated prolonged procedure	• ↑ initial failure rate for placement • Difficulty with positioning, midline and epidural space identification, ↑ risk of catheter migration and dislodgement • May need multiple attempts at epidural placement (>3) • ↑ risk of unilateral block • Slow onset of action
CSE	• ↓ failure rate of epidural catheter • Clear confirmation of success (CSF) • Rapid onset of action (spinal component) • Able to extend block (epidural component) • Similar risk of headache when compared to an epidural • Preferred technique for elective caesarean delivery in the morbidly obese parturient	• Untested epidural catheter: can fail (inadequate analgesia) when intrathecal block is resolved, ↑ risk of conversion to a general anaesthetic • May need longer time for placement compared to a spinal anaesthetic
CSA	• See below in table	• See below in table
Anaesthesia for caesarean section		
Epidural	• See above in table	• See above in table
Single-shot spinal	• Fast, reliable, dense, and predictable block • Clear confirmation of success (CSF)	• Technically difficult placement, need different needle sizes and length • Short duration given ↑ risk of prolonged surgical procedure with obesity • Difficult titration of spinal medications for adequate surgical block and duration • More profound hypotension
CSE	• See above in table	• See above in table
CSA	• The 'ideal' choice • Rapid, reliable surgical block • Easy titration of medication to desired level and duration at any point during the procedure	• ↑ incidence of infection although rare • ↑ failure rate of the catheters due to dislodgement, inexperience • ↑ rate of PDPH in recent studies • Not a routinely used anaesthetic technique
General anaesthesia	• Controlled and safe placement of ETT • Faster onset (in select patients—where placement of neuraxial block is difficult)—standard of care for emergent caesarean delivery • Controlled surgical field (motionless, speechless patient) • Avoidance of all risks or adverse effects of regional anaesthesia (including significant hypotension, PDPH, nerve injury, total spinal, local anaesthetic toxicity, etc.)	• ↑ risk of difficult airway (ventilation and intubation) • ↑ risk of aspiration of gastric contents • ↑ risk of peripartum haemorrhage • ↑ risk of thromboembolism • No maternal–infant bonding • ↑ exposure of drugs to fetus

CSA, continuous spinal anaesthesia; CSE, combined spinal epidural; CSF, cerebrospinal fluid; ETT, endotracheal tube; PDPH, postdural puncture headache.

when used for caesarean section [53]. However, when not contraindicated, neuraxial anaesthesia remains the preferred gold standard for caesarean delivery in developed countries and is perceived to be safer for the mother and fetus than general anaesthesia—specifically in the obese parturient. Benefits range from better mother–baby bonding, superior intra- and postoperative analgesia with minimal adverse effects, maternal satisfaction, minimal exposure of drugs to the fetus, avoidance of the instrumentation of the airway, and a reduction in both the aspiration and venous thromboembolism risk [8,13,15]. Table 30.2 illustrates the several options for surgical anaesthesia in this patient population.

Elective caesarean delivery Ideally, the preferred anaesthetic technique for an elective caesarean delivery in a morbidly obese parturient is continuous spinal anaesthesia. It produces a rapid, reliable, dense, and predictable surgical block where titration of medication to desired level and duration can occur at any point during the procedure. Nevertheless, due to the widespread unavailability of these catheters, combined spinal epidural and primary epidural anaesthesia remain the other reliable options. With a combined spinal

epidural, anaesthesia can be extended with the epidural catheter for the entire duration of surgery, which could be prolonged. There is, however, a small risk of intraoperative catheter failure (unilateral, inadequate, or absent block) after the resolution of the initial intrathecal block. Although this risk has been shown to be smaller or similar to the risk of failure from a primary epidural technique [13,54], with the primary technique, the anaesthesiologist is able to replace a suboptimal or non-functioning primary epidural catheter until adequate block is achieved prior to initiating surgery.

Urgent or emergent caesarean delivery The anaesthesiologist should be able to rapidly achieve surgical anaesthesia for an anticipated emergent delivery by:

• *Conversion of labour analgesia → surgical anaesthesia*: with a pre-existing *functional* epidural catheter, utilizing 2% lidocaine or 3% chloroprocaine, dosed in small aliquots, to establish a dense block is often adequate for operative delivery [13]. Controversial reports exist on whether to attempt a single-shot spinal anaesthetic after a failed epidural catheter [55,56]. It is important to be aware

Table 30.3 Recommendations for the use of neuraxial analgesia/anaesthesia in the obese parturient

	Recommendations
Timing	1. With extreme obesity, an anticipated or known difficult airway → an epidural catheter should be placed *early* in the labour process. Be *proactive*! 2. An initial airway evaluation and *continuous airway assessments* during active labour is important
Options	See Table 30.2
Placement	1. Identifying landmarks and midline can be easier in the *sitting* rather than the lateral decubitus position although is still challenging 2. ↑ risk of *multiple attempts* prior to successful placement 3. Utilizing *the parturient* to identify midline can be helpful 4. The epidural space may be deeper with obesity but BMI is a poor predictor of distance to the epidural space. Most studies report an *average depth of 8 cm* in the obese parturient 5. The use of an *ultrasound* has been shown to be valuable to identify the midline, localize the epidural space, and measure the skin-to-epidural space distance 6. Due to an increased risk of catheter migration or dislodgement and a higher rate of emergency caesarean delivery, *frequent evaluation* of an adequate sensory level is necessary 7. Have a low threshold to *replace a non-functional or inadequately functioning epidural catheter* in the obese parturient. Positive association between ↑ number of boluses during labour and a failed conversion of epidural analgesia to anaesthesia 8. The prevention of catheter dislodgement can be challenging in the morbidly obese parturient where frequent positioning by the obstetric team is often inevitable 9. With a difficult or questionable insertion, *a deliberate spinal* with a pencil-point spinal needle may be performed through the epidural needle for confirmation of CSF with no intrathecal medications administered 10. Although the epidural requirement of local anaesthesia has been shown to be lower in the obese patient, recent evidence has supported the need for the *same amount of intrathecal local anaesthetic* as the non-obese parturient
Complications	1. With an accidental dural puncture, the epidural catheter can be converted to a *continuous spinal catheter* with extreme caution in dosing 2. Although findings have been inconsistent, some studies indicate a *lower risk of dural puncture headache* in the obese parturient due to the ↑ risk of caesarean delivery in this population. Bearing down in vaginal delivery ↑ risk of PDPH due to ↑ in dural rent and CSF loss 3. ↑↑ risk of *profound hypotension* (refractory to fluids and vasopressors) most likely due to aortocaval compression as optimal positioning is difficult in these patients

CSF, cerebrospinal fluid; PDPH, postdural puncture headache.

of the increased risk of a high block or total spinal anaesthesia necessitating emergent airway intervention when a spinal anaesthetic is performed after a partly functional epidural catheter is bolused and removed [57]. Performing a combined spinal epidural where a much smaller dose than usual is administered and the epidural catheter subsequently used to titrate to adequate anaesthetic levels can be considered a safe intermediate between the two options [13]. Continuous spinal anaesthesia is the practical, safe, and optimal alternative after the failed attempt to convert epidural analgesia to surgical anaesthesia but these catheters are still unavailable in several institutions. With all possible options, the goal of the anaesthesiologist is to quickly achieve surgical anaesthesia while avoiding an unplanned emergent airway intervention in a possible difficult airway.

- *General anaesthesia*: the need for an emergent delivery in the setting of a non-functioning or absent epidural catheter may require the anaesthesiologist to proceed with a general anaesthetic in the obese parturient. In addition, despite an obvious preference for neuraxial anaesthesia for childbirth in the morbidly obese patient, occasionally, general anaesthesia is the *only option* of choice for delivery. In the event that general anaesthesia is required, adequate and detailed preparation is essential for patient care [13]. **Table 30.4** outlines some of the recommendations for the use of general anaesthesia in the obese parturient [3,6,8,9,13,15,46,58–68].

Postpartum care

Monitoring

A review of anaesthesia-related maternal deaths from 1985 to 2003 in Michigan, United States, showed six of the eight anaesthesia-related deaths were in women who were obese or morbidly obese and all airway complications occurred in the postoperative-postextubation period mostly due to lapses in standard monitoring and vigilance [69]. Postpartum monitoring is critical in morbidly obese patients with multiple systemic conditions. It is important to remember that these patients may need more vigilant nursing care and hence staffing ratios should be considered appropriately [3]. Patients with OSA who required continuous positive airway pressure during the antenatal course, need to continue treatment and be monitored closely during the immediate postoperative period.

Postoperative analgesia

Adequate pain control is a major goal for women in the postpartum period. Cautious titration of intravenous opioid to desired effect or vigilant monitoring after the administration of long-acting neuraxial opioid is particularly essential in the obese patient due to increased sensitivity to opioids [30]. Recent studies, however, have failed to demonstrate a higher incidence of respiratory depression in obese parturients who received neuraxial morphine after caesarean delivery [43]. Nonetheless, a multimodal approach involving the use of non-steroidal anti-inflammatory drugs or other opioid-sparing medications may be helpful [8]. Optimal analgesia is needed to improve postoperative pulmonary toileting and prevent associated adverse physiological outcomes such as respiratory impairment, ileus, suboptimal mobilization, tachycardia, hypertension, insulin resistance, or more obvious effects of sleep deprivation, impaired maternal–infant bonding, and consequently longer hospitalization [30].

Thromboprophylaxis

The American Congress of Obstetricians and Gynecologists recommends stratification of pregnant women into risk categories

Table 30.4 Recommendations for the use of general anaesthesia in the obese parturient

	Recommendations
Preparation	1. A sufficiently *stocked difficult airway cart and a clear plan* for surgical airway back-up should be immediately available for every high-risk obstetric unit caring for the morbidly obese parturient 2. *Simulations and drills* should be performed regularly to educate and update all personnel about the implications of general anaesthesia in a morbidly obese parturient. Individuals should be aware of their roles in the event that an unplanned emergent situation occurs 3. An *adequate airway assessment* is essential in all obese pregnant patients. This includes assessment of facial oedema, short neck, neck flexion, mouth opening, dentition (protruding maxillary incisors, missing), oropharyngeal structures (Mallampati classification), mandibular space (thyromental distance), congenital anomalies, etc. 4. *Extreme caution* should be taken to avoid initiating a general anaesthetic in an obese parturient with a known or potential difficult airway for *perceived* fetal indications. An ultrasound should be considered when external indicators of fetal compromise are questionable given high-risk population 5. *Communication about current and possible events* should be maintained during the course of labour between the anaesthesia team, obstetric team, nursing team, and patient
Induction	1. Anti-aspiration prophylaxis with *rapid sequence induction and cricoid pressure* (although efficacy is controversial) is advocated 2. Maximize the chances of success with the initial attempt at intubation. Position with a *ramp or flexed surgical table* for alignment of the EAM with the sternum 3. Cephalad retraction of the heavy panniculus can cause aortocaval compression, maternal hypotension, and fetal distress, and can restrict the ability to effectively secure the airway in the event of an emergency 4. *Early preoxygenation (100% oxygen) for 3 minutes* in the reverse Trendelenburg position or *with 8 VC deep breaths* in emergent situations; is critical for adequate denitrogenation 5. Avoid repeated or massive doses of succinylcholine during induction. Utilize *actual BW* (1–2 mg/kg) up to maximum of 200 mg. For other induction drugs—utilize LBW for drug doses. IBW may result in underdosing
Intubation	1. *Videolaryngoscopes* provide an improved glottic view and may reduce the time to intubation. If not utilized, these gadgets and a difficult airway cart should be present in the operating room or near the vicinity during intubation 2. *Avoid multiple attempts* at intubation due to the risk of irreversible damage 3. If unable to intubate the trachea, institute the rehearsed protocol including the difficult airway algorithm immediately. The *placement of a supraglottic airway device* (ProSeal LMA®) for ventilation with a trans-LMA placement of an endotracheal tube can be attempted while maintaining cricoid pressure. The use of propofol and succinylcholine increases the tendency to resume spontaneous ventilation rapidly. Awaken the parturient and revert to an awake fibreoptic intubation or regional anaesthetic if not contraindicated and fetal indications for delivery are not urgent 4. If fetal indications are still urgent, clinical judgement should be utilized to determine when the management of the mother is *prioritized* over the fetus to avoid two potentially bad outcomes 5. The call for a *surgical airway* should be done very early in the process if concerned (stand-by) 6. Successful endotracheal tube placement should be confirmed with the presence of *end-tidal carbon dioxide* prior to incision or bilateral breath sounds via auscultation 7. An *awake fibreoptic intubation* is strongly encouraged in an obese parturient with a known difficult airway and a contraindication for neuraxial anaesthesia
Maintenance	1. Low-dose benzodiazepines should be administered immediately after the baby is delivered for amnesia. A combination of *inhalational agent, nitrous oxide, opioid, and benzodiazepines* is essential to *minimize the risk of awareness* in this patient population 2. Non-depolarizing muscle relaxants may be required to facilitate surgery

Emergence	1. The parturient *must* fulfil all extubation criteria prior to extubation to:
	  (a) Minimize the risk of re-intubation, which is similar to a failed intubation
	  (b) Minimize the risk of aspiration, which can lead to dire consequences. Consider the placement of an orogastric suction catheter after induction and suction airway prior to extubation
	2. Extubate in semi-upright position and with pressure-support ventilation
	3. *Triage to appropriate recovery area* depending on preoperative and intraoperative events—patient room versus post-anaesthesia care unit versus intensive care unit

EAM, external auditory meatus; IBW, ideal body weight; LMA, laryngeal mask airway; TBW, total body weight; VC, vital capacity.

for thrombosis ranging from low to very high risk. Obese parturients are at higher risk for venous thromboembolism than their non-obese counterparts and the use of low-molecular-weight heparin (dosed using their actual body weight) should be considered in addition to the use of intermittent compression devices [3,8]. It is recommended that neuraxial techniques be avoided within 10–12 hours following and 24 hours prior to the administration of thromboprophylaxis [3,8].

Triage

Both pre-existing comorbidities and intrapartum/intraoperative events should help guide the discharge of morbidly obese patients to the appropriate area for immediate acute or postpartum recovery [8]—with possible areas including the post-anaesthesia care unit on the labour and delivery suite or the intensive care unit.

Conclusion

Given the associated maternal and fetal implications of obesity in pregnancy, it is essential for all anaesthesiologists to have a basic understanding of the general impact of obesity in pregnancy and develop clear and easy-to-follow protocols to first identify those at risk and ultimately, ensure that optimal care is instituted early in the course of labour to avert catastrophe. Obesity in pregnancy remains a public health issue of utmost concern.

CASE REPORT

A 30-year-old primigravida, at 37 weeks' gestation, presents to the pre-anaesthesia clinic for evaluation. She is 165 cm tall, weighs 250 kg, and is super-morbidly obese, with a calculated BMI of 91 kg/m². She reports a 18 kg weight gain in her pregnancy. Her comorbidities include hypertension, OSA (non-compliant with her continuous positive airway pressure mask), type 2 diabetes, and dyslipidaemia. On physical examination, she has diminished breath sounds bilaterally, swollen hands and feet, a class IV airway with a short but large neck, and her lumbar spine is hard to palpate. She has had no prior surgeries. She does have a history of difficult intravenous access.

The obstetricians, due to the fear of her going into labour at an inopportune time, plan to admit her and do an elective caesarean delivery in 2 days. The anaesthesia team is involved in the decision-making along with the neonatologist and obstetrician.

The plan is to try to place an epidural with ultrasound guidance. In case of failure of a regional technique and having to convert to general anaesthesia, the risks increase significantly, especially the risk of an airway disaster. The risk of a lost airway is a constant threat and given the high-risk obstetric case, the results could be disastrous to mother and child. In case of failure of regional technique and needing to deliver via general anaesthesia, the plan is to intubate her using an awake fibreoptic technique.

Two days later, she presents for delivery with a barely working 20-gauge intravenous catheter. The anaesthesiologist decides to place a two-lumen right internal jugular catheter with ultrasound guidance and then proceeds to try to place an epidural using ultrasound technique. The epidural is abandoned after 45 minutes of efforts by three senior anaesthesiologists, who all try and fail. It is then decided to place a continuous spinal and this is accomplished with some difficulty and the case is started after a suitable block is placed. Fortunately, the surgical part of the caesarean section is slow but otherwise uneventful. The baby is delivered with APGAR scores of 7 and 8. The spinal catheter is removed and the mother transferred to an observation unit with pulse oximeter monitoring for 24 hours. On day 3 she is discharged home with a healthy baby.

From an anaesthetic point of view, the problems of securing the airway are preceded by challenges with intravenous access. In this instance, with the first option of a regional anaesthetic for labour, an airway management plan had to be in place. This is a good time to have experienced colleagues as back-ups. The suggestion of a continuous spinal saved the patient the added risks of general anaesthesia and given her size and potential longer time from skin incision to delivery, risks to the newborn as well.

The ultra-obese parturient presents a set of challenges that have to be handled with good forethought, multispecialty planning, and having redundant help for anaesthesia care.

REFERENCES

1. Centers for Disease Control and Prevention (CDC). Vital signs: state-specific obesity prevalence among adults—United States, 2009. MMWR Morb Mortal Wkly Rep. 2010;**59**:951–55.
2. Flegal KM, Carroll MD, Kit BK, et al. Prevalence of obesity and trends in the distribution of body mass index among US adults, 1999–2010. JAMA. 2012,**307**:491–97.
3. Soens MA, Birnbach DJ, Ranasinghe JS, et al. Obstetric anesthesia for the obese and morbidly obese patient: an ounce of prevention is worth more than a pound of treatment. Acta Anaesthesiol Scand. 2008;**52**:6–19.
4. Ogden CL, Carroll MD, Kit BK, et al. Prevalence of childhood and adult obesity in the United States, 2011–2012. JAMA. 2014;**311**:806–14.
5. Lewis G. The Confidential Enquiry into Maternal and Child Health (CEMACH). Saving Mother's Lives: Reviewing Maternal Deaths to Make Motherhood Safer: 2003–2005. The Seventh Report on Confidential Enquiries into Maternal Deaths in the United Kingdom. London: CEMACH; 2007.
6. Roofhooft E. Anesthesia for the morbidly obese parturient. Curr Opin Anaesthesiol. 2009;**22**:341–46.
7. Sturn R. Increases in clinically severe obesity in the United States, 1986–2000. Arch Intern Med. 2003;**163**:2146–48.
8. Loubert C, Fernando R. Cesarean delivery in the obese parturient: anesthestic considerations. Women's Health. 2011;**7**:163–79.
9. Tan T, Sia AT. Anesthesia considerations in the obese gravida. Semin Perinatol. 2011;**35**:350–55.
10. Pan L, Freedman DS, Gillespie CF, et al. Incidences of obesity and extreme obesity among US adults: findings from the 2009 Behavioral Risk Factor Surveillance System. Popul Health Metr. 2011;**9**:56.
11. Institute of Medicine (US) and National Research Council (US) Committee to Reexamine IOM Pregnancy Weight Guidelines. Weight Gain During Pregnancy: Reexamining the Guidelines. Rasmussen KM, Yaktine AL, eds. Washington, DC: National Academies Press (US); 2009.
12. Alanis MC, Villers MS, Law TL, et al. Complications of cesarean delivery in the massively obese parturient. Am J Obstet and Gynecol. 2010;**203**:271.e1–7.
13. Vasudevan A. The obese parturient. Int Anesthesiol Clin. 2013;**51**:136–63.
14. Barash PG, Cullen BF, Stoelting RK, et al. (eds). Clinical Anesthesia. 6th ed. Philadelphia, PA: Lippincott Williams & Wilkins; 2009.
15. Shah N, Latoo Y. Anesthetic management of obese parturient. BLMP. 2008;**1**:15–23.
16. Munnur U, de Boisblanc B, Suresh MS. Airway problems in pregnancy. Crit Care Med. 2005;**33**(Suppl 10):S259–68.
17. Chestnut DH, Wong CA, Tsen LC, et al. Chestnut's Obstetric Anesthesia: Principles and Practice. 5th ed. Philadelphia, PA: Elsevier Saunders; 2014.
18. Bernando PD, Jenkins JG. Failed tracheal intubation in obstetrics: a 6-year review in a UK region. Anaesthesia. 2000;**55**:685–94.
19. Juvin P, Lavaut E, Dupont H, et al. Difficult tracheal intubation is more common in obese than in lean patients. Anesth Analg. 2003;**97**:595–600.
20. Lee JJ, Larsen RH, Buckley JJ, et al. Pulmonary function and its correlation to the degree of obesity in 294 patients. Anesth Rev. 1981;**8**:28–32.
21. Kress JP, Pohlman AS, Alverdy J, et al. The impact of morbid obesity on oxygen cost of breathing at rest. Am J Respir Crit Care Med. 1999;**160**:883–86.
22. Øberg B, Poulsen TD. Obesity: an anaesthetic challenge. Acta Anaesthesiol Scand. 1996;**40**:191–200.
23. Saravanakumar K, Rao SG, Cooper GM. Obesity and obstetric anaesthesia. Anaesthesia. 2006;**61**:36–48.
24. Vellie JC, Hanson R. Obesity, pregnancy, and left ventricular functioning during the third trimester. Am J Obstet Gynecol. 1994;**171**:980–83.
25. Vasan RS. Cardiac function and obesity. Heart. 2003;**89**:1127–29.

26. Abdullah A, Hoq S, Choudhary R, et al. Cardiac performance is impaired in morbidly obese pregnant females. J Obstet Gynaecol Res. 2012;**38**:258–65.

27. Tseuda K, Debrand M, Zeok SS, et al. Obesity supine death syndrome: reports of two morbidly obese patients. Anesth Analg. 1979;**58**:345–47.

28. Tatham K, Hughes-Roberts Y, Davies S, et al. Peripartum cardiac chest pain and troponin rise. Int J Obstet Anesth. 2010;**19**:453–55.

29. Mendelson CL. The aspiration of stomach contents into the lungs during obstetric anesthesia. Am J Obstet Gynaecol. 1945;**52**:191–204.

30. Ogunnaike BO, Whitten CW. Anesthesia and obesity. In: Barash PG, Cullen BF, Stoelting RK, et al., eds. Clinical Anesthesia. 6th ed. Philadelphia: Lippincott Williams & Wilkins, 2009:1230–46.

31. Wong CA, McCarthy RJ, Fitzgerald PC, et al. Gastric emptying of water in obese pregnant women at term. Anesth Analg. 2007;**105**:751–55.

32. Juvin P, Fevre G, Merouche M, et al. Gastric residue is not more copious in obese patients. Anesth Analg 2001;**93**:1621–22.

33. Maltby JR, Pytka S, Watson NC, et al. Drinking 300 ml of clear fluid two hours before surgery has no effect on gastric fluid volume and pH in fasting and nonfasting obese patients. Can J Anaesth 2004;**51**:111–15.

34. Roberts RB, Shirley MA. Reducing the risk of acid aspiration during caesarean section. Anesth Anag. 1974;**53**:859–68.

35. Obrien TG Jr. LOS pressure and oesophageal function in obese humans. J Clin Gastroenterol. 1980;**2**:145–48.

36. Brock Utne JG, Dow TG, Dimopoulos GE, et al. Gastric and lower oesophageal pressure in early pregnancy. Br J Anaeth. 1981;**53**:381–84.

37. Vaughan RW, Bauer S, Wise L. Volume and pH of gastric juice in obese patients. Anesthesiology. 1975;**43**:686–89.

38. Morgan ES, Wilson E, Watkins T, et al. Maternal obesity and venous thromboembolism. Int J Obstet Anesth. 2012;**21**:253–63.

39. Heit JA, Kobbervig CE, James AH, et al. Trends in the incidence of venous thromboembolism during pregnancy or postpartum: a 30-year population based study. Ann Intern Med. 2005;**143**:697–706.

40. Main EK. Maternal mortality: new strategies for measurement and prevention. Curr Opin Obstet Gynecol. 2010;**22**:511–16.

41. Nakata M, Yada T, Soejima N, et al. Leptin promotes aggregation of human platelets via the long form of its receptor. Diabetes. 1999;**48**:426–29.

42. Stewart FM, Freeman DJ, Ramsay JE, et al. Longitudinal assessment of maternal endothelial function and markers of inflammation and platelet function throughout pregnancy in lean and obese mothers. J Clin Endocrinol Metab. 2007;**92**:969–75.

43. Gaiser R. Anesthetic considerations in the obese parturient. Clin Obstet Gynecol. 2016;**59**:193–20

44. American Congress of Obstetricians and Gynecologists (ACOG). Obesity in pregnancy. Committee Opinion No. 549. Obstet Gynecol. 2013:**121**;213–17.

45. Kodali BS, Chandrasekhar S, Bulich LN, et al. Airway changes during labor and delivery. Anesthesiology. 2008;**108**:357–62.

46. Rao DP, Rao VA. Morbidly obese parturient: challenges for the anaesthesiologist, including managing the difficult airway in obstetrics. What is new? Indian J Anaesth. 2010;**54**(6):508–21.

47. Wear D, Aultman JM, Varley JD, et al. Making fun of patients: medical students' perception and use of derogatory and cynical humor in clinical settings. Acad Med. 2006;**81**:454–62.

48. Watts RW. The influence of obesity on the relationship between body mass index and the distance to the epidural space from the skin. Anaesth Intens Care. 1993;**21**:309–310

49. Bauer ME, Kountanis JA, Tsen LC, et al. Risk factors for failed conversion of labor epidural analgesia to cesarean delivery anesthesia: a systematic review and meta-analysis of observational trials. Int J Obstet Anesth. 2012;**21**:294–309.

50. Panni MK, Columb MO. Obese parturients have lower epidural local anaesthetic requirements for analgesia in labour. Br J Anaeth. 2006;**96**:106–110.

51. Carvalho B, Collins J, Drover DR, et al. ED(50) and ED(95) of intrathecal bupivacaine in morbidly obese patients undergoing cesarean delivery. Anesthesiology. 2011;**114**:529–35.

52. Lee Y, Balki M, Parkes R, et al. Dose requirement of intrathecal bupivacaine for cesarean delivery is similar in obese and normal weight women. Rev Bras Anesthesiol. 2009;**59**:674–83.

53. Afolabi BB, Lesi FE. Regional versus general anesthesia for caesarean section. Cochrane Database Syst Rev. 2012;**10**:CD004350.

54. Norris MC, Fogel ST, Conway-Long C. Combined spinal-epidural versus epidural labor analgesia. Anesthesiology. 2001;**95**:913–20.

55. Visser WA, Dijkstra A, Albayrak M, et al. Spinal anesthesia for intrapartum cesarean delivery following epidural labor analgesia: a retrospective cohort study. Can J Anaesth. 2009;**56**:577–83.

56. Portnoy D, Vadhera RB. Mechanisms and management of an incomplete epidural block for cesarean section. Anesthesiol Clin North Am. 2003;**21**:39–57.

57. Kinsella SM. A prospective audit of regional anesthesia failure in 5080 cesarean sections. Anaesthesia. 2008;**63**:822–32.

58. Leung TY, Chung PW, Rogers MS, et al. Urgent cesarean delivery for fetal bradycardia. Obstet Gynecol. 2009;**114**:1023–28.

59. Vanner R. Cricoid pressure. Int J Obstet Anesth. 2009;**18**:103–105.

60. Lebowitz PW, Shay H, Straker T, et al. Shoulder and head elevation improves laryngoscopic view for tracheal intubation in nonobese as well as obese individuals. J Clin Anesth. 2012;**24**:104–108.

61. Baraka AS, Taha SK, Siddik-Sayyid SM, et al. Supplementation of pre-oxygenation in morbidly obese patients using nasopharyngeal oxygen insufflation. Anaesthesia. 2007;**62**:769–73.

62. Rapaport S, Joannes-Boyau O, Bazin R, et al. Comparison of eight deep breaths and tidal volume breathing preoxygenation techniques in morbid obese patients. Ann Fr Anesth Reanim. 2004;**23**(12):1155–59.

63. Bathory I, Granges JC, Frascarolo P, et al. Evaluation of the video intubation unit in morbid obese patients. Acta Anaesthesiol Scand. 2010;**54**:55–58.

64. Jungbauer A, Schumann M, Brunkhorst V, et al. Expected difficult tracheal intubation: a prospective comparison of direct laryngoscopy and video laryngoscopy in 200 patients. Br J Anaesth. 2009;**102**:546–50.

65. Cook TM, Brooks TS, Van der Westhuizen J, et al. The Proseal LMA is a useful rescue device during failed rapid sequence intubation: two additional cases. Can J Anaesth. 2005;**52**:630–33.

66. Kristensen MS. Airway management and morbid obesity. Eur J Anaesthesiol. 2010;**27**:923–27.

67. Combes X, Sauvat S, Leroux B, et al. Intubating laryngeal mask airway in morbidly obese and lean patients: a comparative study. Anesthesiology. 2005;**102**(6):1106–109.

68. Benumof JL. Management of the difficult adult airway with special emphasis on the awake difficult intubation. Anesthesiology. 1991;**75**:1087–110.

69. Mhyre JM, Riesner MN, Polley LS, et al. A series of anesthesia-related maternal deaths in Michigan, 1995–2003. Anesthesiology. 2007;**106**:1096–104.

Enhanced recovery after bariatric surgery

Jon Livelsberger and Alla Spivak

Introduction

The bariatric patient population is unique for the practice of anaesthesia. In addition to the usual anaesthetic concerns, many other factors must be part of the perioperative management of this group. Comorbidities such as hypertension, diabetes, hyperlipidaemia, sleep apnoea, obesity hypoventilation syndrome, and the possibility of cor pulmonale all weigh heavily on the decisions made for these patients starting from their visit to preadmission testing through their postoperative follow-up care. Utilization of the Enhanced Recovery After Surgery (ERAS) Society guidelines have proven to be greatly beneficial by reducing the length of stay and decreasing costs. More recently, bariatric surgery-specific ERAS protocols have been established. By applying the practices set forth in the ERAS guidelines, we are better able to manage these patients, improve overall outcomes, contain cost by decreasing length of stay, and reduce morbidity and mortality.

Preoperative management

Preoperative patient counselling can be beneficial in several ways. Goals and expectations can be addressed early on which have been demonstrated to reduce patient fear and anxiety in addition to allowing for earlier recovery and discharge [1]. This serves to be a time for the patient to receive education on anaesthesia and analgesia via neuraxial and other regional anaesthesia techniques in addition to general techniques [2].

Cessation of smoking and alcohol use

It has been found that smoking cessation 4 weeks prior to surgery improves surgical outcomes [3]. The routine use of cigarettes induces a state of increased oxygen consumption and diminished oxygen delivery, resulting in hypoxia that is most prominent in peripheral tissue. Additionally, there is a decreased immune response. If there is not enough of a time lapse between smoking cessation and surgery, mucus production is still excessive while ciliary function is still diminished. These findings were deduced off of a series of 11 randomized controlled trials with 1194 patients included. It was found that not only did such intervention result in a higher percentage of patients continuing to be non-smokers at the 1-year mark, but there was a lower complication risk in regard to wound healing. Greater rates of non-smoking success were found in patients who received nicotine replacement therapy in addition to counselling [4].

The use of alcohol has also been linked to increased overall morbidity in patients with greater infection risks as well as cardiac, pulmonary, and coagulopathy risks. Arrhythmias are not unusual in the patient population with a strong alcohol use history. Elevated bleeding time can be another challenge in a surgical patient. The ideal time frame is at least 4 weeks of abstinence to minimize most of these risks. An exaggerated stress response is yet another concern. Other studies have argued that great lifestyle change is required of this bariatric surgery population and state that most centres, in patients with significant alcohol use history, require a 2-year period of cessation prior to this significant elective surgery [5,6].

Fluid/carbohydrate loading and fasting guidelines

A long-standing practice exists where patients who are preoperative for surgery are told to restrict fluid and food intake after midnight the day of surgery. The concerns are quite clear when it comes to diminished airway reflexes after induction of anaesthesia with a subsequent aspiration risk [2]. Such risk is taken very seriously as an aspiration event can result in effects ranging from a chemical pneumonitis to fulminant respiratory distress syndrome and even death. It is both the volume and acidity of gastric aspirate that is associated with increased risks.

It has been found that immediate preoperative (8 to 2 hours prior to surgery) drinking decreased a patient's sensation of thirst, anxiety, and hunger without increasing their risk of aspiration and regurgitation [7]. This applies to both water as well as a clear fluid with added carbohydrate. Furthermore, gastric content volume in patients who had taken water was lower than those with a strict 'nothing by mouth after midnight' after midnight approach. The most noteworthy benefit of allowing carbohydrate loading along with fluid pretreatment is a reduction in insulin resistance that normally occurs in true 'nothing by mouth after midnight' patients [2]. At this time, data are lacking to support routine use of this modality in morbidly obese patients as well as in patients with pre-existing gastro-oesophageal reflux.

Currently, it is recommended that clear liquids be allowed until 2 hours preoperatively and solid foods until 6 hours. The recommendation is based on high-grade data when applied to non-diabetic but obese patients [2,6].

Fluid management has been another topic of debate over time. Fluid management goals should aim to target appropriate urine output, maintain normal stroke volume variation, and ultimately allow for end-organ perfusion. This is best achieved with avoidance of hypotension and a goal-directed fluid therapy approach. Liberal fluid management has fallen out of favour for a multitude of reasons, most of which are related to worse outcomes and prolonged hospitalization [8].

Preoperative weight reduction

Analyses of patients undergoing open gastric bypass as well as those undergoing laparoscopic gastric bypass have been conducted to determine the efficacy and benefit of preoperative weight loss for obese patients. The ultimate goal is to determine if weight loss will prevent postoperative complications including wound infections, respiratory failure, bleeding, thromboembolic phenomenon, renal failure, and others [9]. A study conducted at Geisinger Medical Center (Danville, PA, USA) over a 3-year period from 2002 to 2006 which included 884 patients determined that patients who were able to achieve preoperative weight loss in the 5–10% range had a greater success with postoperative weight loss as well as a decreased postoperative length of stay [10,11].

Glucocorticoids

Postoperative nausea and vomiting is one of the commonest reasons for unplanned admissions. A single dose administered within 90 minutes of anaesthesia induction along with use of a serotonin (5-HT$_3$) receptor antagonist has been proven to succeed at reducing nausea and vomiting [12]. Although a concern for hyperglycaemia and steroid use exists, no evidence has been found linking a single dose to any other major surgical risk [13]. Given this possibility, vigilant glucose monitoring and treatment of hyperglycaemia should be part of routine care.

The use of glucocorticoids has further been found to decrease overall length of stay, reduce inflammatory response, lower infection rates, improve pain control, and lead to improved sleep with no evidence of delayed wound healing [13,14].

Neuromuscular blockade

Current recommendations for neuromuscular blockade are to monitor depth of blockade, choose a suitable monitoring device, titrate to maintain response to stimulation, avoid the use of neuromuscular blockade as an adjunct to the depth of anaesthesia, dose anticholinesterases appropriately, and, if possible, use quantitative monitors. It has been estimated that among patients entering the post-anaesthesia care unit, upwards of 25–30% had a train-of-four (TOF) ratio less than 0.9 and even more alarming, 10–15% had a TOF ratio less than 0.7 [15].

Quantitative TOF assessment is far more superior to qualitative monitoring and clinical judgement. Although, traditionally, a TOF of 0.7 at the adductor pollicis was accepted as indicating acceptable recovery, it has been demonstrated that at this level of blockade still on board, weakness and swallowing dysfunction still occur [16]. In addition, hypoxaemia, aspiration, and prolonged recovery occur [6]. Current practice recommends a TOF of at least 0.9.

When it comes to reversal, the use of neostigmine did not decrease postoperative respiratory failure and was associated with a higher incidence of oxygen desaturation. The most optimal reversal strategy is one where TOF count of at least 3 has returned [17]. The effects of inappropriate high-dose neostigmine, greater than 60 mcg/kg, is consistent with increased postoperative atelectasis, increased hospital length of stay, longer time to discharge from the post-anaesthesia care unit, pulmonary oedema, and lower patient satisfaction [17,18].

Of the new agents, sugammadex, a cyclodextrin chelating agent for rocuronium and to a lesser degree vecuronium, has shown great potential for use in the obese population. It has been shown to produce full reversal faster than neostigmine [19].

Airway management

Airway management strategies in bariatric patients involve both a standard airway examination as well as understanding of potential difficulties in this group. Body mass index, neck circumference, poor neck mobility, and sleep apnoea are all red flags during airway assessment [20,21]. It has also been found that mask ventilation tends to be more challenging in this patient group [22,23]. As such, it becomes critical to plan ahead by discussing your concerns with the patient as well as planning and utilizing the difficult airway algorithm if needed.

Body mass index itself has been shown to play a role in Mallampati scoring—a lower body mass index equates with a lower Mallampati class in the same patient in subsequent surgery. Laryngoscopy grading did not have the same reporting [20]. Laryngoscopy difficulty has been closely associated with higher Mallampati scores as well as an increased neck circumference.

Endotracheal intubation is considered the standard for airway management given the strong risk of hypoventilation, aspiration, and potential for loss of natural airway [24–26].

Ventilation strategies

The main culprit that causes postoperative respiratory complications is a change in the chest wall function. There is a loss of muscle coordination in addition to or independent of an absence of muscle tone that results from mechanical ventilation. The net effect is a reduction of both lung volume and capacity. It is estimated that more than 90% of anaesthetized morbidly obese patients have atelectasis independent of age, sex, or anaesthetic used [27].

It has been found that by utilizing a lung protective strategy of low tidal volume and positive end-expiratory pressure, there is diminished expression of alveolar and systemic inflammatory mediators [6]. In general, this approach has been associated with lower rates of atelectasis and better gas exchange with lower reintubation rates [28]. It has been found that patients having received protective ventilation strategies had higher postoperative ratio of partial arterial pressure of oxygen/fraction of inspired oxygen (FiO$_2$) and fewer complications [29].

If inappropriately large tidal volumes are utilized, acute lung injury ensues. Factors leading to development of lung injury included large tidal volume ventilation, transfusion of blood products, anaemia, and a history of having restrictive lung disease such as that with an obese patient. It was also found that females were often ventilated with larger volume strategies and subsequently developed lung injury more often [30]. Similar outcomes were reported in pneumonectomy patients having received larger tidal volumes (8.3 vs 6.7 mL/kg) [31].

Laparoscopy

Although surgical technique is not dependent on the anaesthesiologist, the anaesthesiologist does depend on the surgical technique implemented. Laparoscopy has proven itself to be favourable over open procedures for a multitude of reasons. Common benefits included shorter hospitalizations, less occurrence of incisional hernias, decreased blood loss, faster recovery time, and improved pain control [6]. It becomes obvious that such outcomes achieve the goals defined previously and lead to improved patient outcomes as well as decreased cost of care. While there is an argument that laparoscopy is more expensive, the reduction in complications as well as hospital stay more than compensate for additional expenses accrued using these techniques [32]. It is important to also bear in mind surgical skill and speed as these can compound the cost of the procedure. There may also be an increased patient risk if time under anaesthesia is significantly longer than average.

Nasogastric tubes

Routine use of nasogastric tubes has fallen out of favour when it comes to abdominal surgery. They have actually been found to do more harm than good and have been implicated in worse respiratory outcomes and delaying return of gastric motility [33]. A more detailed look at their use in the bariatric surgery population falls in line with these findings as well. Aside from increased pain and decreased participation in deep breathing from discomfort, there is also an induced gastro-oesophageal reflux [34]. The use of a nasogastric tube in and of itself, for reasons of induced reflux, creates an open pathway for aspiration and subsequent pneumonia [35].

It is important to bear in mind that although routine use is not indicated, selective use remains at the discretion of the team caring for the patient. It may become necessary to use a nasogastric tube.

Chemical and mechanical deep vein thrombosis prophylaxis

Thromboembolism in the form of deep vein thrombosis and pulmonary embolism remains a major threat to surgical patients. It is one of the leading causes of preventable death [36,37].

Utilization of the Caprini scoring system can help with risk stratification. Points are given for various comorbidities including age, surgery type (open versus laparoscopic, orthopaedic fractures), BMI, current ambulation ability, recent stroke, history of coagulopathic state (lupus anticoagulant, self or family history of venous thromboembolism, thrombophilia, etc.), malignancy, central venous cannulation, and myocardial infarction to name a few. Risk is graded on a numeric scale based on zero indicating a very low risk and 5 or more points correlating to a high-risk group [38].

The most optimal situation is one in which chemical and/or mechanical prophylaxis is initiated during hospitalization (before or shortly after surgery) and continued, at the very least, until the patient is fully ambulatory [39]. Additionally, short surgical time, early ambulation, and mechanical compression devices can serve to

be greatly beneficial as well and may even decrease the need to use chemical prophylaxis [40,41].

Current guidelines for obesity surgery are derived from limited studies, but, however, do favour low-molecular-weight heparin over unfractionated heparin [41,42]. This intervention was not noted to have increased bleeding risk.

Postoperative nausea and vomiting–multimodal approach

Well-established risk factors exist when it comes to identifying those at elevated risk for postoperative nausea and vomiting. The categories can be patient factors, surgical factors, and anaesthetic factors. The commonly known risk factors include young age (<50 years old), female sex, non-smokers, the use of volatile anaesthesia, longer duration of anaesthesia, postoperative opioid use, and a personal history of postoperative nausea and vomiting or motion sickness [43]. Apart from recommendations for the general at-risk group, strong recommendations exist for prophylaxis in the obese patient population, especially those undergoing bariatric surgery. When looking at the risk involved, it becomes evident that these patients often meet many of the above-mentioned risk factors.

Less traditionally, hypotension and bradycardia have been linked to triggering emesis. Ephedrine has been found to be beneficial in reducing postoperative nausea and vomiting in this category of patients as it has effects similar to droperidol (without the accompanying sedation) [44].

Propofol has been noted to have a decreased incidence of early postoperative nausea and vomiting when compared with volatile anaesthetics [45]. Opioid-free anaesthesia has been found to be more favourable when looking at postoperative nausea and vomiting [44]. Along these same lines, research on gabalin and pregabalin has been conducted as a part of a multimodal pain approach with the additional promise of decreasing nausea and vomiting in the first 24 hours after surgery [46]. Liberal crystalloid administration is favourable in reducing postoperative nausea and vomiting [47]. This should be considered and weighed against the risk of overly aggressive fluid management as that, in and of itself, can have detrimental effects.

A standard approach involves identifying at-risk patients and providing early prophylaxis. First-line agents are the $5-HT_3$ antagonists, steroids, phenothiazines, phenylethylamine, butyrophenones, antihistamines, and anticholinergics. More recently studied agents include neurokinin and opioid antagonists [44,48].

Current recommendations are strong for prophylaxis and endorse a multimodal approach, most notably studied in patients undergoing laparoscopic sleeve gastrectomy, with a combination of haloperidol, dexamethasone, and ondansetron [49].

Postoperative pain management strategies

Enhancing recovery after surgery in regard to pain management should begin in the preoperative setting. This includes a discussion with the patient concerning the type of surgery they are about to have and the expectations of how their pain will be managed. It is at this time where opioid-sparing techniques such as regional or neuraxial anaesthesia should be introduced. The key factor in bariatric pain management is a multimodal approach.

Multimodal analgesia

Whenever possible, especially in the bariatric population, the treatment of pain should maximize efficacy and minimize opioids. The prevalence of obstructive sleep apnoea (OSA) in the obese patient is well documented, as is the detrimental effect of opioids on this disease state [50,51]. As the name implies, more than one modality should be used in the treatment of pain. Non-opioids options include the use of non-steroidal anti-inflammatory drugs and/or the use of acetaminophen (paracetamol). These medications should be administered regularly or at least until the patient's pain is well controlled. It is important to assess the patient's pain severity and take a step-wise approach to treating it. Acetaminophen, regardless of delivery route, has been shown to lower total opioid consumption and possibly decrease length of stay [52–55]. Non-steroidal anti-inflammatory drugs such as ketorolac have been shown to be highly effective in limiting the use of opioids, decreasing pain scores, and reducing postoperative nausea and vomiting [56]. Gabapentin/pregabalin may be effective adjuvants at reducing opioid consumption and decreasing pain scores; however, they should be used with caution due to their sedative effects [57,58]. Administration of preoperative gabapentin has also been shown to decrease postoperative pain scores in obese patients receiving gastric bypass [59]. Ketamine, via bolus or infusion, may also reduce opioid consumption [60]. In the obese population, when combined as part of opioid-free total intravenous anaesthesia, ketamine has also been shown to aid in decreasing postoperative nausea and vomiting [61]. The efficacy of intravenous lidocaine infusions has been accepted as part of ERAS protocols; however, no clear guidelines exist for dosing in the obese patient [62]. A lidocaine bolus followed by infusion has been shown to improve the quality of recovery after laparoscopic bariatric surgery [63].

Opioid analgesics

As stated previously, the use of opioids in the treatment of pain for the obese patient presents a unique set of challenges, especially in the first 24 hours after surgery. Practitioners frequently undertreat pain in the morbidly obese patient out of concern for adverse respiratory effects of these medications [64]. First of all, it is important to avoid an opioid-centred treatment protocol. Second, when resorting to using an opioid to treat pain, it is best to use shorter-acting opioids at the minimum effective dose and titrate to effect [65]. Use of patient-controlled analgesia should be reserved for patients with moderate to severe pain who are unable to receive oral opioid therapy. Basal/continuous patient-controlled analgesia rates should be avoided. If OSA is suspected in the patient requiring opioid patient-controlled analgesia, respiratory status should be monitored closely [53].

Regional/neuraxial anaesthesia

The use of perineural local anaesthetic to minimize pain and analgesic consumption has been well recognized. The obese patient, however, may present difficulties in performing these techniques resulting in an increased failure rate [66]. Regardless of a patient's BMI, when appropriate, regional/neuraxial anaesthesia should be offered and attempted as part of the multimodal approach. Compared to general anaesthesia, neuraxial anaesthesia in high-risk patients has been shown to decrease the risk of pneumonia as well as 0–30-day mortality [67]. The addition of ultrasound scanning may increase the efficacy of the regional anaesthesia procedure [68]. In the obese patient, ultrasound guidance has also been shown to decrease procedural time as well as procedure-related pain [69]. When combined as part of a multimodal approach, transverse abdominis plane blocks have been shown to improve pain scores, decrease sedation, promote early ambulation, and improve satisfaction in morbidly obese patients undergoing laparoscopic bariatric surgery [70]. Peripheral nerve blockade can also be extended by the use of adjuvants and/or the introduction of an indwelling catheter [71,72].

Dosing

Drug dosing for the treatment of pain in the obese patient may also be problematic. Typical recommendations centre on weight-based dosing. The physiological changes associated with obesity coupled with the altered pharmacokinetics of commonly used drugs results in an uncertain approach. Additionally, few guidelines exist for the appropriate dosing of pain medications. In general, medications should be dosed largely based on ideal body weight and titrated to effect [73]. For more details on drug dosing, see Chapter 4 and Chapter 5.

Protocol

ERAS is often instituted as a protocol that varies based on individual institution. When implemented effectively, an ERAS protocol can lead to decreased length of hospital stay and possibly a decrease in morbidity. It is important that this protocol be the result of a multidisciplinary approach that places the patient at its focus [74].

Additional postoperative considerations

Nutrition and glucose management

The discussion of nutritional goals should be started prior to surgery itself and can be discussed at preoperative surgical planning visits. Nutrition markers should be obtained via blood work for baseline values. These markers should be repeated to successfully trend subsequent changes [75]. Early goals are timely initiation of clear liquids within hours after surgery and subsequent advancement of diet, which is based on both surgery type and patient tolerance [6].

Significant concerns for malnutrition exist for this group of patients, thereby making a consultation with a nutritionist a high-priority task. Protein goals should be high priority as patients with malabsorption are at higher risk of adverse events. Additional supplementation in the forms of vitamins and minerals is also advisable [76]. Malnutrition should be taken very seriously and close patient follow-up and guidance are needed to ensure postoperative success.

Aside from nutritional deficiencies, one of the common risks remains weight regain. While some degree of weight regain is expected over time in a vast majority of patients, there are ways to decrease the risk of this occurrence. Needless to say, diet and lifestyle are significant contributors; however, surgical failure should not be overlooked [77]. This again leads us back to the significance of a team that can guide the patient through both preoperative and postoperative goals and expectations.

It is recommended to maintain normoglycaemia. The current goals are to aim for a glycated haemoglobin concentration less than 7%, fasting glucose less than 110 mg/dL, and postprandial glucose less than 180 mg/dL [6,78]. Additionally, patients who are insulin dependent should be maintained on their insulin regimen [77]. While strict glucose control is important, it is also necessary to remember that many of these patients will have significant changes in their insulin requirements as early as a few weeks after surgery [79,80] with promising long-term results.

Postoperative oxygenation and non-invasive ventilation

The clinician caring for an obese patient should maintain a high suspicion for OSA in their patient regardless of prior diagnosis. Additionally, these patients have a reduced functional residual capacity and are at increased risk of persistent atelectasis postoperatively [81]. The impact of preoperative incentive spirometry on postoperative atelectasis has been questioned in the past; however, a meta-analysis did not show a meaningful benefit in regard to improved oxygenation [82]. Additionally, the site of surgery as well as the degree of associated pain has been shown to have a direct negative impact on lung volumes [83]. This further supports the use of neuraxial or peripheral nerve blockade to reduce pain and possibly improve respiratory function.

Oxygen supplementation in the postoperative setting should be provided on a patient-to-patient basis. Although each patient may vary, it is important to realize that there exists an increased risk of pulmonary complications in the obese patient and be prepared to treat accordingly. No evidence exists to support a minimum duration for the supplementation of oxygenation. In contrast, the head-elevated position has been shown to minimize pulmonary atelectasis [84]. Pulse oximetry and respiratory rate should be monitored at minimum. For patients with a prior diagnosis of OSA, supplemental oxygen therapy has been shown to improve oxygen saturation, but one should use the lowest required FiO_2 [85]. High FiO_2 when utilized postoperatively in the morbidly obese patient population has been shown to increase the risk of hypopnea and apnoea [85].

Given the increased risk of OSA in the obese population, it is important to note that obese patients often benefit more from supportive positive pressure ventilation than from therapeutic oxygen alone [86]. Examples include continuous positive airway pressure (CPAP) as well as bi-level positive airway pressure (BiPAP). Care can further be directed by a preoperative STOP-Bang score which has been shown to have a high OSA predictive value. Positive pressure support is recommended for those patients with a moderate to high risk score [87]. For the positive pressure 'naïve' patient, it is recommended that CPAP should be first started at 5 cmH$_2$O and increased as needed and tolerated. There is a lack of published evidence to support the use of BiPAP unless previously required by the patient or in the setting of obesity hypoventilation syndrome. Patients with obesity hypoventilation syndrome are especially sensitive to the respiratory depressive effects of opioids and have been shown to benefit from prophylactic nasal BiPAP for at least 24 hours postoperatively [88].

For the patient who carries a diagnosis of OSA and is either non-compliant or not yet receiving CPAP therapy, it is important to consider factors that may increase their postoperative need for non-invasive positive pressure ventilation. These factors include age greater than 50 years, male sex, BMI greater than 60 kg/m^2, moderate to severe OSA, pulmonary comorbidity, open surgery, and the need for reoperation [6]. In the setting of these risk factors as well as inadequate ventilation or oxygen saturation less than 90%, one should consider early and liberal use of CPAP [89].

Patients who carry a previous diagnosis of OSA who are compliant should be continued on their home CPAP settings in the postoperative area. It is important to consider the detrimental effects of anaesthesia as well as surgery when fine-tuning these settings. Studies have shown that these patients may initially require slightly higher CPAP settings than those required outside the perioperative setting [90].

REFERENCES

1. Halaszynski TM, Juda R, Silverman DG. Optimizing postoperative outcomes with efficient preoperative assessment and management. Crit Care Med. 2004;**32**:S76–86.
2. Nygren J, Thacker J, Carli F, et al. Guidelines for perioperative care in elective rectal/pelvic surgery: enhanced recovery after surgery (ERAS®) Society recommendations. World J Surg. 2013;**37**:285–305.
3. Mastracci TM, Carli F, Finley RJ, et al. Effect of preoperative smoking cessation interventions on postoperative complications. J Am Coll Surg. 2011;**212**:1094–96.
4. Tonnesen H, Nielsen PR, Lauritzen JB, et al. Smoking and alcohol intervention before surgery: evidence for best practice. Br J Anaesth. 2009;**102**:297–306.
5. Ostlund MP, Backman O, Marsk R et al. Increased admission for alcohol dependence after gastric bypass surgery compared with restrictive bariatric surgery. JAMA Surg. 2013;**148**:374–77.
6. Thorell A, MacCormick AD, Awad S, et al. Guidelines for perioperative care in bariatric surgery: Enhanced Recovery After Surgery (ERAS) Society recommendations. World J Surg. 2016;**40**:2065–83.
7. Brady M, Kinn S, Stuart P. Preoperative fasting for adults to prevent perioperative complications. Cochrane Database Syst Rev 2009;**4**:CD005285.
8. Varadhan KK, Lobo DN. A meta-analysis of randomised controlled trials of intravenous fluid therapy in major elective open abdominal surgery: getting the balance right. Proc Nutr Soc. 2010;**69**:488–98.
9. Benotti PN, Still CD, Wood GC, et al. Preoperative weight loss before bariatric surgery. Arch Surg. 2009;**144**:1150–55.
10. Still CD, Benotti P, Wood GC, et al. Outcomes of preoperative weight loss in high-risk patients undergoing gastric bypass surgery. Arch Surg. 2007;**142**:994–98.
11. Gerber P, Anderin C, Gustafsson UO, Thorell A. Weight loss before gastric bypass and postoperative weight change: data from the Scandinavian Obesity Registry (SOReg). Surg Obes Relat Dis. 2016;**12**:556–62.
12. Henzi I, Walder B, Tramer MR. Dexamethasone for the prevention of postoperative nausea and vomiting: a quantitative systematic review. Anesth Analg. 2000;**90**:186–94.
13. Srinivasa S, Kahokehr AA, Yu TC, et al. Preoperative glucocorticoid use in major abdominal surgery: systematic review and meta-analysis of randomized trials. Ann Surg. 2011;**254**:183–91.
14. Zargar-Shoshtari K, Sammour T, Kahokehr A, Connolly AB, Hill AG. Randomized clinical trial of the effect of glucocorticoids on peritoneal inflammation and postoperative recovery after colectomy. Br J Surg. 2009;**96**:1253–61.

15. Lien CA, Kopman AF. Current recommendations for monitoring depth of neuromuscular blockade. Curr Opin Anaesthesiol. 2014;**27**:616–22.

16. Murphy GS, Szokol JW, Marymont JH et al. Intraoperative acceleromyographic monitoring reduces the risk of residual neuromuscular blockade and adverse respiratory events in the postanesthesia care unit. Anesthesiology. 2008;**109**:389–98.

17. Sasaki N, Meyer M, Malviya S, et al. Effects of neostigmine reversal of nondepolarizing neuromuscular blocking agents on postoperative respiratory outcomes: a prospective study. Anesthesiology. 2014;**121**:959–68.

18. Fortier LP, McKeen D, Turner K et al. The RECITE Study: a Canadian prospective multicenter study of the incidence and severity of residual neuromuscular blockade. Anesth Analg. 2015;**121**:366–72.

19. Blobner M, Eriksson LI, Scholz J, et al. Reversal of rocuronium-induced neuromuscular blockade with sugammadex compared with neostigmine during sevoflurane anaesthesia: results of a randomised, controlled trial. Eur J Anaesthesiol. 2010;**27**:874–81.

20. Shimonov M, Schechter P, Boaz M, Waintrob R, Ezri T. Does body mass index reduction by bariatric surgery affect laryngoscopy difficulty during subsequent anesthesia? Obes Surg. 2017;2016;**27**:737–39.

21. De Jong A, Molinari N, Pouzeratte Y, et al. Difficult intubation in obese patients: incidence, risk factors, and complications in the operating theatre and in intensive care units. Br J Anaesth. 2015;**114**:297–306.

22. Acikgoz AO, Karagoz H, Yilbas AA, Akca B, Uzumcugil F, Pamuk G. Difficult airway and risk factors in bariatric surgery patients. Bariatr Surg Pract Patient Care. 2015;**10**:145–49.

23. Cattano D, Katsiampoura A, Corso RM, Killoran PV, Cai C, Hagberg CA. Predictive factors for difficult mask ventilation in the obese surgical population. F1000Res. 2014;**3**:239.

24. Nicholson A, Cook TM, Smith AF, et al. Supraglottic airway devices versus tracheal intubation for airway management during general anaesthesia in obese patients. Cochrane Database Syst Rev 2013;**9**:CD010105.

25. Murphy C, Wong DT. Airway management and oxygenation in obese patients. Canadian Journal of Anesthesia. 2013;**60**:929–45.

26. Brodsky JB, Lemmens HJM, Brock-Utne JG, Vierra M, Saidman LJ. Morbid obesity and tracheal intubation. Anesth Analg. 2002;**94**:732–36.

27. Tusman G, Böhm SH, Warner DO, Sprung J. Atelectasis and perioperative pulmonary complications in high-risk patients. Curr Opin Anaesthesiol. 2012;**25**:1–10.

28. Futier E, Constantin JM, Paugam-Burtz C et al. A trial of intraoperative low-tidal-volume ventilation in abdominal surgery. N Engl J Med. 2013;**369**:428–37.

29. Yang M, Ahn HJ, Kim K, et al. Does a protective ventilation strategy reduce the risk of pulmonary complications after lung cancer surgery? A randomized controlled trial. Chest. 2011;**139**:530–37.

30. Gajic O, Dara SI, Mendez JL, et al. Ventilator-associated lung injury in patients without acute lung injury at the onset of mechanical ventilation. Crit Care Med. 2004;**32**:1817–24.

31. Fernández-Pérez ER, Keegan MT, Brown DR, Hubmayr RD, Gajic O. Intraoperative tidal volume as a risk factor for respiratory failure after pneumonectomy. Anesthesiology. 2006;**105**:14–18.

32. Sussenbach S, Silva E, Pufal M, Casagrande D, Padoin A, Mottin C. Systematic review of economic evaluation of laparotomy versus laparoscopy for patients submitted to Roux-en-Y gastric bypass. PLoS One. 2014;**9**:e99976.

33. Lawrence VA, Cornell JE, Smetana GW, American College of Physicians. Strategies to reduce postoperative pulmonary complications after noncardiothoracic surgery: systematic review for the American College of Physicians. Ann Internal Med. 2006;**144**:596–608.

34. Manning BJ, Winter DC, McGreal G, Kirwan WO, Redmond HP. Nasogastric intubation causes gastroesophageal reflux in patients undergoing elective laparotomy. Surgery. 2001;**130**:788–91.

35. Huerta S, Arteaga JR, Sawicki MP, Liu CD, Livingston EH. Assessment of routine elimination of postoperative nasogastric decompression after Roux-en-Y gastric bypass. Surgery. 2002;**132**:844–48.

36. Clagett GP, Reisch JS. Prevention of venous thromboembolism in general surgical patients. Results of meta-analysis. Annals of Surgery. 1988;**208**(2):227–40.

37. Kreutzer L, Minami C, Yang A. Preventing venous thromboembolism after surgery. JAMA. 2016;**315**:2136.

38. Bilgi K, Muthusamy A, Subair M, et al. Assessing the risk for development of venous thromboembolism (VTE) in surgical patients using adapted Caprini scoring system. Int J Surg. 2016;**30**:68–73.

39. Hull RD, Pineo GF, Stein PD, et al. Timing of initial administration of low-molecular-weight heparin prophylaxis against deep vein thrombosis in patients following elective hip arthroplasty. Arch Intern Med. 2001;**161**:1952–60.

40. Gonzalez QH, Tishler DS, Plata-Munoz JJ, et al. Incidence of clinically evident deep venous thrombosis after laparoscopic Roux-en-Y gastric bypass. Surg Endosc. 2004;**18**:1082–84.

41. American Society for Metabolic and Bariatric Surgery Clinical Issues Committee. ASMBS updated position statement on prophylactic measures to reduce the risk of venous thromboembolism in bariatric surgery patients. Surg Obes Relat Dis. 2013;**9**:493–97.

42. Birkmeyer NJO, Finks JF, Carlin AM, et al. Comparative effectiveness of unfractionated and low-molecular-weight heparin for prevention of venous thromboembolism following bariatric surgery. Arch Surg. 2012;**147**:994–98.

43. Apfel CC, Heidrich FM, Jukar-Rao S, et al. Evidence-based analysis of risk factors for postoperative nausea and vomiting. Br J Anaesth. 2012;**109**:742–53.

44. Obrink E, Jildenstal P, Oddby E, Jakobsson J. Post-operative nausea and vomiting: update on predicting the probability and ways to minimize its occurrence, with focus on ambulatory surgery. Int J Surg. 2015;**15**:100–106.

45. Kumar G, Stendall C, Mistry R, Gurusamy K, Walker D. A comparison of total intravenous anaesthesia using propofol with sevoflurane or desflurane in ambulatory surgery: systematic review and meta-analysis. Anaesthesia. 2014;**69**:1138–50.

46. Grant MC, Betz M, Hulse M, et al. The effect of preoperative pregabalin on postoperative nausea and vomiting: a meta-analysis. Anesth Analg. 2016;**123**:1100–107.

47. Apfel CC, Meyer A, Orhan-Sungur M, Jalota L, Whelan RP, Jukar-Rao S. Supplemental intravenous crystalloids for the prevention of postoperative nausea and vomiting: quantitative review. Br J Anaesth. 2012;**108**:893–902.

48. Gan TJ, Apfel CC, Kovac A, et al. A randomized, double-blind comparison of the NK1 antagonist, aprepitant, versus

ondansetron for the prevention of postoperative nausea and vomiting. Anesth Analg. 2007;**104**:1082–89.

49. Benevides ML, Oliveira SS, de Aguilar-Nascimento JE. The combination of haloperidol, dexamethasone, and ondansetron for prevention of postoperative nausea and vomiting in laparoscopic sleeve gastrectomy: a randomized double-blind trial. Obes Surg. 2013;**23**:1389–96.

50. Schug SA, Raymann A. Postoperative pain management of the obese patient. Best Pract Res Clin Anaesthesiol. 2011;**25**:73–81.

51. Schumann R, Jones SB, Cooper B, et al. Update on best practice recommendations for anesthetic perioperative care and pain management in weight loss surgery, 2004–2007. Obesity. 2009;**17**:889–94.

52. Schumann R. Anaesthesia for bariatric surgery. Best Pract Res Clin Anaesthesiol. 2011;**25**:83–93.

53. Budiansky AS, Margarson MP, Eipe N. Acute pain management in morbid obesity—an evidence based clinical update. Surg Obes Relat Dis. 2017;**13**:523–32.

54. Ziemann-Gimmel P, Hensel P, Koppman J, Marema R. Multimodal analgesia reduces narcotic requirements and antiemetic rescue medication in laparoscopic Roux-en-Y gastric bypass surgery. Surg Obes Relat Dis. 2013;**9**:975–80.

55. Song K, Melroy MJ, Whipple OC. Optimizing multimodal analgesia with intravenous acetaminophen and opioids in postoperative bariatric patients. Pharmacotherapy. 2014;**34**(Suppl 1):S14–21.

56. Govindarajan R, Ghosh B, Sathyamoorthy MK, et al. Efficacy of ketorolac in lieu of narcotics in the operative management of laparoscopic surgery for morbid obesity. Surg Obes Relat Dis. 2005;**1**:530–35.

57. Mishriky BM, Waldron NH, Habib AS. Impact of pregabalin on acute and persistent postoperative pain: a systematic review and meta-analysis. Br J Anaesth, 2015;**114**:10–31.

58. Ho KY, Gan TJ, Habib AS. Gabapentin and postoperative pain—a systematic review of randomized controlled trials. Pain. 2006;**126**:91–101.

59. Hassani V, Pazouki A, Nikoubakht N, Chaichian S, Sayarifard A, Shakib Khankandi A. The effect of gabapentin on reducing pain after laparoscopic gastric bypass surgery in patients with morbid obesity: a randomized clinical trial. Anesth Pain Med. 2015;**5**:e22372.

60. Sollazzi L, Modesti C, Vitale F, et al. Preinductive use of clonidine and ketamine improves recovery and reduces postoperative pain after bariatric surgery. Surg Obes Relat Dis. 2009;**5**:67–71.

61. Ziemann-Gimmel P, Goldfarb AA, Koppman J, Marema RT. Opioid-free total intravenous anaesthesia reduces postoperative nausea and vomiting in bariatric surgery beyond triple prophylaxis. Br J Anaesth. 2014;**112**:906–11.

62. Vigneault L, Turgeon AF, Cote D, et al. Perioperative intravenous lidocaine infusion for postoperative pain control: a meta-analysis of randomized controlled trials. Can J Anaesth. 2011;**58**:22–37.

63. De Oliveira GS, Duncan K, Fitzgerald P, et al. Systemic lidocaine to improve quality of recovery after laparoscopic bariatric surgery: a randomized double-blinded placebo-controlled trial. Obes Surg. 2014;**24**:212–18.

64. Kaw R, Chung F, Pasupuleti V, Mehta J, Gay PC, Hernandez AV. Meta-analysis of the association between obstructive sleep apnoea and postoperative outcome. Br J Anaesth. 2012;**109**:897–906.

65. Porhomayon J, Leissner KB, El-Solh AA, Nader ND. Strategies in postoperative analgesia in the obese obstructive sleep apnea patient. Clin J Pain. 2013;**29**:998–1005.

66. Nielsen KC, Guller U, Steele SM, Klein SM, Greengrass RA, Pietrobon R. Influence of obesity on surgical regional anesthesia in the ambulatory setting: an analysis of 9,038 blocks. Anesthesiology. 2005;**102**:181–87.

67. Guay J, Choi P, Suresh S, Albert N, Kopp S, Pace NL. Neuraxial blockade for the prevention of postoperative mortality and major morbidity: an overview of Cochrane systematic reviews. Cochrane Database Syst Rev. 2014;**1**:CD010108.

68. Soberón JR, McInnis C, Bland KS, et al. Ultrasound-guided popliteal sciatic nerve blockade in the severely and morbidly obese: a prospective and randomized study. J Anesth. 2016;**30**:397–404.

69. Lam NCK, Petersen TR, Gerstein NS, Yen T, Starr B, Mariano ER. A randomized clinical trial comparing the effectiveness of ultrasound guidance versus nerve stimulation for lateral popliteal-sciatic nerve blocks in obese patients. J Ultrasound Med. 2014;**33**:1057–63.

70. Sinha A, Jayaraman L, Punhani D. Efficacy of ultrasound-guided transversus abdominis plane block after laparoscopic bariatric surgery: a double blind, controlled study. Obes Surg. 2013;**23**:548–53.

71. Brattwall M, Jildenstål P, Warrén Stomberg M, Jakobsson JG. Upper extremity nerve block: how can benefit, duration, and safety be improved? An update. F1000Res. 2016;**5**:907.

72. Aguirre J, Del Moral A, Cobo I, Borgeat A, Blumenthal S. The role of continuous peripheral nerve blocks. Anesthesiol Res Pract. 2012;**2012**:560879.

73. Leykin Y, Miotto L, Pellis T. Pharmacokinetic considerations in the obese. Best Pract Res Clin Anaesthesiol. 2011;**25**:27–36.

74. Małczak P, Pisarska M, Piotr M, Wysocki M, Budzyński A, Pędziwiatr M. Enhanced recovery after bariatric surgery: systematic review and meta-analysis. Obes Surg. 2017;**27**(1):226–35.

75. Brolin RE. Gastric bypass. Surg Clin North Am. 2001;**81**:1077–95.

76. Kushner R. Managing the obese patient after bariatric surgery: a case report of severe malnutrition and review of the literature. JPEN J Parenter Enteral Nutr. 2000;**24**:126–32.

77. Heber D, Greenway FL, Kaplan LM, et al. Endocrine and nutritional management of the post-bariatric surgery patient: an Endocrine Society Clinical Practice Guideline. J Clin Endocrinol Metab. 2010;**95**:4823–43.

78. Finfer S, Bellomi R, Blair D, et al. Intensive versus conventional glucose control in critically ill patients. N Engl J Med. 2009;**360**:1283–97.

79. Rubino F, Gagner M, Gentileschi P, et al. The early effect of the Roux-en-Y gastric bypass on hormones involved in body weight regulation and glucose metabolism. Ann Surg. 2004;**240**:236–42.

80. Peterli R, Steinert RE, Woelnerhanssen B, et al. Metabolic and hormonal changes after laparoscopic Roux-en-Y gastric bypass and sleeve gastrectomy: a randomized, prospective trial. Obes Surg. 2012;**22**:740–48.

81. Eichenberger A, Proietti S, Wicky S, et al. Morbid obesity and postoperative pulmonary atelectasis: an underestimated problem. Anesth Analg. 2002;**95**:1788–92.

82. do Nascimento Junior P, Módolo NS, Andrade S, Guimarães MM, Braz LG, El Dib R. Incentive spirometry for prevention of postoperative pulmonary complications in upper abdominal surgery. Cochrane Database Syst Rev 2014;**2**:CD006058.

83. von Ungern-Sternberg BS, Regli A, Schneider MC, et al. Effect of obesity and site of surgery on perioperative lung volumes. Br J Anaesth. 2004;**92**:202–207.

84. Mehta V, Vasu TS, Phillips B, et al. Obstructive sleep apnea and oxygen therapy: a systematic review of the literature and meta-analysis. J Clin Sleep Med. 2013;**9**:271–79.

85. Giles TL, Lasserson TJ, Smith BJ, et al. Continuous positive airways pressure for obstructive sleep apnoea in adults. Cochrane Database Syst Rev. 2006;**1**:CD001106.

86. Wong DT, Adly E, Ip HY, et al. A comparison between the Boussignac continuous positive airway pressure mask and the venturi mask in terms of improvement in the PaO2/F(I)O2 ratio in morbidly obese patients undergoing bariatric surgery: a randomized controlled trial. Can J Anaesth. 2011;**58**:532–39.

87. Chung F, Subramanyam R, Liao P, et al. High STOP-Bang score indicates a high probability of obstructive sleep apnoea. Br J Anaesth. 2012;**108**:768–75.

88. Macintyre PE, Loadsman JA, Scott DA. Opioids, ventilation and acute pain management. Anaesth Intensive Care. 2011;**39**:545–55.

89. Mutter TC, Chateau D, Moffatt M, et al. A matched cohort study of postoperative outcomes in obstructive sleep apnea: could preoperative diagnosis and treatment prevent complications? Anesthesiology. 2014;**121**:707–18.

90. Bolden N, Smith CE, Auckley D, et al. Perioperative complications during use of an obstructive sleep apnea protocol following surgery and anesthesia. Anesth Analg. 2007;**105**:1869–70.

Obesity and non-operating room anaesthesia

Akshat Gargya, Matthew Troum, and Marc Goldberg

Introduction

Obesity, the modern-day epidemic, comes with many physiological consequences that make the job of an anaesthesiologist challenging. When an obese patient presents to your operating room you need to take many different variables into account. These variables include, but are not limited to, airway management, co-morbid conditions, safest anaesthetic technique, physiological and mechanical changes that occur in the obese patient, positioning, and postoperative care. When a similar patient presents for anaesthetic care outside the operating room, sometimes called 'out-of-operating room anaesthesia' or 'non- operating room anaesthesia', these factors are compounded for multiple reasons. These include distance from the 'mother ship' (the main operating room), colleagues who can provide back-up, and availability of all emergency equipment, among others.

The World Health Organization defines morbid obesity as a body mass index (BMI) of at least 40 kg/m^2 or at least 35 kg/m^2 in the presence of obesity-related comorbidities. Obesity (BMI ≥30 kg/m^2) is associated with multiple comorbidities including coronary artery disease, hypertension, type 2 diabetes, obstructive sleep apnoea, thromboembolism, gall bladder disease, liver disease, reduced wound healing, and psychosocial impairment. BMI, which is the patient's weight in kilograms divided by the square of the patient's height in metres, is the scale used to measure a patient's obesity (Table 32.1).

Table 32.1 Classification of obesity

Classification	BMI (kg/m^2)
Underweight	<18.5
Normal	18.5–24.9
Overweight	25.0–29.9
Obesity:	≥30.0
Class 1	30.0–34.9
Class 2	35.0–39.9
Class 3/extreme obesity	≥40.0

There are many variables that need to be considered when planning for an obese patient in the operating room. What about in a non-operating room setting? There is plenty of ambiguity and controversy among anaesthesiologists about the selection of patients who can be anaesthetized outside of the operating room. Whether they are presenting in the gastroenterology suite, bronchoscopy suite, electrophysiology laboratory, or an ambulatory surgery centre, important preparation and education must take place to ensure safe anaesthesia care. This chapter will explore points that need to be considered when deciding whether or not it is appropriate to perform an anaesthetic outside of the operating room.

Preoperative assessment/physiological changes in obesity

The physiological changes should be carefully considered and their importance is greatly heightened in obese patients when performing anaesthesia care in non-operating room settings. Improper knowledge of these changes could make performing an anaesthetic a catastrophe.

Airway

The multiple changes that occur in the airway of an obese patient should be the first concern of the anaesthesiologist taking care of a patient outside of the operating room. Patients will have an increased neck circumference, often accompanied by an increase of soft tissue surrounding the upper airway [1]. The increase in soft tissue makes collapse of the airway more likely in these patients with the induction of anaesthesia as well as during emergence. Whether or not you are performing a general anaesthetic with airway manipulation or a monitored anaesthesia care technique, the potential upper airway obstruction must be addressed prior to the induction phase of the anaesthetic. This is particularly important as obese patients more often are difficult to mask ventilate due to extra facial adipose tissue. An obese patient can present with a large tongue and decreased mandibular and cervical mobility, further complicating airway manipulation [1]. Since obese patients should be considered a potential difficult airway, preparations must be made for appropriately positioning these patients. The term used among anaesthesiologists is the 'sniffing' position, which aligns the pharyngeal and laryngeal axes, making intubation less challenging and also aids in ventilation. Perhaps even better than the sniffing position is the head-elevated laryngoscopy position (HELP) position, in which the patient's head is at a 30-degree elevation from the horizontal axis. This position decreases the sense of unease felt by patients who have difficulty lying flat and drops the patient's pannus away from the diaphragm, increasing ease of mask ventilation and improving alignment of oral, pharyngeal, and laryngeal axes. The Mallampati score is another tool used by anaesthesiologists to predict a difficult airway. Obese patients may present with Mallampati 3 (soft palate visualized) or Mallampati 4 (only hard palate visualized) and these are sensitive and specific indicators for a potential difficult airway [2]. The anaesthesiologist must elicit a full history and perform a physical exam prior to surgery to try and identify patients who could have a difficult airway. What is possibly most relevant in the history is a prior history of difficult intubation and when appropriately documented, can indicate what did and didn't work at the last attempt of airway instrumentation. Anther relevant factor is how long ago was the airway instrumented and has the patient's weight changed since then. With every potential difficult airway, especially in non-operating room settings, the anaesthesiologist must be prepared for a challenging start to the case. Different-sized endotracheal tubes, different sizes of laryngeal mask airways, videolaryngoscopes, fibre-optic intubation equipment, short-acting paralytics, and induction agents should be readily available. A checked and fully functional anaesthesia machine should always be present in the non-operating room setting as well as a backup Ambu bag for any emergency situation that may arise. A common fear among anaesthesiologists in the non-operating room settings is the amount of support from anaesthesia colleagues available to you. Any concern that the airway of a patient you are about to anaesthetize will be difficult to secure, in the absence of trained anaesthesia help nearby and immediately available mandates the procedure to be delayed until appropriate resources become available, or relocated to another setting [3,4].

Respiratory changes

Obesity has detrimental effects on the respiratory system that greatly affect administering of anaesthesia. Obesity causes a proportional increase in oxygen consumption as well as an increase in carbon dioxide production. This should be taken into account in patients who need more oxygen supply to their vital organs, such as patients with cardiovascular disease [5]. Obese patients typically have restrictive lung pathology even when their intrinsic lung function is normal. This is seen by a reduction of forced expiratory volume in 1 second (FEV_1) and forced vital capacity (FVC) with a relatively normal FEV_1/FVC ratio. Perhaps the most important respiratory effect is a reduction in functional residual capacity (FRC) and an increase in closing capacity. The significance of these reductions is a closure of the smaller airways in the lungs resulting in rapid atelectasis and consequent desaturation [6].

When performing a non-operating room anaesthetic in a morbidly obese patient, these parameters need to be considered. The induction of anaesthesia further exacerbates these decreases in lung volumes which quickly become apparent when obese patients rapidly desaturate from their increased demand and decreased reserve of oxygen. Obese patients continue to decrease their oxygen saturation when there is a significant time period between induction and intubation. It is important to keep in mind that atelectasis begins when the patient is settled on the operating room table in the supine position and continues long after the patient is extubated. Atelectasis in the obese patient can be managed with a multitude of techniques. Preoxygenation with a fraction of inspired oxygen of 1.0 along with continuous positive airway pressure (CPAP) could reduce the amount of atelectasis seen with induction [7]. Intraoperatively, positive end-expiratory pressure (PEEP) and the reverse Trendelenburg position could also benefit oxygenation and ventilation. Recruitment manoeuvres are a useful intraoperative tool to increase oxygen saturation.

Thorough preoperative assessment of pulmonary function should be ascertained prior to a non-operating room anaesthetic. Assess for comorbid conditions such as asthma, chronic obstructive pulmonary disease, and obstructive sleep apnoea. Assess the patient's exercise capacity. A resting pulse oximeter value of less than 96% while breathing room air, in the absence of known irreversible pathology, should create consideration for further cardiorespiratory workup in a patient prior to an elective procedure [8]. Arterial blood gas analysis as well as pulmonary function testing may show that the patient has severe restrictive lung disease requiring optimization prior to elective surgery. All of these parameters should be considered when deciding which patients are appropriate for outpatient surgery and which are not [9].

Cardiovascular changes

Cardiovascular changes in the obese patient pose an interesting challenge to anaesthesiologists. Cardiac output increases linearly with increasing body weight. This increases the preload and afterload [10]. The increase in afterload may be quite concerning in an obese patient who must have an adequate perfusion pressure to perfuse the coronary arteries. As many as half of obese patients have at least moderate hypertension as well as significant coronary artery disease, myocardial infarctions, and cerebrovascular accidents [6]. Many obese patients who present for surgery are taking a variety of cardiovascular medications. This is highly significant to the administration of anaesthesia practice, as it makes the management of a patient's haemodynamics more challenging.

When deciding whether a patient is appropriate and optimized for outpatient surgery, the visit to a preadmission testing centre is the first opportunity to obtain all necessary information and materials needed to perform safe anaesthesia care. One of the most important predictors of intraoperative cardiac events is a patient's ability to exercise [11]. If the patient has limited exercise capability, it may be worthwhile to obtain an exercise stress test or a pharmacological stress test to look for ischaemic heart disease in high-risk patients. An echocardiogram may be useful to look for evidence of pulmonary hypertension and right ventricular function [12]. Basic information of right heart function can also be gleaned from a 12-lead electrocardiogram by identifying signs of right ventricular strain, which in the absence of an echocardiogram, since most patients will not present with one, is a great screening tool in the 'proceed or delay' decision in an out-of-operating room scenario.

Gastrointestinal and endocrine changes

Obese patients present other concerns for the anaesthesiologist. Obese patients have substantially increased abdominal pressure, making them highly susceptible to diaphragmatic hernias as well as, by some studies, an increased risk for aspiration [13]. Precautions need to be taken for these patients to prevent aspiration. Oral sodium bicitrate as well as intravenous H_2 blockers and proton pump inhibitors have been employed with some documented success [14]. Insulin resistance as well as elevated cholesterol, triglycerides, and liver enzymes may also be seen in these patients [15].

Mechanical challenges for non-operating room anaesthesia

In non-operating room settings, much needs to go into the care of an obese patient outside of the patient themselves. Patient transfer is a problem encountered with many obese patients in outpatient surgical settings. Outpatient surgical settings should be equipped with the necessary tools needed to move a patient to the operating room table [16]. There are multiple available devices allowing two people to move any obese patient without sustaining any injuries. These devices need be employed at all remote surgical locations as well, where availability of ancillary staff may be limited.

Another concern in non-operating room settings is the maximum weight that the surgical table can hold safely. All surgical tables are labelled with a maximum weight and this should be checked to ensure that the weight of the patient does not exceed the maximum weight capacity of the table. Skytron (Grand Rapids, MI, USA) produces operating room tables that allow for a maximum patient weight of about 545 kg (1200 lbs) when flat and 365 kg (800 lbs) when articulated. For optimal outcomes, meticulous planning and extra attention to detail are required from all professionals involved in providing a safe anaesthetic to a morbidly obese patient in a location outside of the operating room [17].

Special equipment is also needed by anaesthesiologists when performing an anaesthetic outside of the operating room. These special tools allow for reassurance and back-up in case of an emergency. This equipment includes, but is not limited to, videolaryngoscopes as well as fibreoptic bronchoscopes for difficult airway management (**Box 32.1**) [18].

Intraoperative considerations in obese patients

Obese patients come with their unique set of problems and it requires a team effort from the surgical, anaesthesiology, and ancillary staff to optimize the surgical outcome. Along with the patient's functional status and associated comorbidities, the intraoperative anaesthetic plan must be appropriate for the type and urgency of surgery. The importance of a well-performed pre-anaesthetic assessment and identification of high-risk patients ahead of time cannot be overstated.

Choice of anaesthesia

Various factors should be taken into consideration when deciding the type of anaesthesia suitable for the surgery. These include, but are not limited to, type of surgical procedure, patient positioning during surgery, and anticipated difficult airway. Laparoscopic

---

Box 32.1 Equipment for managing obese surgical patients

Ward equipment
- Specialized electrically operated beds that can raise a patient to standing without the need for manual handling with a pressure-relieving mattress.
- Suitable bathrooms with floor-mounted toilets, suitable commodes.
- Large blood pressure measuring cuffs.
- Extra-large gowns.
- Suitably sized compression stockings and intermittent compression devices.
- Larger chairs, wheelchairs, and trolleys all marked with the maximum recommended weight.
- Scales capable of weighing up to 300 kg.
- On-site blood gas analysis.

Operating room equipment
- Bariatric operating table—this should be able to incorporate arm boards and table extensions, attachments for positioning such as leg supports for the lithotomy position, and shoulder and foot supports.
- Gel pads and padding for pressure points.
- Wide Velcro strapping to secure the patient to the operating table.
- Ramping device/pillows.
- Raised step for the anaesthetist.
- Large tourniquets.
- Readily available difficult airway equipment.
- Anaesthetic ventilator capable of PEEP and pressure modalities.
- Hover mattress or slide sheet.
- Portable ultrasound machine.
- Depth of anaesthesia monitoring to minimize residual sedation.
- Neuromuscular monitor.
- Long spinal and epidural needles.
- Long arterial lines if femoral access is necessary.

Adapted with permission from Griffiths, R., Popat, M.T., Pandit J. J., et al. Peri-operative management of the obese surgical patient 2015. *Anaesthesia*, 70(7): 859–876. © 2015 The Authors. Anaesthesia published by John Wiley & Sons Ltd on behalf of Association of Anaesthetists of Great Britain and Ireland.

---

procedures, trauma surgery, and thoracotomy warrant the use of general anaesthesia with an endotracheal tube compared to procedures such as knee replacement, orthopaedic procedures, and various podiatry procedures which are often performed under either spinal or regional anaesthesia techniques. Regional anaesthesia is generally preferred over general anaesthesia (when feasible) as it is associated with lesser incidence of postoperative pulmonary complications, earlier recovery of bowel function, and better pain control [19]. However, appropriate patient positioning and identification of anatomical landmarks may become difficult in obese patients. Failure of regional anaesthetic techniques is also more frequently seen in this patient population which makes the prior preparation for general anaesthesia vital [20]. Appropriate measures for an anticipated difficult airway and intubation should be in place.

Patient positioning

Placing an obese patient in the Trendelenburg or even the supine position can cause a significant reduction in FRC and a decrease in venous return due to inferior vena cava compression, which—accompanied by a high metabolic oxygen requirement—can cause rapid desaturation [5,6]. In comparison, patients with their backs up/reverse Trendelenburg position are easier to ventilate and have better alignment of pharyngeal, laryngeal, and oral axes, all aiding to improve intubation success.

The prone position has been shown to improve lung function, ventilation, and oxygenation. A patient in the prone position has less cephalad displacement of the diaphragm, causing a decrease in atelectasis. These patients are found to have higher respiratory capacities and better lung compliance [17,21]. Facial pressure ulcers, postoperative vision loss, and endotracheal tube dislodgement are more commonly associated with a prone patient [22].

Physiologically, the lateral position increases the ventilation in the non-dependent lung and perfusion in the dependent lung causing V/Q mismatch. Laterally placed patients are prone to radial and saphenous nerve injury and hence forearm support and leg paddings are imperative to prevent nerve injury. In this position, since the endotracheal tube is on the side of the patient and the position of the patient's arm is on the top, it can make adequate head positioning challenging. Chest rolls and gel pads to support the thorax and to maintain the head in a neutral position are often required. Anaesthesiologists must check the eyes regularly during the case for compression.

Surgeons may be forced to deploy the lithotomy position for various gynaecological and urological procedures and hence knowing the lithotomy-related complications in obese patients is essential. Compartment syndrome should always be considered in the postoperative period if a patient complains of pain out of proportion to tissue trauma after surgery in the lithotomy position. Venous thrombosis is also more common due to obstruction of venous drainage in this position and hence sequential compression devices should be placed prior to surgical draping.

Appropriate positioning of obese patients requires careful identification of pressure points, bony prominences, and adequate padding to reduce nerve injury and pressure ulcers. Safety straps often supplemented by silk tapes should be used to prevent unnecessary movement.

Intravenous access

Ultrasound is a handy tool to find the correct location of veins and their depth both in the holding area as well as intraoperatively, as finding a vein in deep subcutaneous fat can be challenging. Placing a central line comes with its own challenges of positioning a patient in the Trendelenburg position. Aside from finding the anatomical landmark in a thick neck, placing a patient in the Trendelenburg position also exacerbates other comorbidities in obese patients. For example, positioning an obese patient in a Trendelenburg position causes pressure on the vena cava due to weight. This decreases the venous return, causing hypotension and possibly cardiovascular compromise. Due to displacement of the abdominal contents towards the thorax, FRC decreases and increases speed and depth of desaturation, and hence central line placement should be avoided unless absolutely necessary. In any case, knowledge of the potential sites and anatomical landmarks can improve the success rate for an intravenous line placement in the obese. Other devices, including those utilizing light as a vein-identifying technology, are available, but their utility in this patient population may be limited.

Airway management and ventilation

Airway management in obese patients requires proper planning and emergency preparedness for situations such as difficult mask ventilation and difficult intubation. Consequently, proper positioning of

a patient is essential. Flexion of the neck on the body and extension of the head on the neck can be achieved by elevating the patient's upper body, head, and neck. Preoxygenation with a bag-valve mask is always beneficial as once apnoeic, obese patients desaturate rapidly. As previously discussed, the reason for this is a reduced FRC in obese patients causing a reduction in oxygen reserve. Due to increased oxygen requirements, it causes a rapid mismatch in oxygen demand and supply. Bag-valve mask use in the obese patient is often difficult due to the complexity in securing a seal at the mouth, reduced chest wall compliance, and the redundant supraglottic tissue. Use of nasal and oral airways, when applied carefully, is always beneficial and often two-person bag-mask ventilation becomes necessary. In case of emergency, positive pressure may be applied with CPAP masks, which can also be connected to standard ventilators, or by using a PEEP valve on a standard bag mask [4]. Even passive or apnoeic oxygenation utilizing a nasal cannula at high flow (approximately 10 L/min) may increase apnoea time and allow a careful and deliberate approach to the challenging airway.

Obese patients have a higher risk of aspiration but the preferential use of rapid sequence induction in these patients to avoid aspiration is a controversial topic with a large meta-analysis failing to find enough support to encourage or discourage the use of rapid sequence induction [13]. In case of a failed ventilation and failed intubation, rescue devices (e.g. a laryngeal mask airway) can be lifesaving at a critical point of the case although they do not protect against aspiration.

Awake intubation with topical anaesthesia and aerosol sprays is one possible technique when a difficult laryngoscopy is anticipated ahead of time. Patients with a disproportionally large tongue, a neck circumference greater than 50 cm, a history of obstructive sleep apnoea, and Mallampati grade 3 or 4 are generally the candidates in whom the possibility of awake intubation should be considered and discussed [1,2]. Once the patient is on a ventilator, PEEP can be used as an effective tool to cause a greater increase in lung volume and subsequently partial pressure of oxygen in comparison to giving obese patients a larger tidal volume [7,23]. In addition, PEEP has also been found to diminish atelectasis which is another factor causing decreased gas exchange in obese patients [14]. After any recruitment manoeuvre application of PEEP, approximately 8–10 cm H_2O and tidal volumes of 6–10 mL/kg (based on ideal body weight) are generally recommended until the patient becomes haemodynamically stable [24].

Induction agents

Knowledge of dosing of commonly used induction and maintenance drugs based on ideal, lean, or total body weight is critical as the difference between ideal and total body weight in obese patients can be significant (for details of pharmacology in obese patients, see Chapter 4). The general consensus is to use lean body weight for most anaesthetic drugs, except non-depolarizing neuromuscular blocking drugs where ideal body weight is appropriate [24]. The volume of distribution of lipophilic drugs increases in obese patients due to accumulation of drugs in the fat store of the body and hence an increased dose of lipophilic drugs such as fentanyl will be required. Dose requirements of hydrophilic drugs are generally not affected. **Table 32.2** summarizes the accepted drug guidelines for commonly used drugs.

Table 32.2 Dosing of some commonly used anaesthetic drugs

Drug dosing based on ideal body weight (IBW) in kg: males = height in cm − 100, females = height in cm − 110	Drug dosing based on lean body weight (LBW) in kg: males = 50 + 0.9 kg for every cm over 150 cm, females = 45 + 0.9 kg for every cm over 150 cm	Drug dosing based on total body weight (TBW)
Cisatracurium (0.15–0.2 mg/kg) Midazolam (0.15–3.0 mg/kg) Rocuronium (0.6–1.2 mg/kg) Vecuronium (0.10–0.12 mg/kg)	Etomidate (0.2 mg/kg) Fentanyl (2–3 mcg/kg) Ketamine (1–2 mg/kg) Morphine (0.05–0.10 mg/kg) Remifentanil (0.2–2.0 mcg/kg/min infusion) Sufentanil (1–2 mcg/kg) Propofol (induction dose 1.5–2.5 mg/kg)	Enoxaparin (0.5 mg/kg) Succinylcholine (1–1.5 mg/kg) Propofol (maintenance dose) Neostigmine (0.05 mg/kg)

Fluid management

Intraoperative fluid management in obese patients is controversial but the concept of goal-directed therapy appears to be the most promising approach. A patient's haemodynamic assessment based on vital signs, central venous pressure, or urine output lacks accuracy as these parameters do not correlate with cardiac output [10,12,25]. Fluid administration based on these parameters can cause inadequate resuscitation and have been proven to increase mortality and mortality in obese patients. Furthermore, aggressive fluid management and positive fluid balance strategies have the potential to cause multiple organ dysfunctions including pulmonary and myocardial oedema, hepatic congestion, and a decrease in renal blood flow and glomerular filtration rate [25]. Goal-directed therapy is a target-driven fluid resuscitation method which focuses on measuring outcomes of fluid therapy via parameters such as stroke volume, cardiac index, and mixed venous oxygen saturation by use of oesophageal Doppler or pulse contour analysis.

Emergence from anaesthesia and extubation

Extubation is generally performed in a semi-recumbent or sitting position to allow maximal diaphragmatic excursion. It should be ensured that neuromuscular blocking drugs are adequately reversed. It is generally preferred that patient is awake. Airway obstruction is one of the main causes of extubation failure and hence it becomes necessary to suction the airway prior to taking the endotracheal tube to prevent aspiration of oral secretions [26]. In patients with obstructive sleep apnoea, insertion of a nasal trumpet is an easier and quick method of decreasing airway obstruction at emergence.

Postoperative care in obese patients

Some guidelines for managing an obese patient in the postoperative period have been summarized in **Box 32.2**.

Box 32.2 Postoperative care in obese patients.

- In patients with a history of obstructive sleep apnoea, placing the patient on 100% oxygen will help decrease the number of desaturation episodes [27].
- Bariatric surgery patients should have CPAP immediately after extubation as it reduces the risk of airway obstruction and improves lung function [28].
- Early mobilization and incentive spirometry should be encouraged.
- After surgery, obese patients should be placed either in the sitting position or with head-end elevated to around 30–45 degrees to help improve FRC.
- Early use of patient-controlled analgesia along with multimodal pain control techniques are advocated. Adequate pain control also decreases the rate of pulmonary complications in obese patients by enhancing a patient's capability to breathe deeply. Basal rates in patient-controlled analgesia are generally avoided to decrease oversedation. Intramuscular or subcutaneous analgesics should be avoided due to variable absorption rates in obese patients due to poor subcutaneous blood supply [29].
- Obese patients have a higher risk of pulmonary embolism and a new onset of tachycardia or episode of desaturation should always be evaluated with a high degree of suspicion. Evaluating an arterial blood gas with serum lactate levels can help evaluate a diagnosis.
- Patients can be discharged when arterial oxygen saturation returns to the preoperative values and other institution-specific discharge criteria are met.

CASE REPORT

Mr Smith presents for a colonoscopy in an outpatient surgery centre. He is 55 years old with a BMI of 58 kg/m². His past medical history includes hypertension, hyperlipidaemia, diabetes type 2, obstructive sleep apnoea for which he uses a CPAP device at night, and prior myocardial infarction at age 52 for which he had a bare metal stent placed. He is 'mostly compliant' with his CPAP mask at night but does not know his settings. He has been off clopidogrel for 3 years but continues to take a daily aspirin along with his insulin regimen, lisinopril, metoprolol, amlodipine, atorvastatin, and a daily vitamin. His last set of laboratory tests revealed a mild anaemia with haemoglobin of 9.8 mg/dL and a platelet count of 220,000/mm³. His coagulation studies were normal. His last echocardiogram, 7 months ago, showed an ejection fraction of 50% with no regional wall abnormalities and no valvular disease.

With obesity rates steadily increasing among the general population, this case scenario is commonly seen by anaesthesiologists in both the operating room and in non-operating room settings. The question, therefore, is—whether or not this is being done in an outpatient surgery centre or in a hospital in a remote location—is it safe to perform an anaesthetic in this patient outside and away from the operating room?

REFERENCES

1. Ezri T, Gewürtz G, Sessler D, Medalion B, Szmuk P, Hagberg C, et al. Prediction of difficult laryngoscopy in obese patients by ultrasound quantification of anterior neck soft tissue. Anaesthesia. 2003;**58**(11):1111–14.

2. Voyagis G, Kyriakis K, Dimitriou V, Vrettou I. Value of oropharyngeal Mallampati classification in predicting difficult laryngoscopy among obese patients. European Journal of Anaesthesiology. 1998;**15**(3):330–34.

3. Levine A, DeMaria S. An updated report by the American Society of Anesthesiologists Task Force on Management of the Difficult Airway. Anesthesiology. 2013;**119**(3):731–32.

4. Weingart S, Levitan R. Preoxygenation and prevention of desaturation during emergency airway management. Annals of Emergency Medicine. 2012;**59**(3):165–75.

5. Yap JC, Watson RA, Gilbey S, Pride NB. Effects of posture on respiratory mechanics in obesity. Journal of Applied Physiology 1995;**79**(4):1199–205.

6. Paul D, Hoyt J, Boutros A. Cardiovascular and respiratory changes in response to change of posture in the very obese. Anesthesiology. 1976;**45**(1):73–78.

7. Pelosi P, Ravagnan I, Giurati G, Panigada M, Bottino N, Tredici S, et al. Positive end-expiratory pressure improves respiratory function in obese but not in normal subjects during anesthesia and paralysis. Survey of Anesthesiology. 2000;**44**(6):360–61.

8. Shenkman Z, Shir Y, Brodsky J. Perioperative management of the obese patient. British Journal of Anaesthesia. 1993;**70**(3):349–59.

9. Forgiarini Júnior L, Rezende J, Forgiarini S. Alveolar recruitment maneuver and perioperative ventilatory support in obese patients undergoing abdominal surgery. Revista Brasileira de Terapia Intensiva. 2013;**25**(4):312–18.

10. Küntscher M, Germann G, Hartmann B. Correlations between cardiac output, stroke volume, central venous pressure, intra-abdominal pressure and total circulating blood volume in resuscitation of major burns. Resuscitation. 2006;**70**(1):37–43.

11. Hernandez A, Whellan D, Stroud S, Sun J, O'Connor C, Jollis J. Outcomes in heart failure patients after major noncardiac surgery. ACC Current Journal Review. 2005;**14**(1):37.

12. Marik P, Baram M, Vahid B. Does central venous pressure predict fluid responsiveness? A systematic review of the literature and the tale of seven mares. Chest. 2008;**134**(1):172–78.

13. Neilipovitz D, Crosby E. No evidence for decreased incidence of aspiration after rapid sequence induction. Canadian Journal of Anesthesia. 2007;**54**(9):748–64.

14. American Society of Anesthesiologists Committee on Standards and Practice Parameters. Practice guidelines for preoperative fasting and the use of pharmacologic agents to reduce the risk of pulmonary aspiration: application to healthy patients undergoing elective procedures. Anesthesiology. 2011;**114**(3):495–511.

15. Cheah M, Kam P. Obesity: basic science and medical aspects relevant to anaesthetists. Anaesthesia. 2005;**60**(10):1009–21.

16. Metzner J, Domino K. Risks of anesthesia or sedation outside the operating room: the role of the anesthesia care provider. Current Opinion in Anaesthesiology. 2010;**23**(4):523–31.

17. Boyce J, Ness T, Castroman P, Gleysteen J. A preliminary study of the optimal anesthesia positioning for the morbidly obese patient. Obesity Surgery. 2003;**13**(1):4–9.

18. Nightingale C, Margarson M, Shearer E, Redman J, Lucas D, Cousins J, et al. Peri-operative management of the obese surgical patient 2015. Anaesthesia. 2015;**70**(7):859–76.

19. Neuman M, Silber J, Elkassabany N, Ludwig J, Fleisher L. Comparative effectiveness of regional versus general anesthesia for hip fracture surgery in Adults. Anesthesiology. 2012;**117**(1):72–92.

20. Ingrande J, Brodsky J, Lemmens H. Regional anesthesia and obesity. Current Opinion in Anaesthesiology. 2009;**22**(5):683–86.

21. Lai-Fook SJ, Rodarte JR. Pleural pressure distribution and its relationship to lung volume and interstitial pressure. Journal of Applied Physiology. 1991;**70**(3):967–78.

22. Kwee M, Ho Y, Rozen W. The prone position during surgery and its complications: a systematic review and evidence-based guidelines. International Surgery. 2015;**100**(2):292–303.

23. Katz J, Ozanne G, Zinn S, Fairley H. Time course and mechanisms of lung-volume increase with PEEP in acute pulmonary failure. Anesthesiology. 1981;**54**(1):9–16.

24. Ingrande J, Lemmens H. Dose adjustment of anaesthetics in the morbidly obese. British Journal of Anaesthesia. 2010;**105**(Suppl 1):i16–23.

25. Prowle J, Echeverri J, Ligabo E, Ronco C, Bellomo R. Fluid balance and acute kidney injury. Nature Reviews Nephrology. 2009;**6**(2):107–15.

26. Cavallone L, Vannucci A. Extubation of the difficult airway and extubation failure. Survey of Anesthesiology. 2013;**57**(6):312–13.

27. Mehta V, Vasu T, Phillips B, Chung F. Obstructive sleep apnea and oxygen therapy: a systematic review of the literature and meta-analysis. Journal of Clinical Sleep Medicine. 2013;**9**(3):271–79.

28. Neligan P, Malhotra G, Fraser M, Williams N, Greenblatt E, Cereda M, et al. Continuous positive airway pressure via the Boussignac system immediately after extubation improves lung function in morbidly obese patients with obstructive sleep apnea undergoing laparoscopic bariatric surgery. Anesthesiology. 2009;**110**(4):878–84.

29. Garimella V, Cellini C. Postoperative pain control. Clinics in Colon and Rectal Surgery. 2013;**26**(3):191–96.

33

Intensive care

Andrea L. Tsai and Roman Schumann

Introduction

Care of the intensive care unit (ICU) patient with obesity presents clinical and logistical challenges. Obesity is often a constellation of disease processes associated with perturbations across multiple organ systems, and care of these patients must be appropriately tailored. Unfortunately, there is a lack of robust data to establish best practices, and thus most recommendations are based predominantly on small trials and expert opinion. In this chapter, we review best practices by organ system in the care of the ICU patient with obesity and discuss outcome data for these patients.

Neurological

The most recent critical care guidelines recommend targeting light sedation when needed, avoiding benzodiazepine use, and striving for early mobilization [1]. These recommendations may be specifically important for the obese population, although they certainly present clinical and logistical challenges. We present dosing recommendations for sedative agents and other neurotropic drugs where available and discuss the challenges involved in efforts at mobilizing the critical care patient with obesity.

The patient with obesity may be at increased risk for respiratory failure in the context of sedation [2,3]. The aetiology of this respiratory compromise is likely multifactorial and includes an increased baseline risk for sleep-disordered breathing (and diseases within this spectrum such as obstructive sleep apnoea, obesity hypoventilation syndrome, etc.) [4] and their restrictive pulmonary physiology [2,3,5,6]. Careful dose titration of sedative agents therefore is needed, particularly in non-intubated patients with obesity.

A comprehensive discussion of drug pharmacokinetics is presented elsewhere in this volume (see Chapter 4), and this discussion focuses on practical 'rules of thumb' and specific drugs commonly encountered in the ICU. In the absence of robust detailed data for dosing in different weight categories of obesity for many drugs, some authors advocate to use total body weight (TBW)-based dosing for patients with a body mass index (BMI) less than 35 kg/m², because these patients are typically included in drug approval studies [7]. For patients with a BMI greater than 35 kg/m², in the absence of

drug-specific data guiding weight-based dosing, several options exist; see Table 33.1 [6].

Guidelines recommend dosing by titration to effect for necessary sedation in all critically ill patients and suggest use of either the Richmond Agitation-Sedation Scale [8] or the Riker Sedation-Agitation Scale [9] as a tool for appropriate drug titration to the level of desired sedation [1]. However, in circumstances where a weight-based dosing option is used, the choice of that option for patients with a BMI greater than 35 kg/m² must balance the risks and benefits of potential sub- and supratherapeutic drug levels. If subtherapeutic dosing carries a more favourable risk:benefit profile, then dosing based on ideal body weight (IBW), adjusted body weight (ABW), or lean body weight (LBW) may be preferred. If supratherapeutic dosing carries a more favourable risk:benefit profile, then dosing based on TBW may be preferred. Drugs with a volume of distribution less than 1 L/kg with primarily renal clearance may preferably be dosed based on LBW [7,10], as creatinine clearance is underestimated by IBW and overestimated by TBW in patients with obesity [11].

Table 33.1 Dosing options

Dosing strategy	Formula
Dosing based on ideal body weight (IBW)	IBW = • Men (kg) = 50 kg + 2.3 kg for each inch in height over 60 inches • Women (kg) = 45.5 kg + 2.3 kg for each inch in height over 60 inches
Dosing based on adjusted body weight (ABW)	ABW (kg) = IBW + 0.4 (TBW − IBW)
Dosing based on lean body weight (LBW)	LBW = • Men (kg) = (1.1 × weight in kg) − 120 (weight in kg/height in cm)² • Women (kg) = (1.07 × weight in kg) − 148 (weight in kg/height in cm)²
Dosing based on total body weight (TBW)	Not applicable
Non-weight-based dosing	Not applicable
Titration to effect	Not applicable

Regarding specific sedatives, dexmedetomidine and ketamine are attractive options in the obese population for their lack of associated respiratory depression and their usefulness as adjuncts to analgesia, though pharmacokinetic data in critically ill patients with severe obesity are largely unavailable [3]. A propofol infusion regimen was studied in a small population ($n = 8$) of morbidly obese patients undergoing elective surgeries and dosing based on TBW was found to be appropriate [12]. In contrast, for the majority of alternative ICU sedative and paralytic agents including midazolam, diazepam, remifentanil, atracurium, rocuronium, and vecuronium, dosing based on IBW is generally suggested [3,7]. Finally, studies on the anticonvulsant phenytoin suggest a loading regimen of 14 mg/kg IBW plus 19 mg/kg for additional weight over IBW, with a loading dose cap of 2 g; further maintenance dosing should be based on conventional dosing or IBW [7].

Early mobilization of the critically ill patient is safe [13,14] and now part of critical care guidelines because it is associated with improved muscle strength, functional mobility, quality of life, and decreased incidence and duration of delirium, hospital and ICU length of stay, and duration of mechanical ventilation [1,15]. Obese patients are at increased risk for adverse sequelae from immobility [16,17] while simultaneously presenting caregiver workload and equipment limitation challenges to mobilization potentially affecting both clinician and patient safety [16,18–20]. For example, in a patient weighing 136 kg (300 lbs), one leg can weigh approximately 22 kg (48 lbs) [16]. In a study of ICU nursing workload, a trend towards greater workload was found as patients' obesity increased from World Health Organization (WHO) class I (BMI 30–34.9 kg/m^2) to class II (BMI 35–39.9 kg/m^2), becoming statistically significant when WHO class III obesity was present (BMI ≥40 kg/m^2) [18]. To prevent injury to patient and healthcare personnel, the American Nurses Association as well as the National Association of Bariatric Nurses recommend use of assistive equipment and devices when mobilizing these patients [16]. However, even with appropriate staffing and the assistance of devices such as air mattresses, lifts, slings, and so on, mobilization and care of patients at the extremes of obesity can be hampered by equipment limitations. The safe working load of standard equipment ranges from 181–227 kg for stretchers, 159–200 kg for carry chairs, 178–191 kg for hospital beds, to 140–190 kg for hoists [20]. Specialized lifts exist with weight capacities of up to 227–318 kg [16].

Radiographic studies can be similarly limited in obese patients. In addition to attenuation of ultrasound energy, X-rays, and photons from body habitus, some patients at the extremes of obesity may exceed the diameter or weight limit of radiographic equipment [21,22]. Energy attenuation by excess soft tissue results in lower-quality ultrasound, plain film, fluoroscopic, computed tomography (CT) and magnetic resonance imaging (MRI) images [21,22]. Additionally, table weight limits and bore diameter of scanners may further limit imaging efforts. The maximum table loads for different radiodiagnostic modalities are as follows: 217 kg for plain films on typical radiographic tables (no weight limitation if patient is standing, and no table is needed) with a field of view of 36 × 43 cm, 160–200 kg for a CT scanner table with a typical bore diameter of 70 cm, 147–200 kg for an MRI table with a bore diameter of 60 cm, 160–181 kg for a nuclear medicine scanner, 159–204 kg for a fluoroscopy table, and 159–181 kg for interventional procedure surfaces including angiography,

mammography, and so on [19,21–23]. Specialized CT scanner tables are available that support patients up to 279–299 kg with bore diameters of 80–90 cm [21]. Anecdotal reports exist of the use of zoo or veterinary hospital scanners for imaging patients with extreme obesity; however, this is unlikely to be a feasible option [23]. Many zoos and veterinary hospitals do not have large capacity scanners, and the majority of those that do, have policies prohibiting the imaging of human patients [23]. Ultra-low-field MRI is an emerging technology with potential application in the obese population due to a wider scanner bore diameter [24]. Though still in development, it is an exciting and promising technology for the future.

Cardiovascular

The cardiovascular critical care challenges of patients with obesity include their increased risk for complications following cardiac surgeries, the pharmacokinetic considerations for appropriate inodilator and vasoactive drug dosing, as well as obtaining vascular access and invasive monitoring.

Patients with obesity undergoing cardiac surgery are at increased risk for complications, particularly for those with a BMI of 40 kg/m^2 or greater. In a systematic review and meta-analysis, obese (BMI ≥30 kg/m^2) cardiac surgical patients had an increased risk for new-onset postoperative atrial fibrillation compared to their non-obese (BMI <30 kg/m^2) counterparts (odds ratio (OR) 1.12, 95% confidence interval (CI) 1.04–1.21) [25]. A multivariate analysis of the American College of Surgeons National Surgical Quality Improvement Program (ACS-NSQIP) data showed that coronary artery bypass grafting in patients with a BMI of at least 40 kg/m^2 had significantly increased odds of postoperative cardiac arrest and myocardial infarction (OR 2.35, 95% CI 1.01–5.47) [26]. The same analysis also reported increased complications across all organ systems in these patients, including a higher odds of pulmonary (pneumonia, postoperative reintubation, and ventilatory support >48 hours, OR 1.81, 95% CI 1.10–2.98), thromboembolic (deep venous thrombosis or pulmonary embolism, OR 4.58, 95% CI 1.74–12.1), septic (sepsis and septic shock, OR 2.74, 95% CI 1.27–5.92), renal (new or progressive renal insufficiency, OR 2.74, 95% CI 1.27–5.89) and wound (OR 4.73, 95% CI 2.48–9.01) complications [26]. Patients with a BMI of 40 kg/m^2 or greater undergoing cardiac valve replacement or repair surgeries also experienced increased pulmonary (OR 2.37, 95% CI 1.50–3.74), renal (OR 2.46, 95% CI 1.25–4.83), and wound (OR 6.40, 95% CI 2.66–15.4) complications [26].

For treating arrhythmias in patients with obesity, consideration of obesity-induced alterations of the pharmacokinetic profile of therapeutic agents is again of importance. Some authors suggest a conservative blanket approach that includes dosing of cardiovascular medications according to standard regimens or otherwise based on IBW [7]. This is supported by pharmacokinetic studies in obese patients for drugs including digoxin, procainamide, propranolol, nebivolol, and labetalol [7]. In contrast, pharmacokinetic profiles of drugs such as lidocaine and verapamil that have been studied in obese patients suggest that at least initial loading doses should be TBW based, with subsequent maintenance dosing according to non-weight-based dosing [6]. For the lipophilic drug amiodarone, with its large volume of distribution, one would expect larger than usual doses to initially be needed in the obese population. Unfortunately, to our knowledge, only one study addresses amiodarone's pharmacodynamics in adults including some with obesity. The investigation was conducted in 23 Japanese patients with a BMI of 17.6–31.4 kg/m² (where obesity was defined according to Japanese standards: a body fat percentage >23% for males or >28% for females, or BMI >25 kg/m²) [27]. This study found a reduced clearance of amiodarone as BMI increased to above 25 kg/m² as well as highly variable inter-individual pharmacodynamics [27]. In the absence of more definitive data, it appears reasonable that the current best practice includes initial amiodarone dosing based on standard regimens (e.g. 150 mg intravenously over 10 minutes followed by 360 mg over next 6 hours, then 540 mg over the remaining 18 hours) [27,28].

In addition to more frequent complications following cardiac surgery and the special dosing considerations for cardiac drugs, patients with obesity frequently present technical challenges for vascular access and haemodynamic monitoring. Peripheral intravenous access can be more time-consuming and difficult, and central venous catheters (CVCs) are often necessary [19,29]. However, CVC placement in obese patients is not a trivial task either due to obfuscation of anatomical landmarks, greater skin-to-vessel distance, and short, stubby necks [29–31]. Ultrasound guidance can be used to assist with vessel cannulation and may increase the success rate and decrease the complication rate in obese patients requiring internal jugular CVC placement [29,30]. However, ultrasound-guided placement of subclavian CVCs is limited by poor visualization of the subclavian vein at higher BMI ranges [32]. Although more recent data and analyses provide compelling arguments that no difference exists in catheter-related bloodstream infection rates between the internal jugular, subclavian, and femoral vein CVC sites [33,34], subgroup analysis demonstrates that patients with higher BMI (28.4–45 kg/m²) have an increased CVC colonization risk at the femoral vein site compared to the internal jugular vein site. This evidence makes femoral CVC placement in individuals with obesity highly undesirable [35].

Given the likelihood of difficulties with vascular access procedures, establishing extracorporeal membrane oxygenation (ECMO) in critically ill patients with obesity could be highly morbid. Indeed, obesity is currently listed as a relative contraindication for venoarterial ECMO by the Extracorporeal Life Support Organization guidelines for adult cardiac failure [36]. This relative contraindication may also be due to the higher resting cardiac outputs of obese individuals [29,37] and the limitations encountered when attempting to achieve higher ECMO flows (e.g. suction events, haemolysis, etc.). However, multiple case series describe successful venovenous ECMO for respiratory support in patients with obesity [37,38]. These case series included patients with BMIs of up to 88.6 kg/m² [38]. The majority of patients were percutaneously cannulated with a femoral venous drainage cannula and a right internal jugular return cannula [37,38]. Only a minority of patients received dual-lumen single cannulae due to the weight limitations of the table needed for fluoroscopic guidance of catheter placement [37,38]. Despite logistical and personnel challenges (e.g. two to four people to retract the panniculus to facilitate cannulation, four to six assistants for patient repositioning, etc.) [38], successful weaning from ECMO and survival was similar in obese and non-obese groups, leading the authors to conclude that venovenous ECMO is feasible and potentially lifesaving for these critically ill patients [37,38].

Pulmonary

Compared to the non-obese, patients with obesity are at baseline higher risk for pulmonary comorbidities including sleep-disordered breathing, hyper-reactive airway diseases, and pulmonary hypertension [6]. Furthermore, ICU patients with obesity appear to also have a higher incidence of acute respiratory distress syndrome (ARDS) [31,39]. The pathophysiology engaging pulmonary morbidity in these patients is multifactorial and complex. Hormonal changes, including leptin resistance, may play a role [4,29,40]. Obesity is a chronic proinflammatory state, which may predispose patients to hyper-reactive airway diseases, though the possible link to acute lung injury is unclear [31]. Mechanical and physiological pulmonary changes from obesity are also key factors, including decreased compliance [41,42], increased airway resistance [4,29], increased work of breathing [41,43], higher oxygen consumption (VO_2), and carbon dioxide production (VCO_2) [29,40], and reductions in expiratory reserve volume, forced vital capacity, forced expiratory volume in 1 second, functional residual capacity, total lung capacity, and maximum voluntary ventilation [4,5,40,41,43]. These changes are exacerbated by supine positioning [4,41] and a central pattern of obesity, that is, an increased waist-to-hip ratio and increased neck circumference [40]. All of these factors when combined, result in challenging airway management and mechanical ventilation in the ICU patient with obesity.

A BMI greater than 26 kg/m² is an independent risk factor for difficult mask ventilation [5], and some consider increased BMI to be associated with difficult intubation [5,44,45]. Indeed, prospective observational studies of intubations in ICU patients with a BMI of at least 30 kg/m² and at least 35 kg/m² showed a 16.3% and 15% incidence of difficult intubation, respectively [44,45]. Predictors of difficult intubation for ICU patients with obesity included Mallampati score III or IV, obstructive sleep apnoea, severe hypoxaemia (<80%), and coma [44]. Difficult intubation in the ICU was associated with an increased risk of severe life-threatening complications (relative risk 1.5, 95% CI 1.1–2.0 for severe hypoxaemia, severe cardiovascular collapse, cardiac arrest, and death) [44]. Thoughtful anticipation and preparation whenever possible is recommended to facilitate intubation in the ICU, particularly since patient repositioning can be difficult. Back-up airway equipment (e.g. bougie introducer, video laryngoscope, fibreoptic scope, etc.) was used more often to facilitate intubation in ICU patients with a BMI of at least 30 kg/m² compared with a similar patient cohort in the operating room [44]. Positioning in a 'sniffing' (cervical flexion, head extension), 'ramped' (where sternal notch and external auditory meatus are at the same horizontal level), or reverse Trendelenburg position facilitates laryngeal exposure and potentially improves pulmonary mechanics [5,29,31,46]. Comparisons of a 'sniffing' to a 'ramped' position in bariatric surgery patients with a BMI of 40 kg/m² or greater suggest an improvement in grade of laryngoscopic view with 'ramped' positioning [46]. If there is sufficient concern over the difficulty of a patient's airway, a practitioner experienced in airway management should be sought and an awake intubation should be considered [5,31].

Patients with obesity present mechanical ventilation challenges as well. The ARDS Network has established that lung protective ventilation strategies include limiting tidal volumes (V_T) to less than or equal to 6 mL/kg IBW and plateau pressures (P_{plat}) to less than or equal to 30 cmH₂O [47,48]. Analysis of a cohort of mechanically ventilated patients showed, however, that patients with obesity were more likely to receive high V_T based on IBW, potentially leading to harmful over-distention of alveoli and ventilator-induced lung injury [39]. Because of the obesity-induced restrictive pulmonary physiology, P_{plat} may exceed levels recommended for lung protective ventilation, and positive end-expiratory pressure (PEEP) titration is unclear.

A protective ventilation strategy using transpulmonary pressures (P_{tp}) rather than airway pressures (P_{aw}) has been examined in obese ICU patients [43]. Evidence suggests that P_{tp}, not P_{aw}, may be the culprit for lung injury [48]. Generally speaking, P_{tp} is equal to P_{aw} minus pleural pressure (P_{pl}) (**Fig. 33.1**). P_{pl} is positive in sedated and mechanically ventilated patients with obesity [41,43]; therefore, even in the presence of elevated P_{aw}, P_{tp} may be negative, potentially resulting in airway collapse and atelectrauma [42,48]. Furthermore, elevated P_{plat}, in the presence of elevated P_{pl}, may not actually be injurious, as much of the ventilator pressure is dissipated in the expansion of the chest wall rather than the lung (**Fig. 33.1**) [48].

Determination of P_{pl} is complex, but it can be approximated by oesophageal pressure (P_{es}) [31,48]. Compared to the ARDS Network PEEP titration protocol, a P_{es}-guided protocol in medical and surgical ICU patients with ARDS ($n = 61$) resulted in a sustained improvement in PaO_2 as well as a significant reduction in 28-day adjusted mortality (relative risk 0.46, 95% CI 0.19–1.0) [49]. Though this trial did not focus specifically on patients with obesity, a separate smaller trial ($n = 14$) examining patients with a BMI of 35.2–91.8 kg/m² using P_{es}-guided PEEP titration similarly resulted in improved oxygenation, lung volumes, and respiratory system elastance [43]. These studies suggest using P_{es} to up-titrate PEEP and P_{plat} to achieve

an end-expiratory P_{tp} of 0–10 cmH₂O and an end-inspiratory P_{tp} less than 25 cmH₂O. The mean PEEP in these trials ranged from 17 to 21 cmH₂O (standard deviation 4–6) [43,49]. Based on these insights, a phase II trial of P_{tp}-guided mechanical ventilation in patients with ARDS (EPVent2) is underway at the time of writing this chapter and may change ventilation strategies including for the ICU patient with obesity [50].

A decremental PEEP trial is an alternative method for titration when P_{es} is not available [43]. In a decremental PEEP trial, after a recruitment manoeuvre (RM), PEEP is set at a high level (e.g. 25 cmH₂O), then progressively reduced (e.g. in 2 cmH₂O increments every 2 minutes) while delta pressure ($P_{plat} − PEEP$) is measured [43]. The best PEEP corresponds to the PEEP with the lowest delta pressure. PEEP determined in this fashion was found to have good correlation with PEEP determined by P_{es} [43].

Other strategies for improving pulmonary function in mechanically ventilated patients with obesity include RMs (e.g. applying $P_{aw} = 40$ cmH₂O for a brief period) [31,43], elevation of the head of bed (HOB) [5,31,43,51], and prone positioning [52]. Data for RM use in the obese ICU population are nascent. A small study indicates that RMs improve lung volumes, elastance, and oxygenation, even when compared to increased PEEP without RMs [43]. RMs were well tolerated with 5 of 14 patients studied experiencing a transient systolic blood pressure decrease (<90 mmHg) [43]. PROBESE, an ongoing trial comparing intraoperative ventilation with PEEP of at least 12 and RMs to PEEP of 4 without RMs in patients with a BMI of at least 35 kg/m², may provide further guidance applicable to the ICU as well [6,53].

The use of HOB elevation to improve pulmonary function appears intuitive: particularly in the obese population, it should lead to decreased transdiaphragmatic pressure, decreased atelectasis, and improved gas exchange [31,51]. A study of intubated, spontaneously breathing patients with abdominal distention, ascites, or obesity demonstrated larger V_T and lower respiratory rates in a

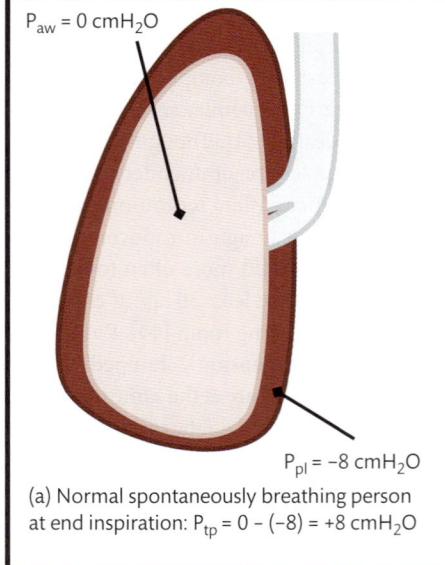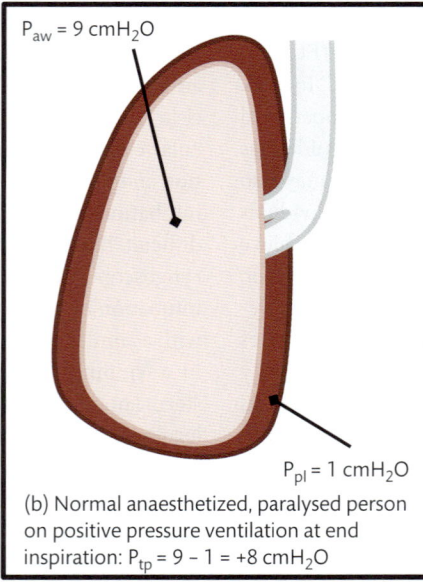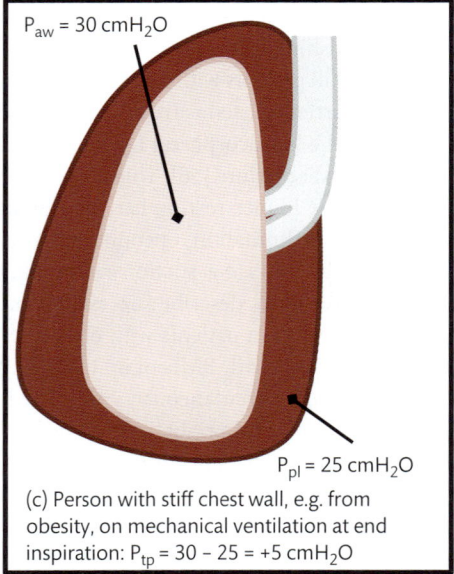

$P_{aw} = 0$ cmH₂O	$P_{aw} = 9$ cmH₂O	$P_{aw} = 30$ cmH₂O
$P_{pl} = −8$ cmH₂O	$P_{pl} = 1$ cmH₂O	$P_{pl} = 25$ cmH₂O
(a) Normal spontaneously breathing person at end inspiration: $P_{tp} = 0 − (−8) = +8$ cmH₂O	(b) Normal anaesthetized, paralysed person on positive pressure ventilation at end inspiration: $P_{tp} = 9 − 1 = +8$ cmH₂O	(c) Person with stiff chest wall, e.g. from obesity, on mechanical ventilation at end inspiration: $P_{tp} = 30 − 25 = +5$ cmH₂O

Fig. 33.1 Airway, pleural, and transpulmonary pressures in (a) spontaneously breathing patient. (b) Same patient as in (a), now on positive pressure ventilation. (c) Patient with stiff chest wall from obesity on positive pressure ventilation.

Adapted with permission from Slutsky, A.S., and Ranieri, V. M., Ventilator-Induced Lung Injury. *New England Journal of Medicine*, 369:2126–2136. Copyright (2013) Massachusetts Medical Society. DOI: 10.1056/NEJMra1208707

45-degree reverse Trendelenburg position, potentially facilitating ventilator weaning [54]. Two additional studies in mechanically ventilated patients with obesity support these findings. One study (BMI >35 kg/m²) showed that HOB elevation improved lung volumes and decreased optimal PEEP requirements [43]. Another trial (BMI >45 kg/m²) determined that the sitting position relieved expiratory flow limitation, auto-PEEP, and P_{plat} [51]. In both studies, HOB elevation was well tolerated and feasible.

Prone positioning has been extensively studied in ARDS [31,52,55] and is thought to improve oxygenation by promoting homogeneous lung inflation and improving ventilation and perfusion matching, compliance, and functional residual capacity [31,52]. When applied early (e.g. within 36 hours of the onset of mechanical ventilation) for prolonged durations (e.g. 12–20 hours) to select patients with moderate to severe ARDS, prone positioning significantly decreased 28-day and 90-day mortality [55]. This technique presents obvious technical challenges for the patient with obesity. However, a recent case–control study demonstrated prone positioning to be safe in patients with obesity (BMI ≥35 kg/m²) and appeared to improve their oxygenation to a greater degree than in comparable non-obese patients (**Fig. 33.2**) [52]. The authors suggested that patients with obesity may be uniquely suited to benefit from prone positioning in ARDS [52].

Gastrointestinal

Critical care specific gastrointestinal considerations for patients with obesity include the incidence and management of intra-abdominal hypertension and abdominal compartment syndrome as well as nutritional considerations. intra-abdominal hypertension is defined by the World Society of the Abdominal Compartment Syndrome as a sustained or repeated pathological elevation in intra-abdominal pressure (IAP) greater than or equal to 12 mmHg, whereas abdominal compartment syndrome is a sustained IAP of at least 20 mmHg associated with new organ dysfunction or failure [56]. Obesity (BMI >30 kg/m²) is an independent risk factor for intra-abdominal hypertension in the ICU [56–58]; however, it is unclear if the standard definition of intra-abdominal hypertension should apply to obese individuals. In 62 bariatric patients (BMI 37.1–62.6 kg/m²) undergoing elective surgery, mean IAP was 14 mmHg (range 10–18 mmHg), with a positive direct correlation between BMI and IAP [59]. The mechanism for this increase in IAP is thought to be due to a direct mass effect from visceral adiposity [60]. Studies suggest that obese patients have a chronically elevated IAP, leading some to conclude that 'normal' IAP in obese individuals ranges from 7 to 14 mmHg, although whether this leads to a change in the threshold for developing abdominal compartment syndrome remains to be determined [60]. There are no obesity-specific treatment recommendations for abdominal compartment syndrome at this time.

In 2016, the Society of Critical Care Medicine (SCCM) and the American Society for Parenteral and Enteral Nutrition (ASPEN) released updated guidelines for the nutritional support of adult ICU patients, with special provisions for obese patients as outlined here. Guidelines recommend initiating enteral nutrition within 24–48 hours of ICU admission for all patients who cannot sustain volitional intake, including those with obesity [61]. Nutritional support is often delayed in obese critically ill patients, perhaps out of the misconception that these patients have adequate nutritional reserves [62]. In fact, a study in ICU patients with polytrauma demonstrated that those with a BMI greater than 30 kg/m² derived proportionately

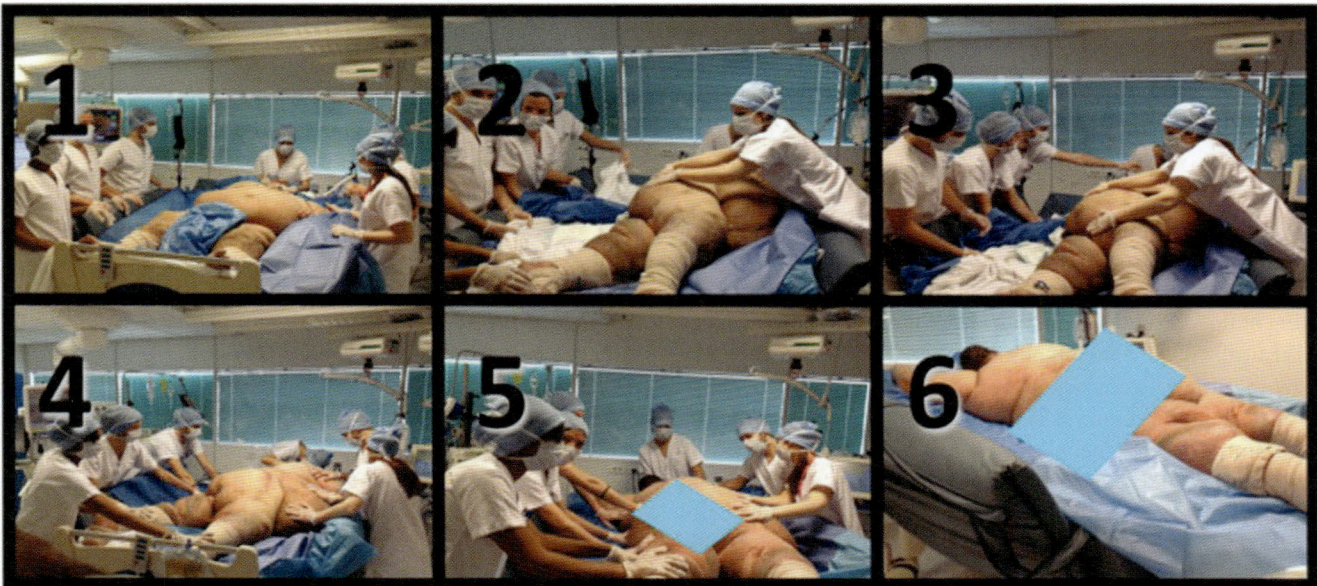

Fig. 33.2 Stepwise repositioning from supine to prone of an ICU patient with obesity. Step 1: the patient is supine and deeply sedated. One operator is at the head of the patient to secure the airway access, three operators are on the right, two on the left, and one is moving to help the others. Step 2: monitors are checked prior to patient movement. The patient is then turned on the left side first. Step 3: the patient is then moved to the other side of the bed to prepare for proning. Step 4: the patient is turned into the prone position. Step 5: upper chest and pelvic supports are placed to ensure free abdominal movements. Step 6: the patient is prone positioned, with a regular checking of compression points, and the head is turned every 2 hours.

more of their energy from protein rather than fat metabolism compared to their lean counterparts, placing obese patients at higher risk for loss of lean body mass [63]. Nutrition is critical for maintaining lean body mass; furthermore, nutritional support provides multiple non-nutritive benefits, such as maintaining gut integrity, decreasing bacterial translocation, and modulating the stress and immune response [61].

For parenteral and enteral nutrition in ICU patients with obesity, SCCM and ASPEN guidelines recommend a high-protein, hypocaloric regimen, with the goal of preserving lean body mass, mobilizing adipose tissue, and minimizing complications from overfeeding [61]. To determine energy requirements, while indirect calorimetry is preferred for all patients regardless of BMI, for patients with obesity, the recommended caloric goal is no more than 65–70% of that determined by indirect calorimetry [61]. If indirect calorimetry is unavailable, guidelines suggest using weight-based calculations to estimate energy requirements: 11–14 kcal/kg TBW/day for patients with a BMI of 30–50 kg/m^2, and 22–25 kcal/kg IBW/day for patients with a BMI greater than 50 kg/m^2 [61]. Protein should be dosed at 2.0 g/kg IBW/day for patients with a BMI of 30–40 kg/m^2 and 2.5 g/kg IBW/day for patients with a BMI of 40 kg/m^2 or greater [61]. No recommendation was made in support of or against any predictive equation, except to note that these equations are less accurate in obese patients [61]. No recommendations were made in support of any immune-modulating nutritional formula or supplement due to a lack of data; however, guidelines do recommend that in patients with a history of bariatric surgery, thiamine supplementation precedes any dextrose administration and that evaluation for commonly associated micronutrient deficiencies (calcium, thiamine, vitamin B$_{12}$, fat-soluble vitamins (A, D, E, K), folate, iron, selenium, zinc, copper) is considered [61].

Renal

An independent association between obesity and acute kidney injury has been noted across a range of critically ill patients, including trauma [64], mixed [65,66], and ARDS patients [67]. The reason for this is unclear but may be related to the chronic inflammatory state of obese individuals, their elevated IAP predisposing them to abdominal compartment syndrome, or an exacerbation of subclinical obesity-related nephropathy [10,68]. The current understanding of the prevention and management of acute kidney injury in the critically ill patient with obesity suffers from insufficient data to draw meaningful conclusions at this time. Therefore, management of acute kidney injury is similar to that of normal-weight patients: optimization of renal perfusion, avoidance or careful dosing of nephrotoxins, and renal replacement therapy as needed. When estimating creatinine clearance in obese patients, using LBW and the Cockcroft–Gault equation appear to be the most accurate unless a timed urine collection is performed [7,10].

Haematology

Obesity and critical illness are recognized independent risk factors for venous thromboembolism (VTE) [6,69–72]. Guidelines were updated in 2012 for the prevention of VTE in orthopaedic surgical

[73], non-orthopaedic surgical [74], and non-surgical patients [75]. For non-surgical patients, the Padua Prediction Score [76] is used to risk stratify patients into low or high risk for VTE; many medical ICU patients with obesity meet criteria for the high-risk category due to their BMI (≥30 kg/m^2) and reduced mobility [75]. For determining VTE risk in surgical patients, the Caprini [72] or the Rogers [77] scores are used in the 2012 guidelines [74], and the Caprini score classifies a BMI greater than 25 kg/m^2 as a risk factor for the development of VTE. Pharmacological VTE prophylaxis is recommended for surgical ICU patients at high VTE risk and medical ICU patients at increased VTE risk, with the addition of mechanical prophylaxis (e.g. sequential compression devices) in the case of post-surgical patients [73–75]. Notably, 2013 guidelines for bariatric surgical patients recommend dual (chemical and mechanical) VTE prophylaxis for all bariatric patients [78]. Guidelines suggest that dosing of enoxaparin, dalteparin, or tinzaparin should be based upon TBW up to a weight of 144 kg, 190 kg, and 165 kg, respectively [79]. Routine ultrasound VTE screening or prophylactic inferior vena cava filter placement a priori is not recommended [74,78].

Infectious disease

For critical care patients with obesity, infectious complications are of particular concern. Patients with a BMI of at least 40 kg/m^2 appear to have an increased risk for the development of pressure ulcers in the ICU [80]. ACS-NSQIP data from 16 major cardiovascular, orthopaedic, and oncological procedure categories revealed that a BMI of at least 40 kg/m^2 significantly increased the odds for wound complications in all surgeries analysed except for pneumonectomy [26]. An increase in infectious complications in surgical patients with obesity has been found across several analyses, including bariatric [81], general surgery [82], and major and minor orthopaedic procedures [83–86]. Potential strategies to minimize infectious complications of surgery include use of minimally invasive approaches when possible, layered closure of incisions, and weight-adjusted antibiotic dosing [26,78,81].

Regarding antimicrobial dosing, as with the dosing of most medications in the critically ill and obese population, due to the limited data available, recommendations are based largely on extrapolation [87]. An excellent 2016 review of the effects of obesity on the pharmacokinetics of antimicrobials in critically ill patients concluded that in general, standard dosing regimens would suffice to achieve pharmacodynamic goals, but that therapeutic drug monitoring should be utilized whenever possible [87]. If weight-based dosing is employed, then LBW is suggested for lipophilic drugs such as fluoroquinolones, glycylcyclines, oxazolidinones, and macrolides and LBW or ABW is suggested for hydrophilic drugs such as beta-lactams, aminoglycosides, glycopeptides (with the exception of using TBW for the loading dose of vancomycin), polymyxins, lipopeptides, and fluconazole [87].

Endocrine

Obesity commonly coexists with metabolic syndrome: a constellation of hypertension, dyslipidaemia, and dysglycaemia [6]. In 2009, multiple national and international organizations released a statement in an attempt to unify the definition of metabolic syndrome to at least three of the following five criteria: elevated waist circumference (no specific cut-off listed as this metric varies by sex, ethnicity, and region); triglyceride levels of at least 150 mg/dL; high-density lipoprotein concentration less than 40 mg/dL in men or less than 50 mg/dL in women; systolic blood pressure of at least 130 mmHg and/or diastolic blood pressure of at least 85 mmHg; and fasting glucose concentration of at least 100 mg/dL [88]. SCCM and ASPEN guidelines recommend assessing obese ICU patients for central adiposity, metabolic syndrome, sarcopenia, BMI greater than 40 kg/m², and the systemic inflammatory response syndrome [61]. It is recommended that obese ICU patients receiving supplemental nutrition should be monitored for worsening of hyperglycaemia, hyperlipidaemia, hypercapnia, fluid overload, and hepatic fat accumulation [61].

Outcomes

Despite evidence of increased complications in critically ill patients with obesity, the relationship between obesity and mortality is unclear. Reports have indicated a range of outcomes from no association [39,89–91], a positive association [92–94], an inverse association [95], to a 'U'- or 'J'-shaped association (where mortality is highest for patients with a BMI <25 kg/m² and ≥40 kg/m² and lowest for patients with a BMI of 25–39.9 kg/m²) [96,97]. The conflicting nature of these findings suggests that additional variables may need to be accounted for, in the analysis of outcomes data.

The cause of ICU admission seems to influence outcomes for patients with obesity, with trauma being linked most closely to increased mortality [94,97]. Other variables affecting survival, such as increased age or disease severity, positive smoking status, and recent weight loss, are often correlated with a decreased BMI, yet are not always considered in analyses [6]. Multivariate analyses may help account for these variables. Research strategies to provide clarity include a more refined BMI stratification or definition of obesity and limiting analyses to long-term survival to avoid reverse causation (where decreased BMI is not inherently associated with decreased survival, but rather is a marker of disease severity, poor prognosis, and decreased survival) [6]. Although BMI is a convenient tool by which to measure obesity, stratifying obesity by the presence or absence of abdominal (versus peripheral) obesity and/or metabolic syndrome may be more appropriate and useful for outcomes research [6]. Several studies demonstrate that measures of central obesity such as waist circumference, sagittal diameter, waist-to-hip ratio, or CT scans have a stronger association with ICU mortality [94,97]. Using these measures may help allocate resources for patients at highest risk for poor outcomes and clarify associations between obesity and mortality in future studies in this patient population.

CASE REPORT

A 47-year-old morbidly obese (BMI 72 kg/m²) woman is admitted to the surgical intensive care unit (SICU) after intramedullary nailing of a femoral fracture sustained 1 day ago after a fall from standing in the shower. The intraoperative course was complicated by hypoxia necessitating a fraction of inspired oxygen (FiO₂) of 100% on 5 cmH₂O of PEEP for an oxygen saturation of 95%. Due to hypoxia, the patient was left intubated postoperatively and was admitted to the SICU.

On postoperative day 1, the patient developed bilateral patchy pulmonary opacities on chest X-ray and continued to have pulmonary difficulties. She had been mechanically ventilated using volume-controlled ventilation with V_T of 4 mL/kg IBW, P_{plat} of 30 cmH₂O, PEEP of 14 cmH₂O, and FiO₂ of 80% resulting in an arterial blood gas (ABG) showing pH 7.22, PaCO₂ 70 mmHg, PaO₂ 61 mmHg. An oesophageal balloon was placed and pleural pressures were measured at 25 cmH₂O; based on these results, PEEP was uptitrated to 25 cmH₂O and V_T was increased to 6 mL/kg IBW with resulting P_{plat} = 47 cmH₂O.

By postoperative day 2 the patient's ventilator settings were volume-controlled ventilation, V_T 6 mL/kg IBW, P_{plat} 45 cmH₂O, FiO₂ 60%, PEEP 25 cmH₂O, ABG showing pH 7.38, PaCO₂ 49 mmHg, PaO₂ 60 mmHg. On postoperative day 3, patient ABG and ventilator settings remained stable and oesophageal pressures remained at 25 cmH₂O. In attempt to further wean FiO₂, PEEP was increased to 30 cmH₂O. Over the course of the day, FiO₂ was able to be weaned to 40%; however, urine output, which had previously been within normal limits, decreased to 10 mL/hour with a concomitant increase in serum creatinine from 0.9 mg/dL to 1.6 mg/dL. Due to the temporal association between the increase in PEEP and the development of oliguria, abdominal compartment syndrome from high intrathoracic pressures was strongly suspected. In response, on postoperative day 4, PEEP was decreased to 20 cmH₂O. The patient remained stable from a respiratory standpoint with ABG 7.39, PaCO₂ 47 mmHg, PaO₂ 68 mmHg on FiO₂ 40% on V_T 6 mL/kg IBW, and urine output increased to greater than 30 mL/hour with concomitant decrease in serum creatinine to 1.4 mg/dL. Throughout the course of postoperative day 5, the patient tolerated a PEEP wean to 7 cmH₂O and renal function continued to return to baseline. On postoperative day 6, after a successful spontaneous breathing trial on pressure support ventilation at 7 cmH₂O of inspiratory pressure, 5 cmH₂O of PEEP and FiO₂ 40%, the patient was extubated successfully to nasal cannula.

REFERENCES

1. Devlin JW, Skrobik Y, Gelinas C, Needham DM, Slooter AJC, Pandharipande PP, et al. Clinical practice guidelines for the prevention and management of pain, agitation/sedation, delirium, immobility, and sleep disruption in adult patients in the ICU. Crit Care Med. 2018;**46**(9):825–873.
2. King DR, Velmahos GC. Difficulties in managing the surgical patient who is morbidly obese. Crit Care Med. 2010;**38**(9 Suppl):S478–82.
3. Aantaa R, Tonner P, Conti G, Longrois D, Mantz J, Mulier JP. Sedation options for the morbidly obese intensive care unit patient: a concise survey and an agenda for development. Multidiscip Respir Med. 2015;**10**(1):8.
4. Crummy F, Piper AJ, Naughton MT. Obesity and the lung: 2. Obesity and sleep-disordered breathing. Thorax. 2008;**63**(8):738–46.
5. Walz JM, Zayaruzny M, Heard SO. Airway management in critical illness. Chest. 2007;**131**(2):608–20.
6. Tsai A, Schumann R. Morbid obesity and perioperative complications. Curr Opin Anaesthesiol. 2016;**29**(1):103–108.

7. Erstad BL. Designing drug regimens for special intensive care unit populations. Pediatr Crit Care Med. 2015;**4**(2):139–51.

8. Ely EW, Truman B, Shintani A, Thomason JWW, Wheeler AP, Gordon S, et al. Monitoring sedation status over time in ICU patients: reliability and validity of the Richmond Agitation-Sedation Scale (RASS). JAMA. 2003;**289**(22):2983–91.

9. Riker RR, Fraser GL, Simmons LE, Wilkins ML. Validating the Sedation-Agitation Scale with the Bispectral Index and Visual Analog Scale in adult ICU patients after cardiac surgery. Intensive Care Med. 2001;**27**(5):853–58.

10. Bucaloiu ID, Perkins RM, DiFilippo W, Yahya T, Norfolk E. Acute kidney injury in the critically ill, morbidly obese patient: diagnostic and therapeutic challenges in a unique patient population. Crit Care Clin. 2010;**26**(4):607–24.

11. Brown DL, Masselink AJ, Lalla CD. Functional range of creatinine clearance for renal drug dosing: a practical solution to the controversy of which weight to use in the Cockcroft-Gault equation. Ann Pharmacother. 2013;**47**(7–8):1039–44.

12. Servin F, Farinotti R, Haberer JP, Desmonts JM. Propofol infusion for maintenance of anesthesia in morbidly obese patients receiving nitrous oxide. A clinical and pharmacokinetic study. Anesthesiology. 1993;**78**(4):657–65.

13. Adler J, Malone D. Early mobilization in the intensive care unit: a systematic review. Cardiopulm Phys Ther J. 2012;**23**(1):5–13.

14. Parker A, Needham D. The Importance of Early Rehabilitation and Mobility in the ICU. Society of Critical Care Medicine, 2013. http://www.sccm.org/Communications/Critical-Connections/Archives/Pages/Importance-Early-Rehabilitation-Mobility-ICU.aspx

15. Society of Critical Care Medicine. The Importance of Early Rehabilitation and Mobility in the ICU. Critical Connections. August/September 2013. http://vhms.com/wp-content/uploads/2015/04/BArticle%20-%20Mobility%20in%20the%20ICU%204-8-15.pdf

16. Arnold M, Roe E, Williams D. A pictorial overview of technology-assisted care options for bariatric patients: one hospital's experience. Ostomy Wound Manage. 2014;**60**(1):36–42.

17. Newell MA, Bard MR, Goettler CE, Toschlog EA, Schenarts PJ, Sagraves SG, et al. Body mass index and outcomes in critically injured blunt trauma patients: weighing the impact. J Am Coll Surg. 2007;**204**(5):1056–61.

18. Carrara FSA, Zanei SSV, Cremasco MF, Whitaker IY. Outcomes and nursing workload related to obese patients in the intensive care unit. Intensive Crit Care Nurs. 2016;**35**:45–51.

19. Davidson JE, Callery C. Care of the obesity surgery patient requiring immediate-level care or intensive care. Obes Surg. 2001;**11**(1):93–97.

20. Hignett S, Griffiths P. Manual handling risks in the bariatric (obese) patient pathway in acute sector, community and ambulance care and treatment. Work. 2009;**33**(2):175–80.

21. Modica MJ, Kanal KM, Gunn ML. The obese emergency patient: imaging challenges and solutions. Radiographics. 2011;**31**(3):811–23.

22. Radiology Rounds. Imaging and obese patients. July 2005. http://www.mghradrounds.org/clientuploads/july_2005/july_2005.pdf

23. Ginde AA, Foianini A, Renner DM, Valley M, Camargo CA Jr. The challenge of CT and MRI imaging of obese individuals who present to the emergency department: a national survey. Obesity. 2008;**16**(11):2549–51.

24. Sarracanie M, LaPierre CD, Salameh N, Waddington DEJ, Witzel T, Rosen MS. Low-cost high-performance MRI. Sci Rep. 2015;**5**:15177.

25. Hernandez AV, Kaw R, Pasupuleti V, Bina P, Ioannidis JPA, Bueno H, et al. Association between obesity and postoperative atrial fibrillation in patients undergoing cardiac operations: a systematic review and meta-analysis. Ann Thorac Surg. 2013;**96**(3):1104–16.

26. Sood A, Abdollah F, Sammon JD, Majumder K, Schmid M, Peabody JO, et al. The effect of body mass index on perioperative outcomes after major surgery: results from the National Surgical Quality Improvement Program (ACS-NSQIP) 2005–2011. World J Surg. 2015;**39**(10):2376–85.

27. Fukuchi H, Nakashima M, Araki R, Komiya N, Hayano M, Yano K, et al. Effect of obesity on serum amiodarone concentration in Japanese patients: population pharmacokinetic investigation by multiple trough screen analysis. J Clin Pharm Ther. 2009;**34**(3):329–36.

28. Erstad BL. Dosing of medications in morbidly obese patients in the intensive care unit setting. Intensive Care Med. 2004;**30**(1):18–32.

29. Varon J, Marik P. Management of the obese critically ill patient. Crit Care Clin. 2001;**17**(1):187–200.

30. Brusasco C, Corradi F, Zattoni PL, Launo C, Leykin Y, Palermo S. Ultrasound-guided central venous cannulation in bariatric patients. Obes Surg. 2009;**19**(10):1365–70.

31. Hibbert K, Rice M, Malhotra A. Obesity and ARDS. Chest. 2012;**142**(3):785–90.

32. McGrath TM, Farabaugh EA, Pickett MJ, Wagner DK, Griswold-Theodorson S. Obesity hinders ultrasound visualization of the subclavian vein: implications for central venous access. J Vasc Access. 2012;**13**(2):246–50.

33. Lipshutz AKM, Gropper MA. Central venous catheters: follow the evidence, not the guidelines. Crit Care Med. 2012;**40**(8):2528–29.

34. Marik PE, Flemmer M, Harrison W. The risk of catheter-related bloodstream infection with femoral venous catheters as compared to subclavian and internal jugular venous catheters: a systematic review of the literature and meta-analysis. Crit Care Med. 2012;**40**(8):2479–85.

35. Parienti J-J, Thirion M, Mégarbane B, Souweine B, Ouchikhe A, Polito A, et al. Femoral vs jugular venous catheterization and risk of nosocomial events in adults requiring acute renal replacement therapy: a randomized controlled trial. JAMA. 2008;**299**(20):2413–22.

36. Extracorporeal Life Support Organization. Guidelines. ECMO and ECLS. http://www.elso.org/resources/Guidelines.aspx

37. Kon ZN, Dahi S, Evans CF, Byrnes KA, Bittle GJ, Wehman B, et al. Class III obesity is not a contraindication to venovenous extracorporeal membrane oxygenation support. Ann Thorac Surg. 2015;**100**(5):1855–60.

38. Swol J, Buchwald D, Dudda M, Strauch J, Schildhauer TA. Veno-venous extracorporeal membrane oxygenation in obese surgical patients with hypercapnic lung failure. Acta Anaesthesiol Scand. 2014;**58**(5):534–38.

39. Anzueto A, Frutos-Vivar F, Esteban A, Bensalami N, Marks D, Raymondos K, et al. Influence of body mass index on outcome of the mechanically ventilated patients. Thorax. 2011;**66**(1):66–73.

40. Jones SF, Brito V, Ghamande S. Obesity hypoventilation syndrome in the critically ill. Crit Care Clin. 2015;**31**(3):419–34.

41. Behazin N, Jones SB, Cohen RI, Loring SH. Respiratory restriction and elevated pleural and esophageal pressures in morbid obesity. J Appl Physiol. 2010;**108**(1):212–18.

42. Talmor DS, Fessler HE. Are esophageal pressure measurements important in clinical decision-making in mechanically ventilated patients? Respir Care. 2010;55(2):162–72.

43. Pirrone M, Fisher D, Chipman D, Imber DAE, Corona J, Mietto C, et al. Recruitment maneuvers and positive end-expiratory pressure titration in morbidly obese ICU patients. Crit Care Med. 2016;44(2):300–307.

44. De Jong A, Molinari N, Pouzeratte Y, Verzilli D, Chanques G, Jung B, et al. Difficult intubation in obese patients: incidence, risk factors, and complications in the operating theatre and in intensive care units. Br J Anaesth. 2015;114(2):297–306.

45. Frat J-P, Gissot V, Ragot S, Desachy A, Runge I, Lebert C, et al. Impact of obesity in mechanically ventilated patients: a prospective study. Intensive Care Med. 2008;34(11):1991–98.

46. Collins JS, Lemmens HJM, Brodsky JB, Brock-Utne JG, Levitan RM. Laryngoscopy and morbid obesity: a comparison of the 'sniff' and 'ramped' positions. Obes Surg. 2004;14(9):1171–75.

47. Network TARDS. Ventilation with lower tidal volumes as compared with traditional tidal volumes for acute lung injury and the acute respiratory distress syndrome. N Engl J Med. 2000;342(18):1301–308.

48. Slutsky AS, Ranieri VM. Ventilator-induced lung injury. N Engl J Med. 2013;369(22):2126–36.

49. Talmor D, Sarge T, Malhotra A, O'Donnell CR, Ritz R, Lisbon A, et al. Mechanical ventilation guided by esophageal pressure in acute lung injury. N Engl J Med. 2008;359(20):2095–104.

50. Fish E, Novack V, Banner-Goodspeed VM, Sarge T, Loring S, Talmor D. The Esophageal Pressure-Guided Ventilation 2 (EPVent2) trial protocol: a multicentre, randomised clinical trial of mechanical ventilation guided by transpulmonary pressure. BMJ Open. 2014;4(9):e006356.

51. Lemyze M, Mallat J, Duhamel A, Pepy F, Gasan G, Barrailler S, et al. Effects of sitting position and applied positive end-expiratory pressure on respiratory mechanics of critically ill obese patients receiving mechanical ventilation. Crit Care Med. 2013;41(11):2592–99.

52. De Jong A, Molinari N, Sebbane M, Prades A, Futier E, Jung B, et al. Feasibility and effectiveness of prone position in morbidly obese patients with ARDS: a case-control clinical study. Chest. 2013;143(6):1554–61.

53. ClinicalTrials.gov. Protective ventilation with higher versus lower PEEP during general anesthesia for surgery in obese patients. ClinicalTrials.gov Identifier: NCT02148692. https://clinicaltrials.gov/ct2/show/NCT02148692

54. Burns SM, Egloff MB, Ryan B, Carpenter R, Burns JE. Effect of body position on spontaneous respiratory rate and tidal volume in patients with obesity, abdominal distension and ascites. Am J Crit Care. 1994;3(2):102–106.

55. Guérin C, Reignier J, Richard J-C, Beuret P, Gacouin A, Boulain T, et al. Prone positioning in severe acute respiratory distress syndrome. N Engl J Med. 2013;368(23):2159–68.

56. Kirkpatrick AW, Roberts DJ, De Waele J, Jaeschke R, Malbrain MLNG, De Keulenaer B, et al. Intra-abdominal hypertension and the abdominal compartment syndrome: updated consensus definitions and clinical practice guidelines from the World Society of the Abdominal Compartment Syndrome. Intensive Care Med. 2013;39(7):1190–206.

57. Iyer D, Rastogi P, Åneman A, D'Amours S. Early screening to identify patients at risk of developing intra-abdominal hypertension and abdominal compartment syndrome. Acta Anaesthesiol Scand. 2014;58(10):1267–75.

58. Holodinsky JK, Roberts DJ, Ball CG, Blaser AR, Starkopf J, Zygun DA, et al. Risk factors for intra-abdominal hypertension and abdominal compartment syndrome among adult intensive care unit patients: a systematic review and meta-analysis. Crit Care. 2013;17(5):R249.

59. Frezza EE, Shebani KO, Robertson J, Wachtel MS. Morbid obesity causes chronic increase of intraabdominal pressure. Dig Dis Sci. 2007;52(4):1038–41.

60. Malbrain MLNG, De Keulenaer BL, Oda J, De Laet I, De Waele JJ, Roberts DJ, et al. Intra-abdominal hypertension and abdominal compartment syndrome in burns, obesity, pregnancy, and general medicine. Anaesthesiol Intensive Ther. 2015;47(3):228–40.

61. Taylor BE, Mc Clave SA, Martindale RG, Warren MM, Johnson DR, Braunschweig C, et al. Guidelines for the provision and assessment of nutrition support therapy in the adult critically ill patient: Society of Critical Care Medicine (SCCM) and American Society for Parenteral and Enteral Nutrition (A.S.P.E.N.). Crit Care Med. 2016;44(2):390–438.

62. Borel A-L, Schwebel C, Planquette B, Vésin A, Garrouste-Orgeas M, Adrie C, et al. Initiation of nutritional support is delayed in critically ill obese patients: a multicenter cohort study. Am J Clin Nutr. 2014;100(3):859–66.

63. Jeevanandam M, Young DH, Schiller WR. Obesity and the metabolic response to severe multiple trauma in man. J Clin Invest. 1991;87(1):262–69.

64. Shashaty MGS, Meyer NJ, Localio AR, Gallop R, Bellamy SL, Holena DN, et al. African American race, obesity, and blood product transfusion are risk factors for acute kidney injury in critically ill trauma patients. J Crit Care. 2012;27(5):496–504.

65. Druml W, Metnitz B, Schaden E, Bauer P, Metnitz PG. Impact of body mass on incidence and prognosis of acute kidney injury requiring renal replacement therapy. Intensive Care Med. 2010;36(7):1221–28.

66. Danziger J, Chen KP, Lee J, Feng M, Mark RG, Celi LA, et al. Obesity, acute kidney injury, and mortality in critical illness. Crit Care Med. 2016;44(2):328–34.

67. Soto GJ, Frank AJ, Christiani DC, Gong MN. Body mass index and acute kidney injury in the acute respiratory distress syndrome. Crit Care Med. 2012;40(9):2601–608.

68. Shashaty MGS, Kalkan E, Bellamy SL, Reilly JP, Holena DN, Cummins K, et al. Computed tomography-defined abdominal adiposity is associated with acute kidney injury in critically ill trauma patients. Crit Care Med. 2014;42(7):1619–28.

69. Fontaine GV, Vigil E, Wohlt PD, Lloyd JF, Evans RS, Collingridge DS, et al. Venous thromboembolism in critically ill medical patients receiving chemoprophylaxis: a focus on obesity and other risk factors. Clin Appl Thromb Hemost. 2016;22(3):265–73.

70. Wang L, Pryor AD, Altieri MS, L. Romeiser J, Talamini MA, Shroyer L, et al. Perioperative rates of deep vein thrombosis and pulmonary embolism in normal weight vs obese and morbidly obese surgical patients in the era post venous thromboembolism prophylaxis guidelines. Am J Surg. 2015;210(5):859–63.

71. Vandiver JW, Ritz LI, Lalama JT. Chemical prophylaxis to prevent venous thromboembolism in morbid obesity: literature review and dosing recommendations. J Thromb Thrombolysis. 2016;41(3):475–81.

72. Caprini JA. Thrombosis risk assessment as a guide to quality patient care. Dis Mon. 2005;51(2–3):70–78.

73. Falck-Ytter Y, Francis CW, Johanson NA, Curley C, Dahl OE, Schulman S, et al. Prevention of VTE in orthopedic surgery patients: Antithrombotic Therapy and Prevention of Thrombosis, 9th ed: American College of Chest Physicians

Evidence-Based Clinical Practice Guidelines. Chest. 2012;**141**(2 Suppl):e278S–325S.

74. Gould MK, Garcia DA, Wren SM, Karanicolas PJ, Arcelus JI, Heit JA, et al. Prevention of VTE in nonorthopedic surgical patients: Antithrombotic Therapy and Prevention of Thrombosis, 9th ed: American College of Chest Physicians Evidence-Based Clinical Practice Guidelines. Chest. 2012;**141**(2 Suppl):e227S–77S.

75. Kahn SR, Lim W, Dunn AS, Cushman M, Dentali F, Akl EA, et al. Prevention of VTE in nonsurgical patients: Antithrombotic Therapy and Prevention of Thrombosis, 9th ed: American College of Chest Physicians Evidence-Based Clinical Practice Guidelines. Chest. 2012;**141**(2 Suppl):e195S–226S.

76. Barbar S, Noventa F, Rossetto V, Ferrari A, Brandolin B, Perlati M, et al. A risk assessment model for the identification of hospitalized medical patients at risk for venous thromboembolism: the Padua Prediction Score. J Thromb Haemost. 2010;**8**(11):2450–57.

77. Rogers SO Jr, Kilaru RK, Hosokawa P, Henderson WG, Zinner MJ, Khuri SF. Multivariable predictors of postoperative venous thromboembolic events after general and vascular surgery: results from the patient safety in surgery study. J Am Coll Surg. 2007;**204**(6):1211–21.

78. Mechanick JI, Youdim A, Jones DB, Garvey WT, Hurley DL, McMahon MM, et al. Clinical practice guidelines for the perioperative nutritional, metabolic, and nonsurgical support of the bariatric surgery patient--2013 update: cosponsored by American Association of Clinical Endocrinologists, the Obesity Society, and American Society for Metabolic & Bariatric Surgery. Endocr Pract. 2013;**19**(2):337–72.

79. Garcia DA, Baglin TP, Weitz JI, Samama MM, American College of Chest Physicians. Parenteral anticoagulants: Antithrombotic Therapy and Prevention of Thrombosis, 9th ed: American College of Chest Physicians Evidence-Based Clinical Practice Guidelines. Chest. 2012;**141**(2 Suppl):e24S–43S.

80. Hyun S, Li X, Vermillion B, Newton C, Fall M, Kaewprag P, et al. Body mass index and pressure ulcers: improved predictability of pressure ulcers in intensive care patients. Am J Crit Care. 2014;**23**(6):494–500.

81. Chen SY, Stem M, Schweitzer MA, Magnuson TH, Lidor AO. Assessment of postdischarge complications after bariatric surgery: a National Surgical Quality Improvement Program analysis. Surgery. 2015;**158**(3):777–86.

82. Tjeertes EEKM, Hoeks SSE, Beks SSBJC, Valentijn TTM, Hoofwijk AAGM, Stolker RJRJ. Obesity—a risk factor for postoperative complications in general surgery? BMC Anesthesiol. 2015;**15**:112.

83. Ward DT, Metz LN, Horst PK, Kim HT, Kuo AC. Complications of Morbid Obesity in total joint arthroplasty: risk stratification based on BMI. J Arthroplasty. 2015;**30**(9 Suppl):42–46.

84. Werner BC, Burrus MT, Looney AM, Park JS, Perumal V, Cooper MT. Obesity is associated with increased complications after

operative management of end-stage ankle arthritis. Foot Ankle Int. 2015;**36**(8):863–70.

85. Werner BC, Burrus MT, Browne JA, Brockmeier SF. Superobesity (body mass index >50 kg/m(2)) and complications after total shoulder arthroplasty: an incremental effect of increasing body mass index. J Shoulder Elbow Surg. 2015;**24**(12):1868–75.

86. Werner BC, Griffin JW, Yang S, Brockmeier SF, Gwathmey FW. Obesity is associated with increased postoperative complications after operative management of proximal humerus fractures. J Shoulder Elbow Surg. 2015;**24**(4):593–600.

87. Alobaid AS, Hites M, Lipman J, Taccone FS, Roberts JA. Effect of obesity on the pharmacokinetics of antimicrobials in critically ill patients: a structured review. Int J Antimicrob Agents. 2016;**47**(4):259–68.

88. Alberti KGMM, Eckel RH, Grundy SM, Zimmet PZ, Cleeman JI, Donato KA, et al. Harmonizing the metabolic syndrome: a joint interim statement of the International Diabetes Federation Task Force on Epidemiology and Prevention; National Heart, Lung, and Blood Institute; American Heart Association; World Heart Federation; International Atherosclerosis Society; and International Association for the Study of Obesity. Circulation. 2009;**120**(16):1640–45.

89. Wardell S, Wall A, Bryce R, Gjevre JA, Laframboise K, Reid JK. The association between obesity and outcomes in critically ill patients. Can Respir J. 2015;**22**(1):23–30.

90. Lee CK, Tefera E, Colice G. The effect of obesity on outcomes in mechanically ventilated patients in a medical intensive care unit. Respiration. 2014;**87**(3):219–26.

91. Devarajan J, Vydyanathan A, You J, Xu M, Sessler DI, Sabik JF, et al. The association between body mass index and outcome after coronary artery bypass grafting operations. Eur J Cardiothorac Surg. 2016;**50**(2):344–49.

92. Kumar G, Majumdar T, Jacobs ER, Danesh V, Dagar G, Deshmukh A, et al. Outcomes of morbidly obese patients receiving invasive mechanical ventilation: a nationwide analysis. Chest. 2013;**144**(1):48–54.

93. Joseph B, Hadeed S, Haider AA, Ditillo M, Joseph A, Pandit V, et al. Obesity and trauma mortality: Sizing up the risks in motor vehicle crashes. Obes Res Clin Pract. 2017;**11**(1):72–78.

94. Joseph B, Zangbar B, Haider AA, Kulvatunyou N, Khalil M, Tang A, et al. Hips don't lie: Waist-to-hip ratio in trauma patients. J Trauma Acute Care Surg. 2015;**79**(6):1055–61.

95. Ray JJ, Satahoo SS, Meizoso JP, Allen CJ, Teisch LF, Proctor KG, et al. Does obesity affect outcomes of adult burn patients? J Surg Res. 2015;**198**(2):450–55.

96. Pickkers P, de Keizer N, Dusseljee J, Weerheijm D, van der Hoeven JG, Peek N. Body mass index is associated with hospital mortality in critically ill patients: an observational cohort study. Crit Care Med. 2013;**41**(8):1878–83.

97. Gharib M, Kaul S, LoCurto J, Perez M, Hajri T. The obesity factor in critical illness: between consensus and controversy. J Trauma Acute Care Surg. 2015;**78**(4):866–73.

Obesity and trauma

Maureen McCunn, Justin Richards, and Karla Greco .

Introduction

According to the United States Centers for Disease Control and Prevention, more than one-third of adults are obese [1] and over the next 20 years, a 33% increase in obesity and a 130% increase in severe obesity prevalence are predicted [2]. As the percentage of obese Americans escalates, the number of injuries this population experiences will increase. Conflicting data exist as to whether or not obesity is a true risk factor that increases mortality following trauma. A meta-analysis concluded that the overall mortality for obese trauma patients was 7.7% and for non-obese patients only 4.7%. This study also found a higher incidence of acute respiratory distress syndrome, acute kidney injury, and multiorgan failure in obese trauma patients [3]. In yet another study, obese trauma patients experience a higher mortality rate, increased number of hospital days, and multiple comorbidities [4]. Conversely, a retrospective study that analysed patients with a body mass index (BMI) greater than or equal to 40 kg/m² compared with a BMI less than 40 kg/m² did not find a link between morbid obesity and mortality in critically ill trauma patients [5,6]. What we currently know about the effect obesity has on traumatic injury is based on retrospective analysis and registry data. Anaesthesiologists must be familiar with common coexisting comorbidities in the obese and be able to tailor care accordingly.

Traumatic injury and complications

Many single-centre studies have been conducted to determine the impact obesity has on the morbidity and mortality of critically injured trauma patients. Although there is limited literature to suggest obese patients demonstrate a certain pattern of injuries, those who are obese suffer lower incidences of intracranial and intra-abdominal injuries compared to higher incidences of pulmonary contusions, rib fractures, and pelvic fractures [7]. Bochicchio et al. demonstrated in a prospective study of 1167 patients admitted to the intensive care unit (ICU), that obese patients developed almost twice as many urinary tract infections, central line-associated bloodstream infections, and pneumonia compared to those who were non-obese [7]. Additionally, they found a statistically significant increase in hospital length of stay (25 vs 15 days) and ICU

length of stay (19 vs 11 days) in the obese versus non-obese groups, respectively [7]. These findings were supported by Ciesla et al.'s study that demonstrated multiorgan failure was 1.8 times more likely to develop in obese patients compared to non-obese patients, but they did not have a higher mortality rate [8]. Most multiorgan failure develops within 72 hours of a trauma, which the authors proposed is a result of the proinflammatory response incited by the trauma [8].

Trauma patients often arrive in a state of shock, most commonly as a result of hypovolaemia due to haemorrhage. Obese patients in haemorrhagic shock after blunt injury do poorly. Those with a BMI greater than 40 kg/m² tend to develop acute respiratory distress syndrome and are more likely to have a cardiac arrest compared to normal-weight patients. A BMI greater than 40 kg/m² is an independent risk factor for mortality after blunt traumatic haemorrhagic shock [9].

When it comes to penetrating injuries, obesity may have a protective effect. Based on a review of 249 patients over 12 years with abdominal stab, violation of peritoneum, injury to visceral organ, and injury requiring surgery all varied based on BMI. The abbreviated injury score for both chest and abdomen and the overall injury severity score decreased as BMI increased in stab wounds. Patients with a BMI less than 18.5 kg/m² were three times more likely to need surgery, suggesting that the additional adipose tissue may offer a protective and survival benefit.

Inflammation

Obesity is associated with elevated baseline levels of inflammatory mediators such as tumour necrosis factor (TNF) alpha, interleukin (IL)-6, and leptin, which are secreted by adipose tissue [10]. A positive correlation can be seen in the severity of inflammation and BMI [11]. This proinflammatory state is exacerbated after a traumatic injury with elevations in proinflammatory cytokines such as IL-1, IL-2, IL-6, IL-12, and TNF alpha, potentially leading to a multiorgan dysfunction or failure [12]. This proinflammatory state leads to an increase in the conversion of good M1 macrophages to harmful M2 macrophages and good helper T cells to harmful helper T-17 cells and is exacerbated by traumatic injury [13]. Ciesla et al.'s study demonstrated that early multiorgan failure (within 72 hours of injury) developed in 73% of obese patients versus only 48% of non-obese patients, supporting the idea that the hyperinflammatory state of obesity is worsened after trauma [8]. The higher incidence of infection may be related not only to the proinflammatory environment, but the altered neutrophil function associated with impaired glucose metabolism and insulin resistance that affects obese patients [8]. Despite the possible protective effect of obesity following penetrating trauma, it has been reported that obese patients are 1.6–5.6 times more likely to suffer mortality than non-obese trauma patients overall in all injury patterns [8].

C-reactive protein (CRP), an acute phase protein produced by hepatocytes, is an inflammatory marker that decreases the production of adiponectin, an anti-inflammatory mediator [14,15]. CRP, used to determine systemic inflammation [15], has been shown to be elevated in obese patients with a maximum rise on day 4 after injury [15]. Though CRP levels between obese and non-obese trauma patient were not statistically significant, highest levels were noted in obese patients [14]. Obese patients have also been shown to have significant elevations IL-6 levels on admission to the trauma centre compared to those who are not obese [14]. Both elevated IL=6 levels and CRP levels have a positive correlation with an increased incidence in developing multiorgan dysfunction [14].

Traumatic brain injury

Based on records of blunt injury analysed by Boulanger et al., obese patients were less likely to suffer from severe brain injury [16]. However, a retrospective study looking at motor vehicle crash data from the Crashworthiness Data System (part of the National Automotive Sampling System in the United States) refutes this. Front-seat obese patients are more likely to suffer from severe head trauma and have almost double the risk of mortality as a non-obese front-seat passenger [17]. A proposed suggestion is that restraint systems are designed for average weight males, not obese passengers—therefore, this may put them at increased risk for bodily harm. In another study, obese patients with traumatic brain injury were found to have higher rates of mortality than non-obese patients; however, stepwise logistic regression did not find obesity to be a risk factor for mortality [18].

Orthopaedic injuries

In high-velocity trauma, the odds of sustaining an injury are 48% greater in the morbidly obese [19]. In motor vehicle crashes, energy is transferred from the abdomen to the pelvis, resulting in pelvic ring injuries. In obese patients, this surgical repair has a 6.8 times higher complication rate and 4.7 times higher need for surgical reoperation rate for patients with a BMI greater than 30 kg/m² compared to those with a BMI less than 30kg/m² [20]. Increased BMI is associated with a twofold increase in upper extremity injuries [21].

In a retrospective case–control study by Weinlein et al., morbidly obese patients who had undergone a reamed intramedullary nailing of a closed femoral shaft fracture had increased odds of developing acute respiratory distress syndrome and sepsis. The overall mortality rate for a closed femoral fracture was 1.6%, but in the morbidly obese with an injury severity score greater than 17, the mortality rate was 20% [22]. (The injury severity score is a score that assesses trauma severity which correlates with morbidity, mortality, and hospitalization. A score greater than 15 is considered major trauma [23].)

Initial assessment

The initial assessment of the obese trauma patient usually begins with the first responders such as emergency medical services. Anaesthesiologists are not customarily a part of the first response pre-hospital team in the United States (as they are in Europe) and at many trauma centres, may not meet the patient until arrival in the operating room [24]. It is important to have an understanding of pre-hospital protocols in order to appreciate the challenges that emergency medical services may have while caring for an obese patient. Physically moving patients, establishing and maintaining cervical spine precautions, and placing intravenous (IV) access can all be arduous. Ambulances have weight restrictions on their stretchers and helicopters may not be able to transport morbidly obese patients when the barometric pressure is high [25]. Having appropriate-sized equipment such as blood pressure measurement devices, tourniquets, traction devices, and temporary splints is essential for emergency preparedness.

Once the patient arrives in the trauma bay, initial assessment by the medical team begins with the doctrines of the Advanced Trauma Life Support® (ATLS®) programme. The primary survey identifies life-threatening injuries while focusing on airway, breathing, circulation, neurological status, and resuscitation [5]. Once complete, the secondary survey begins with a medical history when feasible and full physical examination, which includes evaluating skin folds for lacerations, punctures, and soft tissue swelling. Identifying injuries in both the physical examination and radiographic acquisition can be limited due to body habitus. Motor and sensory function can be challenging to assess; therefore, it is recommended that symmetry be used as a tool to identify discrepancies and any irregularities need to be further evaluated.

Many obese patients have multiple comorbidities such as hypertension, diabetes mellitus, and obstructive sleep apnoea (OSA)—each can compromise the cardiac, pulmonary, gastrointestinal, and endocrine systems. Any of these can restrict full physiological compensation to haemorrhage or severe traumatic injury. The obese can have increased cardiac output and lower peripheral resistance compared to normal-weight patients [26]. Over time, excessive blood volume leads to left ventricle hypertrophy [27]. Fat can infiltrate the heart, causing conduction system disturbances [28]. Patients who have had a myocardial infarction are often put on an angiotensin-converting enzyme inhibitor, which disrupts the renin–angiotensin feedback loop, further altering the impaired cardiovascular status [29–31]. In response to a stressful traumatic event, cortisol levels increase causing hyperglycaemia [32]. Stress-induced hyperglycaemia is associated with a higher mortality rate in trauma [33]. Obese patients can also suffer from obesity hypoventilation syndrome and OSA. In extreme cases, this can lead to right heart failure [34]. Cardiac rhythm disturbances, decreased cardiac output, metabolic anomalies, and pulmonary disturbances may be further affected by anaesthesia. A young, healthy patient may tolerate such disturbances, but a critically ill patient may not have the cardiac or pulmonary reserve to compensate. This is important to keep in mind when trying to decide what is an acceptable blood pressure and heart rate for perfusing organs and what ventilator settings may be most appropriate in such circumstances.

Airway management

There are a variety of medical personnel that may be the first to assess the airway. Preparation and anticipation for a potentially difficult airway in the obese trauma patient is necessary in order to optimize a successful first attempt intubation. There should be clear and established communication between involved providers. The initial airway assessment should include a brief, yet focused physical examination, concentrating on neck circumference, facial hair, thyromental distance, and Mallampati score. Confirmation of past medical history and physical examination may provide valuable information prior to airway intervention. The mnemonic 'AMPLE' (Allergies, Medications, Past medical history, Last meal, Events surrounding the traumatic incident) [5] is often helpful, and it may be insightful to ask, 'Have you ever been told you had a difficult airway with prior operations?'

Management of the airway in a patient following traumatic injury can be challenging due to the presence of a cervical collar, the frequent need to emergently intubate a patient with a 'full' stomach, and the need to choose appropriate doses of induction agents in a haemodynamically unstable patient. Airways in the obese patient can be precarious due to the fact that BMI is the most important risk factor for difficult mask ventilation [3]. While BMI may not be a predictor for a difficult intubation by itself [35,36], in conjunction with other factors (Mallampati grade III/IV, male sex, large neck circumference, reduced thyromental distance, or history of previous difficult intubation) a difficult intubation should be anticipated [37]. Of note, obesity is a known risk factor for difficult mask ventilation [38] and patients who are difficult to mask ventilate are more likely to be difficult to intubate [5]. Characteristics associated with difficult mask ventilation (age >55 years, beard, edentulous, BMI >26 kg/m², and a history of snoring) [39] can be identified even in unresponsive patients, with the exception of snoring.

When a difficult airway is anticipated—but securing the airway is imperative—the provider should refer to the American Society of Anesthesiologists (ASA) Committee on Trauma and Emergency Preparedness difficult airway algorithm modified for trauma [40]. The decision to wake a patient is rarely an option and a skilled provider who can perform a surgical airway must be available in the 'cannot ventilate, cannot intubate' scenario. Indications for awake or asleep fibreoptic bronchoscopic intubation in trauma patients are similar to non-trauma patients but may be more difficult due to altered mental status, blood and/or secretions in the airway, and the demand for expedient transport from the trauma bay to the operating room. The presence of a known or suspected cervical spine injury does not necessarily dictate a fibreoptic bronchoscopic intubation; intubation can be safely performed—and without the risk of worsening a cervical spine deficit—with rapid sequence induction/intubation (RSI) and manual in-line stabilization of the cervical spine [41] or with video laryngoscopy [42]. Cervical collars (and cricoid pressure, see later) can make bag-mask ventilation—when performing a *modified* RSI—and intubation more difficult [43]. A modified RSI adds mask ventilation to the application of cricoid

pressure and manual inline stabilization and may help to delay the onset of desaturation; mask ventilation should be done gently, with small tidal volumes, to prevent gastric distension. If difficult mask ventilation or difficult laryngoscopy occurs, in-line stabilization with removal of the anterior portion of the cervical collar may be utilized in order to facilitate these processes.

Body positioning is critical during intubation of the obese trauma patient. Building a 'ramp' under the patient on the operating room table in order to align the external auditory meatus with the sternal notch, called 'HELP' or 'head-elevated laryngoscopy position', aligns the oral axis, pharyngeal axis, and tracheal axis (**Fig. 34.1**). However, certain injury patterns, such as an unstable cervical spine or spinal column injury, may preclude such positioning. Even with suspected spinal cord injury, it is often permissible to position the operating room table in a head-up reverse Trendelenburg position to improve pulmonary mechanics by offloading the thoracic cavity of abdominal contents and allowing further diaphragmatic excursion, thereby reducing the work of breathing and prolonging the safe apnoea period during anaesthetic induction [44,45].

Prior to RSI in an obese trauma patient, preoxygenation is an essential component to minimize rapid desaturation in patients with already compromised pulmonary reserve. This may be provided through a nasal cannula, a non-re-breather mask, or optimally via the operating room ventilator circuit whereby tidal volumes and inspired and expired oxygen concentrations may be monitored. Application of positive end-expiratory pressure (PEEP)

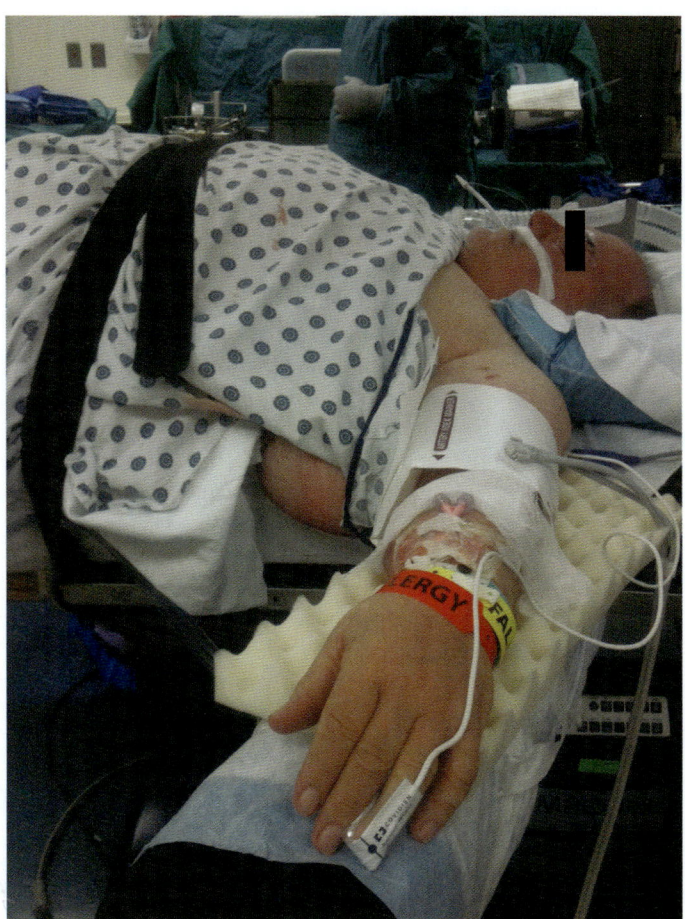

Fig. 34.1 Poor patient positioning.

with non-invasive means has also been demonstrated to improve oxygenation in the morbidly obese patient [46]. In time=sensitive situations, prolonged preoxygenation may not be possible and therefore, in awake patients, having the patient inspire eight vital capacity breaths may be useful to optimize oxygenation in clinically urgent scenarios [47].

All trauma patients are considered to have a full stomach regardless of when they last ate, due to the cessation of gastric and intestinal motility from the time of injury [48]. The traditional technique for RSI includes the use of cricoid pressure, which is now controversial. Cricoid pressure may worsen the laryngoscopic grade of view in up to 30% of patients without providing effective prevention of aspiration, and discontinuing cricoid pressure facilitates intubation in most cases without worsening the grade of laryngoscopic view [49–51]. For these reasons, the Eastern Association for the Surgery of Trauma Practice Management Guidelines for emergency tracheal intubation removed cricoid pressure as a class 1 recommendation. However, a 2014 study demonstrates that *properly* applying cricoid pressure occludes the oesophageal inlet during Glidescope® visualization [52]. What is not clear is whether occlusion occurs during direct laryngoscopy, which involves much more anterior lifting force, or whether inability to intubate the oesophagus correlates with preventing regurgitation of stomach contents. Based on existing evidence, it is reasonable, but not mandatory, to apply cricoid pressure during intubation in non-fasted patients and the pressure can be released if mask ventilation, glottic visualization, or tube placement is difficult.

Induction

Choosing the appropriate medications and dosage for induction is vital in a trauma patient: in a volume-depleted patient with shock, induction agents can lead to severe hypotension or cardiac arrest that can affect long-term morbidity and mortality. Medications are likely to have altered pharmacokinetics in the obese patient as a result of volume of distribution, protein binding, and renal and hepatic clearance [53]. Obese patients have increased cardiac output, total blood volume, and regional blood flow changes, each of which can affect peak plasma concentration, clearance, and half-life of induction agents [54]. Attention to dosing of medications is important as some are based on ideal body weight whereas others on actual body weight. In an obese trauma patient, haemodynamic consequences can occur if the standard dosage is delivered in a haemodynamically unstable patient. Mortality rates double when the systolic blood pressure is less than 100 mmHg for blunt trauma patients and less than 90 mmHg for penetrating injuries [55,56]. Sikorski et al. provide a thorough summary of induction medications and neuromuscular blockade drugs commonly used with trauma patients [57]. There is currently no standardized induction protocol for trauma patients. Unless a contraindication exists, succinylcholine is the neuromuscular blockade drug of choice due to the fastest onset of action, which may facilitate a more rapid intubation [58]. This is especially critical in obese patients due to their decreased functional residual capacity (FRC) and propensity to more rapid desaturation [59,60]. Regardless of drug, care must be delivered when deciding upon dosing.

Monitoring

In addition to standard ASA monitors, there may be an indication for invasive monitors in the obese trauma patient. In a patient who requires continuous blood pressure monitoring, frequent blood gases and/or glucose checks, or if a blood pressure cuff is reflecting inaccurate pressures, then an arterial line is suggested. Ultrasound may be helpful in identifying vascular structures; the caveat is that not every extremity may be available for access due to fractures, soft tissue injuries, burns, or vascular disruption. The arterial line can also monitor stroke volume, stroke volume variation, cardiac index, and cardiac output, which can help determine volume status and response to volume therapies.

The ASA recommends the use of the transoesophageal echocardiogram (TOE) when the surgical procedure or the patient's cardiovascular status may result in severe haemodynamic, pulmonary, or neurological impairment, a category I indication [61]. The use of TOE is relatively safe [62]. A TOE study can offer clues about a patient's pathophysiology and can provide real=time information concerning cardiac injury and treatment effectiveness. Memtsoudis et al. demonstrated that a TOE helped diagnose the cause of cardiac arrest in 19 out of 22 cases [63]. Causes identified were pulmonary embolus, tamponade, left ventricle or right ventricle dysfunction, and hypovolaemia. There are few contraindications to placing a TOE, but it should be noted that all trauma patients are considered to have high gastric contents, therefore decompression with an oral or nasal gastric tube is recommended prior to placement of the TOE. Two absolute contraindications are unstable cervical spine and viscous tear [64].

Access

Obtaining IV access can be a challenge in a corpulent patient due to their habitus (**Fig. 34.2**). A peripheral IV catheter is typically adequate for induction, but insufficient for massive resuscitation. Central venous catheterization with a large-bore, single lumen may be warranted. Several anatomical locations are available and the use of ultrasound may expedite access such as in the femoral or internal jugular vein, remembering that for patients in a cervical collar, internal jugular access may be difficult as are the femoral vessels in a pelvic or femur fracture. The subclavian vein is an option; however, if it takes many attempts to access due to habitus, the increased skin punctures puts the patient at increased risk of infection and thrombosis [65].

An option for quick access is intraosseous (IO) placement, which the American Heart Association advocates for during cardiopulmonary resuscitation if IV access is unattainable [66]. During hypovolaemic shock, peripheral veins can collapse making access impossible, but the IO space is non-collapsible. Several studies have demonstrated that it is faster to place an IO line than a central line and has minimal complications (10.7 vs 1.2 minutes) [67]. This same study showed that first-pass attempts at IO placement were significantly higher than attempts during central venous cannulation (90.3% vs 37.5%) [67]. The IO catheter can be placed in an awake patient who simply has poor access. The same fluids and medicines that can be delivered through an IV catheter can also be delivered

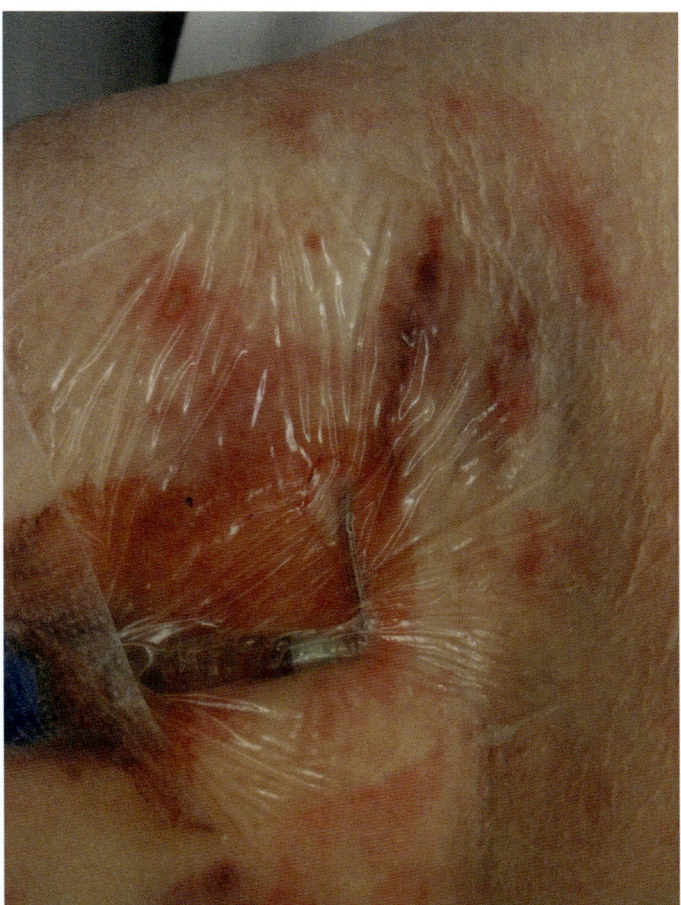

Fig. 34.2 Intravenous access.

through an IO line (with the exception of total parenteral nutrition and chemotherapeutic agents) [68]. This includes the use of induction agents and resuscitation drugs such as epinephrine, atropine, and blood products. An IO line can be used temporarily to induce anaesthesia or begin resuscitation until a larger bore catheter is attained. Flow rates for various sizes of IV catheters and for IO lines are listed in Table 34.1 [69,70].

Positioning

The responsibility of positioning the obese patient lies with both the anaesthesia and the surgical team and will be dictated by the location of the surgery. The maximum weight that the operating room

Table 34.1 Comparison of flow rates for intravenous and intraosseous catheters

Type of catheter	Flow rate
18 G IV	103 mL/min
16 G IV[a]	236 mL/min
14 G IV	270 mL/min
15 G IO (humerus)	500 mL/min (pressure bag)
15 G IO (tibia)	150 mL/min (pressure bag)
8.5 F cordis introducer	200 mL/min (pressure bag)

[a] 16 G × 2 parallel 500 mL/min (pressure bag).

table will accommodate must be known. Typical positions include supine, lateral, lithotomy, and prone. As reviewed in other chapters, the use of neuromuscular blockade in an obese patient in the supine position affects ventilation by shunting blood, decreasing compliance and FRC, and increasing atelectasis. Use of the lateral position helps displace the pannus, taking pressure off the thorax. Prone positioning can improve the intrapulmonary shunt because the lungs are ventilated in areas that are preferentially perfused (posterior, along the dorsum) as compared to the supine position. It is important to have the abdomen free so that the diaphragm has room to expand and contract, and all pressure points need to be padded appropriately as patients are at higher risk for nerve injury. For patients in the prone position during surgery, ischaemic optic neuritis is of clinical concern in patients who are prone. Obesity has been linked as a risk factor for optic ischaemic neuritis, which can cause blindness [71].

Maintenance of anaesthesia and ventilation

Once the airway has been secured and endotracheal positioning confirmed, adequate sedation and analgesia is necessary. In the operative setting, this is usually provided with a volatile anaesthetic. Previous investigations have demonstrated that sevoflurane and desflurane provide similar haemodynamic effects in the obese patient (albeit not in a trauma setting) [72]. Certain injury patterns and operative interventions may necessitate alternative anaesthetic considerations, such as total IV anaesthesia or regional anaesthetics. It should be mentioned that while nitrous oxide may appear to have haemodynamic benefits, this agent could potentially exacerbate underlying pulmonary hypertension and has the propensity to fill air spaces; therefore, it should be avoided in those suspected of having a pneumothorax or pneumocephalus.

Management of ventilation in the obese trauma patient has been evaluated in small studies in the literature. The application of lung protective ventilation strategies in order to minimize ventilation/perfusion mismatch is a reasonable approach. A prospective, randomized study demonstrated the benefits of low tidal volume ventilation (6–8 mL/kg ideal body weight) in patients undergoing elective abdominal operations [73]. With the addition of greater amounts of PEEP (10–15 cm H_2O), this approach aims to maximize FRC and optimize oxygenation. It must also be considered that this strategy typically results in permissive hypercapnia, whereby a partial pressure of carbon dioxide is tolerated to levels of 45–50 mmHg. In obese patients with underlying pulmonary hypertension, or with an increase in intracranial pressure, normocapnia should be the goal. It is valuable to obtain frequent arterial blood gas measurements to ensure appropriate oxygenation and ventilation. Adjusting the inspiratory:expiratory ratio of delivered tidal volume to 1:1.5, or even 1:1, may assist in achieving an open-lung ventilation strategy and optimize oxygenation. The use of recruitment manoeuvres (i.e. interval application of 40–55 cmH_2O plateau pressure for a period of 6–8 seconds) has been described to maintain FRC, compliance, and oxygenation [74]. This should be used with caution in patients who have haemodynamic decompensation following trauma, as positive pressure ventilation worsens hypotension.

Several meta-analyses have shown a beneficial effect of higher PEEP: it has been associated with decreased rates of postoperative pulmonary complications (PPCs) [75] and reduced postoperative atelectasis [76]. However, this was not confirmed in the large PROtective Ventilation (PROVE) Network trial comparing high (12 cmH$_2$O) versus low (2 cmH$_2$O) PEEP in the operating room [77]. The PPCs were similar between the two groups and patients in the high PEEP group had more hypotension and required more vasoactive medications [77]. The largest and most recent meta-analysis sought to clarify the role of intraoperative PEEP and the frequency of PPCs [78]. As previously demonstrated, rates of PPCs were lower in patients assigned to low tidal volume—but there was no statistical difference between PPCs in low tidal volume/high PEEP versus low tidal volume/low PEEP. The optimal level of intraoperative PEEP, therefore, remains unclear. It is worth noting that many of the studies just referenced refer to specific types of surgery (neurosurgery, thoracic surgery, oncological surgery, general surgery) and to patient populations with an increased risk of PPC due to pre-existing comorbidities. There is a paucity of data on the intraoperative management of trauma and acute care surgery patients, and the obese trauma patient.

Fluid management

Adequately resuscitating a patient in shock relies on technology and a series of laboratory values in order to gauge efficacy. To measure tissue perfusion, the lactate and bases excess values are regularly measured. Several studies have demonstrated that targeting a lactate reduces in-hospital mortality [79,80]. Base deficit is used as a marker of clearing acidosis [81] and can help predict transfusion requirements [82].

Two tools used to assess coagulopathies witnessed in trauma are the thromboelastogram (TEG®) and rotational thromboelastometry (ROTEM®). They measure viscoelastic properties from whole blood starting with clot formation, to propagation and stabilization. The TEG® can rapidly diagnose fibrinolysis during early resuscitation, unlike other tests for fibrinolysis, which are time-consuming. Algorithms have been created based on the results of these tests. There is evidence to suggest that the use of TEG® has decreased transfusion of blood products in cardiac and liver transplant surgery. Clot strength correlated with red blood cell, fresh frozen plasma, and platelets transfused during the first 24 hours. Patients with low clot strength were found to have a higher 30-day mortality [83]. It remains to be seen if TEG® and ROTEM® will reduce transfusion requirements. Future studies are needed before it will be known if it is a useful point-of-care tool to guide resuscitative efforts.

Volume resuscitation is the cornerstone of the initial management of many trauma patients. While there is little evidence in the trauma literature to direct haemodynamic resuscitation in obese trauma patient, there are numerous studies documenting the increased operative time and intraoperative blood loss experienced with this patient population. The optimal goal for fluid management in the obese trauma patient should be a euvolemic state. Resuscitation guidance via heart rate, blood pressure, cardiac index, or urine output may grossly misrepresent the actual volume status in an obese patient [84,85]. Haemodynamic parameters such as stroke volume variation or pulse pressure variation may be valuable in goal-directed resuscitation therapy [86]. However, a documented role for these parameters specifically in the traumatically injured obese population is lacking. Consideration of the potential comorbidities is necessary, which may be profoundly impacted by inappropriate volume resuscitation. Overaggressive volume administration in an obese trauma patient with left-sided cardiac dysfunction may result in pulmonary oedema and further respiratory failure; in patients with right-sided heart failure, liver congestion may occur. Inadequate resuscitation may also consequently worsen right heart failure through hypotension and inadequate delivery of oxygen to the right ventricle. These examples are not an inclusive list but rather describe the potential impact of fluid and blood resuscitation in the obese trauma patient.

Obese patients who suffer a traumatic insult may respond differently to therapeutic measures than non-obese patients. Belzberg et al. confirmed haemodynamic abnormalities in obese patients following severe blunt trauma, including lower cardiac index and reduced tissue oxygenation, when compared to non-obese patients [84]. The use of crystalloid has been shown to be detrimental compared to blood products, but the amount of products to administer is unknown. The Pragmatic, Randomized, Optimal Platelet and Plasma Ratios (PROPPR) randomized clinical trial failed to show that there was a decrease in mortality with a 1:1:1 versus 1:1:2 ratio (platelets:fresh frozen plasma:red blood cells), but exsanguination was less within the first 24 hours in the 1:1:1 group [87].

Tranexamic acid can be administered to a patient with traumatic haemorrhagic shock if given within a 3-hour window of the injury. The Clinical Randomisation of an Antifibrinolytic in Significant Haemorrhage (CRASH-2) was a trial that randomized 20,211 adult trauma patients with significant bleeding to receive tranexamic acid or placebo within 8 hours of injury. Tranexamic acid reduced death due to bleeding and all-cause mortality with no increase in vascular occlusive events [88].

Regional anaesthesia

Regional anaesthesia can provide the sole anaesthetic or be offered as an adjunct to general anaesthesia. There are instances when regional anaesthesia may be the preferred technique, such as a known difficult airway. As Brodsky and Mariano point out, regional anaesthesia offers the potential advantage of avoiding difficult airways, the use of inhaled anaesthetics which can be a cardiodepressent and opioids that can impair respiratory drive in a patient prone to obstruct their airway [89]. Regional anaesthesia offers several advantages over analgesics in trauma patients such as decreased sedation, hypoxia, nausea, and vomiting [90]. In addition, regional anaesthesia has been shown to reduce acute pain intensity in trauma injuries [91], but little evidence suggests that use of regional anaesthesia decreases the risk of developing chronic pain.

Regional and specific injuries

Rib fractures

One study showed that patients with three or more rib fractures randomized to either thoracic epidural or opioids were sixfold more likely to develop pneumonia and have a higher number of days on the ventilator if randomized to opioids [92]. In a meta-analysis there was no clear difference in mortality, ICU or hospital length of stay, or duration of mechanical ventilation [93]. Several studies have demonstrated that a femoral nerve block reduces pain intensity following hip fracture and is a valuable adjunct in this population, allowing patients to sit up, move in bed, deep breathe, and cough with reduced pain while awaiting surgery [94–96]. A Cochrane collaboration review of nerve blocks in patients with hip fractures concluded that femoral nerve block resulted in significant reductions in both pain intensity and opioid requirements preoperatively and during surgery [97].

Reimplantation

In patients requiring reimplantation, a continuous brachial plexus block improves outcomes. Regional anaesthesia use here can vasodilate an extremity that has a vasculature injury [98], improving blood flow to at-risk ischaemic limbs, and offer the added benefit of immobilization after the temporary loss of motor function. In one study that randomized patients to continuous supraclavicular block versus parenteral opioids for digit transfer and/or reimplantation, reoperation rates due to vascular insufficiency were 0% versus 29%, respectively [99]. However, a retrospective review failed to show improved survival rates at 6 months with the use of regional anaesthesia [100].

Postoperative management

Extubation

The decision to extubate a trauma patient is dependent upon numerous factors. Frequently, the clinical scenario dictates that the patient remains intubated. When deciding on extubating, the patient should be warm, require minimal to no vasopressor support, have an appropriate acid–base status and pH, be fully awake and responsive, and demonstrate sufficient strength to initiate adequate tidal volume and maintain airway patency. Extubation of an obese trauma patient must also consider the ease with which intubation was initially performed and any massive fluid shifts that may have occurred as a result of resuscitation and contribute to further airway oedema. The decision to extubate should be determined once the patient's haemodynamic, pulmonary, and electrolyte status is optimized to a near-baseline level. As previously described, determination of adequate haemodynamic resuscitation in the obese trauma patient is potentially inaccurate [84,85]. Multiple electrolyte and acid–base abnormalities may be present following severe injury and massive resuscitation. This further complicates the clinical picture in obese patients who may have underlying medical comorbidities, such as a patient with OSA who at a baseline may demonstrate a compensatory respiratory acidosis.

Specific injury patterns also dictate whether an obese trauma patient is suitable for postoperative extubation. Studies have demonstrated that obese patients are more likely to sustain torso and extremity injuries [101,102]. The presence of multiple rib fractures and underlying pulmonary injury may preclude safe extubation, especially in patients with lower extremity injuries in whom early ambulation is not possible. Furthermore, these patients may also require multiple operative procedures in the near future to address extremity and musculoskeletal injuries, which may therefore influence the decision regarding immediate postoperative extubation.

Once extubated, obese trauma patients require aggressive pulmonary therapy in order to maintain FRC, prevent atelectasis and subsequent hypoxia. Emergent reintubation of an obese trauma patient who may be difficult to ventilate and/or intubate is never an optimal situation, regardless of provider experience or comfort. If there is any doubt with regard to patient safety, it is always best for the patient to remain intubated and be transferred to the ICU where extubation may be performed at the appropriate time in a controlled environment. If the patient is successfully extubated postoperatively and transferred to the post-anaesthesia care unit, it is necessary to maintain vigilant monitoring of oxygen saturation. While providing appropriate pain management one should consider the respiratory depressant effects of narcotics, which may prove challenging in addressing optimal pain control in obese patients with underlying pulmonary dysfunction and alterations in respiratory drive, such as occurs in with OSA and obesity hypoventilation syndrome. A useful technique that has recently been demonstrated to provide appropriate oxygenation and reduce emergent reintubation rates is that of non-invasive high-flow oxygen therapy [103].

Intensive care unit management

There is conflicting evidence regarding the impact of obesity and BMI on outcomes in the ICU. Previous studies have documented increased mortality rates in critically ill patients with greater BMI [104,105]. There is general consensus that obesity and increasing BMI are significant risk factors for increased complications and mortality in the trauma population [4,7,106,107]. Prior investigations have documented that in the critically injured trauma patient obesity is associated with prolonged mechanical ventilation, ICU stay, and hospital length of stay [102,108,109]. Furthermore, obese trauma patients are more likely to develop acute kidney injury [108], pneumonia [110], and multiple organ failure [11]. Efforts focused specifically in the orthopaedic trauma population have identified that obesity and BMI are clearly linked with increased wound complications and deep venous thrombosis formation following pelvic and lower extremity long-bone injuries [20,109,111,112]. A study in 2015 even documented that the risk of post-traumatic complications was significantly increased in obese and morbidly obese patients with pelvic and acetabular fractures regardless of whether they required operative intervention [113]. Of particular concern is that obese trauma patients may in fact be hypercoagulable [114] and that pharmacological therapy with weight-based formulations rather than fixed dosing regimens, provides adequate prevention for venous thromboembolic disease [115].

However, some investigations have actually documented an 'obesity paradox' where overweight and obese patients experience a reduction in ICU-related mortality compared to underweight and normal-weight cohorts [116]. A possible explanation for this finding is related to potential hormonal and endocrinological adaptations that offer a survival advantage in critically ill obese patients [11]. Nonetheless, there are numerous challenges in providing ICU care to patients with an elevated BMI, including mobilization of the patient, assessing and preventing decubitus ulcers, obtaining radiological imaging, performing dressing changes, and caring for IV access.

Cardiopulmonary resuscitation

No modifications to the current protocols are recommended for obese patients, although cardiopulmonary resuscitation may present more challenges due to the greater force required for effective compressions. BMI has not been associated with lower survival. Therefore, the American Heart Association has not altered its guidelines for the obese patient [117].

Conclusion

Thorough assessment and treatment of the obese trauma patient are complicated. Due to the nature of emergency cases and the critical status of the patient, past medical history may be unknown. The provider must anticipate common comorbidities seen in this patient population and factor that into treatment options. The obese are at increased risk of longer hospital length of stay, longer ICU length of stay, respiratory failure, surgical site infections, and increased morbidity, and some data suggests mortality. This chapter reviews common problems associated with obese trauma patients such as IV access, intubation techniques, resuscitation strategies, and ventilator management. With proper care and attention to this specific topic and as more research is devoted to the obese trauma patient, morbidity and mortality may decrease.

Key points

- It is important to have an understanding of the pathophysiology obese patient's experience and to apply this knowledge in trauma settings.
- Anticipate difficulty with intubation, access, positioning, imagining, and postoperative extubation.
- Preparation, back-up plans, and resource utilization are essential when caring for an obese trauma patient.

CASE REPORT

A 66-year-old male, weighing 171 kg with a BMI of 58 kg/m², fell from standing and presented with a right trimalleolar fracture. His medical history includes coronary artery disease status post coronary artery bypass graft, atrial fibrillation on coumadin, chronic lymphoedema, gout, hypothyroidism, hyperlipidaemia, supraventricular tachycardia status post cardioversion, chronic kidney disease, OSA, and bilateral knee replacements. Prior to his fall he had a fever but denies syncope and lightheadedness. Initially, the patient went to out-patients with ankle pain, was noted to have an international normalized ratio of 6, and was reversed with vitamin K. Blood cultures grew Gram-negative rods. Physical examination was positive for morbid obesity, Mallampati class III, upper and lower dentures, large neck and tongue, irregular heart rate with systolic murmur, lower extremity lymphoedema, venous stasis, pitting oedema, and swollen right lower ankle. An electrocardiogram showed right bundle branch block and first-degree atrioventricular block. Preoperative vitals included heart rate of 61 beats/min, blood pressure 113/69 mmHg, and oxygen saturation was 91% on room air. Pertinent laboratory results were potassium of 6.0, blood urea nitrogen and creatinine were 77 and 2.29 respectively. Chest X-ray was suggestive of fluid overload.

The patient presented to the operating room for repair of a right trimalleolar fracture with two non-functional peripheral IV catheters. After multiple attempts at peripheral IV catheterization, a 22-gauge catheter was secured in the right antecubital with ultrasound. Sheets were placed behind the patient's shoulders for a ramped position. The patient was preoxygenated for 5 minutes and then induced with fentanyl, propofol, and vecuronium. Dentures were left in place for two-hand mask ventilation, and then removed for intubation. The patient had a grade 1 view during intubation with a Glidescope®. Maintenance of anaesthesia was uneventful. Estimated blood loss was 20 mL and urine output was 575 mL.

Discussion

There were several challenges to this case, all a result of the patient's morbid obesity. The first challenge encountered was the IV access. After several attempts at placing an IV catheter, we had to resort to the ultrasound. Other options would have been an ultrasound-assisted central venous catheter or an IO device, but with the patient's chronic lymphoedema in the lower extremities and adipose tissue in his upper arm, IO access would have been difficult too. The next challenge was securing the airway. More concerning than the intubation was the ability to mask ventilate. The patient's potassium was 6, therefore succinylcholine was not the optimal choice for muscle relaxants, committing us to bag-mask ventilation with a longer-acting neuromuscular blockade drug. Complicating the induction was the patient's room air saturation at 91%. Keeping the dentures in made bag-mask ventilation easier, but an oral airway device and the laryngeal mask airway were readily available. Positioning the patient in a ramp position also improved the view with the Glidescope®. Positioning the patient on the operating room table required several staff and then ample padding was utilized. He was not a regional candidate due to his lymphoedema and poor visualization of the sciatic nerve in the popliteal space on ultrasound. Luckily, the patient tolerated the procedure well and did not require a lot of pain medicine postoperatively. Lastly, with respect to extubation, the patient was moved back to his bed, head up, fully reversed and exhibited strong motor function before extubation. Had the patient not performed well post extubation, bi-level positive airway pressure ventilation was an option for him in the recovery unit. This case highlights several of the difficulties encountered with obese trauma patients. Consistent throughout this case was an alternative plan if initial attempts at procedures failed.

REFERENCES

1. Centers for Disease Control and Prevention. Adult obesity facts. 2020. http://www.cdc.gov/obesity/data/adult.html
2. Finkelstein EA, Khavjou OA, Thompson H, Trogdon JG, Pan L, Sherry B, et al. Obesity and severe obesity forecasts through 2030. Am J Prev Med. 2012;**42**(6):563–70.
3. Liu T, Chen JJ, Bai XJ, Zheng GS, Gao W. The effect of obesity on outcomes in trauma patients: a meta-analysis. Injury. 2013;**44**(9):1145–52.

4. Ditillo M, Pandit V, Rhee P, Aziz H, Hadeed S, Bhattacharya B, et al. Morbid obesity predisposes trauma patients to worse outcomes: a National Trauma Data Bank analysis. J Trauma Acute Care Surg. 2014;**76**(1):176–79.

5. American College of Surgeons Committee on Trauma. ATLS: Advanced Trauma Life Support Program for Doctors. 9th ed. Chicago, IL: American College of Surgeons; 2012.

6. Diaz JJ, Jr, Norris PR, Collier BR, Berkes MB, Ozdas A, May AK, et al. Morbid obesity is not a risk factor for mortality in critically ill trauma patients. J Trauma. 2009;**66**(1):226–31.

7. Bochicchio GV, Joshi M, Bochicchio K, Nehman S, Tracy JK, Scalea TM. Impact of obesity in the critically ill trauma patient: a prospective study. J Am Coll Surg. 2006;**203**(4):533–38.

8. Ciesla DJ, Moore EE, Johnson JL, Burch JM, Cothren CC, Sauaia A. Obesity increases risk of organ failure after severe trauma. J Am Coll Surg. 2006;**203**(4):539–45.

9. Hwabejire JO, Nembhard CE, Obirieze AC, Oyetunji TA, Tran DD, Fullum TM, et al. Body mass index in blunt trauma patients with hemorrhagic shock: opposite ends of the body mass index spectrum portend poor outcome. Am J Surg. 2015;**209**(4):659–65.

10. Docimo S, Jr, Lamparello B, Cohen MF, Kopatsis A, Vinces F. Utilizing quantitative measures of visceral adiposity in evaluating trauma patient outcomes. Int J Surg. 2015;**21**:51–56.

11. Gharib M, Kaul S, LoCurto J, Perez M, Hajri T. The obesity factor in critical illness: between consensus and controversy. J Trauma Acute Care Surg. 2015;**78**(4):866–73.

12. Lenz A, Franklin GA, Cheadle WG. Systemic inflammation after trauma. Injury. 2007;**38**(12):1336–45.

13. Wang C. Obesity, inflammation, and lung injury (OILI): the good. Mediators Inflamm. 2014;**2014**:978463.

14. Andruszkow H, Urner J, Deniz E, Probst C, Grun O, Lohse R, et al. Subjective impact of traumatic brain injury on long-term outcome at a minimum of 10 years after trauma – first results of a survey on 368 patients from a single academic trauma center in Germany. Patient Saf Surg. 2013;**7**(1):32.

15. Ciriello V, Gudipati S, Stavrou PZ, Kanakaris NK, Bellamy MC, Giannoudis PV. Biomarkers predicting sepsis in polytrauma patients: current evidence. Injury. 2013;**44**(12):1680–92.

16. Boulanger BR, Milzman D, Mitchell K, Rodriguez A. Body habitus as a predictor of injury pattern after blunt trauma. J Trauma. 1992;**33**(2):228–32.

17. Tagliaferri F, Compagnone C, Yoganandan N, Gennarelli TA. Traumatic brain injury after frontal crashes: relationship with body mass index. J Trauma. 2009;**66**(3):727–29.

18. Brown CV, Rhee P, Neville AL, Sangthong B, Salim A, Demetriades D. Obesity and traumatic brain injury. J Trauma. 2006;**61**(3):572–76.

19. Finkelstein EA, Chen H, Prabhu M, Trogdon JG, Corso PS. The relationship between obesity and injuries among U.S. adults. Am J Health Promot. 2007;**21**(5):460–68.

20. Sems SA, Johnson M, Cole PA, Byrd CT, Templeman DC, Minnesota Orthopaedic Trauma Group. Elevated body mass index increases early complications of surgical treatment of pelvic ring injuries. J Orthop Trauma. 2010;**24**(5):309–14.

21. Jones CB. Management of upper extremity injuries in obese patients. Orthop Clin North Am. 2011;**42**(1):11–19.

22. Weinlein JC, Deaderick S, Murphy RF. Morbid obesity increases the risk for systemic complications in patients with femoral shaft fractures. J Orthop Trauma. 2015;**29**(3):e91–95.

23. Baker SP, O'Neill B, Haddon W, Jr, Long WB. The injury severity score: a method for describing patients with multiple injuries and evaluating emergency care. J Trauma. 1974;**14**(3):187–96.

24. McCunn M, Vavilala M, Speck RM, Dutton R. ASA trauma care survey: anesthesiology practices demonstrate poor guidelines, implementation and need for education. American Society of Anesthesiology annual meeting, Chicago, IL; October 2011.

25. Federal Aviation Administration. Helicopter performance (chapter 7). In: Helicopter Flying Handbook. Washington, DC: Federal Aviation Administration; 2020. https://www.faa.gov/regulations_policies/handbooks_manuals/aviation/helicopter_flying_handbook/media/hfh_ch07.pdf

26. Alpert MA. Obesity cardiomyopathy: pathophysiology and evolution of the clinical syndrome. Am J Med Sci. 2001;**321**(4):225–36.

27. Messerli FH. Cardiopathy of obesity—a not-so-Victorian disease. N Engl J Med. 1986;**314**(6):378–80.

28. Balsaver AM Morales AR, Whitehouse FW. Fat infiltration of myocardium as a cause of cardiac conduction defect. Am J Cardiol. 1967;**19**:261–65.

29. The SOLVD Investigators. Effect of enalapril on survival in patients with reduced left ventricular ejection fractions and congestive heart failure. N Engl J Med. 1991;**325**(5):293–302.

30. Pfeffer MA, Braunwald E, Moye LA, Basta L, Brown EJ, Jr, Cuddy TE, et al. Effect of captopril on mortality and morbidity in patients with left ventricular dysfunction after myocardial infarction. Results of the survival and ventricular enlargement trial. The SAVE Investigators. N Engl J Med. 1992;**327**(10):669–77.

31. The CONSENSUS Trial Study Group. Effects of enalapril on mortality in severe congestive heart failure. Results of the Cooperative North Scandinavian Enalapril Survival Study (CONSENSUS). N Engl J Med. 1987;**316**(23):1429–35.

32. McCowen KC, Malhotra A, Bistrian BR. Stress-induced hyperglycemia. Crit Care Clin. 2001;**17**(1):107–24.

33. Kerby JD, Griffin RL, MacLennan P, Rue LW, 3rd. Stress-induced hyperglycemia, not diabetic hyperglycemia, is associated with higher mortality in trauma. Ann Surg. 2012;**256**(3):446–52.

34. Kuchta KF. Pathophysiologic changes of obesity. Anesthesiol Clin North Am. 2005;**23**(3):421–29, vi.

35. Brodsky JB, Lemmens HJ, Brock-Utne JG, Vierra M, Saidman LJ. Morbid obesity and tracheal intubation. Anesth Analg. 2002;**94**(3):732–36.

36. Lundstrom LH, Moller AM, Rosenstock C, Astrup G, Wettverslev J. High body mass index is a weak predictor for difficult and failed tracheal intubation: a cohort study of 91,332 consecutive patients scheduled for direct laryngoscopy registered in the Danish Anesthesia Database. Anesthesiology. 2009;**110**(2):266–74.

37. Heinrich S, Birkholz T, Irouschek A, Ackermann A, Schmidt J. Incidences and predictors of difficult laryngoscopy in adult patients undergoing general anesthesia: a single-center analysis of 102,305 cases. J Anesth. 2013;**27**(6):815–21.

38. Kheterpal S, Han R, Tremper KK, Shanks A, Tait AR, O'Reilly M, et al. Incidence and predictors of difficult and impossible mask ventilation. Anesthesiology. 2006;**105**(5):885–91.

39. Langeron O, Masso E, Huraux C, Guggiari M, Bianchi A, Coriat P, et al. Prediction of difficult mask ventilation. Anesthesiology. 2000;**92**(5):1229–36.

40. Hagberg CA, Kaslow O. Difficult airway management algorithm in trauma updated by COTEP. ASA Monitor. 2014;**78**:56–60.

41. Majernick TG, Bieniek R, Houston JB, Hughes HG. Cervical spine movement during orotracheal intubation. Ann Emerg Med. 1986;**15**(4):417–20.

42. Kill C, Risse J, Wallot P, Seidl P, Steinfeldt T, Wulf H. Videolaryngoscopy with glidescope reduces cervical spine

movement in patients with unsecured cervical spine. J Emerg Med. 2013;**44**(4):750–56.

43. Crosby ET. Airway management in adults after cervical spine trauma. Anesthesiology. 2006;**104**(6):1293–318.

44. Boyce JR, Ness T, Castroman P, Gleysteen JJ. A preliminary study of the optimal anesthesia positioning for the morbidly obese patient. Obes Surg. 2003;**13**(1):4–9.

45. Dixon BJ, Dixon JB, Carden JR, Burn AJ, Schachter LM, Playfair JM, et al. Preoxygenation is more effective in the 25 degrees head-up position than in the supine position in severely obese patients: a randomized controlled study. Anesthesiology. 2005;**102**(6):1110–15.

46. Futier E, Constantin JM, Pelosi P, Chanques G, Massone A, Petit A, et al. Noninvasive ventilation and alveolar recruitment maneuver improve respiratory function during and after intubation of morbidly obese patients: a randomized controlled study. Anesthesiology. 2011;**114**(6):1354–63.

47. Pandit JJ, Duncan T, Robbins PA. Total oxygen uptake with two maximal breathing techniques and the tidal volume breathing technique: a physiologic study of preoxygenation. Anesthesiology. 2003;**99**(4):841–46.

48. Stept WJ SP. Rapid induction/intubation for prevention of gastric-content aspiration. Anesth Analg. 1970;**49**:633–36.

49. Levitan RM, Kinkle WC, Levin WJ, Everett WW. Laryngeal view during laryngoscopy: a randomized trial comparing cricoid pressure, backward-upward-rightward pressure, and bimanual laryngoscopy. Ann Emerg Med. 2006;**47**(6):548–55.

50. Ellis DY, Harris T, Zideman D. Cricoid pressure in emergency department rapid sequence tracheal intubations: a risk-benefit analysis. Ann Emerg Med. 2007;**50**(6):653–65.

51. Harris T, Ellis DY, Foster L, Lockey D. Cricoid pressure and laryngeal manipulation in 402 pre-hospital emergency anaesthetics: essential safety measure or a hindrance to rapid safe intubation? Resuscitation. 2010;**81**(7):810–16.

52. Zeidan AM, Salem MR, Mazoit JX, Abdullah MA, Ghattas T, Crystal GJ. The effectiveness of cricoid pressure for occluding the esophageal entrance in anesthetized and paralyzed patients: an experimental and observational Glidescope study. Anesth Analg. 2014;**118**(3):580–86.

53. Casati A, Putzu M. Anesthesia in the obese patient: pharmacokinetic considerations. J Clin Anesth. 2005;**17**(2):134–45.

54. Adams JP, Murphy PG. Obesity in anaesthesia and intensive care. Br J Anaesth. 2000;**85**(1):91–108.

55. Hasler RM, Nuesch E, Juni P, Bouamra O, Exadaktylos AK, Lecky F. Systolic blood pressure below 110 mm Hg is associated with increased mortality in blunt major trauma patients: multicentre cohort study. Resuscitation. 2011;**82**(9):1202–207.

56. Hasler RM, Nuesch E, Juni P, Bouamra O, Exadaktylos AK, Lecky F. Systolic blood pressure below 110 mmHg is associated with increased mortality in penetrating major trauma patients: multicentre cohort study. Resuscitation. 2012;**83**(4):476–81.

57. Sikorski RA, Koerner KA, Fouche Weber LY, Galvagno SM. Choice of general anesthetics for trauma. Curr Anesthesiol Rep. 2014;**4**:225–32.

58. Stollings JL, Diedrich DA, Oyen LJ, Brown DR. Rapid-sequence intubation: a review of the process and considerations when choosing medications. Ann Pharmacother. 2014;**48**(1):62–76.

59. Tanoubi I, Drolet P, Donati F. Optimizing preoxygenation in adults. Can J Anaesth. 2009;**56**(6):449–66.

60. Jense HG, Dubin SA, Silverstein PI, O'Leary-Escolas U. Effect of obesity on safe duration of apnea in anesthetized humans. Anesth Analg. 1991;**72**(1):89–93.

61. American Society of Anesthesiologists, Society of Cardiovascular Anesthesiologists Task Force on Transesophageal Echocardiography. Practice guidelines for perioperative transesophageal echocardiography. An updated report by the American Society of Anesthesiologists and the Society of Cardiovascular Anesthesiologists Task Force on Transesophageal Echocardiography. Anesthesiology. 2010;**112**(5):1084–96.

62. Kallmeyer IJ, Collard CD, Fox JA, Body SC, Shernan SK. The safety of intraoperative transesophageal echocardiography: a case series of 7200 cardiac surgical patients. Anesth Analg. 2001;**92**(5):1126–30.

63. Memtsoudis SG, Rosenberger P, Loffler M, Eltzschig HK, Mizuguchi A, Shernan SK, et al. The usefulness of transesophageal echocardiography during intraoperative cardiac arrest in noncardiac surgery. Anesth Analg. 2006;**102**(6):1653–57.

64. Rebel A, Klimkina O, Hassan ZU. Transesophageal echocardiography for the noncardiac surgical patient. Int Surg. 2012;**97**(1):43–55.

65. Boulanger BR, Milzman DP, Rodriguez A. Obesity. Crit Care Clin. 1994;**10**(3):613–22.

66. Neumar RW, Otto CW, Link MS, Kronick SL, Shuster M, Callaway CW, et al. Part 8: adult advanced cardiovascular life support: 2010 American Heart Association Guidelines for Cardiopulmonary Resuscitation and Emergency Cardiovascular Care. Circulation. 2010;**122**(18 Suppl 3):S729–67.

67. Lee PM, Lee C, Rattner P, Wu X, Gershengorn H, Acquah S. Intraosseous versus central venous catheter utilization and performance during inpatient medical emergencies. Crit Care Med. 2015;**43**(6):1233–38.

68. Science & Clinical Department, Vidacare Corporation. The Science and Fundamentals of Intraosseous Vascular Access Including FAQ. 2nd ed. Shivano Park, TX: Vidacare Corporation; 2013.

69. Harty E. Inserting peripheral intravenous cannulae – tips and tricks. Update Anesth. 2011;**27**(1):22–26.

70. Ngo AS, Oh JJ, Chen Y, Yong D, Ong ME. Intraosseous vascular access in adults using the EZ-IO in an emergency department. Int J Emerg Med. 2009;**2**(3):155–60.

71. Lee LA. Perioperative visual loss and anesthetic management. Curr Opin Anaesthesiol. 2013;**26**(3):375–81.

72. Kaur A, Jain AK, Sehgal R, Sood J. Hemodynamics and early recovery characteristics of desflurane versus sevoflurane in bariatric surgery. J Anaesthesiol Clin Pharmacol. 2013;**29**(1):36–40.

73. Futier E, Constantin JM, Paugam-Burtz C, Pascal J, Eurin M, Neuschwander A, et al. A trial of intraoperative low-tidal-volume ventilation in abdominal surgery. N Engl J Med. 2013;**369**(5):428–37.

74. Aldenkortt M, Lysakowski C, Elia N, Brochard L, Tramer MR. Ventilation strategies in obese patients undergoing surgery: a quantitative systematic review and meta-analysis. Br J Anaesth. 2012;**109**(4):493–502.

75. Hemmes SN, Serpa Neto A, Schultz MJ. Intraoperative ventilatory strategies to prevent postoperative pulmonary complications: a meta-analysis. Curr Opin Anaesthesiol. 2013;**26**(2):126–33.

76. Imberger G, McIlroy D, Pace NL, Wetterslev J, Brok J, Moller AM. Positive end-expiratory pressure (PEEP) during anaesthesia

for the prevention of mortality and postoperative pulmonary complications. Cochrane Database Syst Rev. 2010;9:CD007922.

77. Hemmes SN, de Abreu MG, Pelosi P, Schultz MJ, Severgnini P, Hollmann MW, et al. High versus low positive end-expiratory pressure during general anaesthesia for open abdominal surgery (PROVHILO trial): a multicentre randomised controlled trial. Lancet. 2014;**384**(9942):495–503.

78. Serpa NA, Hemmes S, Barbas C, Beiderlinden M, Biehl M, Binnekade J, et al. Protective versus conventional ventilation for surgery: a systematic review and individual patient data meta-analysis. Anesthesiology. 2015;**123**(1):66–78.

79. Jansen TC, van Bommel J, Schoonderbeek FJ, Sleeswijk Visser SJ, van der Klooster JM, Lima AP, et al. Early lactate-guided therapy in intensive care unit patients: a multicenter, open-label, randomized controlled trial. Am J Respir Crit Care Med. 2010;**182**(6):752–61.

80. Jones AE, Shapiro NI, Trzeciak S, Arnold RC, Claremont HA, Kline JA, et al. Lactate clearance vs central venous oxygen saturation as goals of early sepsis therapy: a randomized clinical trial. JAMA. 2010;**303**(8):739–46.

81. Davis JW, Kaups KL, Parks SN. Base deficit is superior to pH in evaluating clearance of acidosis after traumatic shock. J Trauma. 1998;**44**(1):114–18.

82. Davis JW, Parks SN, Kaups KL, Gladen HE, O'Donnell-Nicol S. Admission base deficit predicts transfusion requirements and risk of complications. J Trauma. 1996;**41**(5):769–74.

83. Nystrup KB, Windelov NA, Thomsen AB, Johansson PI. Reduced clot strength upon admission, evaluated by thrombelastography (TEG), in trauma patients is independently associated with increased 30-day mortality. Scand J Trauma Resusc Emerg Med. 2011;**19**:52.

84. Belzberg H, Wo CC, Demetriades D, Shoemaker WC. Effects of age and obesity on hemodynamics, tissue oxygenation, and outcome after trauma. J Trauma. 2007;**62**(5):1192–200.

85. Winfield RD, Delano MJ, Lottenberg L, Cendan JC, Moldawer LL, Maier RV, et al. Traditional resuscitative practices fail to resolve metabolic acidosis in morbidly obese patients after severe blunt trauma. J Trauma. 2010;**68**(2):317–30.

86. Benes J, Giglio M, Brienza N, Michard F. The effects of goal-directed fluid therapy based on dynamic parameters on post-surgical outcome: a meta-analysis of randomized controlled trials. Crit Care. 2014;**18**(5):584.

87. Holcomb JB, Tilley BC, Baraniuk S, Fox EE, Wade CE, Podbielski JM, et al. Transfusion of plasma, platelets, and red blood cells in a 1:1:1 vs a 1:1:2 ratio and mortality in patients with severe trauma: the PROPPR randomized clinical trial. JAMA. 2015;**313**(5):471–82.

88. CRASH-2 trial collaborators, Shakur H, Roberts I, Bautista R, Caballero J, Coats T, et al. Effects of tranexamic acid on death, vascular occlusive events, and blood transfusion in trauma patients with significant haemorrhage (CRASH-2): a randomised, placebo-controlled trial. Lancet. 2010;**376**(9734):23–32.

89. Brodsky JB, Mariano ER. Regional anaesthesia in the obese patient: lost landmarks and evolving ultrasound guidance. Best Pract Res Clin Anaesthesiol. 2011;**25**(1):61–72.

90. Tezel O, Kaldirim U, Bilgic S, Deniz S, Eyi YE, Ozyurek S, et al. A comparison of suprascapular nerve block and procedural sedation analgesia in shoulder dislocation reduction. Am J Emerg Med. 2014;**32**(6):549–52.

91. Buckenmaier CC 3rd, Rupprecht C, McKnight G, McMillan B, White RL, Gallagher RM, et al. Pain following battlefield injury and evacuation: a survey of 110 casualties from the wars in Iraq and Afghanistan. Pain Med. 2009;**10**(8):1487–96.

92. Bulger EM, Edwards T, Klotz P, Jurkovich GJ. Epidural analgesia improves outcome after multiple rib fractures. Surgery. 2004;**136**(2):426–30.

93. Carrier FM, Turgeon AF, Nicole PC, Trepanier CA, Fergusson DA, Thauvette D, et al. Effect of epidural analgesia in patients with traumatic rib fractures: a systematic review and meta-analysis of randomized controlled trials. Can J Anaesth. 2009;**56**(3):230–42.

94. Beaudoin FL, Nagdev A, Merchant RC, Becker BM. Ultrasound-guided femoral nerve blocks in elderly patients with hip fractures. Am J Emerg Med. 2010;**28**(1):76–81.

95. Watson MJ, Walker E, Rowell S, Halliday S, Lumsden MA, Higgins M, et al. Femoral nerve block for pain relief in hip fracture: a dose finding study. Anaesthesia. 2014;**69**(7):683–86.

96. Temelkovska-Stevanovska M, Durnev V, Jovanovski-Srceva M, Mojsova-Mijovska M, Trpeski S. Continuous femoral nerve block versus fascia iliaca compartment block as postoperative analgesia in patients with hip fracture. Prilozi. 2014;**35**(2):85–94.

97. Parker MJ, Handoll HH, Griffiths R. Anaesthesia for hip fracture surgery in adults. Cochrane Database Syst Rev. 2004;**4**:CD000521.

98. Reynolds TS, Kim KM, Dukkipati R, Nguyen TH, Julka I, Kakazu C, et al. Pre-operative regional block anesthesia enhances operative strategy for arteriovenous fistula creation. J Vasc Access. 2011;**12**(4):336–40.

99. Kurt E, Ozturk S, Isik S, Zor F. Continuous brachial plexus blockade for digital replantations and toe-to-hand transfers. Ann Plast Surg. 2005;**54**(1):24–27.

100. Niazi AU, El-Beheiry H, Ramlogan R, Graham B, von Schroeder HP, Tumber PS. Continuous infraclavicular brachial plexus blockade: effect on survival of replanted digits. Hand Surg. 2013;**18**(3):325–30.

101. Evans DC, Stawicki SP, Davido HT, Eiferman D. Obesity in trauma patients: correlations of body mass index with outcomes, injury patterns, and complications. Am Surg. 2011;**77**(8):1003–1008.

102. Brown CV, Neville AL, Rhee P, Salim A, Velmahos GC, Demetriades D. The impact of obesity on the outcomes of 1,153 critically injured blunt trauma patients. J Trauma. 2005;**59**(5):1048–51.

103. Frat JP, Thille AW, Mercat A, Girault C, Ragot S, Perbet S, et al. High-flow oxygen through nasal cannula in acute hypoxemic respiratory failure. N Engl J Med. 2015;**372**(23):2185–96.

104. Nasraway SA, Jr, Albert M, Donnelly AM, Ruthazer R, Shikora SA, Saltzman E. Morbid obesity is an independent determinant of death among surgical critically ill patients. Crit Care Med. 2006;**34**(4):964–70.

105. Pickkers P, de Keizer N, Dusseljee J, Weerheijm D, van der Hoeven JG, Peek N. Body mass index is associated with hospital mortality in critically ill patients: an observational cohort study. Crit Care Med. 2013;**41**(8):1878–83.

106. Duane TM, Dechert T, Aboutanos MB, Malhotra AK, Ivatury RR. Obesity and outcomes after blunt trauma. J Trauma. 2006;**61**(5):1218–21.

107. Glance LG, Li Y, Osler TM, Mukamel DB, Dick AW. Impact of obesity on mortality and complications in trauma patients. Ann Surg. 2014;**259**(3):576–81.

108. Duchesne JC, Schmieg RE, Jr, Simmons JD, Islam T, McGinness CL, McSwain NE Jr. Impact of obesity in damage control laparotomy patients. J Trauma. 2009;**67**(1):108–12.

109. Childs BR, Nahm NJ, Dolenc AJ, Vallier HA. Obesity is associated with more complications and longer hospital stays after orthopaedic trauma. J Orthop Trauma. 2015;29(11):504–509.

110. Mica L, Keller C, Vomela J, Trentz O, Plecko M, Keel MJ. Obesity and overweight as a risk factor for pneumonia in polytrauma patients: a retrospective cohort study. J Trauma Acute Care Surg. 2013;75(4):693–98.

111. Karunakar MA, Shah SN, Jerabek S. Body mass index as a predictor of complications after operative treatment of acetabular fractures. J Bone Joint Surg Am. 2005;87(7):1498–502.

112. Tucker MC, Schwappach JR, Leighton RK, Coupe K, Ricci WM. Results of femoral intramedullary nailing in patients who are obese versus those who are not obese: a prospective multicenter comparison study. J Orthop Trauma. 2007;21(8):523–29.

113. Morris BJ, Richards JE, Guillamondegui OD, Sweeney KR, Mir HR, Obremskey WT, et al. Obesity increases early complications after high-energy pelvic and acetabular fractures. Orthopedics. 2015;38(10):e881–87.

114. Kornblith LZ, Howard B, Kunitake R, Redick B, Nelson M, Cohen MJ, et al. Obesity and clotting: body mass index independently contributes to hypercoagulability after injury. J Trauma Acute Care Surg. 2015;78(1):30–36.

115. Bickford A, Majercik S, Bledsoe J, Smith K, Johnston R, Dickerson J, et al. Weight-based enoxaparin dosing for venous thromboembolism prophylaxis in the obese trauma patient. Am J Surg. 2013;206(6):847–51.

116. Mullen JT, Moorman DW, Davenport DL. The obesity paradox: body mass index and outcomes in patients undergoing nonbariatric general surgery. Ann Surg. 2009;250(1):166–72.

117. Vanden Hoek TL, Morrison LJ, Shuster M, Donnino M, Sinz E, Lavonas EJ, et al. Part 12: cardiac arrest in special situations: 2010 American Heart Association Guidelines for Cardiopulmonary Resuscitation and Emergency Cardiovascular Care. Circulation. 2010;122(18 Suppl 3):S829–61.

Guidelines and equipment in obese patients

Christian Balabanoff-Acosta, Clint Fleckenstein, and Eric Gewirtz

Introduction

Airway management is often the principal concern of all anaesthesiologists. When presented with an obese patient for general anaesthesia, however, there are even greater challenges to providing sedation. Though many assume that the obese and morbidly obese patient is unique to the United States, the World Health Organization's Global Database on Body Mass Index shows that this is not the case [1]. Anaesthesiologists all over the world are, and will continue to be, encountering more and more obese and morbidly obese patients who require all types of surgery, including, especially, bariatric procedures. At Temple University Hospital (Philadelphia, PA, USA), we are also now experiencing morbidly obese patients who are undergoing robotic and gynaecological surgeries.

Predictors of a difficult airway

As all anaesthesia providers know, it is critical to assess the airway of a patient before she or he undergoes surgery. This is especially important in obese, morbidly obese, and super-morbidly obese patients since they often have additional anatomical and physiological complexities associated with their condition. There are six factors that an anaesthesia provider should consider when evaluating these categories of patients for a potentially difficult airway. No one factor should supersede another; instead, providers should take into account multiple elements to assess their patients fully (it is better to be over-prepared than under-prepared should complications during surgery arise).

1. *Body mass index (BMI).* The National Institutes of Health in the United States defines obesity as an individual whose BMI is greater than 30 kg/m² [2]. Our experience at Temple is that intubating the morbidly obese patient (BMI between 40 and 50 kg/m²) or the super-obese patient (BMI >50 kg/m²) is no more difficult than intubating the obese patient (given this, we will use the term obese to include the morbidly obese and the super-morbidly obese throughout the rest of this chapter). The incidence of difficult intubation in non-obstetric obese patients is roughly 2–8% [3–5].

2. *Mallampati classification.* The Mallampati classification has been considered the gold standard in predicting difficult tracheal intubation since the 1980s [6]. Mallampati scores of 3–4, however, are not all created equally: patients with Mallampati scores of 3–4 who have adequate mouth openings are very different from patients with Mallampati scores of 3–4 with poor mouth openings and very little neck extension.

3. *Neck circumference.* A neck circumference of roughly 40 cm correlates to a 5% probability of difficult intubation, whereas a neck circumference of 60 cm correlates to a 35% probability of difficult intubation [7]. We have also observed clinically that a very large neck circumference is associated with limited neck extension.

4. *Thyromental distance (also known as Patil's test).* Measuring the thyromental distance—the distance from the tip of the cartilage to the tip of the mandible with neck extension—also serves as a possible indicator of a difficult airway [8].

5. *Distance between the lip and the bottom of the chin.* Although rarely described in the published literature, our clinical experience has shown that reduced distance between the lip and the bottom of the prominent chin is a good indicator of a difficult intubation. (The opposite is also true: a greater distance between the lower lip and the bottom of the prominent chin is a good indicator of an easy intubation.) This measurement, especially in association with others described here, has been an excellent predictor of airway difficulty.

6. *Obstructive sleep apnoea (OSA).* Although much more common a diagnosis now than a decade ago, OSA can serve as a predictor of a difficult airway. OSA usually results from soft tissue that collapses during sleep, but in the hands of a skilled anaesthesia provider with proper laryngoscopy skills, this condition is not associated with an increased difficulty for tracheal intubation in the operative setting. There are, however, several other aspects to consider, such as postoperative airway obstruction

and carbon dioxide retention. Also to be considered is preoperative evaluation of right heart failure or unsuspected increases in pulmonary artery pressures when evaluated. This is extremely important if your patient is a carbon dioxide retainer.

General recommendations for airway access during the induction of general anaesthesia

1. It is critical to remember that obese patients often suffer rapid desaturation after standard preoxygenation and induction of general anaesthesia.
2. Many obese patients are on continuous positive airway pressure machines at home, so inducing them with a mask and continuous positive airway pressure support prevents early induction atelectasis and is generally very well tolerated.
3. Having an additional anaesthesia provider available to assist is frequently overlooked and, regrettably, sometimes difficult to have with increasingly busy operating rooms in large academic centres. But arranging for another anaesthesia provider with a skilled set of hands, who understands the airway plan and who can calmly assist you, to be available for managing a difficult airway is of unrecognized importance.

Specific recommendations for airway access during the induction of general anaesthesia

Standard induction

1. Careful attention must be paid to the proper sniffing position. We use many folded blankets at our institution; however, there are foam devices to help create a good positioning.
2. You should have basic equipment readily available, such as the laryngoscope, no. 3 and no. 4 Macintosh blade, as well as a Miller blade.
3. Using an airway bougie is certainly a technique that every anaesthesia provider has to acquire. The anaesthesia provider has to be able to feel the anterior rings of the trachea when using this device, and it is very important to maintain laryngoscopy while the endotracheal tube is inserted over the bougie to avoid cuff rupture, especially given the difficulty of passing the endotracheal tube. If feeling the anterior rings of the trachea is not fully appreciated, important time is wasted and an oesophageal intubation can inflate to the stomach and make aspiration more likely. Using an airway bougie insertion into the trachea is a must in the obese patient because, as mentioned previously, rapid desaturation frequently ensues.
4. Probably the most overlooked item in mask ventilation is the Berman airway—this device has not changed since it was invented. Using the Berman has an almost 100% success rate with four-handed ventilation. On a personal note, Robert A. Berman, a physician, was a prolific inventor who far exceeded his contemporaries in designing and creating assistive airway devices for use within and outside of hospital settings. The senior author for this chapter, Eric Gewirtz, in fact, trained under Berman and finds that many of Berman's theories and devices still hold in the operating room today [9].

5. Supraglottic airways may provide excellent results as a rescue device in obese patients who are not at high risk for gastro-oesophageal reflux. Many anaesthesia providers prefer laryngeal mask airways (LMAs) when ventilating prior to a planned endotracheal intubation. We have a strong preference for using a large no. 4 Berman oral airway first. Placing this prior to ventilating obese patients can help to avoid filling the stomach with air and thus increasing chances of aspiration. If this technique fails and difficulty persists, the use of an intubating LMA is preferred because this offers several other options, if needed, going forward. The 1 to use an intubating LMA are:
   a. There is a better seal because of the rigidity of the device, making it easier to ventilate an obese patient
   b. The anaesthesia provider has the option of proceeding to intubate through the device
   c. The intubating LMA also allows for fibreoptic intubation through the device while having the ability to ventilate and maintain an airway.

The unanticipated difficult airway

Algorithms to manage the unanticipated difficult airway in general surgical patients have been published and revised several times [10,11]. However, in the obese patient the strategy will frequently depend on the experience of the anaesthesia provider and the available equipment.

Surgical airway

Surgical access to an airway is always more difficult technically and is associated with increased risks and an increased chance of failure. So, in managing these difficult airways, special attention must be paid. Ultrasound guidance for percutaneous tracheostomy has been described in critical care units [12], but we have not found ultrasound guidance to be useful in precarious situations where the airway is lost.

Monitoring the anaesthetized patient

The American Society of Anesthesiologists (ASA) recommends five standard monitors for patients undergoing general anaesthesia: end-tidal carbon dioxide, pulse oximetry, blood pressure, electrocardiogram, and temperature monitoring. While there is no reason to deviate from these standard monitors in the obese patient, it must be understood that these recommendations pertain to patients with normal BMIs. Indeed, there is a dearth of information about monitoring the obese patient in the operating room. A review of the literature, however, allows for some discussion of the topic.

Bispectral index monitoring

Traditional monitoring of anaesthetic depth relies on a combination of examining the patient's vital signs and scrutinizing the concentration of exhaled volatile anaesthetics. In recent years, companies have developed newer technologies to monitor the depth of sedation; these technologies are based on a processed electroencephalogram that provides a numerical assessment of the effects of anaesthetics on the brain. The most commonly used and best studied of these modalities is the bispectral index (BIS), which renders a single-digit value for evaluation and decision-making. BIS monitoring has been shown to reduce the incidence of awareness under anaesthesia [13,14]. Additionally, as Luginbühl et al. and Liu have demonstrated, patients undergoing BIS monitoring receive lower doses of both inhaled and intravenous (IV) anaesthetic agents, have shorter recovery times from anaesthesia, and a shorter post-anaesthesia care unit (PACU) stay [15,16]. While Luginbühl et al. and Liu conducted these studies in patients with a normal BMI, Meyhoff et al. and Pandazi et al. saw similar results in morbidly obese patients undergoing bariatric surgery [17,18].

Unfortunately, while there are studies that show reduced amounts of anaesthetic agents, faster times to recovery, and shorter PACU stays with BIS monitoring, the effect of BIS monitoring on postoperative complications has not been formally studied. It is well understood, however, that morbidly obese patients are at an increased risk for postoperative complications including impaired respiratory mechanics and a greater degree of atelectasis [19–21]. It is reasonable to expect, then, that a patient who is more quickly and more completely recovered from anaesthesia may be at a reduced risk for postoperative anaesthetic complications. This idea, coupled with the low risk and cost of BIS monitoring, provides a reasonable argument that BIS monitoring (or other comparable modalities) be employed in morbidly obese patients.

Neuromuscular blockade

Laryngeal muscles, along with other muscles of the oropharynx, are some of the last muscles to recover from neuromuscular blockade (NMB). It is therefore unsurprising that Murphy et al. have identified the residual blockade as a cause of adverse events in the postoperative period [22].

One way to asses NMB is through the use of clinical tests, such as sustained head lift and hand grip strength; these are easily employed and require no special equipment. But while clinical tests are convenient, they are an unreliable means for determining adequate NMB recovery [23]. Despite this, many practitioners rely on such clinical tests and fail to use more sophisticated approaches [24,25].

Using peripheral nerve stimulators, in contrast, provides a reliable means to monitor NMB; they are widely available in practice and are utilized in many clinical settings for qualitative monitoring. These instruments, though, rely on the provider's ability to detect a decrease in strength between successive muscle stimulations, but, as Capron et al. demonstrated, providers are often unable to recognize fade at levels where residual paralysis of laryngeal muscles is present, so practice with the devices is critical [26].

Given the implication of residual NMB on adverse respiratory events and the shortcomings of clinical and qualitative assessments of NMB, a strong argument can clearly be made for the use of quantitative monitoring. This is certainly true in the obese population where respiratory mechanics are already compromised. Fortunately, quantitative peripheral nerve stimulators are commercially available, are relatively easy to use, and can provide a more accurate assessment of NMB when used correctly.

General and specialized equipment

As more and more obese patients have been admitted to hospitals over the years, anaesthesia providers and manufacturers have repurposed old equipment and developed new devices to accommodate the size and the specific and unique needs of these patients. Essential care for obese patients requires, then, that hospitals have specialized equipment available. This equipment must accommodate the greater weights of obese patients without causing any harm to these patients and to the staff responsible for transferring the patient and managing her or his care during surgeries. A list of available and needed equipment should be present in all areas in which obese patients receive care. **Table 35.1** provides an example of such a list. We also present a list of devices in the following sections that anaesthesia providers should consider using for care of the obese patient and our recommendations/cautions about their usage [27].

Operating room tables (general)

Due to the baseline medical issues from which many obese patients suffer, such as diabetes, gastro-oesophageal reflux disease, hypertension, and so on, obese patients have an increased risk of developing postoperative problems if not positioned properly in the operating room—positioning is of the utmost importance.

Most surgical tables today can accommodate the weight of an obese, a morbidly obese, or a super-morbidly obese patient, taking a load of greater than 350 kg. Tables built in the 1990s, however, were not designed with such patients in mind and many can only handle a maximum weight of roughly 225 kg [28]. To deal with such limitations in institutions that do not have access to modern surgical tables, often anaesthesia providers put two of these tables together to increase the total load capacity for the patient and to extend the width of the operating field in order to contain the girth of the patient. While doing this is certainly a necessity when modern tables are unavailable to the anaesthesia provider, using this type of setup significantly limits the provider's ability to change the position of the table to accommodate the needs of the obese patient (e.g. you would not be able to adjust the incline/decline of the head, torso, or legs).

When considering what table to use for obese patients, the procedure table should be capable of articulating, supporting, and

Table 35.1 Sample list of available and needed equipment present in areas in which obese patients receive care

In-patient units	Wide beds Lifting/transferring equipment Wide commodes Wide wheelchairs, stretchers, walkers Wide blood pressure cuffs Oversized sequential compression devices Biphasic defibrillators, emergency airway equipment Wide entrance doors to patient rooms and bathrooms Floor-mounted or reinforced toilets Elevators with wide doors and adequate weight capacity
Operating room	Automated wide operating table with extended weight capacity Lifting/transferring equipment Extra-long instruments, including retractors, laparoscopes, trocars Weight-appropriate equipment in PACU and preoperative holding units

Reproduced from Hammond, K. L. Practical Issues in the Surgical Care of the Obese Patient, *Ochsner Journal*, 13(2): 224–227, 2013. Distributed under the Creative Commons Attribution 4.0 International (CC BY 4.0). https://creativecommons.org/licenses/by/4.0/

lifting patients weighing 363–454 kg and the beds should be wide enough to permit the whole patient to be on the surface of the table, not allowing excess skin to hang over the edge. While the widths of commercially produced tables in not standard, most are available in the 48–53 cm range, and many companies produce accessories that can extend the width by 12 cm.

Even when tables fit within these weight and size parameters, the ability of tables to maintain stability and integrity when articulating patients can vary. For example, when tilting a table, the load capacity may be severely reduced and the centre of gravity for the table/patient combination can shift. In a case reported in the *Journal of the Anesthesia Safety Foundation*, an obese patient weighing 148 kg almost hit his head on the floor of the operating room when the table tipped over after the bed was unlocked and turned [29]. Every anaesthesia provider should be completely familiar with the capabilities of a table should adjustments need to be made during surgery—relying on operating room technicians is not enough.

In addition to the capacities of the table, it is important to make sure that the table mattress provides sufficient support; not doing so can result in the patient developing, for example, decubitus ulcers [30]. Additionally, since the normal capillary interface pressure is 35 mmHg, the Association of Perioperative Registered Nurses suggests padding made of viscoelastic polymers be used to support the patient (these pads are made of AKTON®, commonly known as 'gel pads'); the use of foam supports is not advised since, when compressed against the patient, they do not provide relief of pressure and can cause rapid changes in vital signs in the patient.

Tables (specific)

1. *Orthopaedic tables ('traction tables')*: these tables are an important tool for orthopaedic surgeries, providing a wide range of adaptability for positioning patients. Some of these tables provide tools to traction fractured limbs and some are radiolucent. They come in a wide range of weight capacities, but usually support a maximum weight of 225 kg only. There are some known complications with using these beds, the most common one being ball alignment, but other complications such as neuropraxia and soft tissue injuries can occur. Orthopaedic surgeons recommend the use of a radiolucent, flat-top operating table with free extremity draping to prevent fracture malalignment and malrotation [31].

2. *Jackson orthopaedic tables*: Jackson orthopaedic tables are designed to be open in the middle with two, hinged side rails that allow for supportive pad placement. They are mostly used for prone spinal surgery, anterior/posterior fusions in the cervical, thoracic, lumbar, and sacral regions, surgical correction of deformities, laminectomies, decompressions, kyphoplasties, and osteotomies. The legs of the patient are placed in the centre of the table on a sling, but if the legs of an obese patient are too large, pressure on the lateral aspect of the leg may result. If there is a chance of this occurring, two Jackson tables can be placed side by side to increase support for the legs [32].

   This table also has a 360-degree axis rotational capability and thus facilitates safe and efficient rotation particularly of traumatized patients during combined surgical approaches. It also offers 360 degrees of unobstructed radiolucency for easily obtainable images with either a C-arm or X-ray [33]. The materials used to build these tables vary significantly, thereby affecting the

load they can withstand; some companies offer tables that can support in the range of 225–400 kg.

3. *Hybrid operating room tables*: most of the tables we see in hybrid rooms are designated as 'floating tables', so named because of the seamless flow of motion in all directions, but they lack articulation and the ability to maintain a horizontal position. They are constructed of carbon fibre, making them radiolucent, and most can hold loads of 200–250 kg. New hybrid operating room systems incorporate tables such as the Maquet® Magnus and the TruSystem™ 7500, since these operating room tables can be articulated and the weight load is higher than for floating tables (the Maquet® Magnus system can hold a load up to 250 kg and the TruSystem™ 7500 can hold a load up to 400 kg) [34,35].

4. *C-arm table*: these tables permit the use of the C-arm X-ray device. Much like the hybrid room tables, these are made of radiolucent materials. They can take loads of 225 kg but are unable to be articulated. Some companies do make versions that can take a load up to 450 kg.

5. *Urological and gynaecological tables*: these tables are designed for positioning of the patient in the lithotomy position. Like the C-arm tables, they are made of radiolucent materials that permit the use of a C-arm X-ray or other equipment. The average weight load for these tables ranges from 225 to 275 kg [36].

Bed transfer equipment

There is a variety of equipment available that can be used to transfer obese patients from bed to bed. For example, there are inflatable transfer mattresses, like the Stryker Glide Lateral Air Transfer Patient Transfer System (Stryker®), hover mats (HoverTech®), and transfer boards—transfer boards have been in use for a long time (most of these can be used with smaller obese patients, i.e. those weighing <225 kg, but manufacturers do offer ones that can handle different weight loads).

Patient lifts are also widely used to transfer obese patients. Lifts most commonly found in hospital settings can handle patients weighing 225–325 kg; newer lifts can hold patients weighing up to 450 kg, such as the EZ Way Smart Lift®. The lifts themselves are battery powered and can be moved with the patient on the lift; disposable or washable slings and bags are also available and have weight capacity limits as well.

Blood pressure measurement

Blood pressure cuffs

These vary in size and form. The usual adult cuff size ranges from 22 to 42 cm with even larger sizes available. The correct cuff size for any patient, including an obese one, should be one with a width of 40% of the circumference of the arm [37].

In comparison to radial intra-arterial blood pressure readings, measurements of the upper arm tend to underestimate systolic and overestimate diastolic blood pressure. Measurements using the forearm overestimate systolic and underestimate diastolic blood pressure, but the range difference using this method is much less, which could indicate a more accurate measurement than using the upper arm [38]. Either way you measure blood pressure, the upper arm or forearm has good specificity and sensitivity in comparison to intra-arterial measurements [39]. The American Heart Association recommends that if an adequately sized blood pressure cuff cannot

Table 35.2 Recommended cuff sizes for accurate measurement of blood pressure.

Patient	Recommended cuff size
Adults (by arm circumference)	
22–26 cm	12 × 22 cm (small adult)
27–34 cm	16 × 30 cm (adult)
35–44 cm	16 × 36 cm (large adult)
45–52 cm	16 × 42 cm (adult thigh)
Children (by age)	
Newborns and premature infants	4 × 8 cm
Infants	6 × 12 cm
Older children	9 × 18 cm

Source: Data from Pickering, T. G., Hall, J. E., Appel, L.J. et al. Recommendations for Blood Pressure Measurement in Humans and Experimental Animals, *Circulation*, 111(5): 697–716, 2005, American Heart Association.

be found, blood pressure should be measured, preferably, at the wrist. Upper arm recommendations for different arm circumferences from the American Heart Association can be seen in **Table 35.2** [40].

Finger blood pressure monitors

Finger blood pressure monitors, such as the Nexfin® HD or the Finapres® NOVA, are non-invasive monitors that use a finger pressure cuff and an infrared monitor, which measures the diameter of the arteries at different compressions digitally, in combination to calculate the blood pressure. These devices allow for the continuous measurement of blood pressure (systolic, diastolic, and mean), as well as heart rate, continuous cardiac output, stroke volume, systemic vascular resistance, and an index of left ventricular contractility (dP/dt). These finger monitors can be used to obtain blood pressures if no other method is available.

Intravenous access

IV access in obese patients is the same as in every other patient: it can be easy or difficult. According to observational data, factors associated with difficulty placing a peripheral IV catheter in an adult include obesity, being underweight, the clinician's inexperience, and the clinician's judgement that there is poor peripheral venous access [41]; increased subcutaneous tissue also makes it more difficult to find veins in the arms. There is an arsenal of catheters available for access, and they vary in size and range, from 14 to 24 gauge and lengths from 2 to 15 cm.

There are also a number of tools that you can use to find veins and obtain IV access. The most common (and cheapest) method is to use traditional anatomical structures and landmarks: distally to proximal, there is the hand, which has the metacarpal and dorsal network; the forearm, which has the basilic, cephalic, radial, ulnar, and median basilica; and the antecubital region, which has the cephalic and median cubital. Even more proximal, in the shoulder you can find the cephalic vein and tributaries, and in the neck, the external jugular vein. When all else fails, there are other tools available:

1. *Light transillumination devices*: these devices emit either light, infrared light, or light at different frequencies to detect the veins (at Temple, we have even used a small flashlight placed over the skin of the patient to find veins. Veins found using this method appear dark compared to the pink surrounding). Red-light devices, which emit light at a different frequency, such as the IIlumivein®, Veinlite®, and the IVeye®, can be found from a number of manufacturers. When using these devices, veins are depicted as dark lines that appear inside a halo of red light. A note of caution: there may be difficulty using these devices on dark-skinned patients. More sophisticated devices that use infrared technology, such as VeinViewer® and the AccuVein®, are bulkier but can be used with any type of skin tone. These devices shine an infrared light onto the skin and make deoxygenated blood in the veins visible.

2. *Ultrasound devices*: use of ultrasound technology for peripheral IV access is often the last chosen, but certainly the most effective device available—practitioners are able to locate both superficial veins and those that are located deeper under the skin. The possibility of obtaining one peripheral venous access point is very high using these devices [42]. Ultrasound-guided localization facilitates the navigation and placement of both the catheter and the needle within a vessel, increasing the first-attempt success rate of peripheral venous cannulation in adult obese patients [43]. Training with such devices is fast and should result in fewer punctures to the patient for needle insertion compared to other methods (any personnel, from technicians to physicians, can be trained to use this technology in a short period of time) [44].

Both in-plane and out-of-plane techniques can be used in obese patients. At Temple University Hospital, we first try to gain access at the most distal veins in the upper extremity and work our way up to the most proximal. For distal veins, shorter catheters can be used; for deeper veins, a longer catheter should be used. Practitioners should use an ultrasound depth ruler to choose an appropriately sized catheter; at least a third of the catheter should be in the vessel and the connector should not dent the skin. If none of these techniques work, an ultrasound-guided central line or intraosseous line should be placed.

Arterial line access tools

As with venous access, obtaining arterial access in obese patients is more difficult as compared to patients with normal body habitus; standard locations for arterial punctures are the radial, ulnar, brachial, axillary, femoral, and dorsalis pedis [45–47]. The techniques available for arterial cannulation in obese patients are the same as for non-obese patients, namely palpation, blind insertion, pulse Doppler, ultrasound guided, and the cut-down (all of these techniques can be used in any of the aforementioned locations). The palpation method is the one used most widely and is usually the first (and cheapest) most anaesthesia providers attempt before other more complex techniques.

In the obese patient it may be difficult to palpate the pulse without using an invasive method. This is due to the depth of the artery relative to the skin (using a completely blind technique in an obese patient is not recommended). Should palpation not work, the second most-used techniques to obtain arterial cannulation are an ultrasound-guided or a pulse Doppler approach. Using an ultrasound approach allows the anaesthesia provider to visualize both the artery and the needle while performing the insertion; the pulse Doppler technique consists of placing the pulse Doppler over the chosen arterial site, using the generated sound waves to localize the artery (when the loudest signal is heard), and then inserting the needle blindly, meaning that missing the artery is possible. Some studies that compare the results of the use of the palpation method versus the ultrasound method are mixed, indicating that choosing one technique over the other has little effect on the rates of success on first attempt, failure, or haematoma formation; other studies indicate that ultrasound-guided access has a higher first time success rate than palpation; and even some others indicate that there is also a higher success rate and more rapid access of the arterial catheter using ultrasound over palpation [48,49].

Adjuncts to arterial cannulations are wrist-positioning splints that can be made generically using a bore and gauze or can be purchased from a number of different manufacturers. These devices fix the wrist into an adequate position that allows for the placement of an arterial catheter through the wrist.

When performing femoral cannulations in obese patients, positioning and lifting of the pannus is key. Also, ideally, the patient should be flat. The most common method (and cheapest) is to have a colleague hold the pannus away from the groin. If no one is available to assist, the use of a medical tape is a good alternate choice.

Perioperative guidelines

Preoperative

1. Patients should be evaluated for obesity-related comorbidities including hyperglycaemia, hypertension, metabolic syndrome, and cardiovascular status. Where appropriate, additional tests should be pursued to optimize the patient for surgery.

2. Where undiagnosed OSA is suspected, screening questionnaires, such as STOP-Bang, should be used [50].

3. Consider performing the procedure in an in-patient setting based on factors such as surgical procedure, presence of OSA, patient comorbidities, and the level of post-procedure analgesia expected.

Intraoperative

1. Ensure that appropriate materials are available including:
   a. Instruments/devices for difficult airway management
   b. Oral and nasal airways
   c. Appropriate operating room equipment such as:
      i. Adequately rated/sized operating room table and surgical equipment
      ii. Mechanical venous thromboembolism (VTE) prophylaxis
      iii. Appropriate patient monitors
   d. An ultrasound, especially if difficult IV or epidural access is expected.

2. If a difficult airway is anticipated or there is a known history of it, consider having an additional experienced anaesthesia provider in the room for induction/intubation.

3. Medication dosages titrated to desired effect, generally dosing is based on patient lean body weight.

4. Consider neuromonitoring, such as BIS, to titrate medications [15,17,18,50].

5. Utilize quantitative monitoring of NMB when neuromuscular blocking medications are given [22,26].

6. Consider the use of sugammadex for reversal of NMB [51].

7. Minimize long-acting opioids and sedatives. Consider peripheral nerve blocks, epidurals, or other non-sedating options for postoperative pain management.

8. Consider preventative measures to lessen atelectasis, including the use of recruitment manoeuvres, positive end-expiratory pressure, and oxygen concentrations at less than 40% [52].

9. Consider extubating the patient with the head of the bed elevated by 30 degrees.

Postoperative

1. Limit long-acting opioids and medications that suppress respiratory drive. Employ multimodal pain management strategies.

2. Consider the use of continuous positive airway pressure postoperatively for patients using continuous positive airway pressure regularly prior to surgery.

3. Encourage respiratory physiotherapy, such as incentive spirometry [53].

4. Monitor patients until they are able to maintain a preoperative pulse oximetry level with minimal or no supplemental oxygen while unstimulated.

Conclusion

With an increasing incidence of obesity in our surgical population, management of the airway in these patients has become a must in anaesthesia practice. While there are some additional complexities to the anatomy and physiology of an obese patient, deploying various measures before, during, and after surgery can help to reduce potential complications that arise because of the patient's size and weight. Combining various technologies, such as tables, monitors, and airways, with the skills of an experienced anaesthesia provider will make such a patient's operation and recovery go more smoothly and safely.

REFERENCES

1. World Health Organization. Global database on body mass index. http://www.who.int/topics/obesity/en/

2. National Heart, Lung, and Blood Institute. Assessing your weight and health risk. https://www.nhlbi.nih.gov/health/educational/lose_wt/BMI/bmi_dis.htm

3. Rose D, Cohen M. The airway: problems and predictions in 18,500 patients. 1994;**41**:372–83.

4. Wilson M, Spiegelhalter D, Robertson J, Lesser P. Predicting difficult intubation. Br J Anaesth. 1988;**61**:211–16.

5. Jacobsen J, Jensen E, Waldau T, Poulsen T. Preoperative evaluation of intubation conditions in patients scheduled for elective surgery. Acta Anaesthesiol Scand. 1996;**40**(4):421–24.

6. Mallampati S, Gatt S, Gugino L, Desai S, Waraksa B, Freiberger D, et al. A clinical sign to predict difficult tracheal intubation: a prospective study. Can Anaesth Soc J. 1985;**32**(4):429–34.

7. Riad W, Vaez M, Raveendran R, Tam A, Quereshy F, Chung F, et al. Neck circumference as a predictor of difficult intubation and difficult mask ventilation in morbidly obese patients: a prospective observational study. Eur J Anaesthesiol. 2016;**33**(4):244–49.

8. Patil V, Stehling L, Zauder H. Predicting the difficulty of intubation utilizing an intubation gauge. Anesthesiol Rev. 1983;**10**(8):32–33.

9. Berman J. Robert Alvin Berman, M.D.: Airway inventor (1914–). Am Soc Anesth Newsletter. 1999;**63**(9):17–19.

10. Law J, Broemling N, Cooper R, Drolet, Duggan L, Griesdale D, et al. The difficult airway with recommendations for management. Part 1—difficult tracheal intubation encountered in an unconscious/induced patient. Can J Anaesth. 2013;**60**(11):1089–118.

11. Frerk C, Mitchell V, McNarry A, Mendonca C, Bhagrath R, Patel A, et al. Difficult Airway Society 2015 guidelines for management of unanticipated difficult intubation in adults. Brit J Anaesth. 2015;**115**(6):827–48.

12. Pierre-Grégoire G, Zogheib E, Petiot S, Marienne J, Guerin A, Monet P, et al. Ultrasound-guided percutaneous tracheostomy in critically ill obese patients. Crit Care. 2012;**16**:R40.

13. Myles P, Leslie K, McNeil J, Forbes A, Chan M. Bispectral index monitoring to prevent awareness during anaesthesia: the B-Aware randomised controlled trial. Lancet. 2004;**363**(9423):1757–63.

14. Ekman A, Lindholm M, Lennmarken C, Sandin R. Reduction in the incidence of awareness using BIS monitoring. Acta Anaesthesiol Scand. 2004;**48**(1):20–26.

15. Luginbühl M, Wüthrich S, Petersen-Felix S, Zbinden A, Schnider T. Different benefit of bispectral index (BIS) in desflurane and propofol anesthesia. Acta Anaesthesiol Scand. 2003;**47**(2):165–73.

16. Liu S. Effects of bispectral index monitoring on ambulatory anesthesia: a meta-analysis of randomized controlled trials and a cost analysis. Anesthesiology. 2004;**101**(2):311–15.

17. Meyhoff C, Henneberg S, Jørgensen B, Gätke M, Rasmussen L. Depth of anaesthesia monitoring in obese patients: a randomized study of propofol-remifentanil. Acta Anaesthesiol Scand. 2009;**53**(3):369–75.

18. Pandazi A, Bourlioti A, Kostopanagiotou G. Bispectral index monitoring in obese patients undergoing gastric bypass surgery: experience in 23 patients. Obes Surg. 2005;**15**(1):58–62.

19. Pelosi P, Croci M, Ravagnan I, Cerisara M, Vicardi P, et al. Respiratory system mechanics in sedated, paralyzed, morbidly obese patients. J Appl Physiol. 1997;**82**(3):811–18.

20. Eichenberger A, Proietti S, Wicky S, Frascarolo P, Suter M, Spahn D, et al. Morbid obesity and postoperative pulmonary atelectasis: an underestimated problem. Anesth Analg. 2002;**95**(6):1788–92.

21. Mendonça J, Pereira H, Xará D, Santos A, Abelha F. Obese patients: respiratory complications in the post-anesthesia care unit. Rev Port Pneumol. 2014;**20**(1):12–19.

22. Murphy G, Szokol J, Marymont J, Greenberg S, Avram M, Vender J. Residual neuromuscular blockade and critical respiratory events in the postanesthesia care unit. Anesth Analg. 2008;**107**(1):130–37.

23. Brull S, Murphy G. Residual Nermomuscular block: lessons unlearned. Part II: methods to reduce the risk of residual weakness. Anesth Analg. 2010;**111**(1):129–40.

24. Shah J, Owen-Smith O, Coley S, Rangasami J. A survey of peripheral nerve stimulator (PNS) use. Eur J Anaesth. 2000;**17**(4):273–75.

25. Grayling M, Sweeney B. Recovery from neuromuscular blockade: a survey of practice. Anaesthesia. 2007;**62**(8):806–809.

26. Capron F, Fortier L, Racine S, Donati F. Tactile fade detection with hand or wrist stimulation using train-of-four, double-burst stimulation, 50-hertz tetanus, 100-hertz tetanus, and acceleromyography. Anesth Analg. 2006;**102**(5):1578–84.

27. Hammond K. Practical issues in the surgical care of the obese patient. Ochsner J. 2013;**13**(2):224–27.

28. Buie J. Evolution of operating room tables. http://www.labx.com/article.cfm?articleId=1786/Evolution-of-Operating-Room-Tables/

29. Razavian S, Thurn J. On the tipping point of disaster: operating room surgical table tips with obese patients. APSF J. 2013;**28**(1):1–2.

30. Reddy M, Gill S, Rochon P. Preventing pressure ulcers: a systematic review. JAMA. 2006;**296**(8):974–84.

31. Flierl M, Stahel P, Hak D, Morgan S, Smith W. Traction table-related complications in orthopaedic surgery. J Am Acad Orthop Surg. 2010;**18**(11):668–75.

32. Vaidya R, Sethi A, Lee A, Bartol S, Onwudiwe N, Aebi M. Posterior lumbar spinal fusion and instrumentation in morbidly obese patients using the Synframe retractor system: technical note. Eur Spine J. 2012;**21**(12):2626–32.

33. Schonauer C, Bocchetti A, Barbagallo G, Albanese V, Moraci A. Positioning on surgical table. Eur Spine J. 2004;**13**(Suppl 1):S50–55.

34. Maquet Getinge Group. MAGNUS OR table system. https://www.maquet.com/int/products/magnus/

35. Trumpf Medical. TruSystem™ 7500. https://www.trumpfmedical.com/en/products/or-tables/or-table-systems/trusystem-7500/

36. Surgical Tables Inc. URO-MAX urological tables. http://surgicaltables.com/products/uro-max-urological-tables/

37. Ogedegbe G, Pickering T. Principles and techniques of blood pressure measurement. Cardiol Clin. 2010;**28**(4):571–86.

38. Leblanc M, Croteau S, Ferland A, Bussières J, Cloutier L, Hould F, et al. Blood pressure assessment in severe obesity: validation of a forearm approach. Obesity. 2013;**21**(12):E533–41.

39. Irving G, Holden J, Stevens R, McManus. Which cuff should I use? Indirect blood pressure measurement for the diagnosis of hypertension in patients with obesity: a diagnostic accuracy review. BMJ Open. 2016;**6**(11):e012429.

40. Pickering T, Hall J, Appel L, Falkner B, Graves J, Hill M, et al. Recommendations for blood pressure measurement in humans and experimental animals: part 1: blood pressure measurement in humans: a statement for professionals from the Subcommittee of Professional and Public Education of the AHA Council on High Blood Pressure Research. Circulation. 2005;**111**(5):697–716.

41. Sebbane M, Claret P, Lefebvre S, Mercier G, Rubenovitch J, Jreige R, et al. Predicting peripheral venous access difficulty in the emergency department using body mass index and a clinical evaluation of venous accessibility. J Emerg Med. 2013;**44**(2):299–305.

42. Brandt H, Jepsen C, Hendriksen O, Lindekær A, Skjønnemand M. The use of ultrasound to identify veins for peripheral venous access in morbidly obese patients. Dan Med J. 2016;**63**(2):A5191.

43. Ueda K, Hussey P. Dynamic ultrasound-guided short-axis needle tip navigation technique for facilitating cannulation of peripheral veins in obese patients. Anesth Analg. 2017;**124**(3):831–33.

44. Oliveira L, Lawrence M. Ultrasound-guided peripheral intravenous access program for emergency physicians, nurses, and corpsmen (technicians) at a military hospital. Mil Med. 2016;**181**(3):272–76.

45. Vezzani A, Manca T, Vercelli A, Braghieri A, Magnacavallo A. Ultrasonography as a guide during vascular access procedures and in the diagnosis of complications. J Ultrasound. 2013;**16**(4):161–70.

46. Marik P, Varon J. The obese patient in the ICU. Chest. 1998;**113**(2):492–98.

47. Zaremski L, Quesada R, Kovacs M, Schernthaner M, Uthoff H. Prospective comparison of palpation versus ultrasound-guided radial access for cardiac catheterization. J Invasive Cardiol. 2013;**25**(10):538–42.

48. Peters C, Schwarz S, Yarnold C, Kojic K, Kojic S, Head S. Ultrasound guidance versus direct palpation for radial artery catheterization by expert operators: a randomized trial among Canadian cardiac anesthesiologists. Can J Anaesth. 2015;**62**(11):1161–68.

49. Shiloh A, Savel R, Paulin L, Eisen L. Ultrasound-guided catheterization of the radial artery: a systematic review and meta-analysis of randomized controlled trials. Chest. 2011;**139**(3):524–29.

50. Seet E, Chua M, Liaw C. High STOP-BANG questionnaire scores predict intraoperative and early postoperative adverse events. Singapore Med J. 2015;**56**(4):212–16.

51. Gaszynski T, Szewczyk T, Gaszynski W. Randomized comparison of sugammadex and neostigmine for reversal of rocuronium-induced muscle relaxation in morbidly obese undergoing general anaesthesia. Br J Anaesth. 2012;**108**(2):236–39.

52. Reinius H, Jonsson L, Gustafsson S, Sundbom M, Duvernoy O, Pelosi P, et al. Prevention of atelectasis in morbidly obese patients during general anesthesia and paralysis: a computerized tomography study. Anesthesiology. 2009;**111**(5):979–87.

53. Zoremba M, Dette F, Gerlach L, Wolf U, Wulf H. Short-term respiratory physical therapy treatment in the PACU and influence on postoperative lung function in obese adults. Obes Surg. 2009;**19**(10):1346–54.

Medicolegal issues and the obese patient

Abiona Berkeley, Muhammad Ahmed, and Jose Sosa-Herrera

Introduction

In the United States alone, it is estimated that 15,000–19,000 medical malpractice suits are brought against physicians each year [1]. A retrospective analysis of malpractice claims filed in the United States from 2005 to 2009 uncovered a total of 58,667 claims against American physicians. Of those claims, 96.9% (56,850 claims) were settled with only 3.1% (1817 claims) proceeding to trial [2]. Of those malpractice claims taken to court, obstetrical and surgical claims, as opposed to clinic-based or diagnostic claims, predominated [2] (**Fig. 36.1**). Although data related to unsuccessful claims which were dropped or dismissed prior to trial or in which findings were in favour of the physician have been difficult to quantify, some authors report that these may comprise as many as 50% of all filed legal malpractice actions [3].

A lawsuit is a penultimate marker of disruption of the patient–physician relationship. It brings with it an emotional burden including the stigma of malpractice in the form of delivery of poor medical care and/or unethical behaviour on the part of the physician. For the patient, there is long-standing distrust of the medical system as well as any enduring morbidity and mortality. The burden on the system and all parties involved is substantial in terms of time and financial costs.

The process of litigation itself can be negative and overwhelming, and a clear understanding of the process is often lost on all parties [4]. The Doctors Company, a physician-owned malpractice insurance company, conducted a study of its medical malpractice database from 2007 through 2012 [2]. They uncovered a total of 415 obesity-related claims from a variety of specialties [2]. The field of anaesthesiology, which of necessity intersects with the majority of specialties in the operating room, ranked third in the number of claims filed against a specialty provider [2] (**Fig. 36.2**).

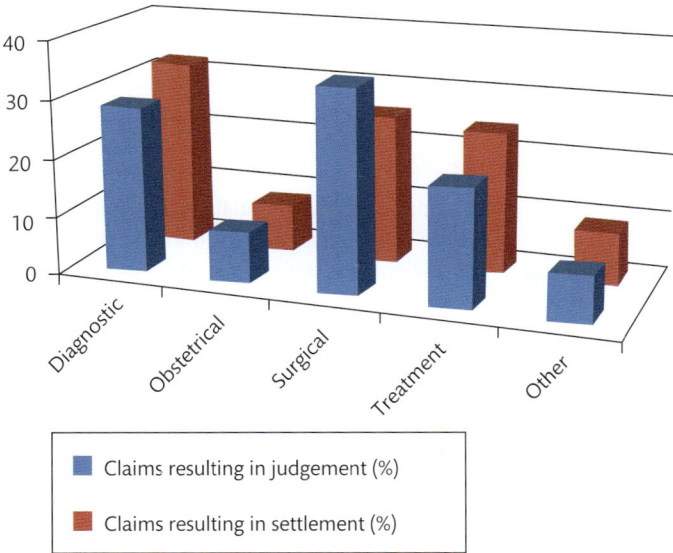

Fig. 36.1 Medical characteristics of claims resulting in judgment and those in settlement.

Source: Data from Rubin, J.B., Bishop, T.F., Characteristics of paid malpractice claims settled in and out of court in the USA: a retrospective analysis, *BMJ Open*, 3(6), 2013, BMJ Publishing Group Ltd.

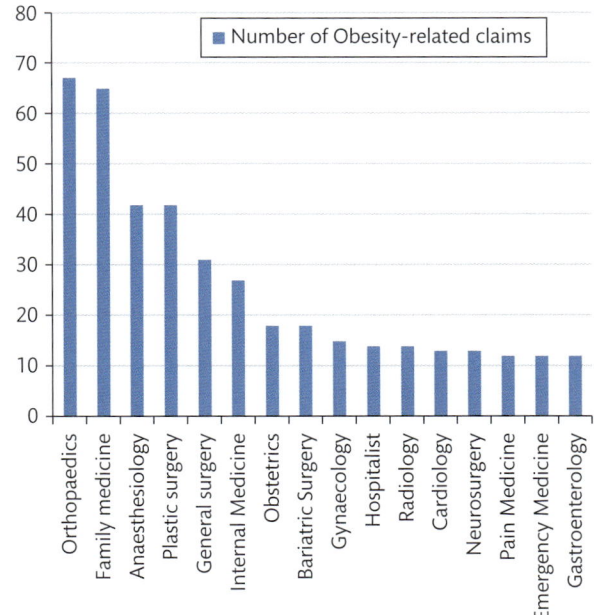

Fig. 36.2 Number of obesity-related claims filed with the Doctors Company from 2007 through 2012.

Source: Data from Doctors Company 'An Overview of Obesity-Related Claims'.

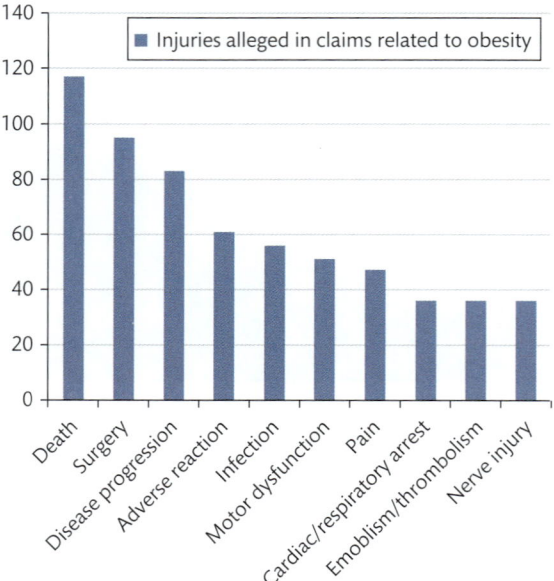

Fig. 36.3 Injuries alleged in claims related to obesity filed with the Doctors Company from 2007 through 2012.
Source: Data from Doctors Company 'An Overview of Obesity-Related Claims'.

The injuries sustained were significant with the most common injury being death in 25% of the claims filed [2] (**Fig. 36.3**).

Principles of medical malpractice claims

Tort law principles

Legal principles define a tort as a civil wrong committed against a person or his or her property. A tort is independent of any contractual obligation owed to that person. The tort may be based on the violation of either a public or private duty or a legal right [5]. In medical malpractice, a tort may occur through wilfulness, negligence, or lack of skill. The tort may be grounded in an entire course of treatment or a single act [6].

To satisfy the requirements of a cause of action, the plaintiff must demonstrate:

a. A duty on the part of the physician/defendant
b. A breach of that duty
c. The physician's breach as the proximate cause of the plaintiff's injuries
d. Damages incurred [7,8].

A duty owed

To demonstrate a medical malpractice claim, the plaintiff has to establish the existence of a plaintiff–doctor relationship. This includes evidence of intent by both parties to enter into this professional relationship. This relationship does not need to be based on a contract. Moreover, the physician does not need to be compensated in order to owe a duty to the patient [7,9]. A doctor who undertakes a patient's treatment for free owes a duty to that patient just as if he or she were to be paid. The Good Samaritan doctrine is an exception to this rule. A physician may volunteer in good faith to respond to an emergency without assuming a duty to the patient. However, the

Good Samaritan doctrine itself may be trumped where that doctor is summoned to aid another doctor who does have a duty to the patient [10].

Breach of duty

A physician is expected to perform with the degree of skill, learning, and care that is expected of an average qualified member of their profession. Based on state requirements, the average physician against whom the physician is compared may be defined by regional or by national standards. Where the physician represents him- or herself as the best in the field, the standard is elevated to meet that claim.

Proximate cause of injury

The plaintiff must demonstrate that the defendant caused his or her injury [11]. The fact that another physician had the opportunity to correct a negligent act is not protective [12].

When several physicians are involved in the management of a case, they are responsible not only for their own mistakes but for the errors of others which they permitted to occur without objection and of which they should have been aware [13].

Damages

The plaintiff must show damages to sustain an action of medical malpractice [14]. When there is no harm or damage, there can be no cause of action. Damage awards may be compensatory or punitive in nature [5]. Compensatory damages awards are intended to reimburse a loss suffered. Punitive damages are awarded to punish and make an example of the defendant for outrageous acts and are awarded above and beyond compensatory damages [5].

Only where each of these elements is demonstrated may a patient prevail in a cause of medical malpractice.

Medical malpractice in patient-specific scenarios

There are several areas within the field of anaesthesiology where medical malpractice has had a significant impact on practice patterns. In all these areas, even when obesity is not directly a factor, the lessons and concerns remain and may be extrapolated.

Obstructive sleep apnoea

The obesity epidemic combined with population longevity has led to the growing prevalence of obstructive sleep apnoea (OSA) within our communities. Surgical patients with either known or suspected OSA are at a heightened risk for perioperative morbidity and mortality [15,16].

In 2016, Fouladpour et al. studied the legal consequences associated with poor outcomes related to OSA in the perioperative setting (**Fig. 36.4**) [1]. They performed searches of three major electronic legal databases for cases adjudicated and with a final decision rendered between 1991 and 2010. The cases all involved surgical patients with known or suspected OSA. Paediatric cases were excluded. Their research uncovered that 92% of those lawsuits were based on elective cases [1]. Almost half of the complications (46%) occurred in the postoperative period on the surgical floors [1], with the fewest complications occurring intraoperatively (21%).

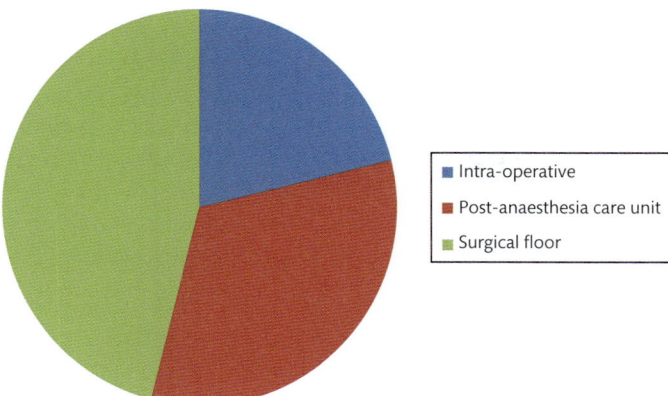

Fig. 36.4 Location of complications sustained by adult surgical patients suspected of or diagnosed with obstructive sleep apnoea.
Source: Data from Fouladpour, N., Jesudoss, R., Bolden, N., Shaman, Z., Auckley, D., Perioperative Complications in Obstructive Sleep Apnea Patients Undergoing Surgery: A Review of the Legal Literature, *Anesthesia & Analgesia*, 122(1):145–51, 2016 International Anesthesia Research Society.

The most common complications were respiratory arrest in unmonitored settings and difficulty in airway management [1]. Immediate adverse outcomes included death (45.6%), anoxic brain injury (45.6%), and upper airway complications (8%). Overall, 71% of the patients died [1]. Verdicts rendered were almost evenly split with a slight predominance in favour of the plaintiff. In those cases in which the plaintiff prevailed, the average financial penalty was US$2.5 million [1].

Perioperative complications related to OSA constitute a growing number of medical malpractice actions. The actual medical, legal, and financial burden is underestimated as most suits are settled out of court.

The paediatric patient

Sleep-disordered breathing and sleep apnoea are often associated with obesity in the paediatric patient [17,18]. Sleep-disordered breathing also constitutes the most common indication for tonsillectomy resulting from airway obstruction [19,20]. The push to conserve medical resources and cost, combined with improving medical techniques, has resulted in an increasing number of these procedures being performed on an outpatient basis. This decreases the number of circumstances in which the anaesthesiologist is able to meet the patient prior to the day of surgery and to observe the patient postoperatively [21]. Tonsillectomy-related malpractice settlements are more common against anaesthesiologists than against surgeons, settling for almost fivefold greater awards due to devastating outcomes [22–24]. Anoxic intraoperative and postoperative events in the paediatric patient have accounted for verdicts as large as US$45 million [21].

Coté et al. analysed data obtained from the American Society of Anesthesiologists Closed Claims Project and an electronic survey performed on more than 2000 members of the Society of Pediatric Anesthesia, identifying adverse events during or after tonsillectomy in children. The cases reported by surgeons and anaesthesiologists included death or neurological injury as complications following tonsillectomy. It appeared that many of these incidents may have been prevented if respiratory monitoring had been continued during first- and second-stage recovery, as well as on the ward

during the first postoperative night. This emphasizes the need for better evaluations and procedures for assessing perioperative risks after surgery in the paediatric patient, in particular, those patients with OSA [21]. Literature also demonstrates that the combination of obesity, OSA, and the need for postoperative opioids significantly increases the potential for adverse postoperative respiratory events in the paediatric patient, creating an increased risk of airway obstruction on the first night of surgery when compared to the preoperative risk, especially those undergoing tonsillectomy with or without adenoidectomy [25,26].

The parturient

Obstetric anaesthesia is an integral part of practice for most anaesthesiologists. For both obstetricians and anaesthesiologists, this area of practice carries a high liability burden [27,28].

Beckmann studied the influence of medicolegal aspects of obstetric anaesthesiology on anaesthetic practice in Australia and New Zealand. Information regarding medical defence organizations and opinions about the current medicolegal trend and demographics were analysed. A total of 95.3% of members of the Australian and New Zealand College of Anaesthetists were concerned about the existing medical indemnity climate and 73.6% expected to have at least one claim against them during their career, spending an average of 8.3% of their income on medical insurance premiums [29]. The study also uncovered that following the preoperative consultation, physicians often made changes to their anaesthetic plan. Some of the changes evidenced a prevalent and growing reluctance to perform neuraxial blocks. Physicians had also become more thorough in their documentation of complications [29].

A study conducted by Crawforth evaluated the anaesthesia care provided during adverse events on the obstetric ward. Malpractice claims filed against nurse anaesthetists for care involving obstetric patients were extracted from the American Association of Nurse Anesthetists Foundation Closed Claim database ($N = 41$). They included events which occurred between 1990 and 1996 and represented anaesthesiology care provided by both anaesthesiologists and nurse anaesthetists. The most prevalent risks factors identified in this study were advanced maternal age and obesity [30].

Treating patients with respect

As anaesthesiologists, we are obligated to discuss with all patients their health issues and associated perioperative risks. Obesity is one such comorbidity. Patients should be counselled in the course of the consent process regarding the impact that their obesity and/or any associated comorbidities may have on their anaesthetic management and care. The consent process should be well documented to reflect the discussion had with the patient.

Issues of professionalism also play a key role in patient care. Patients suffering from obesity perceive weight discrimination as a component of their care with negative ramifications [31]. The negative consequences include not only higher rates of psychiatric conditions, such as depression, but a cycle that includes poorer success at weight loss [32].

In 2013, a patient scheduled for a colonoscopy recorded on his mobile phone conversations occurring between the medical staff and physicians while he was anaesthetized. The mobile phone recordings captured the anaesthesiologist ridiculing and humiliating the patient while he was under her care. The verdict returned in favour of the patient of $500,000 for malpractice, defamation, and punitive damages [33]. Physician attitudes and behaviours play an integral part in both patient care and expectations of professionalism.

Recommendations for the anaesthesiologist

The practice of anaesthesia is a complex discipline that requires a constantly evolving body of knowledge, techniques, and interpersonal skill. An analysis performed in 2013 of over 40,000 physicians cited anaesthesiology as the specialty with the third highest number of open claims [34]. A 2012 study reported that anaesthesiologists feared both financial ruin and the effect on professional reputation among colleagues and patients [35]. This fear persists although some estimate that as many as 80% of malpractice claims settled by jury find in favour of physicians.

Medical malpractice litigation has affected the practice of medicine in all specialties increasing the cost of healthcare in the United States due to direct costs of litigations, the practice of defensive medicine, and a rise in malpractice premiums [36]. This increase is estimated to be in the order of billions of dollars [37]. These sums do not include the social and emotional costs of litigation on the patient, the physician, and society.

It is critical that at a baseline, anaesthesiologists establish respectful relationships with their patients both when the patient is conscious and anaesthetized. Honest interactions with the patient should include a discussion of the anaesthetic risks associated with obesity when applicable. This allows patients to have reasonable expectations regarding possible outcomes prior to engaging in an intervention. The discussion should be well documented particularly where the risks involved are evident. Ensure that the patient is aware of the risks and benefits of the procedure. In the effort to reassure the anxious patient, be certain not to make assurances that cannot be guaranteed. Never be reticent to seek help when needed. In the event of an adverse outcome, contact your risk management team as soon as possible.

CASE REPORT

A 42-year-old, 178 cm, 213 kg (BMI 67 kg/m²) male patient presents for arthroscopic shoulder surgery at the ambulatory surgery centre. His prior medical history includes hypertension, diabetes mellitus, OSA, dyslipidaemia, and degenerative arthritis. The patient is non-compliant with his continuous positive airway pressure mask because he 'can't sleep with the mask on'. His airway exam shows a large patient in relative comfort with a Class III Mallampati exam, a neck circumference of 46 cm, and a full beard. His laboratory values are unimpressive except for an apnoea–hypopnoea index of 60. The surgeon plans to place the patient lateral, because that is how he 'always' does his cases.

The anaesthesiologist is hesitant to upset the surgeon or patient by cancelling the case. The case proceeds to the operating room where the anaesthesiologist fails to intubate the patient with an endotracheal tube and places a supraglottic airway device. The case then proceeds with the patient breathing spontaneously in the lateral

position. At the conclusion of the case, the patient is placed supine and extubated. Shortly thereafter, the anaesthesiologist notices that the patient is no longer breathing. The anaesthesiologist is unable to place any airway device back in the airway. The patient becomes hypoxic, develops a cardiac arrest, is ineffectively coded, and suffers anoxic brain injury. Two days later the patient's care is withdrawn.

The patient's family sues the anaesthesiologist, the surgeon, and the facility. The case is settled against the anaesthesiologist for a very large sum.

REFERENCES

1. Fouladpour N, Jesudoss R, Bolden N, Shaman Z, Auckley D. Perioperative complications in obstructive sleep apnea patients undergoing surgery: a review of the legal literature. Anesth Analg. 2016;**122**(1):145–51.
2. Nagle, P. An overview of obesity-related claims. Doctors Company. 2014. https://www.thedoctors.com/articles/an-overview-of-obesity-related-claims/
3. Rubin JB, Bishop TF. Characteristics of paid malpractice claims settled in and out of court in the USA: a retrospective analysis. BMJ Open. 2013;**3**(6):e002985.
4. Waldman SA, Berkeley A. Medicolegal aspects of epidural steroid injections. Tech Reg Anesth Pain Manag. 2009;**13**(4):272–80.
5. Black H. Black's Law Dictionary. 6 ed. St. Paul, MN: West Publishing Co; 1990.
6. Physicians and Surgeons. CJS. 70 §81 (2008).
7. Physicians and Surgeons. CJS. 70 §82 (2008).
8. Huntoon M, Levy R. How to keep a bad outcome from becoming a lawsuit. Pain Med. 2008;**9**(1):128–32.
9. Physicians and Surgeons. CJS. 70 §103 (2008).
10. Physicians and Surgeons. CJS. 70 §104 (2008).
11. Physicians and Surgeons. CJS. 70 §91 (2008).
12. Physicians and Surgeons. CJS. 70 §90 (2008).
13. Physicians and Surgeons. CJS. 70 §107 (2008).
14. Physicians and Surgeons. CJS. 70 §98 (2008).
15. Memtsoudis S, Liu SS, Ma Y, Chiu YL, Walz JM, Gaber-Baylis LK, et al. Perioperative pulmonary outcomes in patients with sleep apnea after noncardiac surgery. Anesth Analg. 2011;**112**(1):113–21.
16. Mokhlesi B, Hovda MD, Vekhter B, Arora VM, Chung F, Meltzer DO. Sleep-disordered breathing and postoperative outcomes after bariatric surgery: analysis of the nationwide inpatient sample. Obes Surg. 2013;**23**(11):1842–51.
17. Arens R, Muzumdar H. Childhood obesity and obstructive sleep apnea syndrome. J Appl Physiol (1985). 2010;**108**(2):436–44.
18. Carter R 3rd, Watenpaugh DE. Obesity and obstructive sleep apnea: or is it OSA and obesity? Pathophysiology. 2008;**15**(2):71–77.
19. Costa DJ, Mitchell R. Adenotonsillectomy for obstructive sleep apnea in obese children: a meta-analysis. Otolaryngol Head Neck Surg. 2009;**140**(4):455–60.
20. Lumeng JC, Chervin RD. Epidemiology of pediatric obstructive sleep apnea. Proc Am Thorac Soc. 2008;**5**(2):242–52.
21. Coté CJ, Posner KL, Domino KB. Death or neurologic injury after tonsillectomy in children with a focus on obstructive sleep apnea: Houston, we have a problem! Anesth Analg. 2014;**118**(6):1276–83.

22. Simonsen AR, Duncavage JA, Becker SS. A review of malpractice cases after tonsillectomy and adenoidectomy. Int J Pediatr Otorhinolaryngol. 2010;74(9):977–79.

23. Morris LG, Lieberman SM, Reitzen SD, Edelstein DR, Ziff DJ, Katz A, et al. Characteristics and outcomes of malpractice claims after tonsillectomy. Otolaryngol Head Neck Surg. 2008;138(3):315–20.

24. Stevenson AN, Myer CM 3rd, Shuler MD, Singer PS. Complications and legal outcomes of tonsillectomy malpractice claims. Laryngoscope. 2012;122(1):71–74.

25. Brown KA, Morin I, Hickey C, Manoukian JJ, Nixon GM, Brouillette RT. Urgent adenotonsillectomy: an analysis of risk factors associated with postoperative respiratory morbidity. Anesthesiology. 2003;99(3):586–95.

26. Nixon GM, Kermack AS, McGregor CD, Davis GM, Manoukian JJ, Brown KA, et al. Sleep and breathing on the first night after adenotonsillectomy for obstructive sleep apnea. Pediatr Pulmonol. 2005;39(4):332–38.

27. Kuczkowski KM. Anesthetic management of labor pain: what does an obstetrician need to know? Arch Gynecol Obstet. 2005;271(2):97–103.

28. Kuczkowski KM. Medico-legal issues in obstetric anesthesia: what does an obstetrician need to know? Arch Gynecol Obstet. 2008;278(6):503–505.

29. Beckmann LA. The influence of the current medicolegal climate on New South Wales anaesthetic practice. Anaesth Intensive Care. 2005;33(6):762–67.

30. Crawforth K. The AANA Foundation closed malpractice claims study: obstetric anesthesia. AANA J. 2002;70(2):97–104.

31. Spalholz, J, Baer, N, Konig, H, Riedel-Keller, S, Luck-Sikorski, C. Obesity and discrimination—a systematic review and meta-analysis of observational studies. Obes Rev. 2016;17(1):43–55.

32. Hübner C, Schmidt R, Selle J, Köhler H, Müller A, et al. Comparing self-report measures of internalized weight stigma: the weight self-stigma questionnaire versus the weight bias internalization scale. PLoS One 2016;11(10):e0165566.

33. Spargo C. Patient is awarded $500,000 after he secretly recorded his doctor saying she wanted to hit him and joking that he had STD—while he was under anesthesia. Daily Mail. 24 June 2015. http://www.dailymail.co.uk/news/article-3136989/After-five-minutes-wanted-punch-face-Man-wins-500-000-recording-doctor-falsely-saying-STD-hemorrhoids-wants-hit-him.html

34. Seabury SA, Chandra A, Lakdawalla DN, Jena AB. On average, physicians spend nearly 11% of their 40-year careers with an open, unresolved malpractice claim. Health Aff (Millwood). 2013;32(1):111–19.

35. Burkle CM, Martin DP, Keegan MT. Which is feared more: harm to the ego or financial peril? A survey of anesthesiologists' attitudes about medical malpractice. Minn Med. 2012;95(9):46–50.

36. Radvansky BM, Farver WT, Svider PF, Eloy JA, Gubenko YA, Eloy JD. A comparison of plaintiff and defense expert witness qualifications in malpractice litigation in anesthesiology. Anesth Analg. 2015;120(6):1369–74.

37. Anderson GF, Hussey PS, Frogner BK, Waters HR. Health spending in the United States and the rest of the industrialized world. Health Aff (Millwood). 2005;24(4):903–14.

Index

Tables are indicated by an italic *t* following the page number.